ADOLESCENT RHEUMATOLOGY

ADOLESCENT RHEUMATOLOGY

Edited by

DAVID A ISENBERG, MD, FRCP

Arthritis Research Campaign's
Diamond Jubilee
Professor of Rheumatology
University College
London, UK

JOHN J MILLER III, MD, PhD
Emeritus Professor of Paediatrics
Stanford University School of Medicine
California, USA

MARTIN DUNITZ

© Martin Dunitz Ltd 1999

First published in the UK in 1999 by
Martin Dunitz Ltd
The Livery House
7–9 Pratt Street
London NW1 0AE

A CIP catalogue record for this book is available
from the British Library.

ISBN 1-85317-553-6

Distributed in the United States by:
Blackwell Science Inc.
Commerce Place, 350 Main Street
Malden, MA 02148, USA
Tel: 1-800-215-1000

Distributed in Canada by:
Login Brothers Book Company
324 Salteaux Crescent
Winnipeg, Manitoba, R3J 3T2
Canada
Tel: 204-224-4068

Distributed in Brazil by:
Ernesto Richmann Distribuidora de Livros, Ltda
Rua Coronel Marques 335, Tatuape 03440-000
São Paulo
Brazil

Composition by Scribe Design, Gillingham, Kent
Printed and bound in Spain

Contents

List of contributors

Balu H Athreya MD
Pediatric Rheumatology
duPont Hospital for Children
1600 Rockland Road
Wilmington, DE 19899
USA

John Baum MD
Division of Pediatric Immunology, Allergy
and Rheumatology
Department of Pediatrics
University of Rochester
School of Medicine and Dentistry
Rochester, NY
USA

Frank Biro MD
Division of Adolescent Medicine
Children's Hospital Medical Center
3333 Burnet Avenue
Cincinnati, OH 45299–3039
USA

Brian Cohen FRCS(ORTH)
Department of Orthopaedics
Arthur Stanley House
Middlesex Hospital
40–50 Tottenham Street
London
W1P 9PG, UK

Stephen J Drew FRCS(ORTH)
Department of Orthopaedics
Arthur Stanley House
Middlesex Hospital
40–50 Tottenham Street
London
W1P 9PG, UK

Jo CW Edwards MD, FRCP
Centre for Rheumatology
Bloomsbury Rheumatology Unit
University College London
Arthur Stanley House
Middlesex Hospital
40–50 Tottenham Street
London
W1P 9PG, UK

David N Glass MD
Division of Rheumatology
Children's Hospital Medical Center
3333 Burnet Avenue
Cincinnati, OH 45299–3039
USA

Jane Harrington MSc
Unit of Health Psychology
Department of Psychiatry and
Behavioural Science
Bland Sutton Institute
Wolfson Building
Middlesex Hospital
41 Riding House Street
London
W1N 8AA, UK

Philip J Hashkes MD, MSc
Department of Pediatrics
Rebecca Sieff and Poriah Hospitals
Safed and Tiberias
Israel

Carol J Henderson MS, RD, LD
Children's Hospital Medical Center
Rowe Division of Pediatric Rheumatology
3333 Burnet Avenue
Cincinnati, OH 45229–3039
USA

David A Isenberg MD, FRCP
Centre for Rheumatology
Bloomsbury Rheumatology Unit
University College London
Arthur Stanley House
Middlesex Hospital
40–50 Tottenham Street
London
W19 9PG, UK

Adrienne Kirk MSc
Unit of Health Psychology
Department of Psychiatry and
Behavioural Science
Bland Sutton Institute
Wolfson Building
Middlesex Hospital
41 Riding House Street
London
W1N 8AA, UK

Bianca A Lang MD, FRCPS
Department of Pediatrics
Dalhousie University
IWK Grace Health Centre
1850 University Avenue
Halifax
NS B3J 3G9
Canada

Ronald M Laxer MD, FRCP
Department of Pediatrics
University of Toronto
Division of Rheumatology
Hospital for Sick Children
555 University Avenue
Toronto
ON M5G 1X8
Canada

Richard L Levine MD
Department of Pediatrics
Penn State Geisinger Health System
Milton S Hershey Medical Center
Hershey, PA 17033
USA

Carol B Lindsley MD
Department of Paediatrics
University of Kansas City Medical Center
3901 Rainbow Boulevard
Kansas City, KS 66160
USA

Daniel J Lovell MD, MPH
Children's Hospital Medical Center
Rowe Division of Pediatric Rheumatology
3333 Burnet Avenue
Cincinnati, OH 45229–3039
USA

Katherine Martin MRCP
Centre for Paediatric and Adolescent
Rheumatology
Windeyer Institute for Medical Studies
University College London
46 Cleveland Street
London
W1P 6DB, UK

Janet McDonagh MD, MRCP
Department of Rheumatology
The Medical School
University of Birmingham
Birmingham
B15 2TT, UK

Kevin Murray FRACP
Centre for Rheumatology
Bloomsbury Rheumatology Unit
University College London
Arthur Stanley House
Middlesex Hospital
40–50 Tottenham Street
London
W1P 9PG, UK

Stanton Newman D Phil
Unit of Health Psychology
Department of Psychiatry and
Behavioural Science
Bland Sutton Institute
Wolfson Building
Middlesex Hospital
41 Riding House Street
London
W1N 8AA, UK

Barbara E Ostrov MD
Pediatric and Adult Rheumatology
Departments of Pediatrics and Internal
Medicine
Penn State Geisinger Health System
Milton S Hershey Medical Center
Hershey, PA 17033
USA

Lauren M Pachman MD
Department of Pediatrics
Division of Immunology and Rheumatology
Northwestern University Medical School
2300 Children's Plaza
Chicago, IL 60614
USA

Clarissa Pilkington MRCP
Centre for Paediatric and Adolescent
Rheumatology
Windeyer Institute for Medical Studies
University College London
46 Cleveland Street
London
W1P 6DB, UK

Patricia A Rettig RN, MSN, CRNP
duPont Hospital for Children
1600 Rockland Road
Wilmington, DE 19899
USA

David D Sherry MD
Paediatric Rheumatology
Children's Hospital Medical Centre
4800 Sand Point Way NE
Seattle, WA 98105
USA

David Siegel MD, MPH
Division of Pediatric Immunology, Allergy
and Rheumatology
Division of Adolescent Medicine
Department of Pediatrics
University of Rochester
School of Medicine and Dentistry
Rochester, NY
USA

Lori B Tucker MD
British Columbia Children's Hospital
Vancouver
BC V6H 3V4
Canada

Patience H White MD
Division of Adult and Pediatric Rheumatology
George Washington University School of
Medicine and Health Sciences
2300 I Street, NW# 708
Washington, DC 2037
USA

Johan D Witt FRCS(ORTH)
Department of Orthopaedics
Arthur Stanley House
Middlesex Hospital
40–50 Tottenham Street
London
W1P 9PG, UK

Patricia Woo PhD, FRCP
Centre for Paediatric and Adolescent
Rheumatology
Windeyer Institute for Medical Studies
University College London
46 Cleveland Street
London
W1P 6DB, UK

Introduction

A precise definition of adolescence is hard to find, but it clearly represents a tumultuous stage between childhood and adulthood. The considerable physical and psychological developments that take place during the teenage years and early twenties have a profound impact upon the individual, their friends and relatives. Rheumatologists have received little training in understanding how these profound developments affect the adolescent with significant rheumatological disease. It is most important to do so, however, given that a wide variety of these diseases, ranging from ankylosing spondylitis to systemic lupus erythematosus, frequently begin during this period. It is clear that rheumatological diseases in adolescents may significantly impede the development of joints and their adjacent tissues, leading to permanent damage, which in turn affects the ability of an individual to progress through their higher education, to form normal relationships, and to cope with the long-term sequelae of both these diseases and their treatment.

Adolescent medicine, as a discipline, is in its infancy. We acknowledge with gratitude the major efforts made by our chapter authors to seek out relevant source material for their topics, which is scattered among the literature of both paediatrics and internal medicine.

This book analyses a wide variety of rheumatological diseases that affect adolescents. The authors, selected both for their experience and their ability to write well (and to time!), provide a detailed assessment of joint development during adolescence, a discussion of how to assess outcome in these diseases, an analysis of the variety of and forms taken by the major rheumatological disorders, together with a considered view of their management (including surgical requirements) and the impact of these diseases, both psychological and physical.

There is continuing debate among paediatric/adolescent rheumatologists about the preferred nomenclature in juvenile onset arthritis (see Chapter 5 for detailed discussion). In the main, and especially where the disease is being discussed in general, we have used juvenile idiopathic arthritis. However, when our authors are describing particular published studies, the original nomenclature, juvenile chronic arthritis or juvenile rheumatoid arthritis has been used.

David A Isenberg
London
John J Miller III
Woodside, CA

1

Joint development

Jo CW Edwards and Kevin Murray

INTRODUCTION

Anyone interested in joints should spare a little time to study their development. A grasp of how joints form is of great help in understanding their subsequent function, and their capacity for repair. The impact of childhood rheumatic disease, in particular, is inseparable from the growth and development of the skeleton.

Although most qualitative events in joint development occur during fetal and early childhood life, the processes of linear growth and maturation of joint components continue well into the second and even the third decade of life. The years between 10 and 21, nominally representing adolescence, see major changes in the shape and centre of gravity of the growing human, with resultant changes in forces about the bones and joints of the skeleton. While in a healthy individual this proceeds in a more or less coordinated fashion with the attainment of functional skeletal maturity, chronic diseases, in particular those of a rheumatic nature, have a significant and at times catastrophic impact upon this process.

Of further interest, recent studies indicate developmental similarities between synovial and lymphoid tissues. Synovial joints first appeared in evolution in the form of jaw joints in cartilaginous fishes. Both a recognizable major histocompatibility complex (MHC) and antibodies appeared at much the same time (Figure 1.1).[1] Synovium and lymphoid development both have links with splanchnopleura and

the skeleton. Specifically, both tissues make use of the complement regulatory protein delay-accelerating factor (DAF) and the vascular adhesion molecule (VCAM-1)[2,3] to regulate mononuclear leucocyte/stromal cell interactions. These similarities may prove central to an emerging understanding of why joints and entheses are susceptible to chronic immunological disease.

This chapter focuses on recent developments in joint biology at both cellular and molecular levels, and will seek to relate these to issues of clinical importance during the adolescent years of patients who have new onset or ongoing rheumatic disease. Issues will be considered as they apply to the skeleton as a whole; for detailed information on individual sites of ossification and specific congenital abnormalities, paediatric and radiology texts, such as Resnick and Niwayama's *Diagnosis of Bone and Joint Disorders*,[4] should be consulted.

EMBRYOLOGY OF THE SYNOVIAL JOINT

Early events

Early in human embryonic development the cells which will give rise to the skeleton become distinguishable as a dense continuous mesenchymal core or 'blastema' (Figure 1.2a).[5] Within this blastema, cell foci, one for each future bone, take on features of chondrocytes (Figure 1.2b). These chondrocyte foci grow more

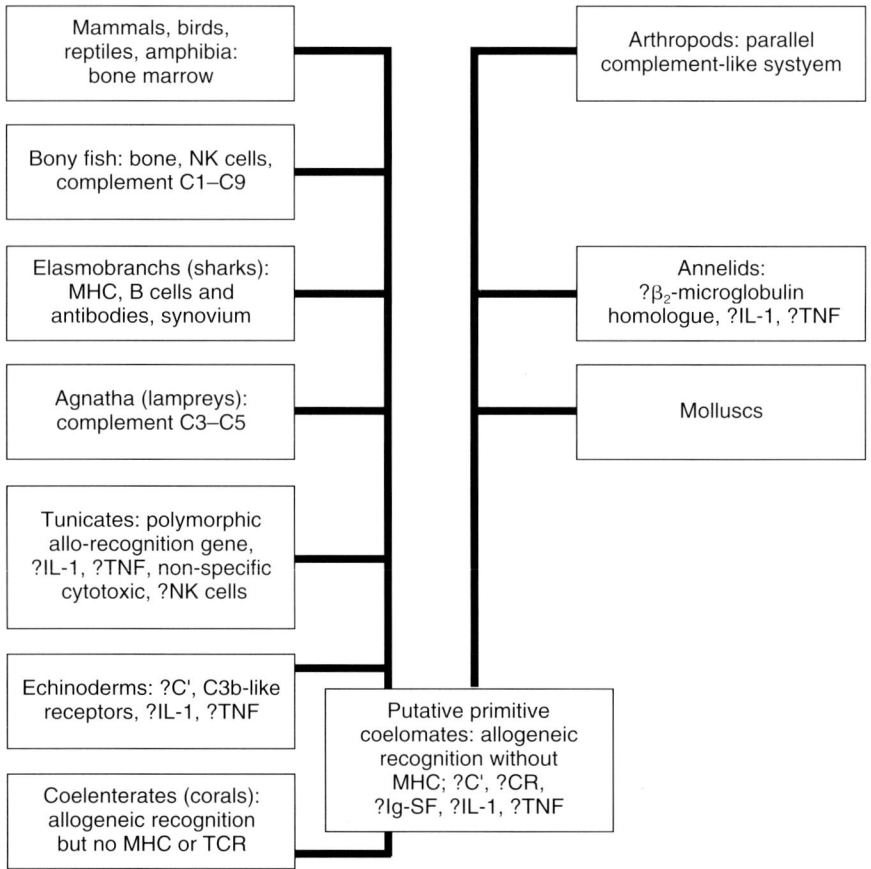

| Mammals, birds, reptiles, amphibia: bone marrow |
| Bony fish: bone, NK cells, complement C1–C9 |
| Elasmobranchs (sharks): MHC, B cells and antibodies, synovium |
| Agnatha (lampreys): complement C3–C5 |
| Tunicates: polymorphic allo-recognition gene, ?IL-1, ?TNF, non-specific cytotoxic, ?NK cells |
| Echinoderms: ?C', C3b-like receptors, ?IL-1, ?TNF |
| Coelenterates (corals): allogeneic recognition but no MHC or TCR |

| Arthropods: parallel complement-like systyem |
| Annelids: ?β$_2$-microglobulin homologue, ?IL-1, ?TNF |
| Molluscs |

| Putative primitive coelomates: allogeneic recognition without MHC; ?C', ?CR, ?Ig-SF, ?IL-1, ?TNF |

Figure 1.1 Simplified schema of where elements of the lymphoid and skeletal systems may have first appeared in evolution. Ig-SF, immunoglobulin superfamily; C', complement system; CR, complement regulatory proteins/receptors; IL, interleukin; MHC, major histocompatibility complex; NK, natural killer; TCR, T-cell receptor; TNF, tumour necrosis factor.

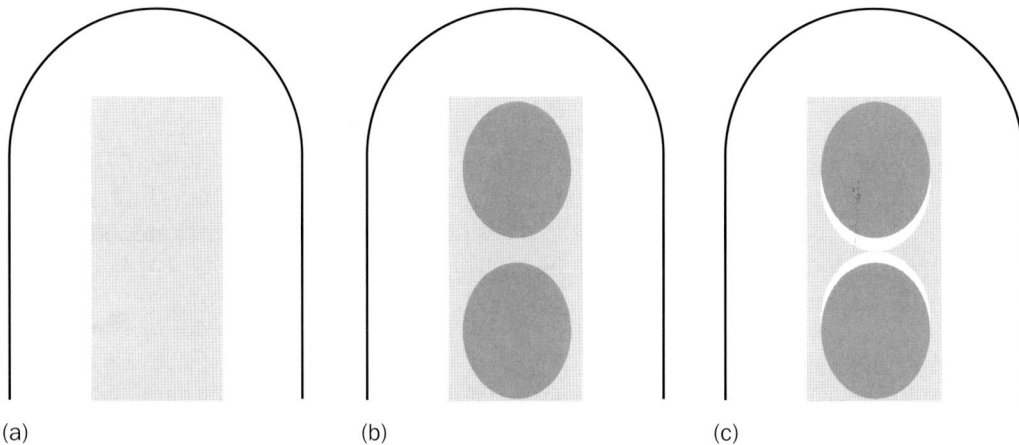

(a) (b) (c)

Figure 1.2 Diagrammatic representation of a developing synovial joint: (a) appearance of a blastemal core; (b) formation of cartilage elements and interzone/perichondrium; (c) formation of a joint cavity.

rapidly, and secrete more matrix than the surrounding cells, so that each cartilage element becomes surrounded by an envelope of flattened cells. Where this envelope surrounds the shafts of cartilage elements it is termed perichondrium. Where it lies between cartilage elements it is termed interzone. At 7 weeks gestation there is no clear demarcation between perichondrium and interzone, the entire envelope staining strongly for the hyaluronan receptor cluster determinant 44 (CD44).[6]

The inner, or chondrogenic, layer of the perichondrial envelope is the probable source of new chondrocytes, to be added to the expanding cartilage element (Figure 1.3). However, cells of the envelope have two other functions, which share some interesting features. The interzone will eventually detach from the articular surfaces of the cartilage element, to form synovium (Figure 1.2c).[5,6] In contrast, perichondrial cells surrounding the mid-shaft of the cartilage element invade the cartilage, together with blood vessels, to form bone marrow.[5] Both these processes are associated with cells expressing, at high level, the adhesion molecule VCAM-1[7] and the complement inhibitory protein DAF.[8] It is interesting to note that synovium precedes bone marrow in evolution, suggesting that the use of these molecules by bone marrow may have been 'borrowed' from synovium.

The factors determining the genesis of the blastema and cartilage elements are poorly understood. However, rules governing limb development have been identified by Wolpert and colleagues.[9,10] In particular, the importance of an apical ectodermal ridge at the apex of the limb bud and a zone of polarizing activity along one side have been established. These determine the number of skeletal rays and the number of bones in each ray. Manipulation of these areas leads to extra or missing rays or elements.

More recently, molecular biological techniques have opened up new levels of understanding of limb development with the identification of homeobox and other genes known to be involved in differentiation.[11] Many of these have homologues in *Drosophila* and have

quaint names such as sonic hedgehog. They regulate transcription of other genes at a very early stage. Other gene products, such as growth/differentiation factor-5 (GDF-5), are expressed later in a specific relationship to sites of joint formation.[12] Their role remains uncertain. What does seem to be emerging is a cascade of regulation of gene transcription that involves gene products which act back within the cell as transcription factors, products which act in an autocrine or paracrine fashion as growth factors (such as bone morphogenetic proteins)[12] and products which are either matrix elements themselves or are involved in synthesis of carbohydrate elements (such as hyaluronan).[13]

It is likely that a clear molecular understanding of joint development is not far off, but it is still difficult to see what the answers will be to questions such as why the surfaces of the hip joint are congruent and those of the knee joint not. Increasing understanding of how joint cavities form suggests that an interplay between gene transcription and physical forces associated with movement contributes to these issues.

The formation of a synovial cavity

Around 8–10 weeks gestational age the interzones between skeletal elements separate from cartilage to form a tongue of synovial tissue and an intervening synovial space (see Figure 1.2c). The site of cavity formation is very precisely programmed. The mechanism of this separation is becoming clear. Prior to cavity formation all interzone cells express CD44.[6] By binding hyaluronan, CD44 can hold cells together.[14] However, just prior to cavity formation, the cells along the line where the cavity is to open up, increase their level of enzymes, such as uridine diphosphoglucose dehydrogenase (UDPGD) and hyaluronan synthase, involved in hyaluronan synthesis.[13] The vicinity becomes rich in free hyaluronan. Excess hyaluronan has the paradoxical effect of saturating CD44 and making cells separate.[14]

This mechanism does not require enzymatic degradation of matrix. Metalloproteinase levels are actually lower at the site of separation than in nearby cartilage.[15] Fibrous matrix elements at the potential joint line run parallel to the line of separation and not across it (Figure 1.4), and therefore do not need to be removed. Nor does separation appear to involve cell death or migration. Apoptotic cells occur scattered through interzones prior to cavity formation, but are not specifically found at the site of separation.[16] The formation of a cavity does not require anything to be taken away. The slow rate of growth of interzone cells in comparison to surrounding chondrocytes (see Figure 1.3) may mean that the interzone is at a slightly negative pressure relative to the surrounding tissue, as is the case in mature joints.[17] Local secretion of hyaluronan allows water to be drawn into the tissue at the joint line and the solid tissue elements to retract, leaving a space. In fact the space is minimal, as in adult life, being no more than 50 μm wide at most sites.

An important part of our understanding of the formation of synovial cavities comes from the effects of immobilization. Paralysed chick embryos fail to show changes in hyaluronan metabolism at the potential joint line, and fail to form synovial cavities.[18,19] This suggests that movement is necessary for the biochemical genesis of the cavity. This may involve links between the cytoskeleton and CD44.[20] As the synovial space forms, cells along the line of the cavity reorientate cytoskeletal elements such as actin and moesin. This may contribute both to the sensing of mechanical stimuli and the subsequent separation of cell layers at the joint line.

In clinical terms, fetuses that have been inhibited from intrauterine movement develop a condition known as arthrogryposis, in which joints are stiff at birth and may remain so.[21] Normal movement during childhood may also be important to both articular surface modelling and range, but evidence is lacking.

Another protein which may be involved in cavity formation is fibrillin-1, which in the human is expressed at the joint line prior to cavity formation (see Figure 1.5). Fibrillin-1 forms extracellular microfibrils, which are prominent in mature synovial intima[22] and other viscoplastic tissue sheets such as amnion and pericardium. Its presence prior to cavity formation may simply indicate anticipation of a future functional requirement. It may, however, provide an anchorage for intimal cells with the required mechanical properties at the time of cavity formation. As will be discussed below, fibrillin-1 is of particular interest in pathogenesis in that in adult synovium it is decorated with DAF.[23] Control of the alternative complement pathway by DAF may be important both in the process of cavity formation and in subsequent tissue function.

Acquisition of the specialized characteristics of synovium

Mature synovium consists of loose connective tissue lined by an intimal cell layer (Figure 1.6).[24] The intima comprises a mixture of fibroblasts and macrophages of specialized phenotype (Figure 1.7) embedded in a specialized matrix.

Specialization of intimal fibroblasts
The earliest documented specialization of synovial cells is the prominent expression of CD44 (approximately 7 weeks).[6] This is shared with perichondrial cells and, prior to cavity formation, is a uniform feature of all interzone cells. Following cavity formation, high level CD44 expression is limited to the intimal layer of synovium, as seen in mature tissue.

High UDPGD activity appears prior to cavity formation (about 8–9 weeks) and is limited to the potential intima in mammalian joints. This high activity persists in intimal fibroblasts in mature tissue, and is important in hyaluronan synthesis by intimal cells. UDPGD converts UDP glucose to UDP glucuronate, which provides monosaccharides for assembly of the hyaluronan polymer by its synthases.

High levels of DAF expression appear before cavity formation and are limited to a mono- or bilayer of cells destined to become synovial intimal fibroblasts. At this stage the potential joint line and the epidermis are the only sites of DAF expression in the fetal limb.[25] The very high level

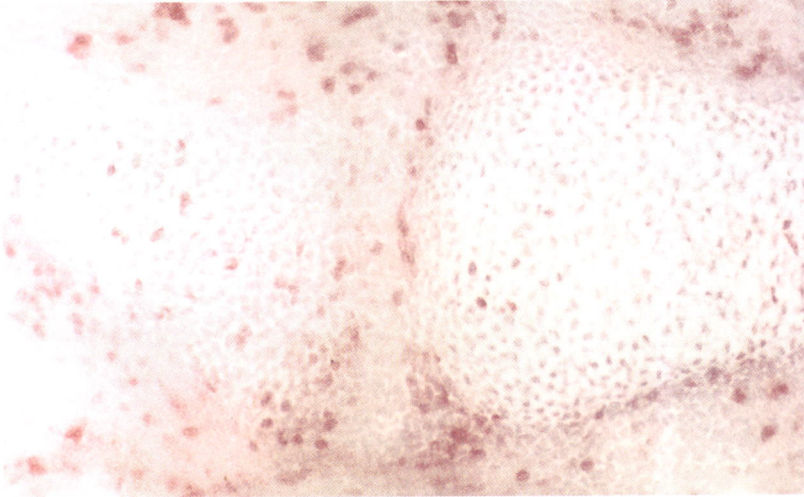

Figure 1.3 Micrograph of fetal human finger joint prior to cavity formation. Dividing cells in the chondrogenic layer of the perichondrial envelope are stained for proliferating nuclear antigen. Division rates within cartilage foci and in the central interzone (down the middle of the picture) are low.

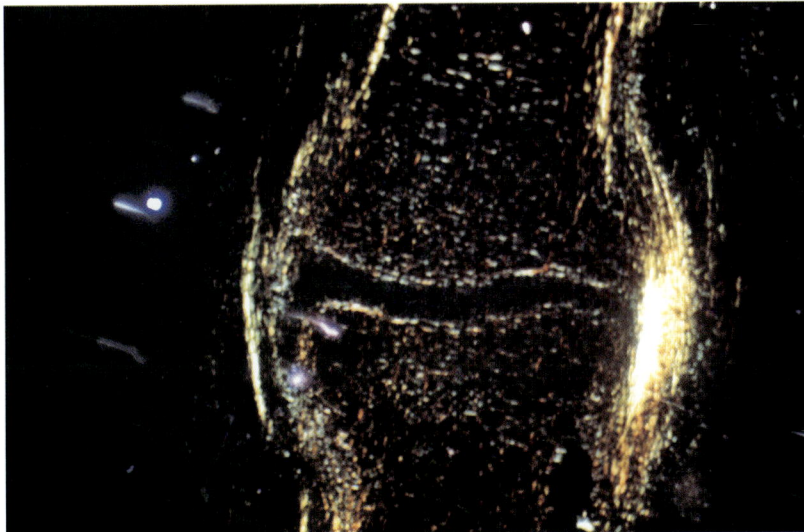

Figure 1.4 Polarized light micrograph of a fetal human finger joint prior to cavity formation. Birefringent collagen fibres are seen in perichondrium and ligament, but do not traverse the interzone, where the cavity is due to form.

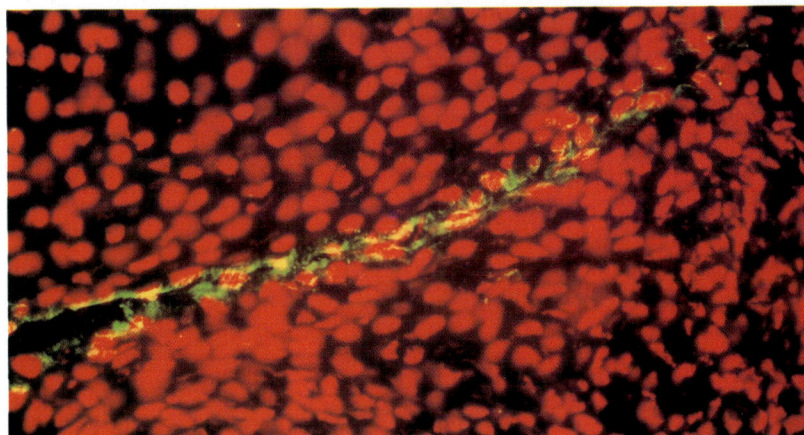

Figure 1.5 Micrograph of a 10-week-old human fetal knee joint showing staining for the immunoglobulin receptor FcγRIIIa (green) at the joint line shortly after the formation of a cavity. Propidium iodide nuclear counterstain (red). The corresponding images for fibrillin-1 and DAF (not shown) are almost identical, and much of the FcγRIIIa seen may be adsorbed on to fibrillin-1-based microfibrils.

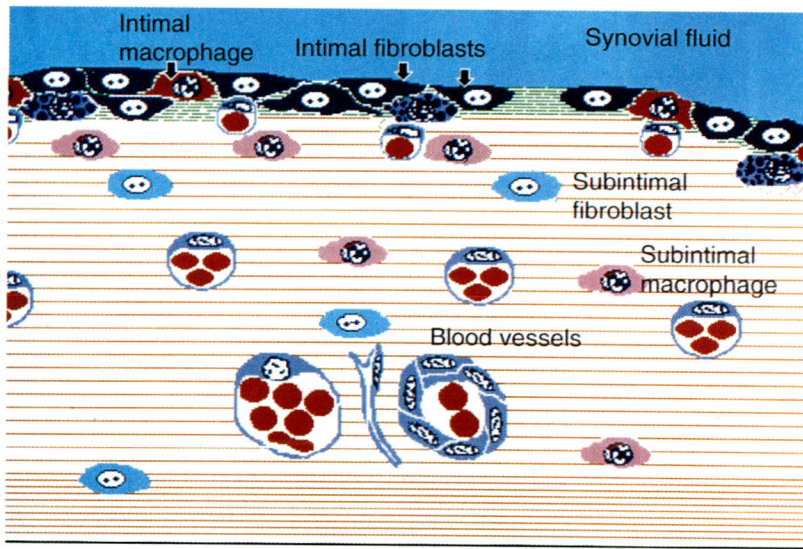

Figure 1.6 Diagrammatic representation of mature synovium. Specialized intimal cell populations are shown in darker colours. The fibrillar intimal matrix is shown in green.

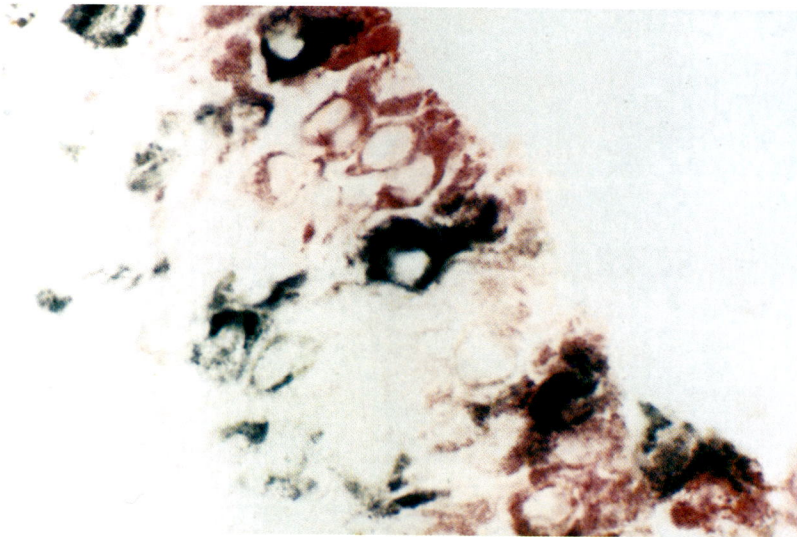

Figure 1.7 Micrograph of mature synovial intima showing fibroblasts expressing DAF (red) and macrophages with non-specific esterase activity (black).

of DAF expression by synovial intimal fibroblasts from this time on is reflected in the fact that the first anti-DAF monoclonal antibody, mAb 67, was initially thought to be synovium specific. As the cavity forms, the DAF-positive cells along the joint line where two cartilage surfaces are apposed separate from the cartilage and are lost. Along synovial surfaces they are retained as intimal fibroblasts.

VCAM-1 expression is a prominent feature of mature synovial intimal fibroblasts. However, fetal joints show no intimal VCAM-1[6] before and for several weeks after cavity formation. The time at which VCAM-1 is acquired remains to be determined. The function of VCAM-1 in synovium is not known, but it is likely to inhibit macrophages and lymphoid cells from entering the synovial space. It may be responsible for the accumulation of macrophages in the intimal layer, although once in the layer macrophages and fibroblasts do not remain in direct contact.

Also prominent in mature synovial intima is β_1 integrin expression – chiefly associated with α chains 3, 5 and 6, but not 4. Preferential intimal expression is seen in fetal joints after the cavity has formed, in a manner similar to that for CD44.

Most mature synovial intimal fibroblasts show all the above features – high UDPGD activity, and high level expression of CD44, DAF, VCAM-1 and β_1 integrins. However, there is incomplete concordance, with some cells expressing some markers and not others. Intriguingly, in the rabbit there are two intimal fibroblast populations: a superficial population with high UDPGD activity and a deeper population expressing VCAM-1.

Specialization of intimal macrophages

Synovial intimal macrophages are true macrophages by all available criteria. They are almost certainly derived from bone marrow.[26] They have a 'mature' phenotype with low CD14 expression.[24] The term 'intimal macrophage' is preferable to 'type A synoviocyte', which is associated with confusion over cell lineage. Nevertheless, intimal macrophages belong to a specific functional subgroup of macrophages which express high levels of the immunoglobulin G Fc receptor FcγRIIIa (see Figure 1.5).[23] Current evidence indicates that a high level of expression is limited to Kupffer cells and synovial intimal, alveolar, serosal, placental and, to a lesser extent, salivary gland and scleral macrophages.

Specialization of intimal matrix

Mature intimal matrix consists of a mat of fibrillar and amorphous proteins surrounding both types of intimal cell, without a basal lamina structure.[27] Laminin and collagen IV are prominent immediately around the fibroblasts. Fibrillin-1 forms a pericellular basketwork which may enclose both types of cell. Collagen VI microfibrils are more loosely arranged, often lying close to the surface. Chondroitin-6-sulphate rich proteoglycans are concentrated at the tissue surface.[28] The contribution of each of these molecules to the filtering and viscoplastic properties of the tissue remain to be established.

Tenascin has also been described in synovium.[29] However, mature synovial intima is not rich in tenascin, but tenascin may occur just beneath the intima. Tenascin is found at junctions between tissues of different types, and in fetal tissues its distribution changes as its development proceeds. It was first identified at the junction between tendon and muscle. It is also present in sectors of perichondrium in early development, some of which may be sites of muscle attachment.

It is not known what signals determine the behaviour of synovial intimal cells and whether they involve interactions between cell types. In vitro studies suggest that the special features of both intimal fibroblasts and macrophages are dependent on their environment. For the fibroblasts, these environmental factors appear to synergize with an embryologically programmed facility to express certain surface molecules. Synovial cell behaviour is probably not determined by chondrocytes, because intimal cells lining blind synovial sacs (bursae) have the same features.

Clues to cellular interactions may come from the times of acquisition of features by one or other cell type. Precise temporal relationships are not known. However, in some human fetal joints, prior to cavity formation a line of DAF positive fibroblasts can be seen at a stage when the few macrophages present are around vessels rather than at the joint line, and do not express FcγRIIIa. This suggests that expression of FcγRIIIa by intimal macrophages may be dependent on arrival at the joint line and contact with DAF-positive fibroblasts. Macrophages carry CD97, a receptor for DAF of as yet unknown function, which may be relevant.

FcγRIIIa has not been observed on dermal macrophages, except at sites of mechanical stress.[30] Since synovium is also a site of stress, it is likely that stress is involved in inducing macrophage FcγRIIIa expression, possibly via transforming growth factor β (TGFβ)[31] or interleukin-10, which induce FcγRIIIa expression in vitro. Movement is implicated in synovial cavity formation, and it may be that the acquisition of DAF by intimal fibroblasts and FcγRIIIa by macrophages occurs in parallel in response to similar mechanical stimuli. Nevertheless, the co-localization of TGFβ-binding proteins and fibrillin-1 in tissues and the very tight restriction of FcγRIIIa expression to the layer of cells surrounded by fibrillin-1 suggest that there may yet be some interplay between the two cells, both during development and in the maintenance of the mature tissue.

The later acquisition of VCAM-1 by intimal fibroblasts would be consistent with a dependence on macrophage-derived tumour necrosis factor-α (TNF-α), which is a potent inducer of VCAM-1. However, cytokine production by resting intimal macrophages is not documented, and further work in this area is needed in order to understand the maintenance of the synovial intimal environment.

Relationship of synovium to other cavity linings
Synovium is embryologically distinct from serosal linings such as pericardium, pleura and peritoneum. The latter derive from invagination of extra-embryonic coelom and carry a true mesothelium of abutting, rather than overlapping, cells resting on a basal lamina. Despite these distinct embryological origins, synovium and serosae share fibrillin-1-based microfibrils decorated with both DAF and FcγRIIIa. It seems that the presence of DAF and FcγRIIIa on microfibrils represents some local immunological adaptation of internal body cavity linings. This adaptation may have originated in evolution at a time before the emergence of immunoglobulin (see Figure 1.1) when complement formed part of a largely non-adaptive immune system. Complement regulation may have been particularly relevant to primitive coelomic cavities, as the first places in which an immune response needed to be mounted in the fluid phase.

Differentiation of articular cartilage, ligaments and entheses

Although rheumatologists like to view hyaline cartilage as adapted to joint movement, this is not borne out by developmental biology. Hyaline cartilage is primarily a growth tissue. Almost the entire skeleton has at some stage been hyaline cartilage. Most adult hyaline cartilage is non-articular (in trachea, ribs, ears, etc.). Hyaline cartilage first evolved in fish without bones or synovial joints. Hyaline cartilage is not even necessary for efficient joint function; birds use it for growth but not for articular surfaces, which are composed of fibrocartilage.

There may, nevertheless, be evidence that joint hyaline cartilage is adapted to articulation. Cartilage matrix is not uniform. Chondrocytes close to articular surfaces are flatter and are surrounded by matrix which is organized differently from that in deeper layers. Type II collagen has two variants, A and B, which are synthesized in different proportions at different sites in growing joints.[16] A variety of other minor collagens, including types III, VI and X, also show variable distribution, as do a number of proteoglycans and the detailed patterns of their sulphated carbohydrate side-chains.[32,33] There is also a suggestion that articular chondrocytes may have a distinct origin from those involved in growth,[34] arising from the chondrogenic layer of the interzone rather than perichondrium proper. Information is limited, but evidence of biochemical diversity of cartilage matrix is increasing.

Ligaments appear as linear condensations of cells alongside developing joints soon after interzones become apparent. These cells become associated with fibrous collagens and elastic fibre components. During growth the ligament is attached to the skeletal element, by either cartilaginous or fibrous tissue.[35,36] The type of tissue varies both with site and stage of development. The detailed changes occurring at different sites in the human during growth and at cessation of growth are not well documented and would merit further study. Mature ligament is largely composed of type I collagen fibres and a variable proportion of elastic fibres, which consist of several proteins. Fibrillins and associated glycoproteins are laid down first as microfibrils. Tropoelastin binds to these microfibrils and is polymerized by lysyl oxidase to mature elastin.

Postnatal events

Most qualitative aspects of skeletal development occur before birth. Postnatal changes are largely quantitative, with changes both in anatomical proportions and biochemical composition of tissues. A few synovial joints do not appear until after birth. The uncovertebral joints of the cervical spine appear in childhood. Changes in synovial compartments may also occur. The suprapatellar pouch usually fuses with the main synovial cavity of the knee in utero, but may persist as a separate compartment during childhood.[37] Bursae may develop de novo at various times during life, especially at unusual sites (adventitious bursae) in response to repeated frictional forces.

Several distinct phases of growth occur during childhood. Relatively rapid growth during infancy is followed by a period of less rapid growth up until the pubertal growth spurt. Cessation of growth is associated with ossification of both growth plate and enthesial cartilage. Detailed accounts of the timing of ossification and closure of epiphyses are given elsewhere.[4] Growth is highly dependent on hormones, including not only growth hormone and thyroxine but also sex steroids. The plasticity of the growth process is demonstrated by abnormal growth in the face of excess defective hormone production. However, the phenomena of 'catch-up and catch-down', in which height regresses to a centile predetermined at birth despite being disturbed by ill health or administration of exogenous hormones, indicates that there is a precise growth programme for each individual, with a built-in clock.

With growth, bone takes up an increasing proportion of the skeleton, and cartilage less. Articular cartilage is relatively thick in infancy and gradually reduces to adult proportions in adolescence. Changes in the congruity of articular surfaces and structure of ligaments are associated with gradual limitation of the extremely mobile state of many infant joints, particularly in

the hindfoot. Natural changes occur in gait and posture, which should not be mistaken for abnormalities. Thus, infantile pes planus commonly disappears by adolescence.

Changes in the vascular architecture in subchondral bone occur with growth and subsequent ageing. The mature subchondral plate is largely impervious to blood-borne nutrients, but nutrient pathways are open in immature bone. The clinical significance of subchondral plate closure is not clear and may only be relevant in adult life. However, in diseased joints changes in vascular supply may be critical to the natural history of disease.

Growth and ageing are associated with shifts in biochemical composition of skeletal tissues. Bone mineral mass increases to a peak in early adult life, which is dependent on effective acquisition in adolescence. Collagen fibril diameter similarly increases until early adult life and then gradually decreases. Cartilage proteoglycan composition changes,[38] with a gradual increase in the keratan sulphate moiety with age,[39] this variously being attributed to increasing mechanical stresses and reducing oxygen tension. Keratan sulphate may also appear in ligament or tendon at sites of high stress.

The key qualitative developmental change during the adolescent period is the cessation of growth with epiphyseal growth plate closure. Important changes probably also occur in ligament, with a cessation of new elastin production, which may be associated with a change in the repertoire of microfibril-associated proteins exhibited to the immune system. These changes may be relevant to the genesis of enthesopathy, as discussed below. However, from the clinical perspective, the importance of developmental changes in adolescence lies more in the shear rate of growth and in potential imbalances in growth rates, which may either induce or be induced by disease. These factors are considered further later in this chapter.

DEFECTS IN DEVELOPMENT

A wide variety of defects can occur in musculoskeletal development, both local abnormalities such as Madelung's deformity and generalized disorders such as osteogenesis imperfecta. The molecular basis of many generalized disorders has now been defined in terms of defects of genes encoding matrix proteins such as collagens and fibrillins[40] or enzymes involved in cross-linkage. Abnormalities of genes controlling growth factor production may contribute to conditions such as cranio-cleido-dysostosis.[41] Understanding of local anatomical abnormalities lags behind, as does our understanding of genes controlling morphogenesis.

Specific developmental abnormalities of joints are uncommon. Most relate to modelling abnormalities of cartilage and bone, as in epiphyseal dysplasias, congenital dislocation of the hip and dyschondroplasia. Modelling abnormalities are increasingly a focus of interest because milder forms may underlie many cases of joint failure in adult life, particularly at the hip.[42] Joint hypermobility also occurs in conditions associated with ligamentous laxity, including Ehlers–Danlos and Marfan syndromes.[40] The main intrinsic developmental problem with synovial joints is a rare condition known as arthrogryposis, in which movement is restricted with or without abnormal modelling of the joint surfaces.

Arthrogryposis is frequently a temporary neonatal problem, but severe forms, known collectively as arthrogryposis multiplex congenita (AMC), produce life-long disability.[19] Arthrogryposis appears to result from reduced intrauterine joint movement. Neonatal arthrogryposis may be associated with oligohydramnios and also with the presence of maternal antibodies to the fetal form of the neuromuscular end-plate.[43] This is thought to induce the intrauterine equivalent of myasthenia gravis. AMC may be due to a range of intrinsic abnormalities of muscle development, which lead to fibrosis.

THE RELEVANCE OF JOINT DEVELOPMENT TO INFLAMMATORY MECHANISMS

The popular perspective on tissue targeting in rheumatic disease is strongly flavoured by the traditional dogma that rheumatic fever is due to a cross-reactivity between bacterial and host tissue-specific (myocardial) antigens. Even in rheumatic fever, however, just how such a mechanism can explain flitting arthritis, erythema annulare, Sydenham's chorea or even the Aschoff node remains unclear.[44] The evidence that either tissue-specific autoantigens or cross-reactivity are relevant to other common rheumatic diseases amounts to little.

An alternative approach is to consider the way different tissues may be differentially susceptible to the arrival, survival and effects of circulating immunological agents such as antibodies, immune complexes, and T, B and natural killer (NK) cells. The obvious example is endothelium, which is exposed to antibodies at a concentration 5- to 10-fold higher than most other cells. As a result it is likely to be susceptible not only to immune-complex-mediated damage, but also to the effects of cell-penetrating antibodies to nuclear antigens such as ribonucleoproteins or topoisomerase-1.

Numerous other factors may be expected to affect tissue susceptibility to immune mediators, many relating to developmental biology. These include differential expression of adhesion molecules (on both endothelial and stromal cells), differential levels of growth factors, differential filtering properties of vessel walls, differential expression of receptors for immunoglobulins E, G and A (IgE, IgG and IgA), local synthesis of complement components, and differential distribution of complement regulatory proteins. There are enough permutations of these factors to explain why almost every organ is the prime target in one or other autoimmune syndrome.

This view of autoimmune rheumatic disease avoids awkward questions about loss of tolerance to tissue-specific antigens. Where autoantigens are involved they are likely to be the ones we are aware of (IgG Fc, C1q, DNA, Ro, topoisomerase-1, etc.). Many of these are essential to the regulation of the immune response, as part of either specific pathways or more general processes such as proliferation and gene transcription. Autoreactivity to these antigens may establish itself because it creates abnormal feedback loops within the immune system. Where no specific antigen has been implicated similar loops may involve non-tissue-specific recognition systems such as MHC class I and killing inhibitory receptors. It remains difficult to be sure which aspects of tissue microenvironments are most relevant in the genesis of any one disorder, but accumulating evidence points to key elements in synovitis, and may also provide clues in enthesitis (see Figure 1.4).

Immunological specialization in synovium

The specialized features of synovial intimal cells are likely to make the tissue susceptible to two pathological events. Macrophage expression of FcγRIIIa should make the tissue a preferential target for immune-complex-mediated inflammation. The facility with which the fibroblasts express DAF and VCAM-1 probably underlies the tendency for ectopic lymphoid follicles to colonize synovium. If those follicles are generating complex-forming immunoglobulins, the two processes are likely to synergize.

Synovium as a target for immune complexes
Most antigens are recognized via more than one epitope and form immune complexes containing several immunoglobulin molecules. As long as these immunoglobulins engage three arms of a C1q molecule,[45] C3b will be generated and, if in the circulation, the complex should be cleared by red cell C3b receptors. Clearance may fail if overloaded, as in meningococcal septicaemia, or with disordered complement regulation, as in systemic lupus.[46] Complement-mediated clearance will also fail if the complexes carry no more than two Fc regions. If such complexes gain access to the extravascular space they are likely to activate macrophages expressing the IgG Fc receptor FcγRIIIa and induce the secretion of inflammatory cytokines, such as TNF-α.[47,48]

FcγRIIIa is only expressed in certain tissues.[23] As indicated in Figure 1.8, binding of complexes to FcγRIIIa should give rise to syndromes which include synovitis, serositis and alveolitis. Activation of Kupffer cells and macrophages in

lymphoid organs may also produce an acute phase response, hepatomegaly, lymphadenopathy, splenomegaly and suppression of erythropoiesis or granulopoiesis. These features are found in adult rheumatoid disease, but are equally characteristic of systemic-onset juvenile chronic arthritis (systemic JCA).[49] The relevant complexes in rheumatoid arthritis are likely to be self-associated IgG rheumatoid factor dimers. The implication is that there are complexes of a similar size in systemic-onset arthritis, but not based on rheumatoid factors. Although complexes have been identified in systemic-onset arthritis, the antigen(s) remains unknown.

In skeletal muscle, synovial intima, pericardium and, to a lesser extent myocardium, FcγRIIIa is present both on cells and adsorbed on to fibrillin-1-based microfibrils.[23] In skeletal muscle, matrix-bound receptor dominates. Attached to extracellular matrix the receptor cannot induce cell signalling, but may act as a sump for small complexes, especially if alternative pathway complement components are engaged. The coexistence of DAF on the same fibres again suggests that the molecules act in some coordinated way. It is not clear what clinical correlate may relate to binding of complexes to microfibril-based FcγRIIIa, but both acute viral myalgia and polymyalgia rheumatica might fit the bill.

Ectopic lymphoid tissue formation in synovium
Histopathologists have remarked that chronic synovitis differs from inflammation in other tissues in the extent of lymphoid follicle formation.[50] A follicle has a central B-cell zone, which in several rheumatic disorders may include a germinal centre. Both the increase in intimal macrophage size and numbers, responsible for what was once termed 'intimal hyperplasia',[50] and the T-cell accumulation seen in chronic synovitis are consistent with any inflammatory stimulus. B-cell accumulation requires a more specific explanation.

The factor in synovium likely to assist B-cell accumulation is the facility with which synovial fibroblasts express VCAM-1 and DAF.[51] Interaction with VCAM-1 is required for

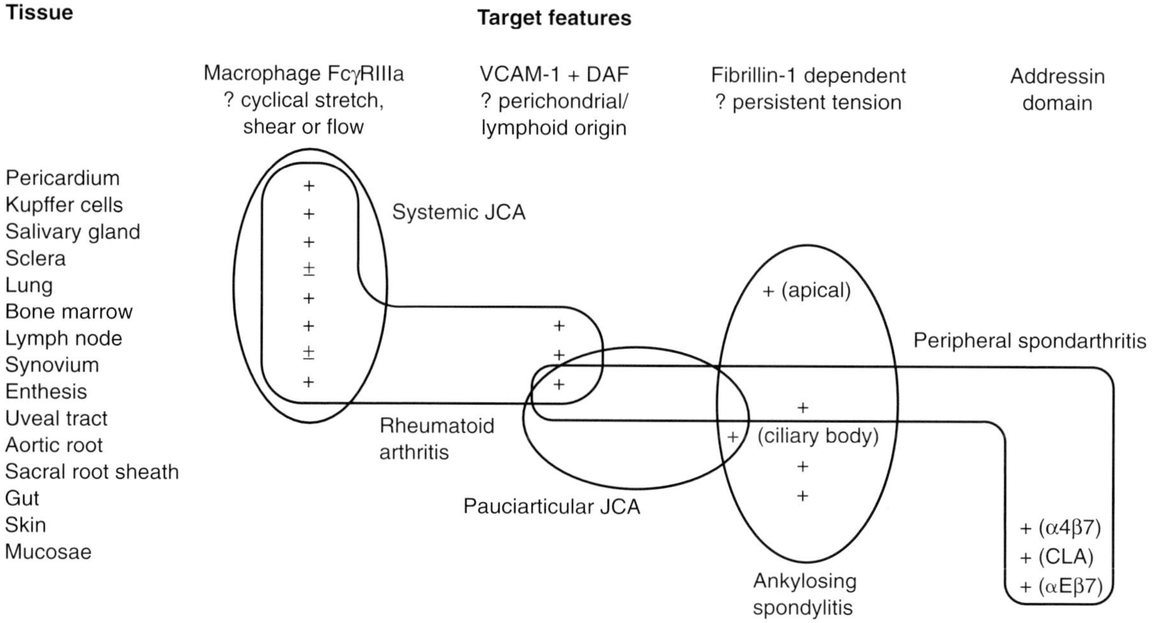

Figure 1.8 Possible targeting factors for autoimmune disease in the immunological microenvironments of connective tissues.

survival at virtually all stages of B lymphocyte life history. DAF is also found at a high level at sites of B lymphocyte survival (bone marrow and follicle centre), and protects against both complement and NK-mediated killing.[52] It also regulates the availability of C3 breakdown products, which are required for antigen presentation to B cells by follicular dendritic cells. Complement receptor CR2 is also essential to B-cell function in follicle centres.[53] It is not present on normal synovial fibroblasts, but the cytokine responsiveness of synovial fibroblasts includes CR2 expression.[51] TNF-α is likely to drive ectopic lymphoid follicle formation, which depends on TNF-receptor ligation.[54]

Normal synovial intimal fibroblasts do not support B-cell survival, probably because they are bathed in excess hyaluronan, with its anti-adhesive effect. If macrophage cytokines such as TNF-α are produced, then VCAM-1 and DAF will be readily induced on subintimal fibroblasts, which are not steeped in hyaluronan.

These cells are then in a good position to support B-cell survival, especially if T cells are available to provide help. An interesting feature of rheumatoid-factor-specific B cells is that they can be helped by a range of T cells recognizing foreign antigens and do not require T cells specific for IgG Fc.

The initial stimulus for the accumulation of lymphocytes in synovium may come from immune complexes or activated T cells. The formation of ectopic lymphoid tissue may be expected to occur in synovium in a range of autoimmune states. This would explain the similar appearance of synovium in seropositive and seronegative arthropathies.

The tissue-targeting mechanism in pauciarticular-onset arthritis[49] is perhaps the most perplexing. The process appears to be systemic, in that several sites are often involved. However, once established, the disease often spreads no further. Autoantibodies are present, most characteristically to the nuclear protein DEK, but there is nothing to suggest a role for immune complexes. Cell penetrating antibodies to DEK, which is an oncoprotein involved in gene transcription and signal transduction in T cells,[55] could disturb control of lymphocyte survival and activation, but in what way? The uveal tract is targeted in anti-DEK-positive individuals, in a way distinct from that seen with human leucocyte antigen B27 (HLA-B27). Susceptibility is associated with both a distinct class I allotype (A2) and a combination of class II allotypes. Bone overgrowth is characteristic of sites involved in pauciarticular arthritis, suggesting that the immune reaction has a specific effect on growth-factor production. None of this seems to add up, but there is a suggestion that autoantibody-producing B-cell clones survive sequestered in a synovium, perhaps because their antibody products interfere with growth control mechanisms affecting both T cells and chondrocytes.

Enthesis

Whereas a number of developmental features have been identified in synovium that may determine susceptibility to autoimmune disease, the situation for enthesis is limited to some tantalising clues. One is the rarity of spinal enthesitis prior to the cessation of growth. HLA-B27-associated disease may present in growing adolescents, but, if so, usually affects peripheral joint synovium or the eye. This suggests that 'autoimmune' enthesitis is dependent on the growth-factor status or responsiveness of the target tissue in some way.

A second clue is the correspondence between the sites of involvement in ankylosing spondylitis and Marfan's syndrome:[56] spinal and peripheral enthesitis, ascending aortitis with valve incompetence, anterior uveitis, apical lung fibrosis, and ectasia of sacral root sheaths, versus scoliosis, ligamentous laxity, ascending aortic dilatation with valve incompetence, ciliary zonule laxity with lens dislocation, apical lung bullae with pneumothorax and ectasia of sacral root sheaths.

Marfan's syndrome is due to abnormalities of the gene for fibrillin-1, which commonly involve the production of protein defective in one of its calcium-binding epidermal-growth-factor-like sequences.[56] Fibrillin-1 is clearly important at all the sites of pathology in Marfan's syndrome, but is in no way limited to these sites. The sites of pathology in Marfan's syndrome are similar to those in defects of other tensile connective-tissue components, as in Ehlers–Danlos syndrome. The significance of these sites would appear to be not that they are rich in fibrillin-1, but that they are sites of persistent tensile stress. Fibrillin-1 is only one of several molecules required for handling such stresses. Thus tissue susceptibility in ankylosing spondylitis is probably only indirectly related to an embryological programme for fibrillin-1 synthesis.

Tensile stresses invoke the secretion of a wide variety of physiological mediators, such as growth factors, prostanoids and nitric oxide. Secretion of these factors is essential to the homeostasis of extracellular matrix, perhaps best documented for bone.[57] Fibrous tissues may be particularly dependent on growth factors such as TGFβ for continual repair. The anterior chamber of the eye is particularly rich in TGFβ.[58]

The most important clue to the genesis of enthesitis must be the association with HLA-B27. This association strongly suggests the involvement of cytotoxic lymphocytes with receptors for MHC class I. These could be CD8/CD3/T-cell receptor complexes, but the function of T-cell receptors is to recognize bound antigenic peptides rather than MHC allotype. Much more likely candidates are class I receptors which downregulate killing (killing inhibitory receptors (KIR) and CD94).[59] These recognize specific allotypes of HLA-A, B or C. B27 confers resistance to conversion of human immunodeficiency virus (HIV) infection to acquired immune deficiency syndrome (AIDS), probably by delaying cytolysis of CD4+ cells.[60] This suggests that B27 gives an unusually potent signal via KIR. It may thereby raise the threshold for killing of unwanted activated lymphoid cells, and skew normal immunoregulation.

Any link between cytotoxic cell surveillance and the enthesis remains speculative. However, the fact that TGFβ is a potent modulator of both class I expression and cytotoxic function may be relevant. Sites such as the anterior chamber of the eye and the spinal entheses may have developed a strategy of local immunoregulation, which is most at risk in the face of an unusual class I/KIR relationship. Another developmental reason to link enthesitis with the control of cytotoxic cell function is the link with lesions in embryologically predetermined addressin domains (see Figure 1.1): the skin in psoriasis, the gut in Crohn's disease and the mucosae in Reiter's syndrome. Each of these domains has its own T-cell population with specialized cytotoxic subsets such as Tγδ and NK cells.

Although enthesitis is often considered a single pathological process in the context of spondarthropathy, it may be necessary to distinguish central (spinal and sacroiliac) from peripheral joint-related enthesitis. The former may be a pure enthesitis. The latter may often involve both enthesis and synovium, as in psoriatic dactylitis and oligoarthritis of the Reiter's type. Synovitis in the latter context may always be associated with enthesitis.[61] This raises the possibility that if a lesion at a peripheral enthesis contiguous with synovium generates cytokines such as TNF-α, then colonization of the adjacent synovium by autoreactive B and/or T cells may occur. The differential susceptibility of central and peripheral entheses remains unexplained, but abnormalities of circulating cytotoxic cells are different in patients with central and peripheral B27 associated disease.[62] It may also be relevant that central enthesitis sites are the sites where haemopoietic marrow is retained following cessation of development.

JOINT DEVELOPMENT IN ADOLESCENCE AND THE IMPACT OF DISEASE

Skeletal development during adolescence is characterized by rapid growth rates and by the achievement of full stature and function through a combination of balanced growth rates in component structures and the timing of growth plate closure. Imbalance in these factors may

either lead to or be caused by pathological change.

Primary developmental problems

A primary imbalance of rates of growth or extracellular matrix deposition has been implicated in a number of adolescent problems, including scoliosis, pneumothorax and disorders of the femoral head. There may be a well-defined underlying connective-tissue abnormality such as Marfan's syndrome, or the reason may be less well defined, perhaps because of polygenic origin.

Among articular structures, the femoral head is the site most susceptible to imbalances in growth. Both Perthes' disease and slipped epiphysis are associated with imbalances in growth rates. Subjects with Perthes' disease often have evidence of developmental abnormalities in other systems. There is frequently evidence for skeletal growth retardation or a catch-up phase prior to the onset of the disease.[63] An imbalance in local skeletal development may therefore be responsible for the vascular changes in the territory of the lateral epiphyseal artery associated with the condition.[64] Perthes' disease usually presents before adolescence, but the potential vulnerability of the femoral head throughout growth is illustrated by a case under the care of one of the authors. A female presented at age 20 years with bilateral femoral head avascular necrosis having developed hypopituitarism at the age of 13 following irradiation of an optic nerve glioma. Although she had received standard corticosteroid replacement, she had not received growth hormone. The growth-plate region was unusually radiodense.

Slipped epiphysis commonly occurs in the early adolescent period. It is associated with an increased slope of the proximal femoral physis, high body weight, and low thyroxine, growth hormone and testosterone.[65]

The impact of disease on development

All chronic diseases with onset in childhood may have major effects upon adolescent development, whether the disease is still active or has wreaked its effects in the early years. Whether the disease is joint specific (e.g. juvenile chronic arthritis) or joint non-specific (e.g. systemic lupus erythematosus (SLE), dermatomyositis or scleroderma), effects upon the musculoskeletal system may be profound. The spectrum of problems encountered is wide, and encompasses the altered body image of the cushingoid child with profound growth failure from corticosteroid use in systemic-onset arthritis, as well as the effects of leg-length discrepancy requiring multiple surgical procedures due to persistent pauciarticular-onset arthritis in the knee. The failure of normal joint development can have profound effects upon the psyche of the adolescent through chronic pain, deformity and loss of function of mobility and upper limb function. These ongoing effects interact directly with the characteristic issues of adolescence, which include the development of social competence and responsibility, emancipation from parents or care-givers with emotional and financial independence. A successful navigation through adolescence is made all the more challenging by abnormal joint development or function. The added issue of difficulties in compliance with medical regimes, which is so typical of the adolescent period, may have major effects upon ongoing already tenuous joint development.

Generalized growth abnormalities
Rheumatic diseases can produce either over- or undergrowth of skeletal elements or the occurrence of deformities specific to the joint in question. All rheumatic diseases with a systemic aspect may suppress linear growth, either temporarily, as in association with delayed puberty, or more commonly with reduction of eventual adult height. Such growth failure is commonplace in juvenile-onset dermatomyositis, and systemic-onset and, to a lesser extent, polyarticular-onset arthritis. This is particularly so in cases where the use of systemic corticosteroids has been mandated by disease uncontrolled by other means. Although such effects are important throughout childhood, it is in adolescence, the time of greatest linear growth

velocity, that the problem manifests itself most clearly and attendant psychological and functional issues become paramount. Recent studies[66] indicate that, although growth hormone therapy may have a role in treatment, patients are not deficient in this factor. The molecular abnormalities may relate to inhibition or deficiency of other factors such as insulin-like growth factor 1 (IGF-1).

Together with the effects on linear growth are the implications for bone mineralization in the maturing skeleton. Adolescence represents the critical time period in the attainment of peak bone mass, and chronic rheumatic diseases and steroid use during this period may have irreversible effects that lower fracture threshold throughout adult life.[67] Poor mineralization of specific weight-bearing joints may be related to the occurrence of avascular necrosis in hips and knees. This is often seen in adolescent patients with systemic forms of rheumatic disease with severe effects on joint integrity and subsequently on linear growth. This effect is undoubtedly magnified by limitations in or abnormal patterns of weight bearing. Given evidence of the probable preventive value of calcium and vitamin D in these instances,[68] the issue of non-compliance in adolescence is of even greater importance.

Localized growth abnormalities
Chronic joint inflammation in childhood or adolescence may have unique sequelae, which are rarely seen in adult-onset rheumatic disease. The growing joint typically has a greater blood supply to the constituting bony epiphyses as compared with later life. It has been suggested that, as a consequence of chronic hyperaemia, an increased, albeit uncoordinated and inappropriate, stimulus is delivered to the joint and elements may overgrow. An alternative possibility is that growth factors are generated as a specific consequence of the immune response within the joint. The occurrence of leg-length discrepancies is typical of arthritis in childhood, particularly early pauciarticular, but also polyarticular, onset forms of the disease. During the rapid growth spurt of adolescence minor

limb-length discrepancies can become magnified, requiring surgical procedures such as osteotomies or epiphyseal stapling to prevent further deformity.[69] The effects of leg-length discrepancy are manifest by altered gait patterns, with subsequent stress on the joints on the contralateral side. If unchecked, these other joints, often also involved in the disease process, can become more painful and eventually at risk of increased inflammatory activity or more rapid degenerative change. In the knee, the medial side of the joint, the femoral and tibial epiphyses, may overgrow relative to the lateral side, producing the typical valgus deformity seen in arthritis in childhood.

Overgrowth may occur in the femoral head relative to the acetabulum. This can result in altered integrity of the joint, with relative uncovering of the lateral margins of the femoral head. In the growing adolescent such an abnormal joint even with quiescent disease is subject to increased risk of altered mechanics and of subsequent degenerative changes.

Overgrowth of components of the elbow joint can lead to great dysfunction with both marked fixed flexion deformity and disabling loss of pronation and supination. The cosmetic implications of such deformity clearly add to the functional disease burden in adolescents.

In contrast, localized growth failure is a feature of some joints affected in generalized arthritis in children. The temporomandibular joint (TMJ) is frequently involved, especially in the polyarticular- and systemic-onset forms of disease.[70] The effects may be symmetric or asymmetric. Symmetrical disease of both joints tends to produce retrognathia or micrognathia due to failure of mandibular development. Disease in the TMJ may be erosive and destructive, with severe limitation of mouth opening and dental malocclusion. The functional consequences may include poor dietary intake secondary to pain and/or reduced mandibular excursion, which may be an added insult to the already parlous catabolic state of many children with severe arthritis. The cosmetic deformity is perhaps the most obvious and distressing feature of the disease in some children with chronic arthritis,

and is particularly prominent during adolescence. Recent surgical and dental techniques, including elongation procedures for the mandible, have produced encouraging results in some patients.[71] In systemic-onset arthritis, TMJ disease tends to produce poor growth of other facial components in concert with the mandible, producing a smaller but more symmetrical facial structure. Asymmetrical disease produces asymmetrical mandibular movement, with pain and secondary problems with chewing and dental malocclusion.

Involvement of the small bones of the hands and feet may produce either over- or undergrowth in an unpredictable fashion. Involvement of the toes can produce marked deformities of the forefoot, with overriding and bizarre valgus and varus postures. Together with deformities such as pes valgoplanus and pes cavus, such effects provide great challenges to the attending podiatrist, and surgery is not infrequently required.[72]

Somewhat paradoxically, epiphyses that have undergone initial overgrowth may fuse prematurely, leading to an overall loss of limb length compared with the expected adult limb length. This adds further to the functional and cosmetic deformities in the adolescent with chronic arthritis.

Joint contractures

A characteristic of joint disease with onset in childhood is the frequency of joint contractures. In part this is because inflamed joints take up a posture of greatest volume, thereby reducing intrasynovial pressure and pain. It is also felt to be the result of spasm of dominant muscle groups about the joint in response to pain and inflammation (such as the adductors and flexors of the hip). As the child grows, such contractures become more obvious and disabling, with contractures of other joints occurring secondarily. Knee contracture frequently follows hip disease, where the flexed posture is initially required to maintain the centre of gravity. This is often balanced above by a lumbar hyperlordosis to re-establish the centre of gravity and an upright trunk. Contractures in the upper limb are also commonplace and can severely interfere with function and the acquisition of new skills, with major consequences in the adolescent. The inability to tie one's own shoelaces or perform adequate toileting represents a great challenge to the teenager attempting to establish independence.

An aggressive approach to physiotherapy programmes and judicious early surgical intervention with soft-tissue releases has gone some way to reduce the impact of contractures, but they often contribute greatly to disability, even when disease has become quiescent.

Repair in the adolescent joint

To a greater or lesser extent the adolescent with a history of arthritis may be emerging from a disease that is no longer actively inflammatory. Long-term prognosis depends on the capacity of articular structures to repair. Synovial tissue has great powers of regeneration, even following surgical removal, and the main limitation on repair is the early establishment of fibrous adhesion with loss of range. Bone shafts also have a great capacity for repair, but articular surfaces do not. At one time the dogma was that hyaline cartilage could not repair. However, chondrocyte cloning and cartilage outgrowth are common in damaged joints. What may remain true is that hyaline cartilage and subchondral bone have a limited capacity to regenerate usefully at load-bearing sites once collagen structure has been disrupted. Damaged hyaline cartilage is usually replaced by fibrocartilage.

Since fibrocartilage has a great capacity for regeneration and forms an effective articular surface in birds, the question arises as to why replacement of hyaline cartilage by fibrocartilage is such a problem. However, hyaline cartilage may be important, at least in long-lived mammals, precisely because of its limited ability to repair. It forms the blueprint for shape in the skeleton and, once development has ceased, may retain 'shape memory' by having a very high threshold for collagen remodelling in response to mechanical stimuli. In this way it retains shape despite joint use. Only under very abnormal stresses will it attempt to remodel, but at the cost of losing shape memory and any chance of perfect restoration of joint function. It may be that all attempts to transplant chondrocytes are doomed to failure, and that in the adult the only way to regenerate the original shape of an articular surface is to regrow the entire limb, as some amphibians can do!

Nevertheless, in childhood and adolescence, there is evidence that 'shape memory' can be restored, at least in part. Almost complete loss of joint space from inflammatory disease in infancy may be followed by a normal joint space in adolescence. The combination of a rather dense, slightly irregular, subchondral plate with overgrowth at the margins and normal joint space is characteristic. Joint failure eventually supervenes in many cases, but often not for another decade. A better understanding of what controls the ability of load-bearing hyaline cartilage to restore itself to a functioning articular surface would be of enormous value in dealing with joint failure. Currently it is often only possible to stand back and see secondary failure supervene. Further insights into joint development might pay great dividends in terms of long-term quality of life.

REFERENCES

1. Horton J, Ratcliffe N. Evolution of immunity. In: *Immunology* (Roitt IM, Brostoff J, Male D, eds), 5th edn. Mosby: London, 1988:199–220.
2. Freedman AS, Munro JM, Rice GE et al. Adhesion of human B cells to germinal centres in vitro involves VLA-4 and INCAM-110. *Science* 1990; **249**:1030–2.
3. Wilkinson LS, Edwards JCW, Poston R, Haskard DO. Cell populations expressing VCAM-1 in normal and diseased synovium. *Lab Invest* 1993; **68**:82–8.
4. Resnick D, Niwayama G. *Diagnosis of Bone and Joint Disorders*, 2nd edn. WB Saunders: Philadelphia, 1988.

5. O'Rahilly R, Gardner E. The embryology of movable joints. In: *The Joints and Synovial Fluid*, vol 1 (Sokoloff L, ed). Academic Press: New York, 1978:105–76.

6. Edwards JCW, Wilkinson LS, Jones HM et al. The formation of human synovial joint cavities: a possible role for hyaluronan and CD44 in altered interzone cohesion. *J Anat* 1994; **185**:355–67.

7. Rice GE, Munro JM, Corless C, Bevilacqua MP. Vascular and non-vascular expression of INCAM-110; a target for mononuclear leucocyte adhesion in normal and inflamed human tissues. *Am J Pathol* 1991; **138**:385–93.

8. Medof ME, Walter EI, Rutgers JL, Knowles DM, Nussenzweig V. Identification of the complement decay accelerating factor on epithelium and glandular cells and in body fluids. *J Exp Med* 1987; **165**:848–64.

9. Wolpert L, Lewis J, Summerbell D. Morphogenesis of the vertebrate limb. *Ciba Found Symp*1975; **29**:91–130.

10. Archer CW, Morrison H, Pitsillides AA. Cellular aspects of the development of diarthrodial joints and articular cartilage. *J Anat* 1994; **184**:447–56.

11. Cohn MJ, Patel K, Krumlauf R, Wilkinson DG, Clarke JD, Tickle C. *Hox9* genes and vertebrate limb specification. *Nature* 1997; **387**:97–101.

12. Francis-West PH, Richardson MK, Bell E et al. The effect of overexpression of BMPs and GDF-5 on the development of chick limb skeletal elements. *Ann NY Acad Sci* 1996; **785**:254–5.

13. Pitsillides AA, Archer CB, Prehm P, Bayliss MT, Edwards JCW. Alterations in hyaluronan synthesis during developing joint cavitation. *J Histochem Cytochem*1995; **43**:263–73.

14. Toole BP, Goldberg RL, Chi-Rosso G, Underhill CB, Orkin RW. Hyaluronate–cell interactions. In: *The Role of Extracellular Matrix in Development* (Trelstad RL, ed). AR Liss: New York, 1984:43–66.

15. Edwards JCW, Wilkinson LS, Soothill P, Hembry R, Reynolds JJ. Matrix metalloproteinases in the formation of human synovial joint cavities. *J Anat* 1996; **188**:355–60.

16. Nalin AM, Greenlee TK Jr, Sandell LJ. Collagen gene expression during development of avian synovial joints: transient expression of types II and XI collagen genes in the joint capsule. *Dev Dynam* 1995; **203**:352–62.

17. Knight AD, Levick JR. Pressure–volume relationships above and below atmospheric pressure in the synovial cavity of the rabbit knee. *J Physiol Lond* 1982; **328**:403–20.

18. Drachman DB, Sokoloff L. The role of movement in embryonic joint development. *Dev Biol* 1996; **14**:401–20.

19. Ward AC, Dowthwaite GP, Edwards JCW, Pitsillides AA. The effect of embryonic limb immobilisation on cavitation associated changes in hyaluronan synthesis and FGF2 and 4 expression during joint development. *Connective Tissue Res* 1996; **36**:104–5.

20. Dowthwaite GP, Edwards JCW, Pitsillides AA. An essential role for the interaction between hyaluronan and hyaluronan binding proteins during joint development. *J Histochem Cytochem* 1998; in press.

21. Hall JG. Arthrogryposis multiplex congenita: etiology, genetics, classification, diagnostic approach, and general aspects. *J Pediatr Orthop B* 1997; **6**:159–66.

22. Waggett AD, Kielty CM, Shuttleworth CA. Microfibrillar elements in the synovial joint: presence of type VI collagen and fibrillin-containing microfibrils. *Ann Rheum Dis* 1993; **52**:449–52.

23. Bhatia A, Blades S, Cambridge G, Edwards JCW. Differential distribution of FcγRIIIa in normal human tissues. *Immunology* 1998; **94**:56–63.

24. Edwards JCW. The synovium. In: *Rheumatology* (Klippel JH, Dieppe PA, eds), 2nd edn. Mosby Year Book: London, 1997:5.6.1–8.

25. Edwards JCW, Wilkinson LS. Distribution in human tissues of the synovial lining associated epitope recognised by monoclonal antibody 67. *J Anat* 1996; **188**:119–27.

26. Edwards JCW, Willoughby DA. Demonstration of bone marrow derived cells in synovial lining by means of giant intracellular granules as genetic markers. *Ann Rheum Dis* 1982; **41**: 177–82.

27. Revell PA, Al-Saffar N, Fish S, Osei D. Extracellular matrix of the synovial intimal cell layer. *Ann Rheum Dis* 1995; **54**:404–7.

28. Worrall JG, Bayliss MT, Edwards JCW. Zonal distribution of sulphated proteoglycans in normal and rheumatoid synovium. *Ann Rheum Dis* 1994; **53**:35–8.

29. McCachren SS, Lightner VA. Expression of human tenascin in synovitis and its regulation by interleukin-1. *Arthritis Rheum* 1992; **35**: 1185–96.

30. Edwards JCW, Blades S, Cambridge G. Restricted expression of FcγRIII (CD16) in synovium and dermis: implications for tissue targeting in rheumatoid arthritis. *Clin Exp Immunol* 1997; **108**:401–6.

31. Wahl SM, Allen JB, Welch GR, Wong HL. Transforming growth factor-β in synovial fluids modulates FgγRIII (CD16) expression on mononuclear phagocytes. *J Immunol* 1992; **148**:485–90.

32. Morrison EH, Ferguson MW, Bayliss MT, Archer CW. The development of articular cartilage: I. *J Anat* 1996; **189**:9–22.

33. Archer CW, Morrison EH, Bayliss MT, Ferguson MW. The development of articular cartilage: I. *J Anat* 1996; **189**:23–35.

34. Archer CW, Frances West P. The development of joints and articular cartilage. In: *The Biology of the Synovial Joint* (Archer CW, Caterson B, Benjamin M, Ralphs JR, eds). Harwood Academic Press: Reading, 1998, in press.

35. Gao J, Messner K, Ralphs JR, Benjamin M. An immunohistochemical study of enthesis development in the medial collateral ligament of the rat knee joint. *Anat Embryol Berl* 1996; **194**:399–406.

36. Ralphs JR, Benjamin M. The joint capsule: structure, composition, ageing and disease. *J Anat* 1994; **184**:503–9.

37. Zidorn T. Classification of the suprapatellar septum considering ontogenetic development. *Arthroscopy* 1992; **8**:459–64.

38. Bolton MC, Dudhia J, Bayliss MT. Quantification of aggrecan and link protein mRNA in human articular cartilage of different ages by competitive reverse transcriptase-PCR. *Biochem J* 1996; **319**:489–98.

39. Scott J. Keratan sulphate – a 'reserve' polysaccharide? *Eur J Clin Chem Clin Biochem* 1994; **32**:217–23.

40. Tilstra DJ, Byers PH. Molecular basis of hereditary disorders of connective tissue. *Annu Rev Med* 1994; **45**:149–63.

41. Erlebacher A, Derynck R. Increased expression of TGFβII in osteoblasts results in an osteoporosis-like phenotype. *J Cell Biol* 1996; **132**:195–210.

42. Michaeli DA, Murphy SB, Hipp JA. Comparison of predicted and measured contact pressures in normal and dysplastic hips. *Med Eng Phys* 1997;**19**:180–6.

43. Riemersma S, Vincent A, Beeson D et al. Association of arthrogryposis multiplex congenita with maternal antibodies inhibiting fetal acetylcholine receptor function. *J Clin Invest* 1996; **98**:2358–63.

44. Veasy LG, Hill HR. Immunologic and clinical correlations in rheumatic fever and rheumatic heart disease. *Pediatr Infect Dis J* 1997; **16**:400–7.

45. Perkins SJ, Nealis AS, Sutton BJ, Feinstein A. Solution structure of human and mouse immunoglobulin M by synchrotron X-ray scattering and molecular graphics modelling. A possible mechanism for complement activation. *J Mol Biol* 1991; **221**:1345–66.

46. Davies KA, Hird V, Stewart S et al. A study of in vivo immune complex formation and clearance in man. *J Immunol* 1990; **144**:4613–20.

47. Huizinga TW, van Kemenade F, Koenderman L et al. The 40-kDa Fcγ receptor (FcRII) on human neutrophils is essential for the IgG-induced respiratory burst and IgG-induced phagocytosis. *J Immunol* 1989; **142**:2365–9.

48. Edwards JCW. Is rheumatoid factor relevant? In: *Rheumatoid Arthritis, Questions and Uncertainties* (Bird H, Snaith ML, eds). Blackwells: London, 1998, in press.

49. White PH. Juvenile chronic arthritis: clinical features. In: *Rheumatology* (Klippel JH, Dieppe PA, eds), 2nd edn. Mosby Year Book: London, 1997:5.18.1–10.

50. Gardner DL. Rheumatoid arthritis: cell and tissue pathology. In: *Pathological Basis of Connective Tissue Diseases* (Gardner DL, ed). Edward Arnold: London, 1992:444–526.

51. Edwards JCW, Leigh RD, Cambridge G. Expression of molecules involved in B lymphocyte survival and differentiation by synovial fibroblasts. *Clin Exp Immunol* 1997; **108**:407–14.

52. Finberg RW, White W, Nicholson-Weller A. Decay-accelerating factor expression on either effector or target cells inhibits cytotoxicity by human natural killer cells. *J Immunol* 1992; **149**:2055–60.

53. Caret RH, Spycher MO, Ng YC, Hoffman R, Fearon DT. Synergistic interaction between complement receptor type 2 and membrane IgM on B lymphocytes. *J Immunol* 1988; **141**:457–63.

54. Fu YX, Molina H, Matsumoto M, Huang G, Min J, Chaplin DD. Lymphotoxin-α (LTα) supports development of splenic follicular structure that is required for IgG responses. *J Exp Med* 1997; **185**:2111–20.

55. Fu GK, Grosveld G, Markovitz DM. DEK, an autoantigen involved in a chromosomal translocation in acute myelogenous leukemia, binds to the HIV-2 enhancer. *Proc Natl Acad Sci USA* 1997; **94**:1811–5.

56. Child AH. Marfan syndrome; current medical and genetic knowledge: how to treat and when. *J Card Surg* 1997; **12**(suppl 2):131–5.

57. Lanyon LE. The physiological basis of training the skeleton. The Sir Frederick Smith Memorial Lecture. *Equine Vet J Suppl* 1990; **9**:8–13.

58. Streilein JW, Takeuchi M, Taylor AW. Immune privilege, T-cell tolerance, and tissue-restricted autoimmunity. *Hum Immunol* 1997; **52**:138–43.

59. Long EO, Burshtyn DN, Clark WP et al. Killer inhibitory receptors: diversity, specificity and function. *Immunol Rev* 1991; **155**:135–44.

60. McNeil AJ, Yap PL, Gore SM et al. Association of HLA types A1-B8-DR3 and B27 with rapid and slow progression of HIV disease. *Q J Med* 1996; **89**:177–85.

61. McGonagle D, Pease C, Green MJ, O'Connor P, Gibbon WW, Emery P. Knee synovitis in reactive arthritis is strongly associated with the presence of knee enthesopathy. *Br J Rheumatol* 1997; **36**(suppl 1):171.

62. Garmendia E, Brito E, Zea A et al. Different distribution of T and NK cell subpopulations in peripheral blood from reactive arthritis and ankylosing spondylitis patients. *Br J Rheumatol* 1997; **36**(suppl 1):127.

63. Kristmundsdottir F, Burwell RG, Harrison MH. Delayed skeletal maturation in Perthe's disease. *Acta Orthop Scand* 1987; **58**:277–9.

64. Ferguson AB. Segmental vascular changes in the femoral head in children and adults. *Clin Orthop* 1985; **200**:291–8.

65. Wilcox PG, Weiner DS, Leighley B. Maturation factors in slipped capital femoral epiphysis. *J Paediatr Orthop* 1988; **8**:196–200.

66. Davies UM, Rooney M, Preece MA, Ansell BM, Woo P. Treatment of growth retardation in juvenile chronic arthritis with recombinant human growth hormone. *J Rheumatol* 1994; **21**:153–8.

67. Hergenroeder AC. Bone mineralization, hypothalamic amenorrhea, and sex steroid therapy in female adolescents and young adults. *J Pediatr* 1995; **126**:683–9.

68. American College of Rheumatology Task Force on Osteoporosis Guidelines. Recommendations for the prevention and treatment of glucocorticoid-induced osteoporosis. *Arthritis Rheum* 1996; **39**:1791–801.

69. Fraser RK, Dickens DR, Cole WG. Medial physeal stapling for primary and secondary genu valgum in late childhood and adolescence. *J Bone Joint Surg Br* 1995; **77**:733–5.

70. Mericle PM, Wilson VK, Moore TL et al. Effects on polyarticular and pauciarticular onset juvenile rheumatoid arthritis on facial and mandibular growth. *J Rheumatol* 1996; **23**:159–65.

71. Pedersen TK, Gronhoj J, Melsen B, Herlin T. Condylar condition and mandibular growth during early functional treatment of children with juvenile chronic arthritis. *Eur J Orthod* 1995; **17**:385–94.

72. Swann M. Management of lower limb deformities. In: *Surgical Management of Juvenile Chronic Polyarthritis* (Arden GP, Ansell BM, eds). Grune & Stratton: New York.

2

Developmental issues in adolescence and the impact of rheumatic disease

Jane Harrington, Adrienne Kirk and Stanton Newman

INTRODUCTION

This chapter examines the findings of studies on the psychological and social impact of arthritic conditions in childhood and adolescence. It only covers the impact on levels of physical functioning where they are related to psychological measures, as physical aspects of juvenile rheumatic disease are covered elsewhere in this volume (see Chapter 3).

THE PROBLEMS OF DEFINING ADOLESCENCE

One of the methodological difficulties of research in this area is exactly how to define 'adolescence'. At a simple descriptive level it can be defined in opposition to childhood and adulthood. Thus the period of adolescence is that which occurs between the beginning of puberty and adulthood. The transition from childhood can also be marked by the onset of puberty. While this biological marker sounds meaningful, its exact onset remains hotly contested. There are also some significant gender differences; for example, most girls have a growth spurt that signals the onset of puberty at about 9.5 years of age, while for boys this growth spurt begins, on average, 2 years later. More importantly, for studies on adolescence there are large individual differences, as some youngsters begin puberty much later than their peers. The transition to adulthood is even more difficult to

establish because there is no biological marker; frequently, researchers have resorted to external criteria such as the transition from full-time education or the independence through work.[1] The important point is that the definition involves both biological and social factors. Furthermore, the problems of applying adolescence as a category for investigation creates confusion about inclusion and exclusion criteria.

The terminology used in studies on 'adolescents' reflects the problem of definition. Authors treat terms such as 'juvenile', 'teenagers', 'young adults'[2] and 'young adulthood'[3] as synonymous with 'adolescents', but only infrequently offer a definition of the term they are using. Most researchers in looking at health and illness and the problems of adolescence have ended up using a broad age range. In many cases the age range applied has been one of convenience, often one which fits around the definition of the 'adolescent' clinic. Even assuming that a chronological age definition successfully captures what the author feels is adolescence, there is no agreed definition of the age parameters, and different researchers use different categories. Eiser and Berrenberg[4] report that in studies of adolescence samples 'are based on very generous definitions of adolescence (somewhere between 8 and 21 years)'. In studies of arthritis the problems of a wide age range are clearly apparent, and in some cases reflect the focus of attention of the researchers. In one study, where the focus was entry into the job market, subjects included were in the age range 16–24 years,[3] while another study used 9–18 years.[5]

Besides the problems of defining the period of adolescence by age, there are problems with assuming that findings can be generalized to the whole period of adolescence. The assumption of homogeneity across the adolescent period has been questioned in a host of psychological research, and is one of the reasons why further developmental divisions have been applied to the rough time-frame of adolescence. Unfortunately, in many clinical research studies the division is not based in psychological theories of development, but often is unspecified and may be chosen largely for statistical reasons, such as for achieving roughly equivalently sized groups. Examples where different divisions of age have been used are: Berry et al,[6] who divided their subjects into age groups of ≤ 10 years and ≥ 11 years; and Daltroy et al,[7] who divided up their 102 subjects into three age groups (4–5, 6–11 and 12–16 years).

Feldman and Elliot[1] focused on the social changes in adolescence. They divided adolescence into three subcategories; early, 10–14 years of age, a time of profound physical and social changes that occur with puberty; middle, 15–17 years of age, which they defined as a time of increasing independence; and late, from 18 to mid-20s, which occurs for those who delay entry into adult roles because of educational goals or other social factors. They used these categories, partly because they fit in with the American school system, and partly because their definition of the end of adolescence is when adult responsibilities such as work or marriage are undertaken. However, taken to its logical conclusion this implies that anyone who stays at university for further study remains an adolescent.

Another approach is to classify periods of adolescence by cognitive development in general and in understanding of illness in particular. One theoretical approach suggests that children's concepts of physical illness evolves in a systematic and predictable sequence consistent with the classical stage theory of cognitive development propounded by Piaget.[8] This maintains that children aged roughly 2–6 years

are at the pre-logical stage of cognitive development. This stage is subdivided into two parts: phenomenonism and contagion. Phenomenism is the most immature explanation for illness, that it is caused by an external phenomenon entirely remote to the child and results in children being unable to explain how these events cause illness. In the contagion stage the child describes the cause of illness as residing in objects or people who are close, but not actually touching the child. Therefore, it is solely proximity that is seen as causal in illness.[9]

The concrete-logical stage spans roughly 7–10 years where the differentiation between self and others increases. Explanations of younger children in this stage are referred to as contamination, where the cause of illness is still located externally in an object or person, but the illness is effected through physical contact resulting in contamination. Older children in this stage offer an explanation of illness referred to as internalization; illness is located within the body, even if its cause may be external. Children at this stage still only describe illness in indistinct, ill-defined terms, illustrating a lack of knowledge about internal organs and their functions.[9]

At about 11 years and older, children enter the formal logical thinking stage. In the earlier part of this stage the children offer a physiological explanation of illness, where external events may be partially responsible for triggering illness, but the cause and nature of illness are internal, such as the non-functioning or misfunctioning of internal organs. The most sophisticated understanding of illness are the psychophysiological explanations, where internal processes are recognized as being important, but psychological factors such as feelings and thoughts can also have an effect on illness. Some support for this stage theory was found by Bibace and Walsh,[9] whose results were congruent with these theoretical expectations.

Many criticisms have been made of the studies supporting the stage approach. Burbach and Peterson[8] point out that there are many methodological weaknesses, such as: poor description of samples, assessment instruments and procedures; lack of control over potential observer bias, expectancy effects and other confounding variables; and minimal attention to reliability and validity issues. Theoretical criticisms of the stage approach include scepticism about the existence of discrete developmental stages, a lack of explanation of the transition between stages and failure to account for environmental, social or cultural factors.[10]

A more functional approach may be better able to explain the developmental differences in children's concepts of illness.[10] Carey (cited in Eiser[10]) claims that children's understanding of illness follows their understanding of the functions of the human body. At about 4 years of age children see the function of the human body in terms of wants and beliefs, and they see illness as punishment for wrong-doing. Older children, with a more sophisticated biological understanding, perceive illness as a result of germs, or the failure of a body organ.

Whatever theoretical position one adopts regarding cognitive development in general and the evolution of understanding illness in particular, it is clear that this changes during the early stages of development, and not all children who may chronologically be classified as being in adolescence will have the same understanding of illness.

It is generally agreed that adolescence is a time when certain tasks are achieved, such as becoming physically and sexually mature, acquiring the skills needed to carry out adult roles, gaining increased autonomy from parents, and realigning social interactions and relationships with members of both the same and opposite sex.[1,4] It is how this is achieved that has been the subject of much dispute. It is commonly believed that the period is a time of 'storm and stress', a time when individuals rebel against adult authority, question conventional norms and sanctions,[1] and is accompanied by great emotion and tension. This view, which originates in work done in the 1950s and 1960s and tends to be reinforced by the media, has in fact little empirical support.[4] Adolescence is not inevitably a time of undue strife, and many adolescents maintain warm and close relationships with their parents.[11]

Given that there are developmental tasks that are carried out during adolescence, the question to be addressed in this chapter is whether the presence of a condition such as chronic arthritis affects the process and achievement of the tasks of adolescence. Before turning to the literature on the impact on rheumatic disease, we wish to address a number of methodological issues specific to studies on adolescence and rheumatological illness that need to be taken into account when considering the research literature in this field.

- *Sample size* is an important factor in research into any form of chronic illness.[12,13] Largely due to the limited numbers of individuals with different arthritic conditions, sample sizes in studies have tended to be small. Besides leading to studies of questionable statistical power, reliance on small samples where all the participants are recruited from a single hospital or clinic and where there is little variability in the severity of the disease severely limits the generalizability of the findings.
- The use of *control groups* in studies of adolescents in arthritis has particular difficulties. It is not uncommon to find studies using the healthy siblings of individuals in a study. Although they have the advantage of attempting to hold genetic and environmental influences relatively constant,[14] the assumption that the sibling is not affected by their brother or sister's illness is questionable.[15] For example, Daniels et al[16] found higher reports of allergies and asthma in siblings of children with rheumatic disease.
- Partly because of the limitation of numbers, studies have tended to define the age of adolescence widely and use *poorly designed studies*. Problems include using retrospective research designs that fail to control for disease duration since diagnosis.[13]
- Some studies have used *inappropriate instruments* to measure chronic illness. For example, the Child Behaviour Checklist (CBCL) has been widely used in adolescent arthritis, but it includes two specific medical conditions (asthma and allergies) and a number of

other items relating to physical symptoms. Thus a high score may directly reflect the illness itself rather than any adjustment problems as a result of the illness. It also may not be sensitive enough to measure the types of mild behavioural difficulties that may be found in children with chronic disease, because the instrument was designed to measure psychopathology. Some of the items in the CBCL assess social accomplishment and participation in physical activities rather than competency of social interactions.[11] Many children/adolescents with chronic illness may not be able to participate in certain activities as a direct result of their illness, but this does not imply that these individuals are less socially able.[17]

- In many studies both parents and adolescent may complete the *same questionnaire* in order that differences between the two can be measured. Although this is in many ways a sensible technique, it is not known whether the parent and adolescent interpret the questions in the same way.
- In some studies the *views of the parents* are assumed to be an accurate representation of those of the adolescent. It is important that the views of the adolescent are taken into account, rather than inferences made from parents' responses.[4]

Given these methodological problems with studies in the area, the remainder of this chapter addresses whether the presence of arthritis during the period of adolescence has a special importance in determining how adolescents understand and respond to their condition. In addition, the way in which rheumatic disease impacts on many facets of the individuals' lives and psychological well-being, and that of their families are also discussed.

THE IMPACT OF ADOLESCENCE ON RHEUMATIC DISEASE

One of the important questions to be addressed is whether adolescents are any different from children on the one hand or adults on the other in the ways in which they interpret, understand and respond to their arthritis and its treatment. Regardless of the disputes as to whether children in their development pass through clear stages in their conception of illness, it is clear that older children tend to have a more sophisticated and differentiated view of illness than do younger children.[9] This finding has been replicated in children with chronic arthritis.[6,18] Berry et al[6] assessed children and adolescents aged 7–17 years on their understanding of their juvenile chronic arthritis (JCA). Following Piaget's stage theory of cognitive development, three major categories of explanations of their illness were identified, which reflected increasing differentiation of the self and more sophisticated explanations of cause and internal physiological processes (see earlier discussion). Children's understanding of JCA followed a developmental progression, with older children demonstrating a more sophisticated understanding of their disease than younger children. However, most subjects at the oldest age level answered questions on JCA at the concrete operational stage of cognitive development, despite the expectation that the majority of them would function at the normal operational level, a level that reflects adult levels of understanding and thinking. Another striking finding from this study was the level of inaccuracies and misunderstandings about causes of arthritis, pain and stiffness, despite the fact that many were long-time clinic attenders who had gone through routine clinic educational teachings.

Adherence to treatment recommendations is seen as a central, and in many ways the most important, issue in most medical interventions. In the context of arthritis it has implications for the relief of symptoms, quality of life, disease progression as well as the costs of treatment.[19] Such adherence is influenced by many factors, including the understanding the individual has of their illness. Inaccurate understanding of the illness is likely to affect adherence, although this has been subjected to only limited study,[6,20] and relatively little is known about how adolescents' understanding of their arthritis influences adherence.

Adolescents are often perceived to be rather troublesome and non-adherent patients, especially when compared to younger children.[1] Their clinic attendance may become erratic or cease, and there may be a decline in therapeutic adherence and an increase in challenges to adult authority. These behaviours are often explained within a 'storm and stress' view of adolescence. However, as discussed above, adolescence is not inevitably a time of undue strife.[11] It is also important to appreciate that there is no evidence from studies that adolescents who have the most problems with adherence are also those who score highly on measures of rebellion or risk-taking.[21]

Pain is one of the primary symptoms of rheumatic disease. Two early studies[22] suggested that children report much less pain than adults. It was concluded that children with JCA experienced less pain than adults with rheumatoid arthritis. These studies had a number of methodological difficulties and failed to take account of the possible developmental differences between children and adults in conceptualizing pain and illness.[23] Beales et al[24] attempted to account for developmental differences by investigating pain in 6–11 and 12–17 year old patients with JCA. Sensory descriptions of pain were similar in the two groups, with all reporting an 'aching' sensation in their affected joints, and almost half of both groups describing a 'sharp' or 'burning' pain. The meaning and interpretation of the pain differed between the younger and older individuals. Only the older children and adolescents reported that these sensations reminded them of their JCA and subsequent functional limitation. Most of the younger group marked below the midpoint on the visual analogue scales for both sensory unpleasantness and pain severity. In contrast, most of the older group marked above the midpoint. Beales et al[24] came to the conclusion that the meaning children attribute to the painful sensations from involved joints may influence the actual degree of pain that is perceived and/or reported. Thus, as older children and adolescents associate internal sensations with internal pathology and adverse consequences for future goals and activities, they

may be more likely to view these sensations as 'painful', and come to behave more like adults.

IMPACT OF ARTHRITIS ON THE INDIVIDUAL

The impact of juvenile arthritis spans all aspects of functioning. Overall levels of psychosocial functioning have been examined and found to be related to different factors. Billings et al[25] found that the patient's age and the severity of the arthritis were important. Those who were severely affected by their condition were rated by their parents as having more psychological and physical problems. Timko et al[26] found negative events, relating to the context of the adolescents' everyday life that had occurred in the past year, chronic life stressors and stable social resources to be associated with psychosocial functioning.

Although somewhat artificial one can attempt to separate out different aspects of psychosocial functioning. The discussion below attempts to distinguish between the physical, psychological and social aspects of functioning.

The physical manifestations of chronic arthritis have a significant impact on the adolescent's functioning in everyday life. Joint stiffness and pain can cause difficulties with everyday tasks such as washing, hair brushing and dressing, and with tasks that require fine motor coordination, such as doing up buttons and tying shoelaces. Some of the most frequent physical problems that youngsters with arthritis experience at school relate to gross and fine motor functioning due to joint stiffness that interferes with everyday school activities, including handwriting, using door handles and locks, climbing stairs, getting to and from classrooms on time, carrying heavy books around and being unable to participate in all aspects of physical recreation (games, sports, etc.).[27] The last of these problems is of particular importance, as children with polyarticular arthritis have been shown to be less fit than controls, but any lack of fitness was not associated with the activity of the arthritis.[28]

Reporting and measuring disability is an important issue in patients with chronic arthritis. The source of reporting has been considered important and questions have been raised as to whether children and adolescents 'accurately' report their disability. One study[25] found no differences between mothers' and children/adolescent's reports of disability, while in another study[29] the children and adolescents reported more restrictions in day-to-day activities than did their mothers. It is possible that parents' anxiety and mood influence their responses about their children and/or that adolescents may underplay their own psychological distress. Although it is also reasonable to argue that the two groups report accurately on their own experiences of the arthritis, what is important is that if studies use only parental data to determine the effects of the problem the findings will be potentially different to those that would have been reported by the adolescents.

At the extreme end of psychological adjustment is psychiatric disturbance. Although there are major issues of definition and classification, there is clear evidence in adults with arthritis of an increased incidence of depression. However, the levels are no higher than those found in adults with other chronic illness.[30]

The incidence of psychiatric disturbance in adolescents with arthritis needs to be placed in the context of the incidence of psychiatric disturbance (as defined by the Diagnostic and Statistical Manual (DSM) and the Manual of the International Classification of Diseases) found in adolescents in large epidemiological studies. It is also important to appreciate the variability that is introduced by the different criteria of disturbance in instruments used to assess psychiatric disturbance in these studies. Overall, epidemiological studies of children and adolescents report a prevalence rate of psychiatric disturbance of 17.6–22%.[31] A study focusing on 1000 adolescents in Blackburn, UK, found 21% of boys and 14% of girls aged 13–14 years to warrant referral;[32] in the Isle of Wight, UK, an epidemiological study of 2000 adolescents showed the 1-year prevalence to be 10–15%.[33] In epidemiological studies children aged 9–11 years with a chronic illness have been found to have higher levels of psychiatric disturbance than those without chronic illness.[33] Little work has been performed specifically on adolescents

with and without chronic illness, and the results discussed here include data on younger children as well as adolescents (Table 2.1).

Overall, there is large variability in the incidence of psychiatric disturbance, with high levels being reported by McAnarney et al,[34] Vandvick and Eckblad[35] and Wilkinson,[36] while Rimon et al[37] and Baildam et al[38] report lower levels. The incidence found in any one study is highly dependent upon the instrument used. For example, Vandvick[39] found that just over half of the 72 school-age children studied met the criteria for one or more psychiatric diagnoses (as defined by the DSM, 3rd edition) when they were assessed by means of interview. In contrast, when the Child Behaviour Checklist was used only 6.6% were found to be in the range of psychopathology, compared with 4.4% of siblings. This is a similar incidence to that found in epidemiological studies.

Several aspects of having severe rheumatic disease have been found to be associated with a higher number of psychiatric referrals. One is restriction in mobility. Wilkinson[36] identified a number of factors in such patients, and found that some were related to mood in general, difficult behaviour, anxieties about treatment and sexual anxieties. Other variables that correlated with depressive symptoms in adolescence were early age of disease onset (≤ 5 years), lack of family intactness and hospitalization of children and adolescents because of their condition.

Besides considering whether a psychiatric disorder is present or not, an overall assessment of the psychological well-being of adolescents with arthritis provides a more general idea of their level of functioning. These assessments are continuous rather than binary, and assess levels of depressed and anxious mood as well as self-esteem and self-concept.

Billings et al[25] compared children and adolescents (aged 1–18 years) with severe ($n = 43$) and mild ($n = 52$) juvenile arthritis and other forms of rheumatic disease with 93 demographically matched controls. They found significantly higher levels of depressed and anxious mood in the severe group (53% anxious and 68% depressed or 'blue'), compared with the mild

Table 2.1 Incidence of psychiatric disturbance in juvenile idiopathic arthritides

Study	n	Age (years)	Disease duration (months)	Sample characteristics	Instruments	Cases (%)
McAnarney et al[34] (1974)	42	6–17	–	Clinic attenders	Behavioural symptom questionnaire (emotional health)	64
Rimon et al[37] (1977)	54	Mean 9.9	1–108	JRA hospitalized	Semi-structured psychiatric interview Psychiatric symptom profile form	31.5
Vandvik[39] (1990)	72	School age, ≥ 7	1–112	JRA first hospitalization	Child Assessment Schedule (interview)	51
					Child Behaviour Checklist	6.6
Wilkinson[36] (1981)	26	12–19		17 hospital patients, 9 outpatients	Semi-structured psychiatric interview	53 (inpatients), 22 (outpatients)
Baildam et al[38] (1995)	29	7–16	6–168	JCA consecutive clinic attenders	Birleson > 15	3.5
					Birleson > 13	14
					Rutter A (parents) > 13	21
					Rutter B (teachers) > 9	5

JRA, juvenile rheumatic arthritis; JCA, juvenile chronic arthritis.

group (24% and 44%, respectively) and the controls (16% and 34%, respectively) when reports were gathered from the parents. However, it should be noted that the severe group included patients with systemic lupus erythematosus. When the older children (aged >10 years; n = 56) completed self-report measures, no differences were found on mood state between the two severity groups and the control group (Table 2.2). Similar results were noted between mothers and children (aged 7–13 years) with JCA on the level of psychological problems.[29]

Pain is one of the major characteristics of JCA and is extremely distressing in itself, but chronic pain also has longer term psychological consequences. Varni et al[40] demonstrated that in both children and adolescents higher pain intensity was associated with greater emotional distress. The greatest associations were found between pain intensity and depressive symptoms (see Table 2.2).

Table 2.2 Psychological well-being/psychosocial adjustment in adolescents with juvenile chronic arthritis (JCA)

Study	Subjects	Age (years)	n	Measures	Findings
Billings et al[25] (1987)	All rheumatic disease patients (mild and severe)	≥ 10 (mean 13.7)	56	Youth Health and Daily Living Form (self-report)	No significant differences between patient and control group
				Piers–Harris Children's Self-concept Scale	Functioning psychologically at the same levels as healthy control group
Ungerer et al[12] (1988)	JCA patients	High-school age	163	Piers–Harris Children's Self-concept Scale	Demonstrated that lower self-concept was related to poorer psychosocial functioning
Daltroy et al[7] (1992)	JCA outpatients (78% girls)	4–16	102	Child Behaviour Checklist	Average female scores similar to population norms. Males showed a trend in behavioural problems, with older males having more problems than younger males. Overall, 18% were in the clinical range for behaviour problems. Teenagers showed lower social competence than population norms, with 19% in the clinical range. All children scored higher on internalizing than on externalizing on the Checklist
Timko et al[26] (1995)	All rheumatic disease patients	12–23	94	Weinberger Adjustment Inventory Senior High School Questionnaire. Child Behaviour Checklist. LISRES-Y	Patients who experienced more acute negative events reported more depressed mood and deviant behaviour. When negative life events were controlled, chronic interpersonal stressors were related to depressed mood and deviant behaviour. When both acute and chronic stressors were controlled, social resources were still related to depressed mood and social competence
Varni et al[40] (1996)	All rheumatic disease patients	5–16	190	Children's Depression Inventory. State–Trait Anxiety Inventory for Children. Child Behaviour Checklist. Self-perception profile for children	Higher pain intensity was related to greater emotional distress for children and adolescents. Higher adolescent-perceived pain intensity was associated with more depressive symptoms, higher state and trait anxiety, lower self-esteem and higher internalizing and externalizing behaviour problems

JCA, juvenile chronic arthritis.

Daltroy et al[7] studied behavioural problems in juvenile arthritis, using the Child Behaviour Checklist which is completed by parents. The 102 subjects were divided into three age groups (4–5, 6–11 and 12–16 years) (see Table 2.2). They found that behavioural problems in girls did not differ from population norms, and only the oldest group of males had more than average behavioural problems, although this finding was not significant. A higher level of disease activity as estimated by the parents was associated with greater levels of behavioural problems. In contrast, Billings et al[25] examined 95 children with a mean age of 10.7 years (range 1–18) who were divided into those with severe ($n = 43$) and those with mild ($n = 52$) disease and compared with a demographically matched control group ($n = 93$). No effects were found of the severity of illness or behavioural problems as assessed by the Health and Daily Living Form.

The way in which adolescents perceive their self-image in relation to their peer group has an impact on and influences how well they cope with their condition. Children and adolescents suffering from arthritis, especially if the disease is severe, may be treated with corticosteroid drugs on a daily basis. One of the long-term consequences of this type of drug therapy is slowing of growth. In a relatively small sample of 28 adolescents, approximately half fell below the 10th percentile in terms of height. Shorter stature tends to be related to increased depressive symptoms, especially in girls. One of the adolescents' major complaints was that being shorter than others resulted in others treating them like children.[36] Being treated like a child is likely to pose problems for the adolescent, given that one of the major developmental tasks of adolescence is achieving autonomy.

Disease severity has also been linked with poorer self-concept. Ungerer et al[12] found that, in a group of 163 adolescents, those with more severe disease had lower scores on measures of self-concept. The adolescents with the lowest self-concept scores were more likely to spend their spare time in the company of their families rather than with friends. Generally, their social lives were more impoverished; they reported feeling lonely more often, having fewer close friends and going out on dates less often. Greater disease severity has also been related to children's athletic competence and perceived physical attractiveness, and perceptions of the disease experience were related to athletic competence, physical attractiveness, social acceptance and global self-worth.[29] In a further study, two-thirds of a high-school group held the belief that their arthritis affected them in a negative way, by lowering their self-confidence and changing their physical appearance, thereby making them different from others. It is important, however, that others thought that their arthritis resulted in some benefits, such as becoming more understanding and making them more determined to have a positive outlook on life.[12]

IMPACT OF ARTHRITIS ON THE TASKS OF ADOLESCENCE

It has only relatively recently been acknowledged that adolescents with chronic diseases, such as rheumatic disease, face special difficulties in their attempts to attain independence. The adolescent with rheumatic disease may meet obstacles, such as a very real dependence on parents for help in administering treatment, or with transport to hospital appointments; and there may be parental anxiety about the disease that is so intense that they impose restrictions that are seen to be unnecessary by the adolescent. It is not uncommon for clinicians to suggest that parents underestimate their adolescents' abilities and thus impose restrictions that are unreasonable, although some studies suggest parents' estimations may be accurate.[7] However, it is clear that adolescents with arthritis do have more restricted lives. Billings et al[25] found that adolescents with low self-concepts also felt discriminated against in both social and work situations, and were more inclined to believe that impairment of physical appearance, restricted activity and feeling different to others, made the development of relationships with others outside the family more difficult.

When considering the impact of rheumatic disease on adolescents there is another important area to be taken into account. The whole area of schooling is one where adolescents with rheumatic disease can experience considerable difficulties, including physical, social and educational difficulties and their implications for the longer term. Some of the problems that may arise may relate to the length of the school day, as it may be too long for young people with rheumatic disease, given that fatigue is a feature of the condition. Fatigue may also compromise school achievement, as may side-effects of medication and distractibility, as a consequence of stiffness, joint inflammation or pain.[41] These issues are potentially compounded by a lack of understanding of their condition by others.[27,42]

Absences from school are inevitable for any adolescent with a chronic condition due to doctor or hospital appointments, or the condition itself. Interestingly, a study looking at disease-specific absences found that all arthritis patients missed an average of 2.7 days over a 2-month period, compared with a national average of 1.1 days per 2-month period. Those with systemic-onset arthritis missed an average of 3.3 days, and those with polyarticular onset missed 3.4 days; the lowest rate was for those with pauciarticular-onset disease (1.4 days over 2 months). When all the rheumatic diseases were considered together, a third have absence rates significantly above the national average.[43] Billings et al[25] found that the amount of absence was related to the severity of the illness, with 62% of a severe-illness group and 29% of a mild-illness group missing school through illness.

Does absence from school affect academic performance? A study by McAnarney et al[34] suggested that patients with arthritis had lower academic achievement scores in comparison to healthy peers judged to possess similar intellectual abilities. However, it may not just be absenteeism alone that accounts for poorer academic performance. In a group of 5–18 year olds with rheumatic disease, it was shown that absenteeism and fatigue together had a mild impact on academic performance. While this particular group of children had rates of absenteeism that were higher than the national average in the USA, they performed within the average range on standardized achievement tests. Inattention and distractibility were shown to be more closely related to scholastic achievement.[44] Studies that have directly compared absenteeism with scholastic performance have found only low correlations.[25]

One problem of schooling identified by adolescents who spend time in hospital is the poor communication between hospital and school. In addition, few hospitals in the UK offer full-time schooling, although this may not be the case elsewhere. Nevertheless, even a short stay in hospital can result in a significant amount of schoolwork being missed, and in many instances it may be impossible to catch up.

There are, of course, longer term implications of rheumatic disease on the adolescent that extend beyond schooling. Rheumatic disease will inevitably have an impact on the choices of career. Extra problems exist for adolescents who develop arthritis when career decisions have already been made. Not only does the adolescent have to deal with a diagnosis that may lead to problems such as 'anxious preoccupation' or 'helplessness',[46] but they then have to cope with the realization that their choice of career may no longer be possible.[45]

The 'transition from school to the world of work is one of the most important tasks of adolescence and young adulthood'.[3] For adolescents with disabilities, the transition to the workforce can be particularly difficult. A poll conducted in the USA revealed that somewhere in the region of half to three-quarters of young adults with disabilities cannot get work, despite the fact that more than two-thirds of those without jobs wanted employment. Diseases of the musculoskeletal system and connective tissue were found to be the most frequent cause of disability in this group.[3] For further discussion of this aspect, see Chapter 13.

IMPACT OF ADOLESCENT ARTHRITIS ON THE FAMILY

Rheumatic disease does not affect the adolescent in isolation. For those who have to care for someone with a severe and disabling chronic condition, the physical and psychological demands may be considerable.[47] This not only has an impact on family relationships through time pressures, but also on finances, as additional expenses may be incurred, or one parent may be restricted in their ability to work.

The psychological impact on parents with children and adolescents with juvenile arthritis has been examined in a number of studies. Daltroy et al[7] found no evidence for poorer psychological well-being in a study of mothers of 4- to 16-year-old arthritis patients. The level of strain experienced by parents has been found to be related to the level of functional disability and lesser social competence of the individual with arthritis.[48] How parents cope with the pressures of a child with chronic arthritis has been found to influence their psychological well-being. Timko et al[15] found that parents who used avoiding coping strategies were less well adapted. It is important that poorer parental functioning has been found to be related to the patient experiencing more pain, psychosocial problems and greater functional disability. Greater social competence was found in children where mothers were more socially active and fathers maintained more close relationships. Fathers' close relationships were also associated with the patients having fewer behaviour problems.

The effects of an individual with juvenile arthritis can also be experienced by siblings. Some parents have admitted that they do pay more attention to their child with JCA, often at the expense of the rest of the family.[49] Where the individual with arthritis has a high level of psychosocial dysfunction and the mother reports more medical symptoms, siblings have been found to experience greater physical and psychological dysfunction.[16]

CONCLUSION

While there are major problems with the research done on the impact of rheumatological disease on adolescents, not least with regard to definition of the term 'adolescence', it is clear that the effects of this illness are widespread. There is, however, a great need for a systematic study to examine, not only the impact of the arthritis, but also the level of cognitive development and understanding of disease in general and arthritis in particular. To understand these issues and examine them with sufficient statistical power, studies will need to be larger than most that have been performed to date.

REFERENCES

1. Feldman SS, Elliot GR (eds). *At the Threshold: The Developing Adolescent*. Harvard University Press: New Haven, CT, 1990.
2. Petty RE. Children and young adults. In: *Oxford Textbook of Rheumatology* (Maddison PJ, Isenberg DA, Woo P, Glass D, eds), 2nd edn. Oxford University Press: Oxford, 1988:9–22.
3. White PH, Shear ES. Transition/job readiness for adolescents with juvenile arthritis and other chronic illness. *J Rheumatol* 1992; **19**(suppl):23–7.
4. Eiser C, Berrenberg JL. Assessing the impact of chronic disease on the relationship between parents and their adolescents. *J Psychosom Res* 1995; **39**:109–14.
5. Duffy CM, Arsenault L, Duffy KNW. Level of agreement between parents and children in rating dysfunction in juvenile rheumatoid arthritis and juvenile spondyloarthritides. *J Rheumatol* 1993; **20**: 2134–9.
6. Berry SL, Hayford JR, Ross CK et al. Conceptions of illness by children with juvenile rheumatoid arthritis: a cognitive developmental approach. *J Pediatr Psychol* 1993; **18**:83–97.
7. Daltroy LH, Larson MG, Eaton HM et al. Psychosocial adjustment in juvenile arthritis. *J Pediatr Psychol* 1992; **17**:227–89.
8. Burbach DJ, Peterson L. Children's concepts of physical illness: a review and critique of the cognitive developmental literature. *Health Psychol* 1986; **5**:307–25.
9. Bibace R, Walsh M. Development of children's concepts of illness. *Pediatrics* 1980; **66**:912–7.

10. Eiser C. Children's concepts of illness: towards an alternative to the 'stage' approach. *Psychol Health* 1989; **3**:93–101.

11. Eiser C. *Growing up with a Chronic Disease*. Jessica Kingsley: London, 1993.

12. Ungerer JA, Horgan B, Chaitow J, Champion GD. Psychosocial functioning in children and young adults with juvenile arthritis. *Pediatrics* 1988; **81**:195–202.

13. Quirk ME, Young MH. The impact of JRA on children, adolescents and their families: current research and implications for future studies. *Arthritis Care Res* 1990; **3**:36–43.

14. Breslau N. The psychological study of chronically ill and disabled children: are healthy siblings appropriate controls? *J Abnorm Child Psychol* 1983; **11**:379–91.

15. Timko C, Stovel KW, Moos RH, Miller JJ. Adaption to juvenile rheumatic disease: a controlled evaluation of functional disability with a one-year follow-up. *Health Psychol* 1992; **11**:67–76.

16. Daniels D, Miller JJ, Billings AG, Moos RH. Psychosocial functioning of siblings of children with rheumatic disease. *J Paediatr* 1986; **109**:379–83.

17. Perrin CE, Stein RE. Cautions in using the child behaviour checklist: observations based on research about children with chronic illness. *J Pediatr Psychol* 1991; **16**:411–21.

18. Beales JG, Holt PJL, Keen JH, Mellor VP. Children with juvenile chronic arthritis: their beliefs about their illness and therapy. *Ann Rheum Dis* 1983; **42**:481–6.

19. Newman S, Fitzpatrick R, Revenson TA et al. *Understanding Rheumatoid Arthritis*. Routledge: London, 1996.

20. Hayford JR, Ross CK. Medical compliance in juvenile rheumatoid arthritis. *Arthritis Care Res* 1988; **1**:190–7.

21. Bloch CA, Clemmons PS, Sperling MA. Puberty decreases insulin sensitivity. *J Pediatr* 1987; **110**:481–7.

22. Scott PJ, Ansell BM, Huskisson EC. Measurement of pain in juvenile chronic arthritis. *Ann Rheum Dis* 1977; **36**:186–7.

23. Jaworski TM. Juvenile rheumatoid arthritis: pain-related and psychosocial aspects and their relevance for assessment and treatment. *Arthritis Care Res* 1993; **6**:187–96.

24. Beales JG, Keen JH, Holt PJ. The child's perception of the disease and the experience of pain in juvenile chronic arthritis. *J Rheumatol* 1983; **10**:61–5.

25. Billings AG, Moos RH, Miller JJ, Gottlieb JE. Psychosocial adaption in juvenile rheumatic disease: a controlled evaluation. *Health Psychol* 1987; **6**:343–59.

26. Timko C, Stovel KW, Baumgartner M, Moos RH. Acute and chronic stressors, social resources, and functioning among adolescents with juvenile rheumatic disease. *J Res Adolescence* 1995; **5**:361–85.

27. Spencer CH, Fife RZ, Rabinovich CE. The school experience of children with arthritis: coping in the 1990s and transition into adulthood. *Pediatr Clin North Am* 1995; **42**:1285–99.

28. Klepper S, Darbee J, Effgens SK, Singsen BH. Physical fitness levels in children with polyarticular juvenile rheumatoid arthritis. *Arthritis Care Res* 1992; **5**:93–100.

29. Ennett ST, DeVellis BM, Earp JA et al. Disease experience and psychosocial adjustment in children with juvenile rheumatoid arthritis: children's versus mother's reports. *J Pediatr Psychol* 1991; **16**:557–68.

30. DeVellis BM. The physiological impact of arthritis: prevalence of depression. *Arthritis Care Res* 1995; **8**:284–9.

31. Offord DR. Child psychiatric epidemiology: current status and future prospects. *Can J Psychiatry* 1995; **40**:284–8.

32. Leslie SA. Psychiatric disorder in the young adolescents of an industrial town. *Br J Psychiatry* 1974; **250**:113–24.

33. Rutter M, Graham P, Chadwick O, Yule W. Adolescent turmoil: fact or fiction. *J Child Psychol Psychiatry* 1976; **17**:35–6.

34. McAnarney ER, Pless IB, Satterwhite B, Friedman SB. Psychological problems of children with chronic juvenile arthritis. *Pediatrics* 1974; **53**:523–8.

35. Vandvik IH, Eckblad G. Relationship between pain, disease severity and psychosocial function in patients with juvenile chronic arthritis (JCA). *Scand J Rheumatol* 1990; **19**:295–302.

36. Wilkinson VA. Juvenile chronic arthritis in adolescence: facing the reality. *Intl Rehab Med* 1981; **3**:11–7.

37. Rimon R, Belmaker RH, Ebstein R. Psychosomatic aspects of juvenile rheumatoid arthritis. *Scand J Rheumatol* 1977; **6**:1–10.

38. Baildam EM, Holt PJL, Conway SC, Morton MJS. The association between physical function

and psychological problems in children with juvenile chronic arthritis. *Br J Rheumatol* 1995; **34**:470–7.

39. Vandvik IH. Mental health and psychosocial functioning in children with recent onset of rheumatic disease. *J Child Psychol Psychiatry* 1990; **31**:961–71.

40. Varni JW, Rapoff MA, Waldron SA et al. Chronic pain and emotional distress in children and adolescents. *J Dev Behav Pediatr* 1996; **17**:154–61.

41. Hagglund KJ. Health psychologists in pediatric rheumatology. *Health Psychol* 1997; **19**:14,22–3.

42. Lineker SC, Badley EM, Dalby DM. Unmet service needs of children with rheumatic disease and their parents in a metropolitan area. *J Rheumatol* 1996; **23**:1054–8.

43. Lovell DJ, Athreya B, Emery HE et al. School attendance and patterns, special services and special needs in pediatric patients with rheumatic diseases. *Arthritis Care Res* 1990; **3**:197–203.

44. Stoff E, Bacon MC, White PH. The effects of fatigue, distractibility, and absenteeism on school achievement in children with rheumatic disease. *Arthritis Care Res* 1989; **2**:49–52.

45. Leak AM. The management of arthritis in adolescents. *Br J Rheumatol* 1994; **33**:882–8.

46. David J, Cooper C, Hickey L et al. The function and psychological outcomes of juvenile chronic arthritis in young adulthood. *Br J Rheumatol* 1994; **33**:876–81.

47. O'Reilly F, Finnan F, Allwright S et al. The effects of caring for a spouse with Parkinson's disease on social, psychological and physical well-being. *Br J Gen Practice* 1996; **46**:507–12.

48. Timko C, Baumgartner M, Moos RH, Miller JJ. Parental risk and resistance factors among children with juvenile rheumatic disease: a four-year predictive study. *J Behav Med* 1993; **16**:571–88.

49. Konkol L, Lineberry J, Gottlieb J et al. Impact of juvenile arthritis on families – an educational assessment. *Arthritis Care Res* 1989; **2**:40–8.

3

Measuring health status and outcome in adolescents with rheumatic disease

Lori B Tucker

INTRODUCTION

Health status and outcomes assessment in paediatric rheumatology is all the rage. Everyone wants to have an outcomes measurement of their very own for their research project or clinical programme. Despite this enthusiasm and excitement, the area of health status and outcomes assessment in paediatric rheumatology is still in its infancy. A number of measurement tools are available, but a solid understanding of their place in research and clinical practice is lacking. In this chapter I discuss important concepts in the area of health-status measurement, review the currently available tools, and discuss the special issues of adolescent health-status measurement.

WHY MEASURE HEALTH STATUS AND OUTCOMES?

Although the answer to the question 'Why measure outcomes?' may seem clear, there are many who question the need for a rigorous scientific approach to something that is already a part of good clinical practice; that is, the assessment by a physician of how the patient is doing (Table 3.1). However, this informal approach to health status and outcome lacks the precision necessary to make accurate assessments across the population of children with rheumatic disease. Measurement of health status and outcome in a standardized method can provide a broad assessment of the impact of chronic

Table 3.1	Why measure health status and outcomes?

- Accurate measurement of patient and family status, and impact of chronic disease
- Determine long-term outcomes of chronic rheumatic conditions
- Assess effectiveness of new therapeutic protocols on quality of life and functional status from patient and family point of view
- Identify predictive factors of outcome
- Justify resource allocation to children with rheumatic disease
- Document quality of care to patients and families

rheumatic disease on the child and family, at a given point in time and over the course of disease. The impact of new therapies on children's well-being, functional status, and quality of life can be investigated, and identification of predictive features of outcome explored. Health-status assessment, which allows comparison of disease impact of children with rheumatic disease to those with other chronic illnesses, will be useful in advocating resource allocation in the current shrinking health-service environment. Health-care administrators and organizations responsible for payment resources in health care are interested in health-status measurement as one method of assessing the quality of care given to patients.[1]

HOW DO WE MEASURE HEALTH STATUS AND OUTCOMES?

Traditional measures of clinical outcome have the highest degree of familiarity among physicians. These measures are nearly always assessments generated from the physician rather than the child and family, and reflect clinically measurable signs and symptoms indicative of disease severity and activity. In childhood rheumatic diseases, although there are a number of generally accepted clinical markers that indicate the degree of disease activity and severity, little work has been done to develop and validate standard disease activity indices. For children with juvenile rheumatoid arthritis (JRA), Giannini et al[2] have developed and tested a core set of outcome variables to be used. These include physician global assessment, patient/parent global assessment, degree of pain, numbers of joints with active arthritis, functional assessment and erythrocyte sedimentation rate. Other clinical measures of disease severity and activity might include the presence of clinical symptoms such as fever and rash, and joint erosions by radiograph in children with arthritis, renal function or abnormal autoimmune serology in systemic lupus erythematosus, or muscle strength and serum muscle enzyme levels in dermatomyositis.

It has been recognized for some time now that reliance solely on clinical signs and symptoms and physician assessment of disease outcome is inadequate for understanding the impact of an illness and its treatments on a patient's life and functioning. One important measure of outcome in rheumatic disease is patient functional status; that is, how well patients can function in their usual tasks of daily living. Measurement of functional status can be reliably obtained from patient report questionnaires which ask the respondent to rate difficulty in doing a variety of listed tasks. Although there are many valid functional assessment tools in rheumatology, there

are fewer designed for use in children. The measurement of functional status in children is complicated by changing developmental levels over time. In particular, adolescents have different functional tasks and interests than adults; for example, the ability to attend school and function in a school environment is important in adolescence, as compared to the work environment for adults. Therefore, functional assessment questionnaires that ask about work and ability to care for one's home are not applicable to adolescents.

Functional status is only one aspect of patients' overall well-being. Clinical researchers have become increasingly interested in understanding the impact of disease on health-related quality of life (HRQOL). A recent World Health Organization–International League Against Rheumatism (WHO-ILAR) taskforce defined HRQOL as 'the physical, emotional, and social aspects of quality of life influenced by an individual's disease and its treatment. Our goal, as health care professionals, is to maintain or improve health-related quality of life as affected by musculoskeletal disorders'.[3] HRQOL is a complex, multi-dimensional concept, which encompasses: functional status; social or role functioning in home, neighbourhood and school; peer and family relationships; and mental health, including behaviour, self-esteem, depression and anxiety. There are a number of well-validated health assessment measures used in rheumatology which incorporate some measures of HRQOL. Some of the most popular and well-known of these measures, which have been developed for, and tested in, adults, include the Arthritis Impact Measurement Scales (AIMS),[4] Health Assessment Questionnaire (HAQ),[5] and the McMaster Arthritis Patient Preference Questionnaire (MACTAR).[6] The utility of these measures in adolescents have, for the most part, not been tested. One study examined the potential utility of the AIMS in childhood using only a portion of the instrument addressing pain and physical disability.[7] Reliability, sensitivity, and discriminant validity of the modified AIMS for childhood were disappointing. Therefore, paediatric rheumatologists were convinced that measures specifically developed for use in children were needed. There now are a number of such measures which assess functional status in children and adolescents; only a few of them address the issue of HRQOL as well. These instruments are described in detail in the following section.

Measures of health status can be generic (applicable to healthy individuals and those with any illness) or disease-specific. Generic measures are useful in determining burden of illness compared with healthy controls, and allow comparisons between different disease groups. However, sensitivity to small yet important clinical changes for a specific disease may be poor. Disease-specific measures are designed to capture these small and important clinical changes, and allow improved sensitivity in measuring differencesd among patients with a particular disease or condition.[8]

An outcomes assessment measure cannot be all things to all people. One of the most important steps in application of outcomes assessment to clinical research is the selection of the best and most appropriate instrument for a particular situation. The qualities of a good health status instrument are shown in Table 3.2. Validity and reliability are key qualities to be shown by developers before an instrument can be adopted for use by others; does this instrument measure what it says it measures? In many situations, clinical researchers would like an instrument which is responsive and sensitive to clinically important change. This is particularly important in treatment studies. The instrument should be practical, not too long (low respondent burden), understandable by the target population (appropriate reading level and language), and easy to score. Most importantly, the scores must be interpretable; that is, the scores should make clinical sense in relationship to understandable clinical situations.

HEALTH-STATUS MEASUREMENT TOOLS AVAILABLE IN PAEDIATRIC RHEUMATOLOGY

In the following section, the currently available measurement instruments developed for use in paediatric rheumatic disease are described. The focus of work to date has been in the area of idiopathic arthritides of childhood (juvenile rheumatoid arthritis (JRA) or juvenile chronic arthritis (JCA)); with one exception, there has been minimal work to date to develop methods of assessment for children with other rheumatic diseases. A comparison of the available instruments is given in Table 3.3.

Childhood Health Assessment Questionnaire (CHAQ)

The CHAQ was developed from the adult Health Assessment Questionnaire (HAQ) and modified for use in childhood.[10] The CHAQ is a parent or child self-report questionnaire that measures functional status in eight domains: dressing/grooming, eating, walking, arising from a bed in the morning, hygiene, grip, reach and general activities. In addition, there is a question to assess the amount of pain (using a visual analogue scale), global assessment of overall status, and a question to assess impact of uveitis if present. The CHAQ modifications include at least one question in each domain applicable to children of every developmental level; therefore, the CHAQ is applicable to children of any age. Of particular importance for adolescents, the CHAQ is sufficiently comparable to the adult HAQ that one could use both questionnaires over time in a long-term study as patients move into adult ages, and compare results easily, making long-term follow-up studies possible.

Table 3.2   Qualities of a good health-status instrument

- Valid
- Reliable
- Responsive – sensitive to clinically important change
- Practical
- Interpretable
- Relevant

The CHAQ has shown good internal reliability and convergent validity in pilot testing on 72 patients with JRA and 22 controls.[11] The CHAQ is scored to give a disability index and a discomfort index; scores range from 0 (completely well) to 3 (severe disability or discomfort). Although the CHAQ is quick to administer, simple to use and easy to score, there is some concern about ceiling effects among populations of patients with arthritis using this instrument. Further use in large patient groups over time is needed to answer these concerns.

The CHAQ has been translated into several languages other than English. There have been a number of long-term follow-up studies of children with JRA that have used the CHAQ as an outcomes measure of disability. Andersson Gare and Fasth[12] re-assessed 124 patients with JCA (median age 17.7 years; median disease duration 7.1 years). They found a relatively low median disability score for this group (0.19; range 0–2.75), and a median pain index of 0.24 (range 0–2.8). A higher CHAQ score seemed to be related to impact of JRA on role function in school, social life and future plans (as assessed by a separate questionnaire), suggesting that the CHAQ accurately assesses disability, which translates into impact on HRQOL. It is important to note that the CHAQ does not itself measure HRQOL.

Ruperto et al[13] examined a population of 227 patients with idiopathic arthritis of childhood from Italy or Cincinnati, USA, with a mean disease duration of 15 years at the time of assessment. Again, CHAQ scores for the group as a whole were relatively low (85% of patients scoring 0–0.5). The investigators showed a moderate correlation

Table 3.3   Comparison of health-status measures developed for children/adolescent with arthritis

Instrument	Description	Domains	Valid	Available
CHAQ	Parent or child self-report	Functional disability Pain Global assessment	Yes	Yes
JAFAR	Parent or child self-report	Functional disability	Yes	Yes
JAQQ	Parent	Functional disability Pain Psychosocial	Yes	Yes
JASI	Parent or child self-report/interview	Self-care Mobility School Domestic	Yes	Yes
CAHP	Parent and child	Functional disability Pain Psychosocial Global assessment	Yes (pilot)	Test

CAHP, Childhood Arthritis Health Profile; CHAQ, Childhood Health Assessment Questionnaire; JAFAR, Juvenile Arthritis Function Assessment Report; JAQQ, Juvenile Arthritis Quality of Life Questionnaire; JASI, Juvenile Arthritis Self-report Index.

between CHAQ scores and scores on a separate quality-of-life scale ($R = 0.49$). Of interest, this study was the first time that the CHAQ and the HAQ had been used in the same study, and the investigators pooled results from the two instruments, demonstrating the utility of the HAQ for this type of research.

Although the CHAQ has primarily been used to assess outcome in children with arthritis, Feldman et al[14] have examined its use in children with juvenile dermatomyositis, finding good responsiveness to clinical change. The CHAQ, therefore, may be useful in evaluating children with any rheumatic condition with a significant component of physical functional disability.

Juvenile Arthritis Functional Assessment Report (JAFAR)

The JAFAR was developed by investigators in Cincinnati, USA,[15] to assess functional status in children with arthritis. Initially, an observer assessment scale was published (JAFAS);[15] subsequently both parent self-report (JAFAR-P) and child self-report (JAFAR-C) versions have been developed.[16] The JAFAR measures ability to perform 23 physical tasks, and includes a visual analogue scale for assessing pain and information concerning the use of aids for functional help. It is a brief questionnaire, and therefore easy to use and score. The JAFAR was developed for use in children aged over 7 years; it has shown good reliability and validity among a small test population of 72 children with JRA and 63 controls. There has been one small study using the JAFAR in a clinical trial,[17] which suggested responsiveness to change over time. Although the JAFAR is simple to use and score, it is somewhat limited by its focus on physical functional status alone. Further testing in larger studies will need to be done in order to understand better its role in rheumatology research.

Juvenile Arthritis Quality of Life Questionnaire (JAQQ)

The JAQQ, developed by Duffy et al[19] in Montreal, is an instrument aimed at measuring psychosocial function and quality of life, as well as the physical functional status of children with arthritis. This questionnaire was designed for use in patients of all ages (parent report for younger children and child self-report in those aged over 9 years). The primary aim of the investigators was to develop an instrument that was patient-specific and highly responsive to change over time.

The final version of the JAQQ contains 74 items in four domains; gross motor function, fine motor function, psychosocial function and general symptoms. Although in the JAQQ the respondent is asked to assess the degree of difficulty with a variety of tasks on a Likert scale, similar to other questionnaires, in addition the respondent is asked to select up to five items in each domain with which they are having difficulty. Respondents are able to volunteer their own items if none of the available questions are pertinent. In effect, each patient who answers the JAQQ may be filling in a different questionnaire. An initial evaluation study of the JAQQ with 62 children with JRA showed the instrument to have very good construct validity and excellent responsiveness, correlating well with physician global assessment of change.[19,20] Further follow-up studies, published in abstract form,[21,22] have verified these findings. Therefore, the JAQQ would be ideal for accurate measurement of change over time, and may be very useful in clinical trials. The JAQQ is unique in its identification of important issues specific to each patient, and perhaps approximates measuring quality of life better than other instruments. However, comparisons between patients in a group would be very difficult, as the patients are not all answering the same questions. The JAQQ is a long questionnaire, and respondent burden and difficulty of scoring may limit its use in certain clinical situations.

Juvenile Arthritis Self-report Index (JASI)

The JASI was developed by Wright et al[23] in Toronto. It focuses on measurement of physical functional abilities, the aim being to allow accurate assessment of the impact of rehabilitation.

The questionnaire is long (over 100 items) and designed for children aged over 8 years; some younger children require assistance to complete it. There are two components to the JASI. In Part 1, patients are asked to assess their difficulty in a variety of tasks in domains including self-care, domestic, mobility, school and extracurricular activities. In Part 2, patients are asked to identify five of the tasks that are most difficult. This allows follow-up over time, and improves the responsiveness of the JASI to change. The JASI was shown to have excellent validity and reliability in a study of 36 children with JRA; however, correlation between scores indicating a change in JASI Part 2 and overall global assessment of change was low.[24]

The JASI does not measure health status or quality of life; it measures functional status in a more complete and comprehensive manner than other instruments. The ability of the JASI accurately to measure change requires further study.

Childhood Arthritis Health Profile (CAHP)

The CAHP was developed by Tucker et al[25] to measure the health-related quality of life of children with JRA, and to include measures of physical functional status as well as psychosocial and family functioning. The CAHP incorporates a generic health-status module to measure general health perceptions, mental health and emotional well-being, bodily pain, self-esteem, behaviour, parental impact of disease and family functioning. A JRA-specific module was developed to address domains of gross and fine motor functioning, role activities (including school, play and family), morning stiffness and pain related to arthritis. The questionnaire is arranged to give individual scores for each health domain. The generic core instrument (known as the Child Health Questionnaire when used alone)[26] has been well validated in health care populations as well as in populations of children with chronic illness such as asthma, epilepsy, attention deficit disorder and JRA. The benefit of having the generic questionnaire as part of the CAHP is that comparisons can be made between children with arthritis, healthy children and children

with other chronic illnesses; in contrast, the addition of JRA-specific scales should improve the ability of the instrument to discriminate between children with JRA. The generic scales of the CAHP allow the disease burden of JRA to be compared with that of other illnesses. The CAHP can also be easily adapted for use in other paediatric rheumatic disorders. Development of disease-specific modules for dermatomyositis and systemic lupus erythematosus is currently underway.

A pilot study was carried out to determine the validity and reliability of the newly developed CAHP.[27,28] Seventy-eight patients with JRA (mean age 10.4 years, range 5–16 years) and their parents were included. Physician-assessed global disease severity was mild in 55%, moderate in 36%, and severe in 8% of patients. The health status scores of this pilot population is shown in Table 3.4; possible scores for the CAHP scales range from 0 (worst health status) to 100 (best possible health status). Internal consistency reliability was very good, with a coefficient α of 0.84. Validity and reliability testing of the JRA-specific scales revealed excellent results. The overall means of the generic health scales indicate lower scores on physically orientated scales (general health perceptions, pain and physical functioning) than on psychological health scales (mental health, behaviour problems and self esteem). Social-functioning scale scores indicate that limitations in social activities and schoolwork were greater when attributed to physical health problems than when attributed to emotional or behavioural problems.

Further analysis was done to examine the sensitivity of the CAHP scales to discriminate between disease-severity groups.[29] The physically orientated scales of the generic portion of the CAHP (physical functioning, pain, limitations in role activities due to physical problems, and general health perceptions) showed very good discriminant qualities when tested by general linear models. When the JRA-specific scales were examined, there were excellent correlations of disease severity with all scales. Currently, a large multicentre data-collection project is underway to verify these findings, to

Table 3.4 Childhood arthritis health profile scale scores: Pilot study

Generic health scales	Mean	JRA-specific health scales	Mean
Physical functioning	77	Gross motor functioning	89
Bodily pain	65	Fine motor/ADL functioning	92
Role/social, physical	87	Usual role, recreation	91
General health perceptions	60	Usual role, school	88
Role/social, emotional	93	Morning stiffness	76
Role/social, behaviour	90	Bodily pain	65
Mental health	77	Role/social, physical	87
Behavioural problems	80	Role/social, emotional	93
Self-esteem	82		
Parent impact on emotions	83		
Parent impact on time	87		

JRA, juvenile rheumatoid arthritis

test a newly available adolescent version of the CAHP, and to determine the sensitivity of the CAHP to change over time.

SPECIAL ISSUES OF HEALTH-STATUS MEASUREMENT RELATED TO ADOLESCENTS

The measurement of health status in paediatric patients offers different challenges to those arising in the study of adults. One of the most contentious issues is the question of who is the appropriate reporter of health status – the parent or the child? In adolescence, it seems clear that, in order to have a true understanding of health status and quality of life, information must be obtained from the patient directly. However, one might consider whether information gained from the parent has equal validity and may provide an additional 'window of understanding'. Although several small studies have shown good agreement between parents' and children's ratings of difficulties due to arthritis,[16,30] a careful look at the data reveals some interesting trends. In the study by Duffy et al,[20] 40 children aged over 9 years and their parents were inter-

viewed using an early version of the JAQQ. Although the level of agreement was good on most physical functioning items, there was poor agreement (κ score less than 0.45) on 23% of psychosocial items, including such items as 'interacts poorly with siblings', 'exhibits inappropriate behaviour for age', 'fails to finish things', 'overly demanding', 'feels unloved', and 'does not feel guilty after wrong-doing'. Perhaps asking teenagers to make an assessment of their psychological and emotional faults is not reasonable; parents may be able to provide a more accurate picture of psychosocial functioning. Assessment of physical functional status may be obtained more easily from adolescents alone. Until further definitive studies are done, it may be most useful to obtain information from both parents and adolescents, if possible, when issues of quality of life are involved.

Taal et al[31] recently published a study addressing whether aspects of emotional well-being, which are not measured by functional status instruments such as the HAQ, are important outcomes in young adults with arthritis. They found that depression, loneliness and self-esteem were correlated with functional status and disease symptoms, and concluded that depression appeared to be an important outcome in the assessment of young adults with arthritis. Their work substantiates the need for measurement of HRQOL as well as functional status in young people with idiopathic arthritis.

The impact of chronic rheumatic conditions on adolescents is clearly quite different from that in younger children. Adolescent role functioning differs from that of young school-aged children and adults. Issues of self-esteem, risk-taking behaviour, development of independence from family, peer relationships, emerging sexual behaviour, substance use/abuse and vocational planning all play important roles for adolescents, and can be influenced by the presence of a chronic illness. Health-status instruments that are meant for use with adolescents should include some measure of these role-function domains. As an example, Starfield et al[32] have developed a generic health-status instrument meant for use in adolescents called the Child Health and Illness Profile (CHIP). The CHIP measures all of the above domains, and is a self-administered questionnaire; however, it is extremely long and perhaps more suited to broad epidemiological survey research rather than routine use in the clinical setting. The health-status instruments described above for

use in JRA address adolescent issues to varying degrees. The CAHP and JAQQ are the only instruments that measure psychosocial functioning, and the CAHP is the only instrument to specifically address issues of self-esteem and family functioning. However, no available instrument specifically addresses sexuality, peer relationships or vocational issues.

CONCLUSIONS

The measurement of health status, quality of life and outcome in adolescents with rheumatic conditions is an active area of research. A variety of measurement tools aimed at children with idiopathic arthritis have become available over the recent years. However, much more work needs to be done before the utility of these instruments is known. Investigators must decide what exactly they need to measure before selecting an instrument to use in clinical studies. Examination of the health status of larger populations of adolescents with rheumatic disease using the available tools must be done in order to see if these instruments are appropriate or whether further instruments designed specifically for use with adolescents would be helpful. The predictive value of outcomes assessment to functioning in adulthood is unknown; large long-term studies should be organized to gather such data.

REFERENCES

1. Mason JH. Outcomes measurement in today's health care environment. *Arthritis Care Res* 1998; **10**:355–8.
2. Giannini EH, Ruperto N, Ravelli A, Lovell DJ, Felson DT, Martini A. Preliminary definition of improvement in juvenile arthritis. *Arthritis Rheum* 1997; **40**:1202–9.
3. Strand CV, Russell AS. WHO/ILAR taskforce on quality of life. *J Rheum* 1997; **24**: 1630–3.
4. Meenan RF, Gertman PM, Mason JH. Measuring health status in arthritis. The Arthritis Impact Measurement Scales. *Arthritis Rheum* 1980; **23**:146–52.
5. Fries JF, Spitz PW, Young DY. The dimensions of health outcomes: The Health Assessment Questionnaire, disability and pain scales. *J Rheumatol* 1982; **9**:789–93.
6. Tugwell P, Bombardier C, Buchanan WW, Goldsmith CH, Grace E, Hanna B. The MACTAR Patient Preference Disability Questionnaire – an individualized functional priority approach for assessing improvement in physical disability in clinical trials in rheumatoid arthritis. *J Rheum* 1987; **14**:446–51.
7. Coulton CJ, Zborowsky E, Lipton J, Newman AJ. Assessment of the reliability and validity of the

arthritis impact measurement scales for children with juvenile arthritis. *Arthritis Rheum* 1987; **30**:819–24.

8. Guyatt GH, Veldhuyzen Van Zanten SJO, Feeny DH, Patrick DL. Measuring quality of life in clinical trials: a taxonomy and review. *Can Med Assoc J* 1989; **140**:1441–8.

9. Duffy CM, Duffy KN. Health assessment in the rheumatic diseases of childhood. *Current Opin Rheum* 1997; **9**:440–7.

10. Singh G, Athreya B, Fries J, Goldsmith D. Measurement of health status in children with juvenile rheumatoid arthritis. *Arthritis Rheum* 1994; **37**:1761–9.

11. Singh F, Brown B, Arthreya B. Functional status in juvenile rheumatoid arthritis: sensitivity to change of the childhood health assessment questionnaire. *Arthritis Rheum* 1991; **34**:S81.

12. Andersson Gare B, Fasth A. The natural history of juvenile chronic arthritis: a population based cohort study. II Outcome. *J Rheumatol* 1995; **22**:308–19.

13. Ruperto N, Levinson JE, Ravelli A et al. Long-term health outcomes and quality of life in American and Italian inception cohorts of patients with juvenile rheumatoid arthritis. I. Outcome status. *J Rheumatol* 1997; **24**:945–58.

14. Feldman BM, Ayling-Campos A, Luy L, Stevens D, Silverman ED, Laxer RM. Measuring disability in juvenile dermatomyositis: validity of the Childhood Health Assessment Questionnaire. *J Rheumatol* 1995; **22**:326–31.

15. Lovell DJ, Howe S, Shear ES et al. Development of a disability measurement tool for juvenile rheumatoid arthritis. *Arthritis Rheum* 1989; **32**:1390–5.

16. Howe S, Levinson J, Shear E et al. Development of a disability measurement tool for juvenile rheumatoid arthritis. *Arthritis Rheum* 1991; **34**:873–80.

17. Giannini EH, Lovell DJ, Silverman ED, Sundel RP, Tague BL, Ruperto N, for the Pediatric Rheumatology Collaborative Study Group. Intravenous immunoglobulin in the treatment of polyarticular juvenile rheumatoid arthritis: a Phase I/II study. *J Rheumatol* 1996; **23**:919–24.

18. Murray KJ, Passo MH. Functional measures in children with rheumatic diseases. *Pediatr Clin North Am* 1995; **42**:1127–53.

19. Duffy CM, Arsenault L, Watanabe Duffy KN, Paquin JD, Strawczynski H. The Juvenile Arthritis Quality of Life Questionnaire: development of a

new responsive index for juvenile rheumatoid arthritis. *J Rheumatol* 1997; **24**:738–46.

20. Duffy CM, Arsenault L, Watanabe Duffy KN. Level of agreement between parents and children in rating dysfunction in juvenile rheumatoid arthritis and juvenile spondyloarthropathies. *J Rheumatol* 1993; **20**:2134–9.

21. Duffy CM, Arsenault L, Watanabe Duffy KN, Paquin JD, Strawczynski H. Relative sensitivity to change of the Juvenile Arthritis Quality of Life Questionnaire following a new treatment. *Arthritis Rheum* 1994; **37**:S196.

22. Duffy CM, Arsenault L, Watanabe Duffy KN, Paquin JD, Strawczynski H. Relative sensitivity to change of the Juvenile Arthritis Quality of Life Questionnaire on sequential followup. *Arthritis Rheum* 1995; **38**:S178.

23. Wright VF, Law M, Crombie V, Goldsmith CH, Dent P. Development of a self-report functional status index for juvenile rheumatoid arthritis. *J Rheumatol* 1994; **21**:536–44.

24. Wright VF, Longo Kimber J, Law M, Goldsmith CH, Crombie V, Dent P. The Juvenile Arthritis Functional Status Index (JASI): a validation study. *J Rheum* 1996; **23**:1066–79.

25. Tucker LB, DeNardo BA, Landgraf J et al. Development of a health status measure for children with juvenile rheumatoid arthritis (JRA): The Childhood Arthritis Health Profile (CAHP). *Arthritis Rheum* 1995; **38**:S796.

26. Landgraf J, Abetz L, Ware JE. *The Child Health Questionnaire: A User's Manual*. The Health Institute, New England Medical Center: Boston, MA, 1996.

27. Landgraf JM, Abetz LN, DeNardo BA, Tucker LB. Clinical validity of the Child Health Questionnaire–Parent Form (CHQ-PF) in children with juvenile rheumatoid arthritis. *Arthritis Rheum* 1995; **38**:S795.

28. Tucker LB, DeNardo BA, Abetz LN, Landgraf JM, Schaller JG. The Childhood Arthritis Health Profile (CAHP): validity and reliability of the condition-specific scales. *Arthritis Rheum* 1995; **38**:S185.

29. Tucker LB, DeNardo BA, Schaller JG. The Childhood Arthritis Health Profile: correlations of juvenile rheumatoid arthritis (JRA)-specific scales with disease severity and activity. *Arthritis Rheum* 1996; **39**:S184.

30. Doherty E, Yanni B, Conroy RM, Breshnihan B. A comparison of child and parent ratings of disability and pain in juvenile chronic arthritis. *J Rheumatol* 1993; **20**:1563–6.

31. Taal E, Rasker JJ, Timmers CJ. Measures of physical function and emotional well being for young adults with arthritis. *J Rheumatol* 1997; **24**:994–7.

32. Starfield B, Bergner M, Ensminger M et al. Adolescent health status measurement: development of the Child Health and Illness Profile. *Pediatrics* 1993; **91**:430–5.

4

Infection, arthritis and adolescence

Philip J Hashkes, Frank Biro and David N Glass

INTRODUCTION

The pattern of arthritis related to infectious agents changes significantly during the transition from childhood to adolescence. Behavioural changes, particularly increased sexual activity, as well as physical and immunological maturity, result in a variety of infectious arthritides, and rheumatological sequelae of infections rarely seen in childhood.

The emphasis of this chapter is on those entities seen more frequently during adolescence, rather than a general review of infectious arthritis. We highlight the distinct clinical aspects of common entities as seen in adolescent patients. Many of the studies quoted in this review have clustered adolescent patients with children or young adults; thus it is often difficult to isolate unique features of these diseases in adolescents. Salient clinical features are given in Tables 4.1 and 4.2.

GONOCOCCAL ARTHRITIS

During childhood the main cause of bacterial arthritis is *Staphylococcus aureus*. In adolescence, however, the cause of more than 50% of acute septic arthritis is *Neisseria gonorrhoeae*.[1-3] *Staph. aureus* is responsible for less than one-third of bacterial joint infections in this age group.[1,2]

Epidemiology
N. gonorrhoeae is a Gram-negative diplococcus that typically is sexually transmitted. Infection may result in an asymptomatic carrier state, or cause urethritis, cervicitis, pelvic inflammatory disease, proctitis and, occasionally, pharyngitis. Disseminated disease, including arthritis, develops in approximately 1–3% of patients with symptomatic gonococcal infection and in 0.1–0.3% of asymptomatic carriers.[4]

The highest incidence of uncomplicated gonorrhoea and disseminated disease occurs in males aged 20–24 years, and in females aged 15–19 years.[5] Rare cases of disseminated disease and gonococcal arthritis (GA) are found in infants, children (invariably a consequence of sexual abuse) and in the elderly.[6,7]

In the past most cases of GA were diagnosed in males. At present, however, the female/male ratio is 3 : 1. Part of the reason for the change is the increased diagnosis of asymptomatic gonococcal infection in females, as well as the ability to differentiate between males with GA and those with Reiter's syndrome (see below).[4]

Factors involved in dissemination of *N. gonorrhoeae*
The factors involved in dissemination of *N. gonorrhoeae* are not completely understood. Furthermore, the affinity of *N. gonorrhoeae* for synovial tissue has not been elucidated. However, a combination of host susceptibility, abnormalities of the immune system and qualities related to the organism are implicated.

The timing of infection and the port of entry may influence the development of disseminated disease. In approximately two-thirds of females

Table 4.1	Comparison of clinical features of common bacterial, viral and negative arthridities				
Disease	Sex, age group	Onset	Arthritis type	Arthritis localization	Treatment
Gonorrhoeae: Early	Female >> male; adolescent	Acute	Migratory polyarthritis, tenosynovitis	Lower, upper limbs	Ceftriaxone
Late		Acute	Mono/oligoarthritis	Lower, upper limbs	Ceftriaxone
Bacterial arthritis from other causes	Male > female; infants, young children, elderly	Acute	Monoarthritis	Lower limbs	According to culture
Tuberculosis	Male = female; children (blacks), elderly (whites)	Subacute	Monoarthritis	Lower limbs, spondylitis (Pott's disease), dactylitis	Isoniazid, rifampin, streptomycin
Brucella	Male = female; all ages	Acute, subacute	Mono/oligoarthritis	Lower limbs, sacroiliac	Tetracycline, rifampin
Lyme	Male = female; all ages	Episodic, chronic	Mono/oligoarthritis	Lower limbs	Doxycycline, ceftriaxone
Rubella	Female > Male; adolescents, young adults	Acute	Symmetrical polyarthritis	Fingers, wrists, lower limbs	Self-resolves
Mumps	Male > female; adolescents	Acute	Polyarthritis, often migratory	Upper and lower limbs, fingers	Self-resolves
Parvovirus	Female > male; adults	Acute, subacute, chronic	Symmetrical polyarthritis, oligoarthritis	Upper and lower limbs, fingers	Self-resolves; often lasts for months
Hepatitis B virus	Female = male; adults	Acute	Symmetrical polyarthritis	Small and large joints	Self-resolves
Reiter's syndrome	Male >> female; young adults	Subacute	Oligoarthritis, enthesitis	Lower limbs	Anti-inflammatory drugs, ?tetracyclines
Reactive arthritis	Male > female; adolescents, young adults	Acute, subacute	Oligoarthritis, enthesitis	Lower limbs	Self-resolves, anti-inflammatory drugs
Rheumatic fever	Male = female; children, adolescents	Acute	Migratory polyarthritis, large joints	Lower and upper limbs	Salicylates, corticosteroids for carditis

Table 4.2   Comparison of clinical and laboratory features of common bacterial, viral and negative arthridities

Disease	Fever	Rash	Leucocytosis	Synovial fluid leucocytes	Synovial culture/PCR
Gonorrhoeae:					
Early	+++	++	+++	++	0
Late	+	0	+	+++	++
	±				
Other septic arthritis	+++	+	++++	++++	+++
Tuberculosis	+	0	±	++	+++
Brucella	+++	0	±	+	++
Lyme:					
Early	+	+++	+	±	0
Late	0	+	0	++	+++*
Rubella	+	+++	±	?	+
Mumps	+++	0	++	?	0
Parvovirus	+	++	0	+	++*
Hepatitis B virus	+	+++	0	?	0
Reiter's syndrome	+	++	++	+++	+*
Reactive arthritis	+	0	+	++	+*
Rheumatic fever	+++	+	++	+++	0

*PCR, polymerase chain reaction.

the onset of GA occurs within 1 week of the start of the menstrual cycle, late pregnancy or post-partum.[8] The incomplete mucosal barrier, changes in the acidity of cervical mucus and decreased activity of antibacterial enzymes during menses may increase the invasive ability of the organism. There is debate about whether the risk of dissemination is greater following pharyngeal infections as opposed to genital infections.[9,10]

Specific characteristics have been found in strains of *N. gonorrhoeae* associated with disseminated disease. The colonies of invasive strains appear transparent when cultured, as opposed to the opaque colour of non-invasive strains.[10] Invasive strains often lack the cell membrane protein II, needed for intercellular adhesion between neighbouring organisms. Most strains from patients with disseminated disease have specific nutritional needs of arginine, hypoxanthine and uracil.[11] Strains of *N. gonorrhoeae* that cause disseminated disease express limited serotypes of protein I. These proteins have an ability to form pores in lipid membranes.[10] Several invasive strains were found to bind immunoglobulin G (IgG) antibodies through a lipopolysaccharide, thus blocking specific antibacterial antibody attachment.[12] The sensitivity of invasive strains to penicillin is usually greater than in strains resulting in non-invasive disease.[13]

Resistance to gonococcal disease is dependent on bactericidal complement lysis. Complement deficiencies, especially homozygote deficiencies in C_5 to C_8, are associated with disseminated gonococcal and meningococcal disease. Pelvic inflammatory disease and GA rarely coexist and, conversely, patients with GA often do not have genital symptoms.[4,14] Strong local inflammatory responses at the primary site of infection may prevent gonococcal dissemination.

Clinical manifestations
Three clinical entities of disseminated gonococcal disease have been described. The first is characterized by systemic features, dermatitis, tenosynovitis and migratory polyarthralgia or polyarthritis. Often, blood cultures are positive, whereas cultures from synovial fluid are sterile; thus, this presentation is called the 'bacteraemic' phase. The second entity is often termed the 'septic-joint' phase. In this phase there is a paucity of systemic features and dermatitis. There is progressive localization of joint symptoms and effusions to one or a few joints. Cultures of synovial fluid are frequently positive, while blood cultures are sterile. There is a third presentation with features of both clinical entities, which may represent a transitional phase.

There has been much debate about whether these entities represent a continuum[8,15–17] or different disease processes.[18,19] Regardless of the outcome of this debate, it is clear that some patients progress from the bacteraemic phase to the septic-joint phase, while others may present with only one form or the other. However, only 4% of patients have positive cultures from blood and synovial fluid simultaneously.[17]

SYSTEMIC FEATURES
These usually appear early in the bacteraemic phase, include fever, chills and prostration, and last for 2–7 days. Systemic symptoms are often absent when septic-joint effusions are present.

DERMATITIS
Lesions are characterized by evolution of erythematous macules and papules, to painful vesicles and pustules. Haemorrhagic pustules may progress to bullae, ulceration and necrosis. At first, these lesions appear on the distal upper extremities. Lesions may later spread to the trunk and lower extremities. In general, the number of lesions is few, and they frequently go unnoticed. The rash is present in 75% of patients with positive blood cultures, 33–50% of patients with GA and in only 15% of patients with positive joint cultures.[19–21]

ARTHRITIS AND TENOSYNOVITIS
The onset of musculoskeletal symptoms is almost always acute; symptoms reach a peak within several days of presentation.[22] In prospective studies, the interval from the first sign of disease to the appearance of joint involvement was 3.6–5.3 days.[23] Early in the disease, many patients have migratory polyarthralgia or arthritis, with systemic features, dermatitis and bacteraemia. Localization of purulent effusions to one or a few joints occurs later in the disease.

Forty per cent of patients present with monoarthritis, 30% with oligoarthritis and 30% with polyarticular involvement. The joints most frequently affected are the wrists and hands.[2,22] However, *N. gonorrhoeae* is most often isolated from the knees, due in part to the relative ease of knee aspiration. Other joints frequently affected, in descending order, are the ankles, elbows, shoulders and feet. The hips are rarely affected, as compared to the case in other causes of bacterial arthritis.[1,2] Rare cases of sacroiliac, temporomandibular and spinal joint involvement have been reported.

An important feature of GA is the appearance of asymmetric tenosynovitis in nearly two-thirds of patients, usually during the bacteraemic phase.[15,19] The dorsum of the hands and wrists are most often affected, but ankles and knees are also frequently involved. *N. gonorrhoeae* is rarely isolated from tenosynovitis.

OTHER MANIFESTATIONS
Other less common manifestations of disseminated gonococcal disease include endocarditis, myocarditis, meningitis and intraperitoneal dissemination with adhesion formation (Fitz–Hugh–Curtis syndrome).

Pathology

Skin lesions are characterized by small-vessel vasculitis with perivascular polymorphonuclear cell infiltration. Intraepidermal infiltrations of polymorphonuclear cells are also seen, unlike in leucocytoclastic vasculitis. Debate exists about whether these lesions represent an immune hypersensitivity phenomenon or septic emboli. Supporting the immune theory is the fact that *N. gonorrhoeae* is rarely found in cultures of skin lesions.[8,10,21] Furthermore, the appearance of skin lesions in some patients is similar to erythema multiforme or urticaria, and on immunofluorescence gonococcal antigens are found in the skin in the majority of patients.[24]

Early joint disease is limited to synovial tissue and tenosynovial tissue, with subsequent spread to the joint space, synovial fluid and cartilage.[16] If untreated, pathological changes are similar to those seen in other bacterial joint infections.

Diagnosis

The diagnosis is not difficult when a sexually active, healthy, female adolescent presents with a history of genitourinary symptoms, rash, tenosynovitis and arthritis. However, GA must be suspected in any adolescent patient with an acute onset of mono- or oligoarthritis, regardless of the sexual history. It is often difficult to obtain intimate information from adolescents. The sexual history should be obtained by the primary physician or health professional closest to the patient, rather than by multiple 'random' examiners or consultants.

A classification scheme for grading the reliability of diagnosis has been proposed by Masi and Eisenstein.[21] GA is categorized as proven when *N. gonorrhoeae* is isolated from synovial tissue, synovial fluid, blood or skin lesions. GA is classified as documented when dermatitis accompanies the typical clinical manifestations of GA, with isolation of *N. gonorrhoeae* from a primary infectious site. Presumptive GA is diagnosed when *N. gonorrhoeae* is isolated from a primary infectious site but dermatitis does not accompany the typical clinical manifestations. Possible GA is considered when clinical manifestations are typical of GA, without microbacterial confirmation (partially treated or cultures not obtained properly). However, one must be careful in the diagnosis of GA, even when clinical features are compatible with GA, if appropriately obtained cultures did not demonstrate *N. gonorrhoeae*.

Cultures should be obtained from all possible primary sites of infection – the urethra, cervix, rectum and pharynx, as well as from blood and affected joints. Smears should be plated immediately, preferably in the clinic or at the bedside, on fresh, prewarmed media, and incubated within 15 minutes in a CO_2 rich atmosphere. Cultures from 'sterile' body fluids should be plated on chocolate agar (heated blood agar) without antibiotic-containing selective media. Cultures from heavily colonized areas should be placed on selective Thayer–Martin media. Gram stains of joint fluid and skin lesions should be performed to search for the characteristic kidney-shaped intracellular Gram-negative diplococci. First voided urine in males can be used as an alternative to urethral specimens.

Blood cultures are positive in approximately 4–10% of patients with disseminated gonorrhoeae, cultures of synovial fluid are positive in 33%, endocervix cultures in 50–60%, urethral or rectal cultures in 20%, pharyngeal cultures in 17–57% and cultures of skin specimens in 4–7%. Gram stain of synovial fluid is positive in 22–30% of patients.[19,21] DNA fragments of *N. gonorrhoeae* are found in the synovial fluid, by polymerase chain reaction (PCR), in the majority of patients with GA.[25]

The erythrocyte sedimentation rate (ESR) is increased in more than 90% of patients, and leucocytosis with polymorphonuclear cell predominance are seen in 75% of patients. Analysis of synovial fluid usually reveals a white blood cell count of 50 000–200 000/mm³ with greater than 90% polymorphonuclear cells and low glucose levels.[26]

Radiographs rarely reveal more than soft tissue swelling (Figure 4.1). Occasionally, in long-standing untreated disease, erosions or joint-space narrowing can be seen.

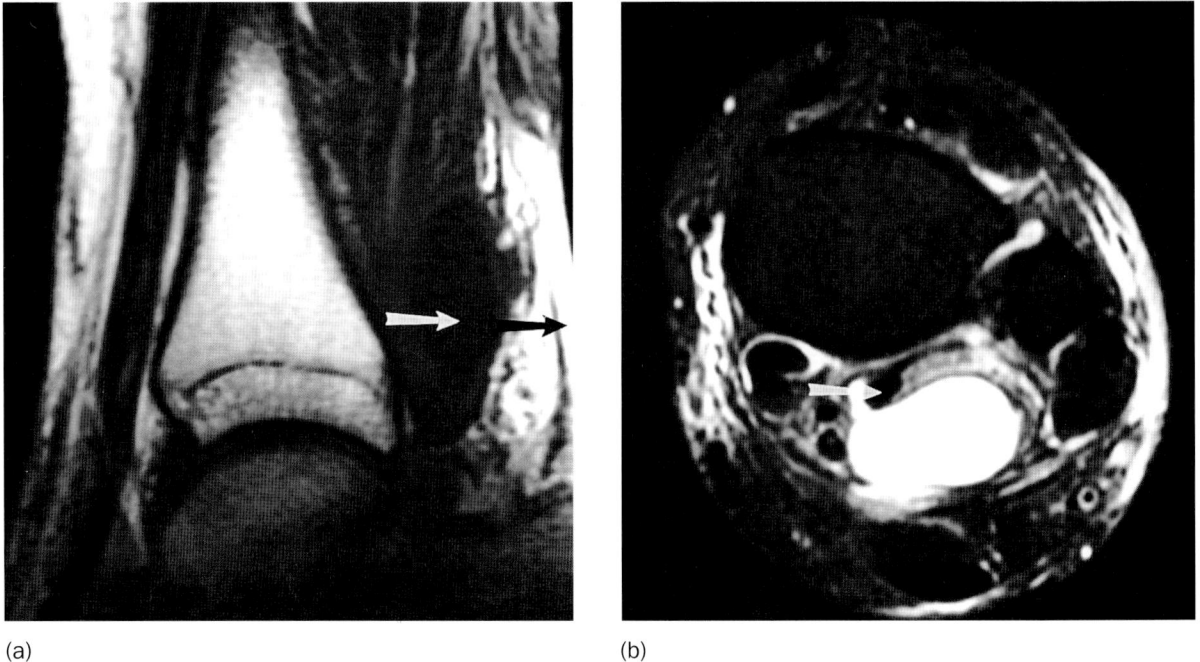

(a)   (b)

Figure 4.1 (a) Sagittal T1-weighted magnetic resonance image (MRI) demonstrates fluid collection (white arrow) of low signal intensity posterior to the tibia and anterior to the Achilles tendon (black arrow). (b) Axial T2-weighted MR image shows the fluid collection (bright signal intensity) is located anterior to the flexor retinaculum and just adjacent to the flexor hallucis longus tendon (white arrow). This adolescent female presented with generalized foot swelling and pain and had a markedly erythrocyte sedimentation rate. Culture of the fluid collection as well as the peripheral blood grew *Neisseria gonorrhoeae*, confirming the diagnosis of gonococcal tenosynovitis.

Differential diagnosis

NON-GONOCOCCAL BACTERIAL ARTHRITIS

Septic arthritis from other causes must be differentiated from GA. Other causes of bacterial arthritis in adolescents include *Staph. aureus* and group A *Streptococcus pyogenes*. Less common organisms include Gram-negative infections, usually seen in intravenous-drug abusers or in immunosuppressed patients, and *Mycobacterium tuberculosis*. Arthritis due to *Brucella* species is common among adolescents in the developing world (see below).

Diagnosis is based on isolation of a particular organism. However, several clinical features can help differentiate GA and non-gonococcal bacterial arthritis.[1–3,21] GA is generally seen in healthy, adolescent females, while non-gonococcal bacterial arthritis is seen in the young, the elderly, more frequently in males and in patients with predisposing comorbidities. These include patients with immunodeficiencies, drug addicts, patients with chronic arthritis, and patients with joint prostheses. Non-gonococcal bacterial arthritis rarely involves more than one joint, and tenosynovitis is less prominent. Lower limb joints and hips are more frequently involved. The response to antibiotics is more rapid and hospitalization shorter in GA.[1]

Cutaneous lesions similar to those in disseminated gonococcal disease can be seen in septic arthritis from *Strep. pyogenes*, *Haemophilus*

Table 4.3   Comparison of Reiter's syndrome and gonococcal arthritis

	Reiter's syndrome	Gonococcal arthritis
Epidemiology	Male, > 20 years	Female, adolescent
Mean interval between genitourinary and joint symptoms (days)	28	6.3
Onset	Gradual	Acute
Fever	Low grade	High; toxic appearance
Localization of arthritis	Lower extremities	Upper and lower extremities
Tenosynovitis	Frequent	Frequent
Conjunctivitis	Frequent	Uncommon
Rash	Keratoderma blenorrhagia; circinate balantis	Vesicular, pustular; mostly upper extremities
Response to antibiotics	Minimal response possible	Prompt

influenzae and staphylococcal arthritis, especially when associated with bacterial endocarditis. In some parts of the USA and Australia, *N. meningitidis* is a more common cause of rash and arthritis in a sexually active adolescent than is *N. gonorrhoeae*. However, patients with meningococcaemia usually have a greater number of skin lesions, with positive throat and skin cultures.[27,28] The maculopapular rash of secondary syphilis, which can be confused with disseminated gonococcal disease, tends to be much more extensive than that seen in *N. gonorrhoeae*. The location of the rash in syphilis, which includes the palms, soles and trunk, and other features such as generalized lymphadenopathy and serological tests, can aid in the correct diagnosis.

Differences in laboratory tests between GA and non-gonococcal bacterial arthritis are less helpful. C-reactive protein levels and synovial neutrophilia are slightly higher in non-gonococcal bacterial arthritis than in GA. Synovial cultures are positive in about 60% of streptococcal arthritis, 40% of staphylococcal arthritis and 57% of arthritis from Gram-negative bacteria, as opposed to 33% in GA.[17]

RHEUMATIC FEVER
The acute onset of fever, rash and migratory arthritis may suggest rheumatic fever (RF) (see later). However, RF usually occurs in younger children. Cardiac manifestations of RF, including endocarditis, are less common in GA. The characteristic rash of RF, erythema marginatum, differs from the rash seen in GA. RF does not respond dramatically to antibiotics. Conversely, GA does not respond well to aspirin. Evidence of prior streptococcal infection is crucial in the diagnosis of RF.

REITER'S SYNDROME
Reiter's syndrome (RS) (see later) or reactive arthritis following non-gonococcal urethritis may be difficult to differentiate from GA (Table 4.3). Cases of RS following *N. gonorrhoeae* infection have been reported.[20,29,30]

Treatment
Until the early 1980s, strains of *N. gonorrhoeae* that caused arthritis were exquisitely sensitive to penicillin. Resolution of GA was reported to occur as soon as 12 hours after penicillin was started.[19]

Recently, however, studies in GA have found penicillin resistance in more than 5% of patients.[31] Therefore, third-generation cephalosporins (typically ceftriaxone) should be used initially until drug susceptibilities are known.[31] Treatment is started immediately after appropriate cultures have been obtained and continued for 7–10 days. Parenteral therapy should be started, and continued until symptoms and signs resolve or significant clinical improvement is demonstrated. Penicillin or ampicillin can be substituted if penicillin sensitivity is established. Tetracycline or doxycycline should be added for treatment of possible coexisting chlamydial infection. Intramuscular spectinomycin is used as the initial drug in patients with allergies to penicillin and cephalosporins. Quinolones can later be substituted in adolescents who have completed their growth, and erythromycin in younger adolescents or pregnant patients.[3]

Admission to hospital is indicated for patients with an uncertain diagnosis, significant purulent effusions or systemic symptoms, and for patients in whom compliance with therapy may be problematic. The mean length of hospital stay for these patients is 5.8 days.[31]

Open drainage is rarely indicated. However, repeated joint aspiration is sometimes needed for treatment of purulent or recurrent effusions. Traction may be beneficial in reduction of pain and muscle spasm.

Prognosis
Prior to the advent of antibiotic therapy, about 25% of the patients developed some degree of permanent joint damage. Today, prompt recovery occurs soon after start of treatment. Unlike other bacterial causes of arthritis, erosive joint changes are rarely seen.

BRUCELLA

Brucella is primarily a zoonotic disease (i.e. an infection naturally transmitted from a vertebrate animal) that is transmitted to humans via contact with infected animals or their secretions. The most common method of infection is through consumption of non-pasteurized goat's milk. Although rarely seen in developed countries, brucellosis is a major cause of septic arthritis in the third world and Middle East, in all age groups, including adolescents.

The disease is caused by small non-motile Gram-negative coccibacilli. There are four species pathogenic to humans, of which the most important is *Brucella melitensis*, found mainly in goats and sheep.

Brucellosis is a multisystem and often prolonged disease. Systemic features include fever, malaise, anorexia, weight loss, lymphadenopathy, hepatosplenomegaly, hepatitis and pancytopenia.

Arthralgia or arthritis are the second most common manifestations of brucellosis, after fever. Arthralgia is seen in 50–75% of patients and arthritis in 33–40%.[32,33] Articular involvement is monoarticular in 70% of cases and oligoarticular in 30%. In adolescents, however, there is a greater frequency of oligoarticular involvement.[34] The hips are affected most frequently (60%), followed by the knees (47%), sacroiliac joints (16–45%), ankles, wrists and elbows. In adolescents, in contrast to adults, the spine and small joints are usually spared.[32] Two common patterns are seen. The first, affecting peripheral joints, is seen more in children. The second pattern, which involves mainly the sacroiliac joint, is seen among adolescents and young adults.[32]

Diagnosis of brucellosis is aided by a careful history of exposure. Cultures of blood, bone marrow and synovial fluid are diagnostic in most patients, and in others *Brucella* is diagnosed by serological demonstration of rising titres. Bone scintigraphy is helpful in the diagnosis of sacroiliac disease. Synovial fluid is inflammatory. However, white cell counts are slightly lower than in other bacterial infections, with a mean of 14 300 cells/mm^3.[32] Cultures of synovial fluid are positive in 50–67% of patients with arthritis. Since *Brucella* is an intracellular pathogen, a higher yield of the organism is obtained from biopsies of synovial tissue. Low titres of rheumatoid factor and antinuclear antibodies are found in 20–25% of patients.

Treatment consists of a 3- to 6-week course of combination trimethoprime–sulfamethoxazole, or tetracycline with rifampin or streptomycin. The articular prognosis is good with an adequate course of antibiotics. Relapses frequently occur if the duration of antibiotic therapy is shorter than 3 weeks.[33,34] Chronic joint damage is rare; most cases have been reported in patients with hip disease or spondylitis.

LYME DISEASE

Lyme disease is caused by fastidious microaerophilic spirochaetes from the *Borrelia* species; they are transmitted to humans by ticks of the *Ixodid* family. In North America the major causative agent is *B. burgdorferi*, which is transmitted primarily by *I. dammini*. In Europe the major causative agents are *B. garinii* or *B. afzelii*, which are transmitted mainly by *I. ricinis*. The larvae and nymphs of these ticks feed on larger mammals, primarily white-tailed deer, mostly during the summer, when the onset of Lyme disease is more frequent.

Lyme disease, first recognized in 1975 in a cluster of children with 'pauciarticular juvenile rheumatoid arthritis' in Lyme, Connecticut, USA, is endemic in the north-east, upper midwest and the northern Pacific coastal states of the USA and in parts of Europe and Asia. The incidence of Lyme disease in the USA in 1994 was 5.2 per 100 000.[35] About one-third of cases occur during childhood and adolescence.[36]

Direct tissue invasion by the spirochaete is responsible for the clinical manifestations. Lyme disease usually begins with erythema migrans, a distinctive skin lesion seen initially at the site of the tick bite. The lesion begins as a red macula and expands peripherally with partial central clearing. Regional lymphadenopathy is common. However, only 20–52% of children and adolescents recall a tick bite.[36–40] Following haematogenic dissemination of the spirochaete, smaller lesions similar to erythema migrans may be seen at other sites.

Disease manifestations are generally divided into early and late manifestations. Early manifestations during the first weeks to months after the tick bite include systemic, neurological, cardiac and musculoskeletal manifestations. Early systemic symptoms include mild flu-like symptoms, mainly fever, fatigue and malaise. Neurological symptoms, seen in 15–20% of children and adolescents, include headaches, aseptic meningitis, encephalitis, seizures, chorea, cranial neuropathies (most commonly Bell's palsy), radiculopathies, mononeuritis multiplex and transverse myelitis.[41] The major early cardiac manifestations include various degrees of atrioventricular blocks and myocarditis, and are seen in 5–10% of patients.[41] In the early stages of disease, patients may complain of migratory pain in joints, muscle, tendons or bone, without objective evidence of joint inflammation. Symptoms in individual joints are generally fleeting, lasting in one location for several hours to days.[42]

The systems predominantly affected in late disease include the nervous system, eyes, skin and joints. Late neurological symptoms include the development of encephalopathy, memory impairment, headaches and fatigue. The major ocular manifestation consists of the uncommon development of keratitis. Atrophic skin lesions termed *acrodermatitis chronica atrophicans* may develop years after infection. These lesions, which are initially plaque-like or nodular with violaceous skin discolouration, later become atrophic. These lesions are seen mainly in European patients, and can be confused with morphea or linear scleroderma.

Lyme arthritis

Several weeks to months after infection, intermittent attacks of arthritis may appear. The prevalence of arthritis in Lyme disease among children and adolescents is 22–60%,[36,37,39,42,43] which is higher than in adults.[36,39,41] In one study the odds ratio of developing arthritis in childhood and adolescence as compared to adults was 1.9.[39] In as many as 50% of children and adolescents in the USA, arthritis is the only manifestation of disease.[37,39,40,44] Careful questioning of adolescent patients will reveal that 50% had a mild flu-like illness several weeks to months prior to the onset of arthritis.[41]

Early flares of arthritis are characterized by brief episodes lasting several days to weeks, with asymptomatic intervals of weeks to months between episodes. The knee is affected in nearly all patients; other sites include elbows, wrists, ankles and hips.[37,38] Arthritis is characterized by large effusions and warmth of the involved joint, without significant pain or erythema. The pattern of arthritis is monoarticular in 70% of patients and oligoarticular in 25%,[45] involving a mean of 2.4 joints.[39]

The natural history of Lyme arthritis in children and adolescents was studied in the 1970s, prior to the advent of antibiotic therapy.[44] During the first year of disease, an average of five arthritic episodes were observed, lasting several days to weeks. The number of flares progressively decreased, with a mean of two episodes observed in the fourth year. The duration of later flares was longer, lasting several weeks to months. There was a direct correlation between the age at disease onset and the total duration of arthritis. In teenagers aged 13–15 years the mean total duration of arthritis was 22 weeks, as compared to only 4 weeks in children aged 2–4 years.[44]

There are other less common forms of arthritis in Lyme disease. An acute onset of monoarthritis resembling septic arthritis, with fever and joint erythema, was seen in one study in about one-third of the children and adolescents.[41] Chronic oligoarticular arthritis, resembling pauciarticular chronic idiopathic arthritis of childhood, was seen in 13%. Many of those patients had low titres of antinuclear antibodies. Lyme arthritis may also present with polyarticular or migratory arthritis.

There is an association between the length and severity of arthritis and the presence of the human leucocyte antigen (HLA) DR4 allele.[44] These patients are at increased risk of developing chronic, erosive arthritis, as seen in 5–10% of children, despite adequate antibiotic treatment.[37,41] Reactive T cells to the outer surface protein A (OspA) of B. burgdorferi have been identified in the synovial fluid of these patients.[46] In one study, patients with prolonged arthritis had increased levels of interleukin-1β in synovial fluid.[47] The synovial pathology of these patients is similar to that of chronic idiopathic arthritis of childhood.[43]

There are several differences between adolescents in North America and Europe, which are perhaps related to the different *Borrelia* species pertaining in the two continents. Erythema migrans is rarely seen in European adolescents with arthritis. In one series, only 1 of 61 patients with arthritis had a history of erythema migrans.[45] Nearly one-third of European children develop chronic arthritis, in contrast to 5% of North American children.[41,45] Antibiotic therapy is less effective among European children, with a treatment failure rate of nearly 20%.[45]

Diagnosis, serologic and laboratory tests

Many problems in the diagnosis of Lyme disease arise from the low specificity of serological tests and the lack of a uniform definition for positive tests using Western-blot assays. Cross-reactivity with other organisms, especially other spirochaetes and the Epstein–Barr virus, as well as high rates of seropositivity in asymptomatic persons living in endemic areas, limit the usefulness of serological tests. Furthermore, it is not possible to distinguish active disease from inactive disease with serological tests. Serological tests for B. burgdorferi may remain positive for more than 1 year after resolution of arthritis.[44] In contrast, patients with only erythema migrans may be seronegative. Therefore, results of serological tests need to correlate with the clinical picture in patients at risk of exposure to B. burgdorferi. It is necessary to confirm by Western blot assay those patients with equivocal or positive IgG antibodies to B. burgdorferi detected by enzyme-linked immunosorbent assay (ELISA). For a positive IgG Western-blot assay, reactivity to at least 5 of 10 common antigen bands is required.[43] The most common bands include the 41 kDA band to flagellar antigen, the 23 kDA band to the OspC, and the 18, 28, 30, 39, 45, 58, 66 and 93 kDA bands. Patients with arthritis usually have high serological titres and respond to more than 10 antigen bands.

PCR can identify the DNA of B. burgdorferi in synovial fluid. In one study, the DNA encoding OspA was identified in the synovial fluid from 70 of 73 patients with Lyme arthritis, but not in patients with synovitis from other causes.[48]

However, PCR is not yet available for routine clinical practice.

T-cell-proliferation assays to *B. burgdorferi* antigens (especially OspA) show increased responsiveness early in the disease process, prior even to the occurrence of a humoral response to the spirochaete. In a study of 17 patients with attenuated Lyme arthritis following inadequate treatment of early Lyme disease, 14 patients had an increased T-cell response, without evidence of antibodies to *B. burgdorferi*.[49]

The ESR and immunoglobulins levels are frequently elevated in Lyme arthritis. Low titres of antinuclear antibodies (ANA) with a homogeneous pattern are seen in 13–30% of children and adolescents.[37,45] In patients with meningitis, cerebrospinal fluid reveals lymphocytic pleocytosis, with an increased protein concentration. Specific IgM and IgG antibodies to *Borrelia* in the spinal fluid are diagnostic of central nervous system disease.

The joint fluid is typically inflammatory, with leucocyte counts ranging from 180 to 100 000, and polymorphonuclear cell predominance. Cultures of joint fluid for *B. burgdorferi* are rarely positive.[50]

Radiological findings generally reveal soft-tissue swelling. In long-lasting disease periarticular osteoporosis is common; joint-space narrowing and erosions may be seen in chronic disease.

Differential diagnosis

Lyme disease needs to be differentiated from other causes (infectious, inflammatory or mechanical) of monoarticular or oligoarticular arthritis. The pattern of Lyme arthritis often resembles pauciarticular chronic idiopathic arthritis of childhood or reactive arthritis, thus delaying the diagnosis of Lyme arthritis.[37,41] In a series of 43 children and adolescents with Lyme arthritis, 15 patients were initially diagnosed with septic arthritis, 12 with juvenile rheumatoid arthritis (JRA; see definition in Chapter 5), and 6 with reactive arthritis. The mean interval between the onset of arthritis and diagnosis was 2 months (range 1 week to 4 years).[38]

Several syndromes that are seen frequently during adolescence are occasionally mistaken for Lyme disease. Fibromyalgia and chronic fatigue syndrome often have a chronological association with erythema migrans or Lyme arthritis. In a study from British Columbia, a non-endemic area, only 2 of 65 children and adolescents referred for evaluation of Lyme disease, did indeed have Lyme arthritis. Eleven patients had fibromyalgia or chronic fatigue syndrome.[51] This problem is compounded by the many false-positive or equivocal serological tests in these patients, which may represent past infection with *B. burgdorferi*. Fibromyalgia is characterized by widespread musculoskeletal pain, sleep disturbances, depression and tender points, but with no objective signs of joint inflammation. Fibromyalgia and chronic fatigue syndrome do not respond to repeated courses of antibiotics, even when the symptoms are associated with the appearance of Lyme disease.

Treatment and outcome

Oral amoxicillin or doxycycline for 30–60 days has been recommended as first-line therapy for Lyme arthritis in adolescent patients in the absence of neurological involvement. In patients with allergy to penicillin or tetracycline, cefuroxime axetil is recommended.[43] A good response has been found in more than 85% of North American patients.[40–42,52] In 10% of children and adolescents, the resolution of arthritis is slow, taking 2–3 months after the completion of the first antibiotic course.[40,53] Intravenous ceftriaxone, 2 g/day for 30 days, is the treatment of choice for patients with neuroborreliosis or for patients with arthritis in whom a course of oral antibiotics has been ineffective.

The prognosis in children and adolescents is better than in adults.[37,40] However, 2–10% of children and adolescents continue to have persistent arthritis despite treatment with intravenous ceftriaxone.[52,54] Patients who express the HLA DR4 allele are at increased risk of this outcome. In most patients with persistent arthritis, *Borrelia* DNA is not detected in synovial fluid.[48] Treatment with anti-inflammatory medications, including non-steroidal anti-inflammatory drugs (NSAIDs), hydroxychloroquine[55] and intra-articular corticosteroid injections, may be warranted for patients who did not respond to two adequate courses of antibiotics.[52] In refractory chronic arthritis, arthroscopic synovectomy may be beneficial.[54,56]

Prophylactic antibiotics after a tick bite in an endemic area is a controversial issue. Most authorities do not recommend universal treatment, since multiple bites are common in tick-infested areas and adverse reactions to antibiotics are not uncommon. However, some advocate treating patients who develop a flu-like illness after a tick bite or patients with asymptomatic seroconversion. It is also recommended to treat pregnant patients, as rare cases of congenital defects after infection with *B. burgdorferi* have been reported.[41]

Some patients continue to have vague symptoms without objective signs of Lyme disease following adequate antibiotic therapy. Brief episodes of arthralgia may occur in 30% of untreated children and adolescents, even as late as 10 years after arthritis has subsided.[42,44] A higher serological response to the spirochaete increases the risk of late arthralgia.[44] Patients may also continue to complain of myalgia, fatigue, palpitations, headache, paraesthesia, concentration defects and weakness. Repeated or prolonged courses of antibiotics do not result in resolution of these symptoms, and occasionally are associated with severe adverse reactions. These phenomena may represent an undefined post-infectious syndrome.[57,58]

Recently a recombinant vaccine to the OspA of *B. burgdorferi* has been developed. A multicentre trial among adults in an endemic area who were less than 60 years old, demonstrated an efficacy of 82% after two doses 1 month apart, and 100% after a third dose 6 months later.[59] There was no excess of joint symptoms in the vaccinated population as compared with the control population. The efficacy in adolescents has not been tested, although a trial is being planned. Clinical indications for use of the vaccine have not yet been developed.

VIRAL ARTHRITIS

Many viruses have been recognized in the pathogenesis of acute and chronic arthritis in childhood and adolescence. Recent advances in the ability to identify viral proteins, DNA and RNA from synovial fluid and tissue have increased the spectrum of viruses implicated in the aetiology of acute infectious arthritis. The musculoskeletal symptoms associated with viral infections are often not observed in prepubertal patients.

Rubella

The togaviruses, mainly rubella, are the most commonly recognized viral-associated cause of arthritis in North America.[60] Musculoskeletal symptoms are more common in females than males and are seen with a greater frequency after natural infection than after vaccination.

Joint symptoms are rarely seen in prepubertal children.[60] In a series of 46 adolescents with natural rubella infection, 52% of the females and 9% of the males developed arthritis. An additional 14% of the girls and 45% of the males developed arthralgia.[61] Following immunization of female adolescents and young adults with the RA 27/3 vaccine, still in current use, only 14% developed arthritis, and 41% developed short-lived arthralgia.[61] Symptoms are generally more severe in female patients.[61,62] An association of arthritis with the menstrual cycle has been observed.[63]

Typically, small joints of the fingers and wrists are affected. Joint symptoms usually appear within 7 days of the beginning of the rash during natural infection, and 14–21 days after immunization. Tenosynovitis of the hand is a frequent occurrence.[62] The arthritis usually resolves within 1 month, but may persist for several months, and occasionally last for years. Tingle et al[61] have reported that joint symptoms persisted for more than 18 months in 30% of female patients and 9% of males following natural infection, but only in 4.5% of females after immunization with the RA 27/3 vaccine.

Mumps

Fifteen per cent of mumps infections occur during adolescence. Joint manifestations are rare (less than 0.5% in one series), but can be severe.[64] Similar to rubella, joint symptoms appear more frequently in adolescence than during childhood.[65] Unlike rubella, joint symptoms are more common in males (3.6 : 1).[65] Arthritis usually appears 1–2 weeks after the complete resolution of parotitis. Rarely, arthritis may precede parotitis by as much as 8 days. Post-vaccination musculoskeletal symptoms have not been reported.[66]

Both large and small joints are affected, frequently in a migratory pattern. Fever, occasionally higher than 40°C, is often present suggesting pyogenic arthritis or systemic-onset chronic idiopathic arthritis of childhood.[67] Nearly 70% of patients with joint symptoms also have orchitis, two to three times the expected rate of testicular involvement.[65]

Laboratory tests reveal an increased ESR, leucocytosis and mild anaemia. Rheumatoid factor is positive in more than 50% of cases.[65] However, in all reported cases, the virus has not been isolated from synovial fluid or tissue; the diagnosis of mumps was through serologic tests.[65] Therefore, it is still unclear whether the pathogenesis of mumps arthritis is by direct viral invasion of synovial tissue or immune mediated.[65,67]

Joint symptoms do not respond well to salicylate therapy.[65,68] A short course of corticosteroids therapy may dramatically improve symptoms. Complete resolution without joint sequela occurs usually within 3 months.

Parvovirus B19

Infection with parvovirus B19 is associated with several clinical syndromes, the most common being erythema infectiosum ('fifth disease'). Studies of young adults and children with musculoskeletal symptoms associated with parvovirus B19 have been reported.[69,70] None have specifically studied adolescents, but several observations can be made from mixed studies of adolescents and children.

Similar to rubella, musculoskeletal symptoms are seen more often in females and adults than in males and children.[69] In less than 50% of patients the typical rash precedes joint symptoms. Two-thirds of patients have a prodrome of mild constitutional symptoms within 1 week of the appearance of joint symptoms. Two major patterns of joint involvement are seen.[69] The majority of adults develop a symmetrical, non-erosive, self-limiting polyarthritis involving the small joints of the fingers, wrists and knees. Laboratory tests are generally normal, and symptoms usually resolve within 4 weeks. About half of the affected children develop a pattern similar to adults, while the other half develop oligoarthritis, mainly of the large joints.[69] One-third of the children have a low to moderate titre of ANA, and nearly 50% have decreased complement activity, attesting to the possible role of immune-complex formation in the pathogenesis of arthritis.[70] The course of arthritis is more prolonged in children, lasting over 2 months in 40% of children, thus fulfilling the criteria for diagnosis of JRA.[70]

Human immunodeficiency virus

Sexual activity and drug use have introduced the human immunodeficiency virus (HIV) into the adolescent population. A variety of musculoskeletal manifestations are recognized in 66–75% of patients with HIV. The most common is mild polyarticular arthralgia, occurring in about 25% of these patients.[71] Incomplete Reiter's syndrome, usually not encompassing the entire triad, is seen in approximately 15% of patients. Most patients do not carry the HLA B27 allele.[71]

A unique inflammatory syndrome consisting of monoarticular or oligoarticular arthritis of large joints is seen in 5–10% of patients. The arthritis is short lived, lasting 1–2 weeks.[71] Other rheumatic disorders include Sjögren's syndrome, psoriatic arthritis, enthesitis and a lupus-like syndrome.

Septic arthritis is seen in 2.5% of patients infected with HIV.[72] Many of these patients have other risk factors, such as intravenous drug use, and are not necessarily immunosuppressed. The most common organism is *Staph. aureus*, but opportunistic infections are seen in nearly one-third of HIV patients with septic arthritis. Other organisms have been identified, including *Candida albicans*, *Histoplasma capsulatum*, *Cryptococcus neoformans*, *Sporothrix schenckii*, *Mucormycosis*, typical and atypical mycobacteria, various staphylococcal species and infections with Gram-negative bacteria.[73]

Hepatitis B virus

During the prodrome period of infection with hepatitis B virus, a disease resembling serum sickness may develop in as many as 20% of adults. Arthralgia is seen in an additional 40% of patients. In adolescence, the incidence is unknown. This entity develops about 12 weeks after exposure to the virus, approximately 2–3 weeks prior to the development of jaundice, and resolves with the appearance of icterus.

The major clinical manifestations include the development of polyarthritis and rash. Both small and large joints are affected in a migratory or additive pattern. A pruritic maculopapular, urticarial or petechial rash may accompany joint symptoms. Symptoms generally last 2 weeks or until the appearance of jaundice. Symptoms can be hard to control, even with the use of anti-inflammatory medication.[74]

The pathogenesis is related to immune-complex deposition in blood vessel walls. Immune complexes containing hepatitis B surface antigen, IgM and C_3 are seen in biopsy specimens of skin lesions, and decreased levels of complement can be found. Haematuria is seen in nearly 50% of cases.[75] In one report, hepatitis B surface antigen was found in synovial tissue.[76] Abnormalities in liver enzymes and the presence of hepatitis B surface antigen are helpful to differentiate this entity from other causes of acute polyarthritis.[73]

Other viruses

Other viruses are associated less frequently with the development of arthritis. These include the Epstein–Barr virus, cytomegalovirus, coxsackie-B virus, adenovirus 7, herpes simplex, varicella-zoster, echoviruses and viruses from the alphavirus family. Few data are available regarding the specific clinical pattern of these viruses in the adolescent age group.

REACTIVE ARTHRITIS

Reactive arthritis describes a sterile synovitis that occurs in association with an infection elsewhere in the body, usually in the gastrointestinal or genitourinary tract. Unlike adults, most cases of reactive arthritis in children and adolescents occur after gastrointestinal rather than genitourinary disease.[77,78] In children, reactive arthritis may also follow upper respiratory disease. The major organisms involved in reactive arthritis include *Chlamydia trachomatis*, *Shigella flexeri*, *Yersinia enterocolitica*, *Salmonella enteriditis*, *Salmonella typhimurium* and *Campylobacter*. Other organisms, including *N. gonorrhoeae* (see above), have also been implicated in reactive arthritis.[29]

Reiter's syndrome

The classic presentation of reactive arthritis is Reiter's syndrome (RS). Although RS was first described in 1918 in a 16-year-old male, RS is very uncommon during adolescence.[77–81] It is estimated that less than 3% of patients with RS are younger than 18 years old.[79]

In adolescents, the male/female ratio is 4–5 : 1, which is less than in adults (10 : 1). This ratio is closer to that seen in post-dysenteric RS than in post-venereal RS.[77] Several cases of siblings or parents with RS have been reported. There are no clear racial predominances.

A history of diarrhoea is elicited in more than two-thirds of adolescent patients.[77,81] Isolation of *Shigella flexeri*, *Y. enterocolitica*, *Salm. enteriditis* and *Salm. typhimurium* from the stool, has been reported. Infrequently, a history of sexual activity can be obtained. *Chlamydia trachomatis* has been isolated from synovial fluid and the urethra in several adolescent cases.[77] PCR studies in adults have shown DNA fragments of chlamydia and ureaplasma in joints of patients with RS.[82]

The clinical features are similar to those in adults.[77,78,80] Conjunctivitis is the most common first manifestation (60%), followed by urethritis and arthritis. The complete triad, when present, appears usually within 2–3 weeks from the onset of the first symptom.

Bilateral conjunctivitis, with or without a sterile discharge, is the most common eye manifestation. Rarely, patients may develop iritis, keratitis and even optic neuritis. The long-term prognosis of ocular involvement is excellent.

The most common genitourinary symptom is dysuria, with urethral discharge and pyuria occurring in one-third of patients.

Mucocutaneous manifestations are less common in adolescents than in adults.[78] These include painless oral ulcerations, keratoderma blenorrhagia (mainly on the soles of the feet) and circinate balantis.

The pattern of arthritis in adolescents differs slightly from that seen in adults. In adults, large joints of the lower extremity are affected in an asymmetrical pattern. In adolescents, there is greater involvement of the upper limb, mainly the wrists.[77] Usually more than one joint is affected. Rare cases of temporomandibular joint and cervical spine involvement have been reported. Arthritis may be symmetrical, with a migratory or additive pattern. Similar to adults, enthesitis is common.

Mild systemic features, including low-grade fever, fatigue and anorexia, are common. Rare manifestations reported in adolescents have included myocarditis, pleuritis, lymphadenopathy and splenomegaly. Valvulitis, nephritis and vasculitis, reported in adults, have not been described in adolescent patients.[77]

Laboratory tests are non-specific, with the exception that more than 85% of adolescent patients carry the HLA B27 allele.[77] The ESR is usually greater than 50 mm/hour; leucocytosis and mild anaemia of chronic disease is common. Synovial fluid analysis reveals inflammatory fluid. The mean white blood cell count is 20 000/mm^3, predominantly polymorphonuclear. Glucose levels are usually normal. Complement levels may be elevated.

Common radiographic features include erosions at sites of ligament insertions to the bone, spur formation and osteopenia. Sacro-iliac involvement has been reported in one adolescent.[77]

The differential diagnosis includes psoriatic arthritis, spondyloarthropathies, chronic idiopathic arthritis of childhood, arthritis associated with inflammatory bowel disease and Behçet's disease. Gonococcal arthritis can be mistaken for RS, although clinical features are usually sufficient to differentiate between the two (see Table 4.3).[20,30]

NSAIDs, especially indomethacin, are the treatment of choice for joint symptoms. Despite the association with gastrointestinal or genitourinary infections, the response to antibiotics is not clear. Several studies have suggested that long courses of tetracycline may shorten the course of RS,[83,84] especially when associated with chlamydial infection.[84] A recent study in adults has suggested that early use of antibiotics in venereal disease may prevent recurrence of RS in patients with a previous episode.[85] Judicial intra-articular corticosteroid injection may also be helpful.

The prognosis is usually good, perhaps better than in adults,[78] with resolution of arthritis within a period of several months.[77] However, occasional cases of prolonged joint symptoms or progression to a full-blown spondyloarthropathy have been reported, mainly in adolescents with the HLA B27 antigen.[78,80,86]

Other types of reactive arthritis

Adolescents, mostly male, more commonly develop reactive arthritis, without the complete triad of RS. The character, distribution and prognosis of joint findings are similar to that of RS.

Nearly two-thirds of adults and adolescent patients with reactive arthritis are carriers of the HLA B27 allele.[87] Patients with this allele generally have a more severe and prolonged course, with greater involvement of soft tissues (enthesitis, tenosynovitis). Most patients report prior sexual activity, usually with a new partner. The mean interval between sexual activity and development of joint symptoms is 28 days (range 0–55 days), and 14 days between urethritis and the appearance of joint symptoms. The proportion of adolescents who develop arthritis following a genitourinary infection has not been determined, although in adults 0.8–4.1% of patients with proven chlamydial genitourinary infection develop reactive arthritis.[87,88]

Salmonella

Reactive arthritis follows about 1.9% of gastrointestinal infections caused by all *Salmonella* species, and 2.4% of infections with *Salm. typhimurium*.[89] Diarrhoea usually precedes onset of arthritis by 2 weeks. However, cases of arthritis preceding gastrointestinal symptoms have been described.[90] Arthritis is generally polyarticular, asymmetric and migratory. Small and large joints are affected, with swelling and tenderness more prominent than erythema. Systemic features of disease, fever, fatigue and weight loss may accompany joint symptoms. The diagnosis is usually based on stool cultures or serological tests for *Salmonella*.

Antibiotic treatment of the infection does not affect the duration of arthritis, which may last as long as 10 months. The outcome is invariably good, with complete recovery. Treatment with NSAIDs, especially indomethacin, may be beneficial. Patients with HLA B27 may develop a clinical picture similar to RS.

Yersinia

Cases of reactive arthritis after infection with *Y. enterocolitis* have been reported in adolescents,[91,92] especially in Northern Europe and Scandinavia. Diarrhoea or fever generally precedes the onset of arthritis. Similar to RS, the pattern of arthritis is usually asymmetric, with oligoarticular involvement of the large weight-bearing joints. HLA B27 is found in the majority of adolescent patients. Arthritis usually resolves within several weeks without sequela, but persistent oligoarthritis lasting more than 1 year has been reported in a few adolescent patients.[91]

RHEUMATIC FEVER

Rheumatic fever (RF) is defined as a delayed non-suppurative inflammatory sequela of an untreated pharyngeal infection caused by group A β-haemolytic streptococci. The disease, which affects multiple systems, usually appears 2–3 weeks after the throat infection.

In recent decades there has been a dramatic decline in the incidence of RF in the USA, Western Europe and Japan, although it remains a major cause of morbidity and mortality in the developing world. An initial decline in the incidence from RF was seen prior to the antibiotic era, and was attributed to improvements in socio-economic conditions, less crowding and greater accessibility to medical care.[93] A further dramatic decline was seen after the widespread use of penicillin for primary treatment of pharyngitis and secondary prevention of pharyngitis in patients who have had RF.[94] However, in the 1980s, a resurgence in outbreaks of RF was seen in various locations in the USA.[95–104]

Pathogenesis

Host, environmental and parasite factors are all instrumental in the pathogenesis of RF. RF is seen more commonly among certain ethnic groups, for example the Maoris in New Zealand and the Samoans in Hawaii.[105] Monozygotic twins of patients with RF are at increased risk of developing the disease.[106,107] An association has been found between the presence of HLA DR4 in Caucasians and DR2 in African-Americans and the risk of developing RF.[108] The alloantigen D8/17 has been found on B lymphocytes in more than 90% of RF patients, compared to less than 10% in the general population.[109–111] This finding is consistent among all ethnic groups.

RF is seen more in minority, urban and poor populations. The factors associated with the development of RF in those populations are overcrowding, poor sanitary conditions and lack of access to medical care. Studies from Baltimore have shown a dramatic decrease in the incidence of RF in inner city blacks after implementation of the Medicaid plan.[112] Major epidemics in the past and present occur in crowded military facilities. Rapid transmission of the streptococcus from person to person has been shown to increase the concentration of the M protein in the cell wall, one of the 'rheumatogenic' factors of the streptococcus.[113,114]

The recent changes in the epidemiology of RF may be due to changes in the virulence of the streptococcus. In recent years an increase in severe streptococcal infections has been seen, including invasive soft-tissue infections, toxic shock syndrome, pneumonia and septicaemia.[114,115] 'Rheumatogenic' strains not seen in the last 30 years have reappeared in the last decade. These strains express dense concentrations of specific M protein epitopes: M1, 3, 5, 6 and 18.[114–116] Furthermore, in several recent outbreaks the colonies of these strains were noted to be heavily encapsulated, conferring a 'mucoid' appearance to cultures of these species.[116]

Both humeral and cellular immunity are involved in the pathogenesis of RF. Cross-reactivity of many streptococcal components with host tissue have been found.[117] Antibodies to hyaluronic acid in the streptococcal capsule also react with synovial tissue. Cross-reactivity has been found between streptococcal cell-wall carbohydrate and heart-valve glycoprotein, M protein with heart myosin and sarcolemma, and streptococcal cell membrane proteins with heart myosin and brain tissue. Increased levels of these antibodies are found in patients with RF as compared to patients with uncomplicated pharyngitis.[118] Aggregates of activated T lymphocytes and macrophages to streptococcus have been found in heart tissue.[119] Elements of the streptococcus may act as superantigens and activate T cells from specific V_β families.[120]

Epidemiology

The incidence of RF in the USA has decreased from 100–250 per 10^5 population at the turn of the century to 0.23–1.88 per 10^5 in the 1980s.[95,121,122] Several outbreaks occurred in the mid-1980s, the most noticeable in Salt Lake City, UT, USA.[95] However, hospital admissions for acute RF continued to decrease between 1985 and 1990 by 8.3% per year.[123]

RF follows untreated pharyngitis in about 0.3% of cases. During major streptococcal epidemics the attack rate may increase to as much as 3%. The attack rate increases to 50% in patients with a previous attack of RF, mostly in the first 3 years after the initial episode.[121] More than 80% of the patients with RF are between 5 and 19 years old. Seventeen per cent to 34% of cases occur in adolescents aged 15–19 years.[112]

The epidemiology of RF in the USA has changed during recent outbreaks. Many of the patients were from the middle class, from rural or suburban surroundings, and with adequate access to medical care.[95,97,98] More than 50% of patients did not seek medical care for symptoms of pharyngitis before the presentation of RF.[95] Crowding, however, still remains a risk factor for development of RF. In the Salt Lake City outbreak, the size of families with cases of RF was twice the state average, and 65% of the patients shared a bedroom.[95]

Clinical manifestations

ARTHRITIS

Migratory polyarthritis of the large joints is the classic presentation of RF. In the past, arthritis was the most common manifestation of RF, seen in 75% of the patients. In recent outbreaks, carditis was seen nearly as frequently, and in some series more often than arthritis.[95,103] In contrast to patients with juvenile idiopathic arthritis (JIA) those with RF develop pain which is severe and disproportionate to the physical findings. The pain may be so severe as to cause pseudoparalysis. The knees are most commonly affected, followed by the ankles, elbows and wrists. Involvement of the small joints and spine is uncommon. The findings in an individual joint usually last for 1–5 days in untreated patients, with an overlap between affected joints. Overall, arthritis develops in an average of six joints.

Resolution of arthritis generally occurs within 3–6 weeks, and does not result in permanent damage. Finger deformities, termed Jaccoud's arthropathy, may develop in severe cases of RF.[124] A dramatic decrease in joint symptoms occurs almost immediately after salicylates are started.

Synovial fluid is inflammatory, with white blood cell counts as high as $100\,000/mm^3$, with polymorphonuclear predominance. Glucose levels are usually normal.

CARDITIS

Carditis is the only manifestation of RF that results in short-term mortality and long-term morbidity. In recent outbreaks, carditis was present in 60–70% of patients.[103] Although not considered as carditis by the modified Jones criteria,[125] valvular disease detected on Doppler echocardiograms may be seen in as many as 90% of patients with RF.[95]

The carditis in RF is a pancarditis. However, the occurrence of pericarditis or myocarditis in the absence of endocarditis is rare. Carditis usually appears in the first 3 weeks of RF. Several presentations have been described. The most common is an asymptomatic murmur in patients with significant arthritis. This pattern is seen mainly in older children and adolescents.[121] Younger patients frequently present with congestive heart failure and a relative paucity of joint complaints. Other patients present with chest pain, tachycardia and dyspnoea, and have evidence of pericarditis and myocarditis, in addition to endocarditis.

A new murmur is the most common feature of carditis. Murmurs usually originate from regurgitation of the mitral and/or aortic valves. Signs of myocarditis include resting tachycardia, cardiomegaly, gallop rhythm, oedema, hepatomegaly and rales. Auscultation of a friction rub indicates the presence of pericarditis. Chest radiographs, electrocardiograms and Doppler echocardiography may confirm the clinical signs. However, echocardiography cannot be used as a diagnostic criterion in the absence of clinical signs.[125]

SYDENHAM'S CHOREA

Chorea is seen in about 10–30% of patients with RF, but is less frequent after puberty, with a peak incidence at age 8 years. Females are affected more frequently than males.[121] The latency between pharyngitis and the development of chorea is 1–6 months, which is longer than for other disease manifestations. Often, there is no longer evidence of prior streptococcal infection.

The onset of chorea is usually insidious. Purposeless involuntary movements, emotional and behavioural lability, muscular incoordination and weakness are characteristic of chorea. Facial and extremity muscles are most affected. Marked changes in handwriting are evident, and these changes can be used to monitor disease activity. Chorea is usually bilateral, although one side may be affected more than the other. Movements may be suppressed voluntarily for short periods, and usually disappear during sleep. Stress and fatigue can exacerbate the movement disorder.

Chorea is self-limiting. Improvement is usually seen within 1–2 weeks; resolution may take 2–3 months. Other conditions, including systemic lupus erythematosus, antiphospholipid antibody syndrome, Wilson's disease and Huntington's chorea, need to be excluded when chorea presents as an isolated phenomenon.

OTHER CLINICAL MANIFESTATIONS

Other major clinical signs include erythema marginatum and subcutaneous nodules. These phenomena are relatively uncommon, and are seen in about 5% of patients, usually those with severe carditis.[97,98] Erythema marginatum is characterized by an expanding macule with a clear centre and erythematous margins with a snake-like appearance. The rash may be transient, lasting only several hours. Subcutaneous nodules are firm, non-tender and mobile, and are usually seen over the extensor surfaces of tendons near bony prominences.

Minor clinical signs include the presence of fever and arthralgia in the absence of arthritis. Fever is usually greater than 39°C. Similar to arthritis, arthralgia is migratory, affecting the large joints. Abdominal pain and epistaxis, although not specific to RF, are also common symptoms.

LABORATORY SIGNS

Signs of systemic inflammation are seen in nearly all patients, other than those with isolated chorea. Increased ESR and positive tests for C-reactive protein are supportive of the diagnosis of RF. Leucocytosis and anaemia are also common. P–R interval prolongation is seen on electrocardiography in 35% of patients with RF,

---

Table 4.4 Jones criteria (revised) for guidance in the diagnosis of rheumatic fever

Major manifestations	Minor manifestations	Evidence of streptococcal infection
Carditis	Arthralgia	Throat culture
Migratory polyarthritis	Fever	Rapid streptococcal antigen
Chorea	Acute phase reactants (ESR, CRP)	Streptococcal antibodies (ASO, anti DNase B)
Erythema marginatum	Prolonged P–R interval	
Subcutaneous nodules		

The presence of two major criteria, or of one major and two minor criteria, indicate a high probability of the presence of rheumatic fever, if supported by evidence of a preceding streptococcal infection.

ASO, antistreptolysin; CRP, C-reactive protein; ESR, erythrocyte sedimentation rate.

---

and is also supportive of the diagnosis. The aetiology is still unknown, although not considered to be associated with carditis.[126]

EVIDENCE OF STREPTOCOCCAL INFECTION

Evidence of prior streptococcal infection is crucial for the diagnosis RF. Positive throat cultures are seen in a minority of the patients, as most patients have already cleared the streptococci from the throat. Serological tests for antibodies to extracellular products secreted by streptococci include antistreptolysin O, antideoxyribonuclease B, antistreptokinase and antihyaluronidase. Increased levels are indicative of past infection. In order to determine whether the streptococcal infection was recent, rising titres should be documented on repeat testing 2–4 weeks apart.[125] Elevated levels of antistreptolysin O are seen only in 80% of patients with RF. The addition of another antibody assay increases the sensitivity of detecting past streptococcal infection to 95%.[121] The streptozyme test is not considered reliable evidence of previous streptococcal infection.[125,127] Serological tests are often normal in patients with isolated chorea. In the last revision of the Jones criteria, a history of recent scarlet fever was eliminated from the list of acceptable evidence of past streptococcal infection.[125] The clinical diagnosis of scarlet fever is considered less reliable today than it was in the past, when it was more common.

Diagnosis

Criteria for guidance in the diagnosis of RF were defined by T. Duckett Jones in 1944, and have undergone modifications and revisions in 1955, 1965 and 1992 (Table 4.4).[125] Major and minor criteria were classified according to the relative specificity of the clinical signs to RF. The 1992 revision excluded leucocytosis from minor criteria, and stated that carditis diagnosed only by Doppler echocardiography is not indicative of carditis. However, not every patient who fulfills the criteria has RF. For example, patients with systemic lupus erythematosus, systemic-onset JIA, gonococcal arthritis, serum sickness and malignancy-related arthritis may fulfil the Jones criteria. Conversely, patients with smouldering carditis or isolated chorea may not strictly fulfil the criteria. Some patients clearly have RF but lack evidence of past streptococcal infection. Anti-inflammatory medication should be withheld until the diagnosis is established, as premature use of such medication may mask the development of migratory polyarthritis.

Treatment of acute RF
Once the diagnosis has been confirmed a full course of antibiotic treatment for streptococcus pharyngitis should be administered, regardless of the status of the throat culture.[127] Although the effect of eradicating the streptococcus once RF has begun is not clear, it is thought that viable streptococci may still exist within pharyngeal and tonsillar tissue and continue to stimulate the immune system.

Salicylates are highly effective in the treatment of arthritis, and are also adequate for use in mild to moderate carditis. Treatment is administered for 6–8 weeks until there is resolution of signs of systemic inflammation. In patients with moderate to severe carditis or congestive heart failure, corticosteroid therapy is recommended. Although not proven to be better than salicylates in prevention of long-term sequela, corticosteroids have a more rapid anti-inflammatory effect. Oral prednisone 2 mg/kg/day is given for 2–3 weeks and then gradually tapered off. Salicylates are started as steroids are being weaned to prevent a rebound of clinical signs. In severe cases intravenous methylprednisolone can be used. Digoxin should be used with care, if necessary, as patients with RF may have increased myocardial sensitivity to this drug.[121]

Secondary prophylaxis
The risk of having another episode of RF is much greater in patients who have had RF in the past. Most subsequent attacks resemble the first episode.[128,129] Therefore, the risk of further cardiac damage is greatest in patients who had carditis during their first attack. However, the risk of developing carditis increases with the number of attacks. Therefore, streptococcal infections should be prevented in all patients who have had an episode of RF. The risk of recurrence is greatest in the first 3–5 years after the initial attack, although there is still an increased risk thereafter.

For the majority of patients in whom compliance may be a problem, and for patients with carditis, intramuscular injections of benzathine penicillin 1 200 000 units are recommended.[127] In the USA, injections every 4 weeks are considered

to confer adequate protection against recurrence. In developing countries, an injection every third week is recommended,[130] as penicillin levels may fall below the minimal inhibitory concentrations in the fourth week.[131,132] Oral alternatives include penicillin V, 250 mg twice daily, sulfadiazine 1 g/day (for adolescents), and erythromycin 250 mg, twice daily for patients allergic to both medications.

The duration of prophylaxis is still controversial. The Committee on RF of the Council on Cardiovascular Disease in the Young, and the American Heart Association have issued guidelines.[127] Patients without carditis should receive prophylaxis for 5 years or until age 21, whichever is longer. Patients with carditis but without residual heart disease should receive prophylaxis for at least 10 years. For patients with residual heart disease, prophylaxis is recommended at least until the age of 40, and in some patients life-long prophylaxis is necessary. In a series of adolescents and adults from Chile, a low recurrence rate was found when prophylaxis was stopped after 5 years or at 18 years of age (whichever was the longer interval) in patients without carditis, or after 10 years or at age 25 in patients with mild mitral regurgitation or healed carditis.[133]

Prophylaxis for bacterial endocarditis should be given to all patients with residual valvular disease, as recommended by the American Heart Association, for dental work and surgery.

Post-streptococcal reactive arthritis
This entity refers to the development of post-streptococcal arthritis without fulfillment of the Jones criteria for the diagnosis of RF.[134–139] The features of arthritis in this syndrome may differ from those of RF. Arthritis often develops earlier following streptococcal infection than in RF.[136] Some patients develop prolonged arthritis, which includes the small joints of the hand, and often the arthritis does not respond well to anti-inflammatory treatment. Therefore, debate exists about whether this entity is similar to other types of reactive arthritis,[135] or is part of the spectrum of RF.[134,136–139] There are several reports that some patients have 'silent' carditis or will later develop

carditis.[134,136–138] Therefore, many authorities advocate the use of antibiotic prophylaxis for patients with this entity.[134,137–139] The duration of prophylaxis may be shorter than in RF, with some physicians recommending only 1 year of antibiotics if carditis is not observed.[127] These patients should have periodic echocardiograms to search for evidence of late carditis.

SUMMARY

We have discussed the common entities of infection-related arthriditis in adolescence, with a focus on the specific clinical aspects in this age group. Adolescence represents a transition from childhood to adulthood. Therefore, the spectrum of disease in adolescence encompasses diseases from both age groups. The major differences from childhood are the increased frequency of arthritis related to sexually transmitted diseases. These include bacterial arthritis from *N. gonorrhoeae*, various types of viral-related arthriditis from HIV and hepatitis B, and reactive arthritis from non-gonococcal urethritis. Other entities commonly seen in childhood but not in adulthood, such as RF, are still prevalent in adolescence.

Very few of the studies cited in this chapter were specifically concerned with patients in this age group. It is hoped that future investigations will better define the specific clinical features and the basic immunology related to these diseases in adolescence.

REFERENCES

1. Garcia-Kutzbach A, Masi AT. Acute infectious agent arthritis (IAA): a detailed comparison of proved gonococcal and other blood-borne bacterial arthritis. *J Rheumatol* 1974; **1**:93–101.
2. Manshady BM, Thompson GR, Weiss JJ. Septic arthritis in a general hospital 1966–1977. *J Rheumatol* 1980; **7**:523–30.
3. Scopelitis E, Martinez-Osuna P. Gonococcal arthritis. *Rheum Dis Clin North Am* 1993; **19**:363–77.
4. Eisenstein BE, Masi AT. Disseminated gonococcal infection (DGI) and gonococcal arthritis (GCA). I. Bacteriology, epidemiology, host factors, pathogen factors, and pathology. *Semin Arthritis Rheum* 1981; **10**:155–72.
5. Kerle KK, Mascola JR, Miller TA. Disseminated gonococcal infection. *Am Family Physician* 1992; **45**:209–14.
6. Fink CW. Gonococcal arthritis in childhood. *JAMA* 1965; **194**:237–8.
7. Allue X, Rubio T, Riley HD. Gonococcal infections in infants and children: lessons from fifteen cases. *Clin Pediatr* 1973; **12**:584–88.
8. Holmes KK, Counts GW, Beaty HN. Disseminated gonococcal infection. *Ann Intern Med* 1971; **74**:979–93.
9. Ross P. Disseminated gonococcal infection: the tenosynovitis–dermatitis and suppurative arthritis syndrome. *Cleveland Clin Q* 1985; **52**:161–73.
10. O'Brien JP, Goldenberg DL, Rice PA. Disseminated gonococcal infection: a prospective analysis of 49 patients and review of pathophysiology and immune mechanisms. *Medicine* 1983; **62**:395–406.
11. Knapp JS, Holmes KK. Disseminated gonococcal infections caused by *Neisseria gonorrhoeae* with unique nutritional requirements. *J Infect Dis* 1975; **132**:204–8.
12. Rice PA, Kasper DL. Characterization of serum resistance of *Neisseria gonorrhoeae* that disseminate: roles of blocking antibody and gonococcal outer membrane proteins. *J Clin Invest* 1982; **70**:157–67.
13. Knapp JS, Thornsberry C, Schoolnik GA, Wiesner PJ, Holmes KK, Cooperative Study Group. Phenotypic and epidemiologic correlates of auxotype in *Neisseria gonorrhoeae*. *J Infect Dis* 1978; **138**:160–5.
14. Handsfield HH. Disseminated gonococcal infection. *Clin Obstet Gynecol* 1975; **18**:131–42.
15. Keiser H, Rubin FL, Wolinsky E, Kushner I. Clinical forms of gonococcal arthritis. *N Engl J Med* 1968; **279**:234–40.
16. Gelfand SG, Masi AT, Garcia-Kutzbach A. Spectrum of gonococcal arthritis: evidence for sequential stages and clinical subgroups. *J Rheumatol* 1975; **2**:83–90.
17. Goldman JA. Pattern of gonococcal arthritis. *J Rheumatol* 1981; **8**:707–9.
18. Brandt KD, Cathcart ES, Cohen AS. Gonococcal arthritis. Clinical features correlated with blood,

synovial fluid and genitourinary cultures. *Arthritis Rheum* 1974; **17**:503–10.

19. Brogadir SP, Schimmer BM, Myers AR. Spectrum of the gonococcal arthritis–dermatitis syndrome. *Semin Arthritis Rheum* 1979; **8**:177–83.

20. McCord WC, Nies KM, Louie JS. Acute venereal arthritis: comparative study of acute Reiter syndrome and acute gonococcal arthritis. *Arch Intern Med* 1977; **137**: 858–62.

21. Masi AT, Eisenstein BI. Disseminated gonococcal infection (DGI) and gonococcal arthritis (GCA). II: Clinical manifestations, diagnosis, complications, treatment, and prevention. *Semin Arthritis Rheum* 1981; **10**:173–97.

22. Garcia-Kutzbach A, Dismuke SE, Masi AT. Gonococcal arthritis: clinical features and results of penicillin therapy. *J Rheumatol* 1974; **1**:210–21.

23. Trentham DE, McCravey JW, Masi AT. Low-dose penicillin for gonococcal arthritis. *JAMA* 1976; **236**:2410–2.

24. Barr J, Danielsson D. Septic gonococcal dermatitis. *Br Med J* 1971; **1**:482–5.

25. Liebling MR, Arkfeld PG, Michelini GA et al. Identification of *Neisseria gonorrhoeae* in synovial fluid using the polymerase chain reaction. *Arthritis Rheum* 1994; **37**:702–9.

26. Al-Suleiman SA, Grimes EM, Jonas HS. Disseminated gonococcal infections. *Obstet Gynecol* 1983; **61**:48–51.

27. Jennens ID, O'Reilly M, Yung AP. Chronic meningococcal disease. *Med J Aust* 1990; **153**:556–9.

28. Merry P, Seifert M. Meningococcal infection: diagnostic and therapeutic pitfalls. *Br J Rheumatol* 1992; **31**:141–2.

29. Rosenthal L, Olhagen B, Ek S. Aseptic arthritis after gonorrhoea. *Ann Rheum Dis* 1980; **39**:141–6.

30. Urd R, Johns J, Chubick A. Comparative study of gonococcal arthritis and Reiter's syndrome. *Ann Rheum Dis* 1979; **38**(suppl):55–8.

31. Wise CM, Morris CR, Wasilauskas BL, Salzer WL. Gonococcal arthritis in an era of increasing penicillin resistance. Presentations and outcomes in 41 recent cases (1985–1991). *Arch Intern Med* 1994; **154**:2690–5.

32. Gotuzzo E, Alacron GS, Bocanegra TS et al. Articular involvement in human brucellosis: a retrospective analysis of 304 cases. *Semin Arthritis Rheum* 1982; **12**:245–55.

33. Al-Eissa YA, Kambal AM, Al-Nasser MN, Al-Habib SA, Al-Fawaz IM, Al-Zamil FA. Childhood brucellosis: a study of 102 cases. *Pediatr Infect Dis J* 1990; **9**:74–9.

34. Al-Eissa YA, Kambal AM, Alrabeeah AA, Abdullah AMA, Al-Jurayyan NA, Al-Jishi NM. Osteoarticular brucellosis in children. *Ann Rheum Dis* 1990; **49**:896–900.

35. Anonymous. Lyme disease – United States, 1994. *Morb Mortal Wkly Rep* 1995; **44**:459–62.

36. Petersen LR, Sweeny AH, Checko PJ et al. Epidemiological and clinical features of 1,149 persons with Lyme disease identified by laboratory-based surveillance in Connecticut. *Yale J Biol Med* 1989; **62**:253–62.

37. Eichenfield AH, Goldsmith DP, Benach JL et al. Childhood Lyme arthritis: experience in an endemic area. *J Pediatr* 1986; **109**:753–8.

38. Culp RW, Eichenfield AH, Davidson RS, Drummond DS, Christofersen MR, Goldsmith DP. Lyme disease in children. An orthopaedic perspective. *J Bone Joint Surg* 1987; **69**:96–9.

39. Williams CL, Strobino B, Lee A et al. Lyme disease in childhood: clinical and epidemiologic features of ninety cases. *Pediatr Infect Dis J* 1990; **9**:10–4.

40. Rose CD, Fawcett PT, Eppes SC, Klein JD, Gibney K, Doughty RA. Pediatric Lyme arthritis: clinical spectrum and outcome. *J Pediatr Orthop* 1994; **14**:238–41.

41. Athreya BH, Rose CD. Lyme disease. *Curr Problems Pediatr* 1996; **26**:189–207.

42. Cristofaro RL, Appel MH, Gelb RI, Williams CL. Musculoskeletal manifestations of Lyme disease in children. *J Pediatr Orthop* 1987; **7**:527–30.

43. Steere AC. Diagnosis and treatment of Lyme arthritis. *Med Clin North Am* 1997; **81**:179–94.

44. Szer IS, Taylor E, Steere AC. The long-term course of Lyme arthritis in children. *N Engl J Med* 1991; **325**:159–63.

45. Huppertz HI, Karch H, Suschke HJ et al. Lyme disease in European children and adolescents. *Arthritis Rheum* 1995; **38**:361–8.

46. Lengl-Janssen B, Strauss AF, Steere AC, Kamradt T. The T helper cell response in Lyme arthritis: differential recognition of *Borrelia burgdorferi* outer surface protein A (OspA) in patients with treatment-resistant or treatment-responsive Lyme arthritis. *J Exp Med* 1994; **180**:2069–78.

47. Miller LC, Lynch EA, Isa S, Logan JW, Dinarello CA. Balance of synovial fluid IL-1β and IL-1 receptor antagonist and recovery from Lyme arthritis. *Lancet* 1993; **341**:146–8.

48. Nocton JJ, Dressler F, Rutledge BJ, Rys PN, Persing DH, Steere AC. Detection of *Borrelia burgdorferi* DNA by polymerase chain reaction in

synovial fluid in Lyme arthritis. *N Engl J Med* 1994; **330**:229–34.

49. Dattwyler RJ, Volkman DJ, Luft BJ, Halperin JJ, Thomas J, Golightly MG. Seronegative Lyme disease: dissociation of the specific T- and B-lymphocyte responses to *Borrelia burgdorferi*. *N Engl J Med* 1988; **319**:1441–6.

50. Snydman DR, Schenkein DP, Berardi VP, Lastavica CC, Parsier KM. *Borrelia burgdorferi* in joint fluid in chronic Lyme arthritis. *Ann Intern Med* 1986; **104**:798–800.

51. Sigal LH, Patella SJ. Lyme arthritis as the incorrect diagnosis in pediatric and adolescent fibromyalgia. *Pediatrics* 1992; **90**:523–8.

52. Steere AC, Levin RE, Molloy PJ et al. Treatment of Lyme arthritis. *Arthritis Rheum* 1994; **37**:878–88.

53. Rees DHE, Axford JS. Lyme arthritis. *Ann Rheum Dis* 1994; **53**:553–6.

54. Zemel LS. Lyme disease – a pediatric perspective. *J Rheumatol* 1992; **19**:1–13.

55. Coblyn JS, Taylor P. Treatment of chronic Lyme arthritis with hydroxychloroquine. *Arthritis Rheum* 1981; **24**:1567–9.

56. Schoen RT, Aversa JM, Rahn DW, Steere AC. Treatment of refractory chronic Lyme arthritis with arthroscopic synovectomy. *Arthritis Rheum* 1991; **34**:1056–60.

57. Asch ES, Bujak DI, Weiss M, Peterson MG, Weinstein A. Lyme disease: an infectious and postinfectious syndrome. *J Rheumatol* 1994; **21**:454–61.

58. Sigal LH. Persisting symptoms of Lyme disease – possible explanations and implications for treatment. *J Rheumatol* 1994; **21**:593–5.

59. Sigal LH, Adler-Klein D, Bryant G, Doherty T, Haselby R, Hilton E. Multicenter efficacy trial of a recombinant *Borrelia burgdorferi* (Bb) outer surface protein A (OspA) vaccine for prevention of Lyme disease (LD). *Arthritis Rheum* 1997; **40**(suppl):S173.

60. Petty RE, Tingle AJ. Arthritis and viral infection [editorial]. *J Pediatr* 1983; **113**:948–9.

61. Tingle AJ, Allen M, Petty RE, Kettyls GD, Chantler JK. Rubella-associated arthritis. I. Comparative study of joint manifestations associated with natural rubella infection and RA 27/3 rubella immunization. *Ann Rheum Dis* 1986; **45**:110–4.

62. Ueno Y. Rubella arthritis. An outbreak in Kyoto. *J Rheumatol* 1994; **21**:874–6.

63. Best JM, Banatvala JE, Bowen JM. New Japanese rubella vaccine: comparative trials. *Br Med J* 1974; **3**:221–4.

64. Association for the Study of Infectious Diseases. A retrospective survey of the complications of mumps. *J R Coll Gen Pract* 1974; **24**:552–6.

65. Gordon SC, Lauter CB. Mumps arthritis: a review of the literature. *Rev Infect Dis* 1984; **6**:338–44.

66. Center for Disease Control. Mumps vaccine: recommendations of the Public Health Service Advisory Committee on Immunization Practices. *Ann Intern Med* 1979; **88**:819–20.

67. Bayer AS. Arthritis associated with common viral infections: mumps, coxsackievirus, and adenovirus. *Postgrad Med* 1980; **68**:55–64.

68. Caranasos GL, Felker JR. Mumps arthritis. *Arch Intern Med* 1967; **119**:394–8.

69. Reid DM, Brown T, Reid TMS, Rennie JAN, Eastmond CJ. Human parvovirus-associated arthritis: a clinical and laboratory description. *Lancet* 1985; **i**:422–5.

70. Nocton JJ, Miller LC, Tucker LB, Schaller JG, Human parvovirus B19-associated arthritis in children. *J Pediatr* 1993; **122**:186–90.

71. Berman A, Reboredo G, Spindler A, Lasala ME, Lopez H, Espinoza LR. Rheumatic manifestations in populations at risk for HIV infection: the added effect of HIV. *J Rheumatol* 1991; **18**:1564–7.

72. Fernandez SM, Quiralte J, Del Arco A et al. Osteoarticular infection associated with the human immunodeficiency virus. *Clin Exp Rheumatol* 1991; **9**:489–93.

73. Keat A. Sexually transmitted arthritis syndromes. *Med Clin North Am* 1990; **74**:1617–31.

74. Inman RD. Rheumatic manifestations of hepatitis B infection. *Semin Arthritis Rheum* 1982; **11**:406–20.

75. Alpert E, Isselbacher KJ, Schur PH. The pathogenesis of arthritis associated with viral hepatitis. *N Engl J Med* 1971; **285**:185–9.

76. Schumacher HR, Gall EP. Arthritis in acute hepatitis and chronic active hepatitis: pathology of the synovial membrane with evidence for the presence of Australian antigen in synovial membranes. *Am J Med* 1974; **57**:655–64.

77. Rosenberg AM, Petty RE. Reiter's syndrome in children. *Am J Dis Child* 1979; **133**:394–8.

78. Smith RJ. Evidence for *Chlamydia trachomatis* and *Ureaplasma urealyticum* in a patient with Reiter's disease. *J Adolesc Health Care* 1989; **10**:155–9.

79. Paronen I. Reiter's disease: a study of 344 cases observed in Finland. *Acta Med Scand* 1948; **130**(suppl 212):1–20.

80. Jay MS, Seymore C, Jay WM, Durant RH. Reiter's syndrome in an adolescent female with systemic sequela. *J Adolesc Health Care* 1987; **8**:280–5.

81. Cuttica RJ, Schenines EJ, Garay SM, Del Carme Romanelli M, Maldonado Cocco JA. Juvenile onset Reiter's syndrome: a retrospective study of 26 patients. *Clin Exp Rheumatol* 1992; **10**:285–8.

82. Li F, Bulbul R, Schumacher HR Jr et al. Molecular detection of bacterial DNA in venereal-associated arthritis. *Arthritis Rheum* 1996; **39**:950–8.

83. Panayi GS, Clark B. Minocycline in the treatment of patients with Reiter's syndrome. *Clin Exp Rheumatol* 1989; **7**:100–1.

84. Lauhio A, Lerisalo-Repo M, Lahdevirta J, Siokku P, Repo H. Double-blind placebo-controlled study of three months treatment with lymecycline in reactive arthritis with special reference to chlamydial arthritis. *Arthritis Rheum* 1991; **34**:6–14.

85. Bardin T, Enel C, Cornelis F et al. Antibiotic treatment of venereal disease and Reiter's syndrome in a Greenland population. *Arthritis Rheum* 1992; **35**:190–4.

86. Thomas DG, Roberton DM. Reiter's syndrome in an adolescent girl. *Acta Paediatr* 1994; **83**:339–40.

87. Keat AC, Maini RN, Pegrum GD, Scott JJ. The clinical features and HLA associations of reactive arthritis associated with non-gonococcal urethritis. *Q J Med* 1979; **190**:323–42.

88. Rich E, Hook EW III, Alarcon GS, Moreland LW. Reactive arthritis in patients attending an urban sexually transmitted diseases clinic. *Arthritis Rheum* 1996; **39**:1172–7.

89. Vertiainen J, Hurri L. Arthritis due to *Salmonella typhimurium. Acta Med Scand* 1964; **175**:771–4.

90. Carroll WL, Balistreri WF, Brilli R, Parish RA, Greenfield DJ. Spectrum of *Salmonella*-associated arthritis. *Pediatrics* 1981; **68**:717–20.

91. Dequeker J, Jamar R, Walravens M. HLA B-27, arthritis and *Yersinia enterocolitica* infection. *J Rheumatol* 1980; **7**:706–10.

92. Borg AA, Gray J, Dawes PT. *Yersinia*-related arthritis in the United Kingdom. A report of 12 cases and review of the literature. *Q J Med* 1992; **84**:575–82.

93. Gordis L. The virtual disappearance of rheumatic fever in the United States: lessons in the rise and fall of disease. *Circulation* 1985; **72**:1155–62.

94. Massell BF, Chute CG, Walker AM, Kurland GS. Penicillin and the marked decrease in morbidity and mortality from rheumatic fever in the United States. *N Engl J Med* 1988; **318**:280–6.

95. Veasy LG, Wiedmeier SE, Orsmond GS et al. Resurgence of acute rheumatic fever in the intermountain area of the United States. *N Engl J Med* 1987; **316**:421–7.

96. Wald ER, Dashefsky B, Feidt C, Chiponis D, Byers C. Acute rheumatic fever in Western Pennsylvania and the tristate area. *Pediatrics* 1987; **80**:371–4.

97. Hoiser DM, Craenen JM, Teske DW, Wheller JJ. Resurgence of acute rheumatic fever. *Am J Dis Child* 1987; **141**:730–3.

98. Congeni B, Rizzo C, Congeni J, Sreenivasan VV. Outbreak of acute rheumatic fever in northeast Ohio. *J Pediatr* 1987; **111**:176–9.

99. Wallace MR, Garst PD, Papadimos TJ, Oldfield EC III. The return of acute rheumatic fever in young adults. *JAMA* 1989; **262**:2557–61.

100. Griffens SP, Gersony WM. Acute rheumatic fever in New York City (1969 to 1988); a comparative study of two decades. *J Pediatr* 1990; **116**:882–7.

101. Leggiadro RJ, Birnbaum SE, Chase NA, Myers LK. A resurgence of acute rheumatic fever in a mid-south children's hospital. *South Med J* 1990; **83**:1418–20.

102. Hefelfinger DC. Resurgence of acute rheumatic fever in West Alabama. *South Med J* 1992; **85**:261–5.

103. Veasy LG, Tani LY, Hill HR. Persistence of acute rheumatic fever in the intermountain area of the United States. *J Pediatr* 1994; **124**:9–16.

104. Bisno AL. Group A streptococcal infections and acute rheumatic fever. *N Engl J Med* 1991; **325**:783–93.

105. Pope RM. Rheumatic fever in the 1980s. *Bull Rheum Dis* 1989; **38**:1–8.

106. Taranta A, Torosdag S, Metrakos JD, Jegier W, Ucheida I. Rheumatic fever in monozygotic and dizygotic twins. *Circulation* 1959; **20**:778.

107. Ayoub EM. The search for host determinants of susceptibility to rheumatic fever: the missing link. *Circulation* 1984; **69**:197–201.

108. Ayoub EM, Barrett DJ, Maclaren NK, Krischer JP. Association of class II human histocompatability leukocyte antigens with rheumatic fever. *J Clin Invest* 1986; **77**:2019–26.

109. Patarroyo ME, Winchester RJ, Vejerano A et al. Association of a B-cell alloantigen with susceptibility to rheumatic fever. *Nature* 1979; **278**:173–4.

110. Khanna AK, Buskirk DR, Williams RC Jr, Gibofsky A, Crow MK, Menon A. Presence of a non-HLA B cell antigen in rheumatic fever patients and their families as defined by a monoclonal antibody. *J Clin Invest* 1989; **83**:1710–6.

111. Gibofsky A, Khanna A, Suh E, Zabriskie JB. The genetics of rheumatic fever: relationship to streptococcal infection and autoimmune disease. *J Rheumatol* 1991; **18**(suppl 30):1–5.

112. Gordis L, Lilienfeld A, Rodriguez R. Studies in the epidemiology and preventability of rheumatic fever – I: Demographic factors and the incidence of acute attacks. *J Chron Dis* 1969; **21**:645–54.

113. Rothbard S, Watson RF. Variation occurring in group A streptococci during human infection: progressive loss of M substance correlated with increasing susceptibility to bacteriostasis. *J Exp Med* 1948; **87**:521–33.

114. Stollerman GH. The nature of rheumatogenic streptococci. *Mount Sinai J Med* 1996; **63**:144–58.

115. Bronze MS, Dale JB. The reemergence of serious group A streptococcal infections and acute rheumatic fever. *Am J Med Sci* 1996; **311**:41–54.

116. Johnson DR, Stevens DL, Kaplan EL. Epidemiologic analysis of group A streptococcal serotypes associated with severe systemic infections, rheumatic fever, or uncomplicated pharyngitis. *J Infect Dis* 1992; **166**:374–82.

117. Ayoub EM, Kaplan E. Host–parasite interaction in the pathogenesis of rheumatic fever. *J Rheumatol* 1991; **18**(suppl 30):6–13.

118. Gibofsky A, Zabriskie JB. Rheumatic fever and poststreptococcal reactive arthritis. *Curr Opin Rheumatol* 1995; **7**:299–305.

119. Kememy E, Grieve T, Marcus R, Sareli P, Zabriskie JB. Identification of mononuclear cells and T cell subsets in rheumatic valvulitis. *Clin Immunol Immunopathol* 1989; **52**:225–37.

120. Tomai M, Kotb M, Majumdar G, Beachey EH. Superantigenicity of streptococcal M protein. *J Exp Med* 1990; **172**:359–62.

121. Homer C, Shulman ST. Clinical aspects of acute rheumatic fever. *J Rheumatol* 1991; **18**(suppl 29):2–13.

122. Dajani AS. Current status of nonsuppurative complications of group A streptococci. *Pediatr Infect Dis J* 1991; **10**(suppl):S25–7.

123. Taubert KA, Rowley AH, Shulman ST. Seven-year national survey of Kawasaki disease and acute rheumatic fever. *Pediatr Infect Dis J* 1994; **13**:704–8.

124. Bittl JA, Perloff JK. Chronic post-rheumatic fever arthropathy of Jaccoud. *Am Heart J* 1983; **105**:515–7.

125. Dajani AS, Ayoub E, Bierman FZ et al. Guidelines for the diagnosis of rheumatic fever. Jones criteria, 1992 update. *JAMA* 1992; **268**:2069–73.

126. Mirowski M, Rosenstein BJ, Markowitz M. A comparison of atrioventricular conduction in normal children and in patients with rheumatic fever, glomerulonephritis, and acute febrile illnesses: a quantitative study with determination of the P–R index. *Pediatrics* 1964; **33**:334–40.

127. Dajani A, Taubert K, Ferrieri P et al. Treatment of acute streptococcal pharyngitis and prevention of rheumatic fever: a statement for health professionals. *Pediatrics* 1995; **96**:758–64.

128. Feinstein AR, Spagnuolo M. The clinical patterns of acute rheumatic fever: a reappraisal. *Medicine* 1949; **41**:279–305.

129. Denny FW. T. Duckett Jones and rheumatic fever in 1986. *Circulation* 1987; **76**:963–70.

130. Lue HC, Wu MH, Wang JK, Wu FF, Wu YN. Long-term outcome of patients with rheumatic fever receiving benzathine penicillin G prophylaxis every three weeks versus every four weeks. *J Pediatr* 1994; **125**:812–6.

131. Kaplan EL, Berrios X, Speth J, Siefferman T, Guzman B, Quesny F. Pharmacokinetics of benzathine penicillin G: serum levels during the 28 days after intramuscular injection of 1,200,000 units. *J Pediatr* 1989; **115**:146–50.

132. Ginsburg CM, McCracken GH, Zweighaft TC. Serum penicillin concentration after intramuscular administration of benzathine penicillin in children. *Pediatrics* 1982; **69**:452–4.

133. Berrios X, Del Campo E, Guzman B, Bisno AL. Discontinuing rheumatic fever prophylaxis in selected adolescents and young adults. *Ann Intern Med* 1993; **118**:401–6.

134. De Cunto CL, Giannini EH, Fink CW, Brewer EJ, Person DA. Prognosis of children with poststreptococcal reactive arthritis. *Pediatr Infect Dis J* 1988; **7**:683–8.

135. Arnold MH, Tyndall A. Poststreptococcal reactive arthritis. *Ann Rheum Dis* 1989; **48**:686–8.

136. Fink CW. The role of the streptococcus in poststreptococcal reactive arthritis and childhood polyarteritis nodosa. *J Rheumatol* 1991; **18**(suppl 29):14–20.

137. Schaffer FM, Agarwal R, Helm J, Gingell RL, Roland JMA, O'Neil KM. Poststreptococcal reactive arthritis and silent carditis: a case report and review of the literature. *Pediatrics* 1994; **93**:837–9.

138. Moon RY, Greene MG, Rehe GT, Katona IM. Poststreptococcal reactive arthritis in children: a potential predecessor of rheumatic heart disease. *J Rheumatol* 1995; **22**:529–32.

139. Gibofsky A, McCarty M, Veasy G, Zabriskie JB. 'A rose by any other name . . .'. *J Rheumatol* 1995; **22**:379–81 [editorial].

5

Juvenile idiopathic arthritides

Katherine Martin and Patricia Woo

INTRODUCTION

Idiopathic juvenile arthritis is the most common chronic rheumatic disease of childhood[1] and a frequent cause of physical disability among adolescents.[2] The annual incidence rate of idiopathic juvenile arthritis in the UK is 10 per 100 000,[1] with 27% of these cases presenting between the ages of 10 and 16 years and 15% between the ages of 12 and 16 years (DPM Symmons, personal communication). In addition, many individuals whose arthritis began in earlier childhood have persistent and disabling disease in adolescence and early adult life.

Adolescence is a period of immense physical and psychological upheaval during which the following 'tasks' should be achieved:

- the development of personal identity, including sexual identity
- the achievement of increasing independence from parents
- the development of meaningful emotional relationships outside the family
- the development of abstract reasoning skills
- planning for the future, including finding a vocation.[3]

One of the most important issues for adolescents with chronic disease is the transition from child- to adult-oriented environments, such as moving from the parental home to independent living, from school to work, and from paediatric to adolescent health-care systems.[4] Chronic disease affects the achievement of both the physical and psychological milestones of adolescence, and the normal physical and psychological changes of adolescence profoundly affect the way the disease should be managed. The tasks of the team caring for an adolescent with chronic arthritis are to empower the individual to achieve these milestones despite their disease. This will involve optimal management of the disease process, as well as practical and psychological support for patients and their families.

This chapter considers the diagnosis, differential diagnosis and management of arthritis first occurring in the adolescent years, as well as the ongoing management of chronic arthritis through adolescence. We review the prognosis of juvenile-onset idiopathic arthritis in adolescence and adult years and consider how to optimize the outcome of this chronic disease in our patients.

CLASSIFICATION OF JUVENILE IDIOPATHIC ARTHRITIS

The terminology of chronic arthritis in childhood and adolescence is confusing. In particular, the nomenclature and classification used in Europe and the USA differs, as shown in Table 5.1.

Juvenile chronic arthritis (JCA) is defined in Europe by the European League Against Rheumatism (EULAR) criteria.[5] The term 'juvenile arthritis' (JA) is sometimes used in Europe to include cases that satisfy the EULAR criteria plus those with rheumatoid-factor-positive

Table 5.1 Comparison of classifications of juvenile idiopathic arthritis

	EULAR criteria	ACR criteria
Name	Juvenile chronic arthritis (JCA)	Juvenile rheumatoid arthritis (JRA)
Onset age	< 16 years	< 16 years
Minimum duration of arthritis	3 months	6 weeks
No. of joints affected in first 6 months:		
oligoarticular or pauciarticular	1–4	1–4
polyarticular	> 4	> 4
systemic	Any number	Any number
Exclusions	Rheumatoid-factor-positive disease (alone termed juvenile rheumatoid arthritis (JRA))	Spondyloarthropathies, psoriatic arthritis, arthritis associated with inflammatory bowel disease

ACR, American College of Rheumatology; EULAR, European League Against Rheumatism.

polyarticular disease.[1] Recognized subtypes of JA are described in Table 5.2. All subtypes of JA may present for the first time in adolescence, but rheumatoid-factor-positive polyarticular disease (termed juvenile rheumatoid arthritis (JRA) in the EULAR classification) and the juvenile spondyloarthropathies typically present at this age (see Tables 5.2 and 5.3).

JRA is defined by the American Rheumatism Association (ARA) criteria[6] used widely in North America. In order to define, as far as possible, homogeneous populations of patients to facilitate scientific study across the world, a taskforce of the Pediatric Committee of the International League Against Rheumatism (ILAR) has proposed a further classification[7] (Table 5.4) based on clinical and prognostic features.

The most frequently occurring subtype of idiopathic arthritis in Caucasian children, oligoarticular or pauciarticular arthritis, is primarily a disease of young children, particularly girls (median age of onset 5.2 years[1]), but may occasionally occur de novo in adolescence. The most commonly affected joints are the knees and ankles, and involvement is often asymmetrical. Antinuclear antibodies (ANA) are found in 40–80% of cases and are associated with the development of chronic anterior uveitis. The patterns of immunofluorescence are usually homogeneous or speckled, and the antigen specificities of these ANA are heterogeneous. More than half of an early series (before the era of routine topical steroid treatment) of 83 affected eyes in patients with juvenile arthritis became blind or partially sighted.[8] Chronic anterior uveitis is usually asymptomatic, hence the importance of regular slit lamp examinations in this subgroup of patients. Recommendations for screening for uveitis in children with idiopathic

Table 5.2 Subtypes of juvenile arthritis

Subtype	Proportion of cases* (%)	Median onset age* (years)	Male/ female ratio*	No. of joints involved	Extra-articular features
Oligoarticular/pauciarticular	50	5.2	1 : 2.0	≤ 4	Chronic anterior uveitis
Rheumatoid-factor-negative polyarthritis	17	6.5	1 : 3.0	>4	Low-grade fever
Rheumatoid-factor-positive polyarthritis	3	9.0	1 : 12.8	> 4	Low-grade fever, rheumatoid nodules
Juvenile spondyloarthropathy	8	11.4	1 : 0.3	≤ 4	Enthesitis, acute iritis
Juvenile ankylosing spondylitis	2	12.1	1 : 0.3	Lumbar spine, sacroiliac joints	Acute iritis
Systemic	11	4.3	1 : 1.2	Variable	High spiking remittent fever, evanescent erythematous rash, polyserositis, hepatosplenomegaly, lymphadenopathy
Juvenile psoriatic arthritis	7	10.1	1 : 1.6	Typically ≤ 4 (dactylitis)	Psoriasis, nail pitting
Inflammatory bowel disease (IBO) associated arthritis	1	10.8	1 : 2.0	≤ 4	Erythema nodosum

*Symmons et al.[1]

Table 5.3 Comparison of relative incidence of juvenile arthritis subtypes at different onset ages*

JA subtype	Onset age range (years)		Total (0–16)
	0–10	10–16	
Pauciarticular arthritis	783 (48.4%)	200 (32.8%)	983 (44.1%)
Extended pauciarticular arthritis	154 (9.5%)	18 (3.0%)	172 (7.7%)
Polyarticular arthritis	310 (19.2%)	90 (14.8%)	400 (17.9%)
Systemic arthritis	167 (8.8%)	18 (5.5%)	185 (8.3%)
JRA	23 (1.4%)	23 (3.8%)	46 (2.1%)
Spondyloarthropathies†	100 (6.2%)	159 (26.1%)	255 (11.5%)
Juvenile psoriatic arthritis	84 (5.2%)	75 (12.3%)	159 (7.1%)
IBD associated arthritis	10 (0.6%)	18 (3.0%)	28 (1.4%)
Total	1618	610	2228

*The figures in the table represent the number of patients with each JA subtype presenting within each age range (percentage of total number of JA patients presenting within each age range). Data from British Paediatric Rheumatology Group database and Symmons (personal communication).
†Including juvenile ankylosing spondylitis and Reiter's syndrome.

Table 5.4 Proposed ILAR classification of idiopathic arthritis of childhood*

1. Systemic arthritis
2. Polyarthritis (rheumatoid-factor negative)
3. Polyarthritis (rheumatoid-factor positive)
4. Oligoarthritis:
   (a) persistent
   (b) extended
5. Enthesitis-related arthritis
6. Psoriatic arthritis
7. Other:
   (a) does not meet criteria for any of categories 1–6 or
   (b) meets criteria for more than one of categories 1–6.

*Taken from Petty.[7]

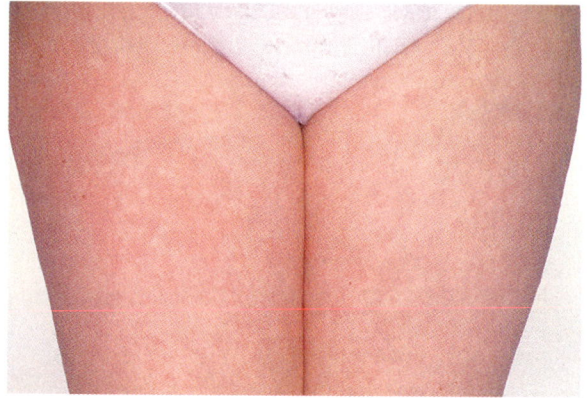

Figure 5.1 The typical evanescent erythematous macular rash of systemic-onset arthritis.

arthritis have been published by the Royal College of Ophthalmologists and the British Paediatric Association.[9]

Polyarticular disease, involving large and small joints, is associated with a greater systemic component than is oligoarticular disease, frequently with low-grade fever, fatigue and malaise. Rheumatoid-factor-negative polyarticular disease may begin at any age throughout childhood and adolescence (median age of onset 6.5 years[1]). In addition, extension of oligoarticular to polyarticular disease may occur after the first 6 months of disease at any time in later childhood or adolescence. Rheumatoid factor positive polyarthritis typically begins in late childhood or adolescence (median age of onset 9 years[1]). This disease is analogous to adult rheumatoid arthritis (RA) and is more than ten times as common in girls as boys. Like adult RA, there is often early erosive arthritis and rheumatoid nodule formation.

Systemic-onset arthritis may occur at any time throughout childhood, but is relatively uncommon in adolescence (median age of onset 4.3 years[1]) and rare in adulthood. Both sexes are affected equally. The disease is characterized by a remittent high-spiking fever and an evanescent erythematous macular rash (Figure 5.1). Arthritis may affect any joint(s) and may not be present ab initio, but may develop later in the disease course. Other features include hepatosplenomegaly, lymphadenitis and polyserositis (pleuritis, pericarditis and abdominal serositis), which may on occasion be life-threatening.

The juvenile-onset spondyloarthropathies (a group of human leucocyte antigen (HLA) B27 related clinical conditions including juvenile ankylosing spondylitis, seronegative enthesopathy and arthropathy (SEA) syndrome, psoriatic and inflammatory bowel disease related spondyloarthritis, and Reiter's syndrome) all have a median age of onset of greater than 10 years,[1] and as a group occur more frequently in boys than girls.[10] These conditions are discussed further in Chapter 6. Juvenile spondyloarthropathy usually presents in adolescent boys as a lower limb asymmetrical large joint arthritis and/or enthesitis. Axial disease and sacroiliitis may not develop until well into adult life.

Arthritis is a common complication of both Crohn's disease and ulcerative colitis. Two patterns of joint inflammation are seen associated with inflammatory bowel disease: peripheral polyarthritis and, less commonly, sacroiliitis.

Juvenile psoriatic arthritis may present in the absence of a typical psoriatic rash. Nail changes, dactylitis or a positive family history of psoriasis may suggest the diagnosis in these cases. The arthritis is most commonly a scattered asymmetrical oligoarthritis affecting both large and small joints.

DIFFERENTIAL DIAGNOSIS OF ARTHRITIS IN ADOLESCENCE

There is a wide differential diagnosis of arthritis in adolescence, and the vast majority of adolescents with limb pain do not have arthritis. Ten per cent to 20% of otherwise healthy school-aged children have recurrent limb pains.[11] Hypermobility of joints is a common finding in children of school age (8% of 11–14 year olds[12]) and is known to be associated with recurrent arthralgia in approximately 40% of cases.[12] The pathogenesis of this pain is unclear, although it may be related to recurrent episodes of subclinical trauma or to the increased muscle tension required to maintain an upright posture in hypermobile individuals.[13]

Idiopathic musculoskeletal pain syndromes (covered in detail in Chapter 10), both localized and diffuse, are also frequently recognized in the adolescent age group, particularly in girls.[14,15] In these patients there may be a past history of other forms of chronic pain, such as abdominal pain or headaches and allodynia (a painful response to a non-noxious stimulus such as light touch) is a characteristic feature. Some patients with a localized idiopathic pain syndrome have additional features of an autonomic disturbance, such as reduced skin temperature, soft-tissue swelling and a purple mottled appearance to the skin. Bizarre posturing of the affected limb and *la belle indifference* complete the picture of reflex sympathetic dystrophy. Diffuse idiopathic pain syndromes include fibromyalgia, which is characterized by the presence of multiple symmetrical soft-tissue limb girdle tender points, and occurs predominantly in teenage girls.[16] Arthralgia or limb pain is also a prominent feature of chronic or post-viral fatigue syndrome or myalgic encephalomyelitis. It is important to recognize these syndromes early, both to institute appropriate therapy, comprising physical rehabilitation and psychological support, and to avoid unnecessary investigation, which may exacerbate symptoms.

The post-infectious arthritides, post-streptococcal, post-enteric and post-viral, are common causes of arthritis throughout childhood and adolescence, and may be suspected from the clinical history of a preceding illness and identified by isolation of the organism or demonstration of a serological response to the organism. Post-viral arthritis, in particular, may be difficult to distinguish clinically from early juvenile idiopathic arthritis and is the rationale behind the EULAR criteria, which require a disease duration of 3 months before making a definite diagnosis of juvenile chronic arthritis.

Neoplasia (including leukaemia and primary bone tumours, such as osteoid osteoma and osteosarcoma) needs to be considered in any adolescent presenting with bone or joint pain. The degree of pain is often greater than in arthritis, with nocturnal prominence and bony tenderness. In acute leukaemia, plain radiographs may show metaphyseal lucencies, and a blood film is usually diagnostic, although in some cases initial blood films and even marrow examination may be normal.[17] Arthritis and arthralgia are common initial symptoms of the autoimmune rheumatic diseases and vasculitides, which, although they are extremely rare in early childhood, are somewhat more frequent in adolescence and early adulthood.

The differential diagnosis of systemic-onset disease is wide, and includes infections, neoplasia (especially leukaemia, lymphoma and neuroblastoma), inflammatory bowel disease, familial Mediterranean fever, haemophagocytic disease, hyperimmunoglobulin D (IgD) syndrome, fever, aphthous stomatitis, pharyngitis and adenitis (FAPA) syndrome, rheumatic fever, other autoimmune rheumatic diseases and vasculitides.

Site-specific conditions

Anterior knee pain is a common symptom in adolescents and may be due to chondromalacia patellae (more frequent in girls), patellar tracking abnormalities or recurrent patellar subluxation. Osteochondritis dissecans of the tibial tuberosity (Osgood–Schlatter disease), which is more common in boys, produces pain and swelling around the tibial tuberosity and is exacerbated by exercise. All these conditions are readily identifiable from the history and examination, and should not be confused with arthritis. Slipped upper femoral epiphysis occurs typically in males in early adolescence and presents with pain, frequently referred to the thigh or knee, a limp and a reduction in range of movement at the hip. The diagnosis is confirmed radiologically.

Hughes et al[18] reviewed 26 adolescents presenting to a juvenile rheumatology clinic with isolated hip pain. Sixteen were found to have non-inflammatory disease, including four with idiopathic protrusio and five with idiopathic chondrolysis. Other diagnoses included undetected hip dysplasia (two cases), avascular necrosis (two cases), idiopathic osteoporosis (one case), slipped epiphysis (one case) and injury (one case).

Back pain is common in adolescents and is reported to affect approximately 8% of 14–15 year olds[19] and 26% of 13–17 year olds.[20] Back pain is only rarely due to arthritis. Other diagnoses that should be considered in this age group include spondylosis/spondylolisthesis, Scheuerman's disease and neoplasia. In spondylosis there is a defect in the pars interarticularis, typically in the lower lumbar vertebrae, particularly L5. Pain is often precipitated by exercise. Bilateral defects may allow the affected vertebral body to shift anteriorly to produce a spondylolisthesis and may result in sciatica. Appropriate radiographs with oblique views will usually identify these lesions. Scheuerman's disease, osteochondritis of the thoracic vertebrae, presents most commonly in the adolescent years and may cause pain, although equally commonly it presents with deformity (kyphosis) in the absence of pain.

AETIOLOGY AND PATHOGENESIS OF JUVENILE IDIOPATHIC ARTHRITIS

Cyclical patterns of incidence of juvenile-onset idiopathic arthritis have been reported in North America,[21,22] but so far no systematic epidemiological studies have been performed to see if an infectious agent can be implicated. Attempts to identify specific infectious agents have shown that streptococcus, mycoplasma, Epstein–Barr virus, rubella, influenza and other upper respiratory viruses can all trigger a flare. However, at onset, no specific infectious agents are usually found. The arthritides are therefore the product of genetic predisposing factors interacting with different environmental triggers.

Progress in molecular genetics has allowed the demonstration of clear genetic associations in the various groups of idiopathic juvenile arthritis. The major histocompatibility gene complex (MHC) is the most studied so far. This is a large group of linked genes, many of which code for proteins involved in processing and presenting foreign antigens to initiate an immune response. The increased associations of these genes with different subtypes of arthritis are summarized in Table 5.5 (preliminary results from the Twelfth International Histocompatibility Workshop and Conference[23]) and are reviewed in Donn et al.[24] Together these genes can exert a significant influence on the likelihood of developing idiopathic arthritis. In one study, the combination of HLA-DRB1*0801, 1101 and DPB1*0201 conferred a relative risk of 236.[25] Since several genes can confer an increased risk of arthritis, it is clear that these diseases are polygenic, and other genes may be involved. A limited genome screen for candidate genes is in progress in the UK and the USA. Of note are the genes that code for cytokines, which mediate cell-to-cell signalling, cell growth and differentiation, and inflammation. Imbalance of cytokines with opposing actions has been shown to be associated with chronic inflammation. A good example is Lyme arthritis, where the infectious agent is known, but the outcome depends on the interleukin-1 (IL-1)/IL-1 receptor agonist (IL-1ra) ratio. The ratio is low in the non-minimally relapsing arthritis subgroup and high in those

Table 5.5 Significant positive HLA associations with different juvenile idiopathic arthritis subtypes*

Arthritis subtype (ILAR proposals)	HLA association	Odds ratio	95% CI
Oligoarthritis	DRB1*01	1.41	1.06–1.90
	DRB1*08	6.23	4.42–8.78
	DRB1*11	3.62	2.97–4.65
	DRB1*13	2.30	1.79–2.98
	DRB1*14	2.09	1.38–3.14
	DPB1*0201	2.59	1.86–3.61
	DQA1*0401	3.84	2.52–5.95
	DQA1*0601	5.13	2.02–12.9
	DQB1*0201	1.53	1.15–2.05
	DQB1*0301	8.31	6.32–10.9
	DQB1*0302	3.92	1.96–7.81
	DQB1*0303	8.10	1.63–40.2
	DQB1*0402	85.56	20.8–351
	DQB1*0603	1.85	1.29–2.67
	DQB1*0604	2.75	1.61–4.69
Extended oligoarthritis	DRB1*08	3.34	2.1–5.23
	DRB1*11	1.70	1.24–2.29
	DQA1*0401	2.28	1.23–4.21
	DQB1*0301	2.36	1.51–3.71
	DQB1*0603	1.85	1.11–3.08
Polyarthritis RF negative, ANA positive	DRB1*08	3.62	1.88–6.97
	DRB1*11	1.84	1.51–2.95
	DQA1*0401	3.67	1.70–7.92
	DQB1*0301	3.37	2.08–5.43
	DQB1*0302	4.65	1.76–12.2
	DQB1*0402	27.47	5.22–141
Polyarthritis RF negative, ANA negative	DRB1*08	1.94	1.11–3.37
	DRB1*14	2.33	1.14–3.85
	DQA1*0401	3.79	2.15–6.71
	DQB1*0301	5.42	3.66–8.04
	DQB1*0302	12.52	6.17–25.41
	DQB1*0402	48.94	10.7–222
Polyarthritis RF positive	DRB1*04	2.16	1.23–3.78
	DQA1*0401	2.89	1.17–7.13
	DQB1*0301	8.45	5.01–14.2
	DQB1*0302	19.37	8.47–44.2
	DQB1*0402	60.87	13.7–349
Juvenile psoriatic arthritis†	DRB1*14	3.11	1.49–6.51
	DPB1*0201	2.67	1.20–4.46
	DQA1*0101	2.38	1.43–3.98
	DQB1*0301	6.95	3.92–12.3

ANA, antinuclear antibody; CI, confidence interval; HLA, human leucocyte antigen; ILAR, International League Against Rheumatism; RF, rheumatoid factor.
*Data from 12th International Histocompatibility Workshop study in JCA.[23]
†Vancouver criteria.

with chronically relapsing arthritis.[26] Genetic polymorphisms have been found in the regulatory regions of a number of these genes, and certain alleles are associated with pathology. A polymorphic variant of the IL-1α gene was found to be associated with uveitis and pauciarticular arthritis in Norwegians,[27] but confirmation in larger studies and other ethnic groups is needed. In systemic arthritis, results from our unit have shown a highly significant association of this subgroup with a lack of an IL-6 genotype that has a low transcription rate under stimulus, i.e. a lack of a 'protective gene' (Fishman D, Faulds G, Jefferey R et al, 1998 unpublished observations).

The initiation of an immune response by HLA molecules involves presentation of peptides, previously processed by the antigen-presenting cell, carried in a groove within the HLA molecule. The combination is recognized by the T-cell receptor of the T lymphocytes, which are subsequently activated if other accessory molecules are also recognized by the T cell. Genetic variations in the complex process of antigen presentation and recognition have been postulated to influence the immune response and contribute to pathology in arthritis. In HLA-B27 transgenic rats arthritis only develops when the rats are reared outside a germ-free environment, suggesting that processing and/or presentation of common germs to the immune system is affected by the presence of B27. In HLA-B27-positive individuals with spondyloarthropathy, T cells have been shown to proliferate in the presence of enteric bacteria, suggesting previous exposure as well as a developed immune response to these bacteria. Studies on HLA-B27-associated later-onset oligoarticular arthritis synovial fluid T cells showed a reaction to a conserved antigen common to bacteria and man, heat shock protein hsp60,[28] and the presence of these clones was found to be associated with a favourable outcome.[29] The converse situation is implied but remains unproven.

MANAGEMENT OF JUVENILE IDIOPATHIC ARTHRITIS

Optimal management of chronic arthritis, particularly in adolescence, requires a multidiscipli-nary approach. Ideally, the team should include a physician and nurses with expertise in adolescent rheumatology, a physiotherapist, occupational therapist, psychologist or psychiatrist, social worker and orthopaedic surgeon. Treatment should be aimed at suppression of inflammation and relief of pain, maintenance of range of joint movement and prevention of deformities and disability. Physiotherapy and splintage to maintain joint position and function are as important as pharmacologic measures. The management of chronic pain must be tailored to the individual, and consider the psychological, emotional and social aspects as well as the sensory component.

Non-steroidal anti-inflammatory drugs (NSAIDs)

NSAIDs are used for the relief of symptoms in arthritis, but have no proven role in influencing the outcome of the disease. The mean time course of response to NSAIDs is 4 weeks and may be as long as 12 weeks.[30] Several drugs may need to be tried, as individual response is unpredictable. Different drugs may suit different children in terms of their efficacy, side-effect profile, dosage regime and formulations. Dosages of NSAIDs per kilogram body weight often need to be higher than in adult rheumatic diseases (Table 5.6), particularly to control fever in systemic-onset arthritis. Slow-release formulations given at night are especially useful in treating early morning stiffness. Although they are sometimes used, there are no data in children or adolescents which show that NSAID combinations are additive or synergistic. NSAIDs appear generally to be better tolerated in children and adolescents than in adults. Gastrointestinal symptoms, such as abdominal pain, nausea and vomiting, are relatively common, but more severe problems such as gastrointestinal haemorrhage are rare in children.[31] Other side-effects include rashes (cutaneous pseudoporphyria,[32,33] particularly in fair children treated with naproxen), central nervous system symptoms (headaches, dizziness, confusion and mood change), asthma, liver toxicity (particularly in

Table 5.6	Doses of NSAIDs used in juvenile idiopathic arthritis		
Drug	Dosage	Maximum daily dose	Formulation
Ibuprofen	20–40 mg/kg/day (three or four times daily) up to 60 mg/kg/day (six daily doses) in systemic disease only	3 g	Tablets, slow-release tablets, suspension, granules (topical spray, cream, gel)
Diclofenac	1–3 mg/kg/day (three times daily)	200 mg	Tablets and capsules, slow-release tablets and capsules, dispersible tablets, suspension, suppositories (topical gel)
Naproxen	10–20 mg/kg/day (twice daily)	1 g	Tables, slow-release tablets, suspension, suppositories
Indomethacin	2–4 mg/kg/day (twice daily)	150 mg	Tablets and capsules, slow-release tablets and capsules, suspension, suppositories

systemic-onset arthritis) and renal toxicity. Salicylates are not now in common usage for juvenile arthritis because of the relatively high incidence of side-effects, the need for multiple daily dosing and the potential association with Reye's syndrome.

Corticosteroids

Intra-articular corticosteroid injections have been shown to be effective in controlling synovitis for prolonged periods in juvenile idiopathic arthritis.[34] They may be used alone as therapy for oligoarticular disease or as an adjunct to other therapies in polyarticular disease. Triamcinolone hexacetonide (approximately 1 mg/kg for large joints, 0.5 mg/kg for small joints) gives the longest lasting effect. The shorter acting hydrocortisone acetate is preferred for injecting tendon sheaths.

Systemic corticosteroids have a limited role in the management of juvenile arthritis because of their long-term side-effects, in particular their deleterious effects on bone metabolism and growth. Indications for systemic corticosteroids are life-threatening systemic disease such as pericarditis, pleuritis or severe anaemia, or persistence of systemic features despite adequate trial of NSAIDs. Doses of oral prednisolone of up to 2 mg/kg/day in divided doses may be required. In addition, oral corticosteroids are sometimes used in lower doses in the initial stages of polyarticular disease, while waiting for a slow-acting antirheumatic drug to take effect. In all cases, the lowest dose that controls the disease should be used and that dose subsequently weaned as soon as possible according to the clinical status of the patient. In some cases, alternate-day administration (or alternate high dose, low dose) may be possible, thus reducing pituitary–adrenal suppression. An additional dose of a NSAID may be helpful on the low/no-dose evening.

Table 5.7 Adverse effects of corticosteroids

- Diabetes mellitus and impaired glucose tolerance
- Osteoporosis
- Avascular necrosis
- Cataracts and glaucoma
- Growth suppression
- Myopathy
- Peptic ulceration
- Mental disturbance, including depression and psychosis
- Increased susceptibility to infection
- Hypertension
- Sodium and water retention
- Potassium loss
- Redistribution of body fat
- Skin changes, including acne and striae

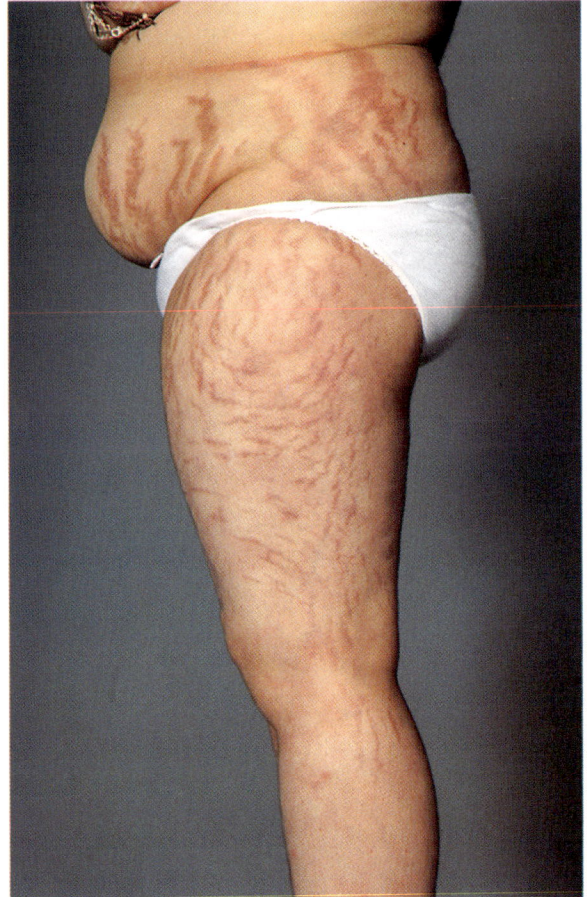

Figure 5.2 Side-effects of long-term corticosteroid therapy: obesity and striae.

Adverse effects associated with corticosteroid therapy are listed in Table 5.7 and illustrated in Figure 5.2. Body image and appearance are of particular importance to adolescents, and the potential development of short stature, obesity, striae, hirsutism and acne should be recognized and discussed. As at any age, the dose of steroids used in adolescents with arthritis should be as low as possible in order to minimize adverse effects, and wherever possible alternative treatment should be considered. Poor compliance with prescribed therapy is well recognized in adolescents with chronic disease. Patients should know that sudden withdrawal of corticosteroid therapy may result in acute adrenal insufficiency, which can be fatal. To improve cooperation and compliance, physicians and therapists need to recognize the young person's increasing need for independence and to involve the young person in the design and organization of their treatment schedule.[35]

Deflazacort, an oxazoline derivative of prednisolone, appears to have a relatively bone-sparing effect.[36,37] In the small randomized study done by Loftus et al,[37] children in a deflazacort treated group showed better maintenance of spine bone mineral content relative to height and weight compared to a prednisolone treated group, with similar anti-inflammatory effect in both groups.

Intermittent pulsed intravenous methylprednisolone is effective at controlling severe systemic symptoms temporarily, and regular intravenous pulses may have less long-term adverse effects than prolonged daily oral dosage.[38] A dose of 30 mg/kg up to a maximum of 1 g intravenous methylprednisolone may be given daily over 2 hours, although an optimal regimen remains to be defined. Side-effects are varied, and include behavioural changes, headache, abdominal complaints, pruritis, transient hypo- or hypertension and anaphylaxis.[39]

Slow-acting antirheumatic drugs (SAARDs)

The traditional philosophy of management of chronic arthritis in childhood (to begin with NSAIDs and move on to SAARDs only if the disease continues to progress) has recently been questioned.[40] Joint damage occurs early in some subtypes of juvenile idiopathic arthritis and may be modified by the earlier use of disease-modifying drugs.[41] We start SAARDs early in those children in whom we suspect a more severe disease course, such as those with rheumatoid-factor-positive disease.

Methotrexate

Methotrexate has been shown in randomized controlled trials to be more efficacious than placebo in polyarticular[42] and extended oligoarticular[43] arthritis and to produce radiological improvement.[41] It is therefore the first-line SAARD for these subtypes of idiopathic arthritis. Low dose (15–20 mg/m^2 body surface area/week) methotrexate was found to be of equivocal benefit in a double-blind placebo controlled study in systemic disease.[43] A starting dose of 10–15 mg/m^2 body surface area/week is indicated by these studies.[42,43] Absorption after a single oral dose is highly variable[44–46] but finite.[45] The oral dose may therefore sometimes need to be elevated to 20–25 mg/m^2 body surface area/week, but further increases in serum levels may only be achieved by parenteral administration. Subcutaneous injections produce similar absorption profiles, in adults with rheumatoid arthritis, but are better tolerated than intramuscular administration.[47] Methotrexate is usually given once a week, although this dosage schedule has never been shown to be optimal in comparative studies. Response may take up to 3 months.

In general, methotrexate is well tolerated by patients with juvenile arthritis.[48] Common adverse effects such as nausea may be limited by the addition of daily oral folic acid (1 mg), splitting the oral dosage over 24 hours or using parenteral administration. Elevation of transaminases usually responds to a temporary reduction or omission of the dose. Longer term hepatic toxicity appears to be mild in juvenile arthritis patients, with none of 12 patients who had received a cumulative dose of 2–3 g methotrexate showing evidence of toxic effects on liver biopsy.[49] Accelerated nodulosis, occurring particularly in patients with rheumatoid-factor-positive polyarticular disease, has been reported.[50] Methotrexate-induced pulmonary disease is exceptionally rare in children. Methotrexate is, however, known to be teratogenic. It is important that this issue is raised with adolescent girls before commencing therapy, and that appropriate contraceptive advice is given where necessary. NSAIDs can alter methotrexate pharmacokinetics,[51] and vice versa,[52] resulting in the potential for increased toxicity in patients receiving the combination. It is not clear when methotrexate should be discontinued after remission has been achieved, although it is known that abrupt discontinuation of methotrexate may lead to a disease flare.[53]

Other SAARDs

Sulphasalazine has also been shown to be efficacious in oligo- and polyarticular arthritis,[54] and may be particularly effective in the HLA-B27-positive arthropathies.[55] Side-effects appear to be more frequent and serious in systemic-onset disease.[56,57] Oligospermia is common among young men taking sulphasalazine,[58] although this is reversible on discontinuing the drug.

Although not shown to be more effective than placebo in a controlled trial,[59] hydroxychloroquine appears anecdotally to be useful in early onset rheumatoid-factor-positive arthritis, particularly where there is relatively mild disease which is not completely controlled by NSAIDs alone. Hydroxychloroquine has a low incidence of adverse effects, and no routine blood tests to monitor for toxicity are required. Clinically significant retinopathy appears to be an extremely rare complication when hydroxy-

Oligoarticular arthritis (persistent)

↓

IA corticosteroid

↓

NSAID + IA corticosteroid

**RF-negative polyarthritis
and extended oligoarticular arthritis**

↓

NSAID ± IA corticosteroid

↓

NSAID + methotrexate

RF-positive polyarthritis (early onset)

↓

NSAID + hydroxychloroquine ± IA corticosteroid

↓

NSAID + methotrexate

RF-positive polyarthritis (later onset)

↓

NSAID + methrotrexate ± IA corticosteroid

Spondyloarthropathies

↓

NSAID ± IA corticosteroid

↓

NSAID + sulphasalazine (up to 3 g/kg)
± intermittent systemic corticosteroid

Systemic disease

↓

NSAID

↙ ↘

NSAID +
IV methylprednisolone
30 mg/kg × 3 doses over
1 week, then oral corticosteroid
(prednisolone 0.5–1 mg/kg/day)

NSAID + oral
corticosteroid
(prednisolone
1–2 mg/kg/day)

↓

NSAID + methotrexate

↓

NSAID + oral
corticosteroid +
methotrexate

↘ ↙

chlorambucil

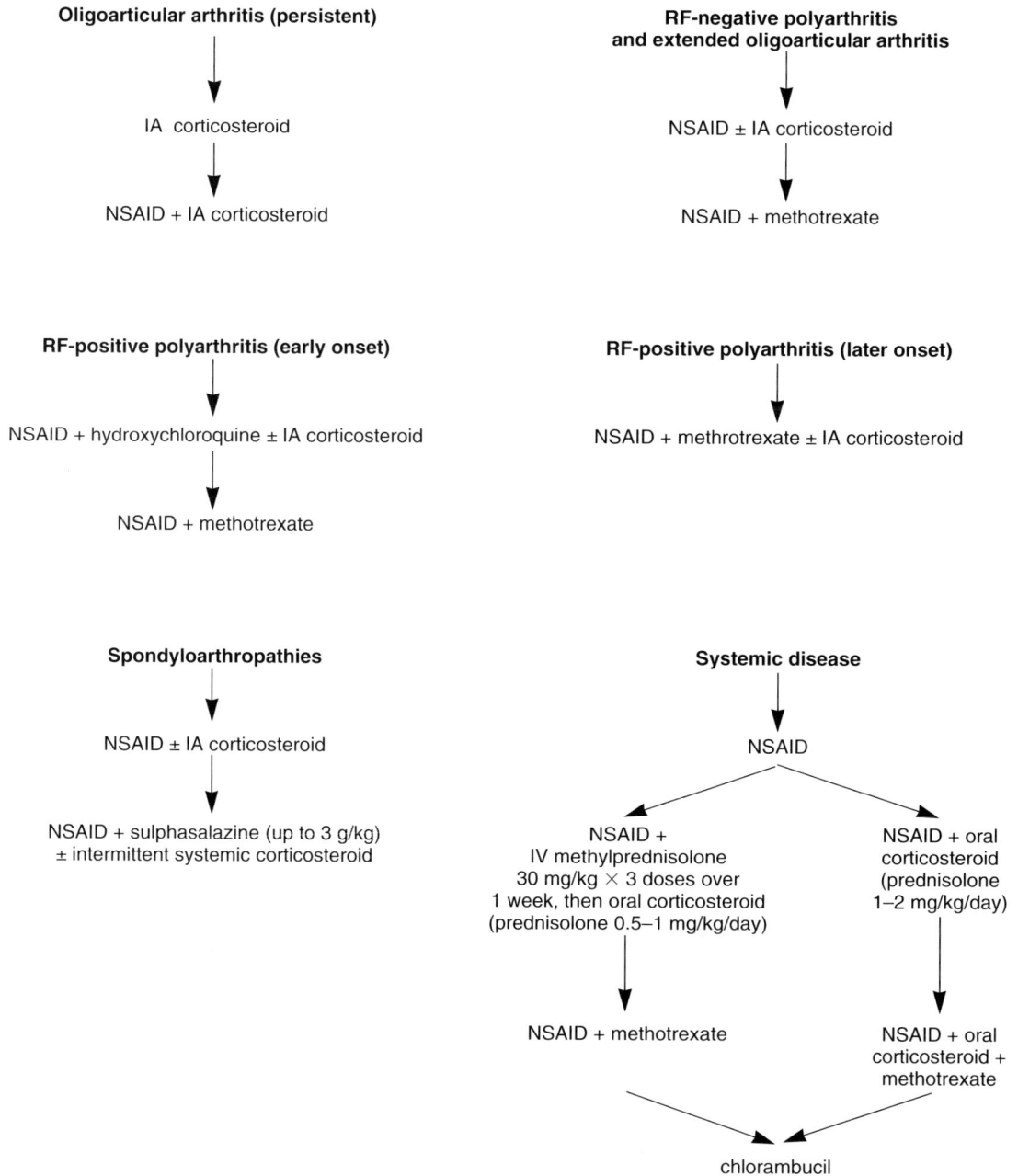

Figure 5.3 Algorithms for the pharmacological management of subtypes of idiopathic arthritis. IA, intra-articular; RF, rheumatoid factor.

chloroquine is used at the currently recommended dosages.[59–61]

Injectable gold (which is known to be toxic during the systemic illness of systemic arthritis) is usually reserved for rheumatoid-factor-positive polyarticular disease. Oral gold, auranofin[62] and penicillamine[59] are not effective in juvenile idiopathic arthritis, and are no longer used. Cyclosporin has been studied only in uncontrolled trials[63,64] and its use remains experimental. It may, however, be the treatment of choice for a rare complication of juvenile-onset arthritis characterized by severe hepatic disease and haemorrhagic and neurological manifestations (the reactive haemophagocytic syndrome).[65] Trials of combinations of SAARDs in idiopathic juvenile arthritis, such as the open study of pulse therapy with methylprednisolone and cyclophosphamide in addition to oral methotrexate by Shaikov et al,[66] are encouraging, but their value is as yet unclear.

Immunosuppressive agents, such as azathioprine, cyclophosphamide and chlorambucil, are occasionally also used in treating severe disease unresponsive to other agents and chlorambucil for systemic amyloidosis. A recent randomized placebo-controlled trial failed to demonstrate any benefit from high-dose intravenous immunoglobulin in systemic-onset arthritis.[67] Monoclonal anti-tumour necrosis factor α (anti-TNF-α) did not improve articular features in a patient with systemic-onset disease.[68]

Algorithms used in our unit for the pharmacological management of the subtypes of juvenile idiopathic arthritis are shown in Figure 5.3.

GROWTH AND DEVELOPMENT IN ADOLESCENTS WITH CHRONIC ARTHRITIS

Acceleration of growth velocity and bone-mass accretion as well as the development of secondary sexual characteristics occur during puberty under the influence of sex hormones and growth hormone. Arthritis in childhood and adolescence may adversely affect growth and development in several ways. Localized epiphyseal disease may result in acceleration of growth velocity followed by premature epiphyseal fusion, resulting in localized growth defects such as limb-length inequalities. Generalized growth retardation is common, particularly in poorly controlled systemic disease (Figure 5.4). Contributing factors include anorexia and poor dietary intake,[69] the effects of circulating proinflammatory cytokines such as IL-1, IL-6 and TNF, and long-term systemic corticosteroid

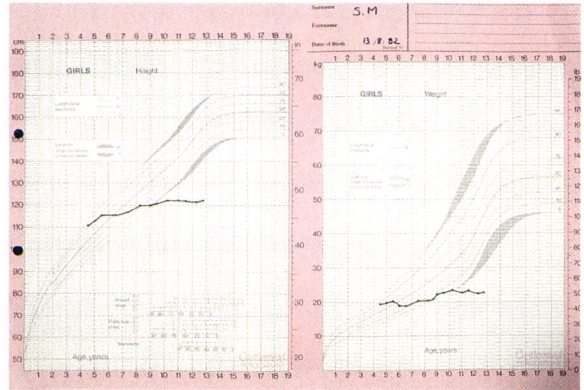

Figure 5.4 A growth chart illustrating severe growth retardation in a girl with resistant systemic-onset arthritis.

medication. Chronic inflammatory disease may also result in delay in sexual maturation and delayed or irregular menstruation in adolescent girls.[70]

Self-confidence is often fragile in adolescents, and delay in growth and development even in healthy individuals (constitutional delay of growth and puberty) may cause considerable psychological distress.[71] In addition, teenagers with arthritis often have other differences from their peer group, such as deformities and relative immobility, to contend with. Strategies to normalize growth velocity and development should be actively pursued. Adequate treatment of disease activity is vital, as it is known that short stature may result from continuing disease activity, even in the absence of corticosteroid therapy, and catch-up growth can occur after remission. Systemic steroid treatment should be avoided in patients in whom alternative therapies are likely to be effective, and where steroids are used the lowest dose that produces adequate control of disease activity should be used.

Treatment with recombinant growth hormone (rGH) in children with idiopathic arthritis produces a significant increase in height velocity.[72] At 5-year follow-up, when some subjects were post-pubertal, this advantage was maintained and no premature epiphyseal fusion or acromegaly was seen (M Rooney, personal communication). Although the effect on final adult height is not yet known, the beneficial psychological effect of increased height in the vulnerable teenage years may be considerable. The increase in height velocity produced by rGH correlates negatively with disease activity,[72] underlining the importance of optimizing disease control before commencing rGH treatment. In the study by Davies et al,[72] however, no correlation was found between steroid dose and response to rGH therapy.

OSTEOPOROSIS IN ADOLESCENTS WITH ARTHRITIS

In healthy individuals bone mass is accumulated progressively from infancy to adolescence and generally parallels linear growth. The greatest increase in bone mineral content during the human life-span occurs between the ages of 11 and 14 years in girls and 13 and 17 years in boys, with an increase in total skeletal mass of approximately 8% per year during the adolescent growth spurt.[73] Increase in bone mineral content stops in the mid-twenties. Any relative impairment in bone formation will have an accentuated effect during the adolescent years, when bone acquisition would normally be at its maximum. Genetics,[74] diet[75,76] and physical activity[77] are known to have important influences on the acquisition of skeletal mass in healthy individuals.

Generalized and periarticular osteoporosis are well described features of juvenile arthritis.[73] Children and adolescents with arthritis have reduced bone mineral density compared to their healthy counterparts,[78,79] and appendicular cortical bone is predominantly affected.[73] Generalized osteoporosis is particularly associated with systemic disease and is a cause of significant morbidity, particularly secondary to vertebral collapse. Depression of markers of bone formation, such as osteocalcin,[80] and the predominance of cortical demineralization indicate that the predominant pathophysiological mechanism is decreased bone formation rather than increased

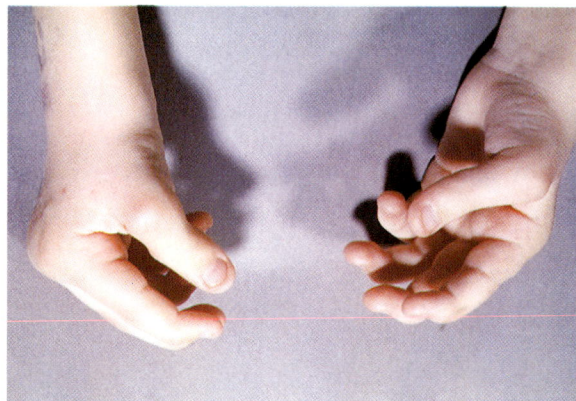

Figure 5.5 The hands of a boy with extended oligoarticular arthritis and 'dry synovitis'.

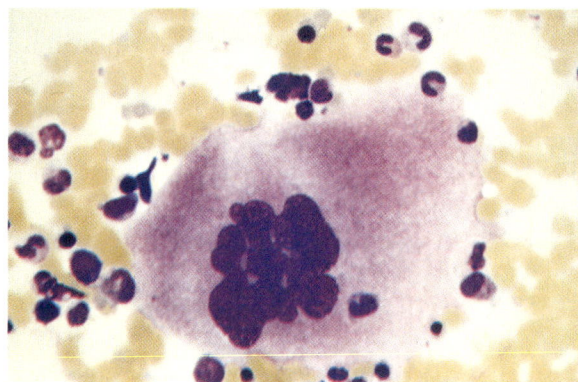

Figure 5.6 Photomicrograph of the bone marrow of a patient with reactive haemophagocytic syndrome, showing a macrophage with multiple nuclei in its cytoplasm.

resorption.[73] In 83 children with arthritis, Reed et al[80] noted a relationship between disease activity and reduced serum osteocalcin levels, suggesting that active inflammation results in reduced bone formation. In a subsequent study, repair of osteopaenia occurred with reduced disease activity,[81] underscoring the importance of suppression of the inflammatory disease in reducing the severity of osteoporosis in chronic arthritis.

Reduced intestinal absorption of calcium has been described in children with chronic arthritis.[82] The active form of vitamin D is required for adequate calcium absorption and decreased plasma levels of 25-hydroxyvitamin D have been described in children with systemic and polyarticular disease on corticosteroid treatment.[83] In addition, corticosteroid therapy is known to reduce calcium absorption. Since calcium[74] and milk[75] supplementation have been shown to increase bone mineral density in placebo-controlled trials in healthy adolescent girls, supplementation may be of value in adolescents with chronic arthritis. Short-term calcium and vitamin D supplementation in 10 corticosteroid treated children with rheumatic disease significantly improved spinal bone density.[84] Although the routine use of a calcium-rich diet and vitamin D supplementation did not prevent the development of reduced bone density in the study done by Fantini et al,[85] the lack of a control group means that it was not possible to determine any ameliorating effect. Our current practice is to give dietary advice on increasing milk intake to all children and adolescents with chronic arthritis and to supplement calcium and vitamin D intake in those on long-term systemic corticosteroids. The importance of weight-bearing activity in the prevention of osteoporosis should be explained. The use of biphosphonates may prove to be of value in treating or preventing osteoporosis in adolescents and children with chronic arthritis. Lepore et al[86] reported a significant improvement in bone density in seven patients treated with disodium clodronate compared with six untreated patients. Falcini et al[87] reported a significant improvement in bone mineral density in 23 patients with connective-tissue diseases treated for 6 months with alendronate. A larger placebo-controlled study is required to investigate this further.

NEW MEDICAL PROBLEMS OCCURRING IN ADOLESCENTS WITH IDIOPATHIC ARTHRITIS

Medical problems that may occur for the first time in adolescents as well as younger children with arthritis include extension of oligoarticular disease, the development of the reactive haemophagocytic syndrome and amyloidosis. Problems that are more specific to the peripubertal age group include reactivation of previously quiescent disease, the apparent lack of efficacy of previously effective drugs and the development of systemic features in juvenile ankylosing spondylitis. In addition, surgical treatment for fixed joint deformities and localized growth disturbances, as well as arthroplasty to replace destroyed joints, may be required in the adolescent and early adult years. Careful counselling is needed prior to any surgery, and consideration should be given to the appropriate timing of any intervention with regard to psychosocial issues as well as medical concerns.

Extension of oligoarticular to polyarticular disease

The course of oligoarticular onset disease is variable. Some children follow a oligoarticular course and may go into remission. In approximately 20% of cases, however, there is progressive increase in the number of joints affected to produce a polyarticular course in later childhood or adolescence (extended oligoarticular arthritis). The arthritis may produce the usual boggy effusions, but in some cases a 'dry synovitis' with progressive stiffening and deformity but with little heat or swelling is seen (Figure 5.5). In our experience, disease progression in these cases may be rapid and aggressive and merits early intervention with SAARDs. Methotrexate at 15–20 mg/m^2 has been shown to be more effective than placebo in a recently conducted multicentre, double-blind, placebo-controlled trial in patients with extended oligoarticular disease.[43]

Reactive haemophagocytic syndrome

The reactive haemophagocytic syndrome or macrophage activation syndrome is a rare but potentially fatal complication occurring particularly in patients with systemic-onset arthritis. The characteristic features at onset include fever, hepatitis, thrombocytopaenia, neutropaenia and hypofibrinogenaemia. Disseminated intravascular coagulation may develop if left untreated. Bone-marrow aspirate reveals macrophages showing active haemophagocytosis with cytoplasmic haematopoietic elements (Figure 5.6). The aetiology of this process is unknown, but it may be triggered by an intercurrent viral infection or by drug therapy. Cyclosporin A appears to be valuable in the management of this serious condition in addition to meticulous supportive therapy.[65]

Amyloidosis

Reactive amyloidosis is a well-recognized complication of long-standing infection or inflammation. High levels of serum amyloid A result in widespread tissue deposition of amyloid fibrils consisting of polypeptide chains derived from this acute-phase protein.[88] The prevalence of reactive amyloidosis in juvenile idiopathic arthritis shows marked geographic variation. Reported figures from Europe vary between 3% and 10%,[89,90] but in the USA the prevalence has been reported to be as low as 0.14%.[91] These differences are probably multifactorial in origin and result at least in part from differences in referral patterns, clinical management and follow-up periods. More recent data from our unit and a study from Finland[92] show that the incidence in Europe is apparently declining, and it is suggested that more effective treatment with SAARDs may be responsible for this.

Severity and chronicity of inflammatory disease are recognized risk factors for the development of amyloidosis, but it is not possible to predict which individuals will be affected. Genetic factors also are likely to be of importance. A restriction fragment polymorphism of the serum amyloid P gene has been identified in UK patients with JIA and amyloidosis.[93] The prevalence of reactive amyloidosis is highest in systemic-onset arthritis although it may occur in all subgroups except monoarticular disease.[90] A retrospective study of 79 juvenile arthritics patients with reactive amyloidosis showed a mean disease duration at diagnosis of amyloidosis of 9.1 years.[94] In an earlier study of 51 patients, the age at onset of amyloidosis ranged from 4 to 30 years.[90]

Amyloidosis is usually suspected when proteinuria and/or loss of renal function is detected. Other features include oedema, hypertension, abdominal pain, hepatosplenomegaly and diarrhoea.[94] No routine laboratory test can identify amyloidosis in patients with idiopathic arthritis, and a high index of suspicion should be maintained in those with persistently active disease. A raised acute-phase response is invariably present, but does not usually contribute to the differential diagnosis. The diagnosis can be confirmed with histology from renal, rectal, gastric, duodenal or fat biopsies. Scintigraphy with a ^{123}I-labelled serum amyloid P component, which has a high affinity for amyloid fibrils and identifies all amyloid deposits, has proved to be valuable in monitoring progression and regression of amyloid deposits.[95]

Chlorambucil has revolutionized the treatment of amyloid A amyloidosis, with 68% of chlorambucil-treated juvenile arthritis patients with amyloid surviving at 15-year review compared with 0% in a non-cytotoxic-treated group.[94] Chlorambucil is used at a dose of 0.1–0.12 mg/kg/day as a single daily oral dose, and is usually well tolerated. Bone-marrow toxicity is usually reversible and rarely necessitates cessation of therapy, but there is an increased risk of malignancy and infertility following treatment, which is correlated with the cumulative dosage. No male patient in the series studied by David et al[94] had fathered a child, but the prognosis for female fertility was more variable. Premature ovarian failure was reported in some women, but there were others who had successful pregnancies. In addition to cytotoxic treatment, renal support (dialysis and/or transplantation), control of hypertension and early treatment of infection are also important in patients with amyloidosis. The commonest cause of death in juvenile-arthritis-associated reactive amyloidosis is renal failure, followed by infection, usually due to bacterial septicaemia.[94]

FERTILITY AND PREGNANCY

Patients with a history of juvenile idiopathic arthritis often express concern about their ability to have a family.[96] They are worried about any adverse effect their disease or its treatment may have on their fertility. Women are concerned about their ability to cope physically with pregnancy and delivery, the effect that pregnancy may have on their disease and the effect that arthritis and its treatment may have on pregnancy and its outcome. As young people with chronic arthritis progress through adolescence, these issues should be considered and discussed with them.

Treatment with cyclophosphamide or chlorambucil may adversely affect fertility and sulphasalazine may produce reversible oligospermia.[58] There is no evidence that the disease itself or treatment with NSAIDs, methotrexate or corticosteroids has any adverse effect on fertility. Improvement in disease activity occurs in about 60% of pregnancies in women with active arthritis,[96] but transient disease flares 3–6 months after delivery are common, even in those with quiescent disease at conception and throughout pregnancy.

Methotrexate, cyclophosphamide and chlorambucil are all known to be teratogenic and should be withdrawn 3–6 months prior to attempting to conceive. Sulphasalazine is not known to have any teratogenic effects. Intra-articular corticosteroids and simple analgesics such as paracetamol are the treatment of choice for arthritis in pregnancy. NSAIDs are also sometimes used, but should be withdrawn in the last trimester because of potential adverse effects on the fetal circulation. Active systemic disease in pregnancy may necessitate systemic corticosteroid treatment, but high doses may produce fetal and neonatal adrenal suppression.

A recent review indicates that most women with juvenile onset arthritis have uneventful pregnancies[96] (see also Chapter 15, where this subject is covered in more detail). Bilateral hip involvement or hip replacement with a reduction in the range of movement may prevent vaginal delivery. Cervical spine and temporomandibular joint involvement may make intubation difficult should a general anaesthetic be required for surgical delivery. It goes without saying that caring for a baby and child may be more difficult for a person with functional impairment and disability.

PROGNOSIS OF JUVENILE IDIOPATHIC ARTHRITIS IN ADOLESCENCE AND ADULTHOOD

Persistent arthritis

We have recently completed a study of patients with juvenile-onset idiopathic arthritis aged 16 years and over who are still attending our follow-up clinic. At a median disease duration of 14.5 years and mean age of 20 years, 45% had persistent arthritis at their last examination and 81% of patients remained on medication for their arthritis. Although our clinic-based population is likely to include patients with more severe or persistent disease than is a population-based study, these figures do not differ greatly from other published studies in disparate populations. Wallace and Levinson[40] summarized six previous studies, and found that 31–55% of patients had active arthritis at least 10 years after disease onset. In our study population, 22% had had joint replacement(s), most commonly hip replacement, and 37% had undergone other orthopaedic operations as a result of their arthritis; 6.7% had a diagnosis of systemic amyloidosis.

Functional outcome

Despite the high incidence of continuing disease activity in our study population, 31% had no measured disability, as assessed by the modified Health Assessment Questionnaire (mHAQ):[97] mHAQ disability index (DI) score = 0. Previous authors who have also used the HAQ or Childhood Health Assessment Questionnaire (CHAQ) in disparate populations have found that up to 60% of patients have a DI score of 0 on prolonged follow-up.[98–101] Most of the earlier published studies on long-term outcome in juvenile-onset chronic arthritis have used the Steinbrocker classification.[102] Wallace and Levinson[40] have summarized the findings from 10 studies. Severe functional limitation (Steinbrocker class III or IV) was found in 9–48% of patients followed for an average of 10 years or more. Length of follow-up, and therefore disease duration, is important when considering outcome of arthritis, there being an increase in functional limitation with time,[40,103] and our study confirmed this, with a significant positive correlation between mHAQ DI and disease duration. Notably, however, in the study by Miller et al,[98] although 45% had measurable disability, 91% stated, when asked directly, that they had little or no disability. In David et al's study,[104] although 74% were disabled (Steinbrocker class II to IV), the distribution of scores on a self-rating problem scale was heavily biased towards experiencing no or very few problems. The development of adaptive coping skills or ways around problems are obviously of great importance to the outcome of disease in terms of quality of life. Assessment of health status and outcome is considered in detail in Chapter 3.

Vision

Chronic anterior uveitis is a particular feature of early onset oligoarthritis, with children who develop uveitis having a mean age of onset of arthritis of 5 years, and uveitis developing within 5 years of onset in 95% of children.[105] The risk of developing eye disease decreases over time but never completely disappears, and cases of uveitis developing for the first time 15–20 years after the onset of arthritis have been described. Regular slit lamp examination is mandatory in oligo-articular-onset disease in particular, as chronic uveitis is usually asymptomatic and can usually be treated successfully with corticosteroid and mydriatic eye drops. A recent follow-up study has shown that 24% of affected eyes develop complications (21% cataracts and 9% glaucoma), but only 15% of affected eyes had impaired vision (corrected acuity 20/50 or worse),[105] compared with the earlier figure of more than 50% before the routine use of topical steroids.[8]

Education and employment

Lovell et al[106] report an average school absence rate for children with chronic arthritis of 12 days per school year, compared with a national average of 5 days per year. In our study population, who were still at school, the mean number of school days missed over the preceding year was 20. Maximizing school attendance and attention to in-hospital education during in-patient stays is obviously of great importance throughout a child's school life, but never more so than during the examination periods of adolescence in the UK. Of course, school attendance is also of importance in the broader social and emotional development of children and adolescents with arthritis and to prevent isolation from their peer groups. In the UK, a statement of special educational needs can empower an individual to obtain extra assistance in the classroom setting. This may include help with mobility around the school site and to and from school, as well as the provision of appropriate equipment, such as a portable word processor or computer for children with difficulties in writing because of hand involvement. Extra time or the provision of a scribe can also be arranged for national school examinations. Specialist careers advice can be arranged at secondary level schooling and, after age 14 years, the Annual Review for a pupil with special educational needs should include a Transition Plan for the move into further education. Educational issues for adolescents with arthritis as they pertain in the USA are described in Chapter 14.

School examination results achieved by our study population were at least as good as the national average. Miller et al[98] found that the last grade of school attained by 50 adults in the USA who had had arthritis in childhood was equal to that of matched siblings, and Peterson et al[100] found that there was no difference in the percentage of arthritis patients versus controls completing high school. Hill et al[107] found that almost twice as many patients completed 1 year of university education than members of the general population of British Columbia. White and Shear[2] conducted a survey of 242 adult patients with juvenile-onset arthritis and other rheumatic diseases, and found that by age 25 years, 27% had completed 4 years or more of university training compared with 7% of the comparable general population of the Cincinnati metropolitan area.

A significantly higher proportion of our study population than the calculated national average described themselves as unemployed, a pattern that has not been described by most other authors. The high unemployment rate in our study population was despite excellent school examination results and was not related to the degree of functional impairment. Unemployment rates similar to the general population[99,107,108] or similar to matched siblings[98] have been found in other studies of juvenile-onset arthritis patients in adulthood. However, in their study of 43 adults with juvenile-onset polyarticular arthritis, David et al[104] found an unemployment rate of 30%. Like us, they were studying a somewhat biased population – those still attending hospital follow-up – and this may account to some degree for the apparent discrepancy between studies.

Shields et al[109] described 'vocational immaturity' in adolescents with rheumatic disease and stressed the importance of early and appropriate career counselling and vocational training schemes. Centres in the USA have instituted programmes of career education and habilitation specifically for children and adolescents with rheumatic disease.[2] In the UK, there is as yet no coordinated effort to address this issue. The support groups Young Arthritis Care and the Children's Chronic Arthritis Association both have embryonic but vital programmes including guidance and, in particular, mentoring for young people with chronic arthritis.

PSYCHOSOCIAL AND SEXUAL ISSUES

The incidence of depression and psychological problems in adolescents with arthritis has not been widely studied. Evidence of psychological dysfunctioning was found by Baildam et al[110] in 8 of 29 children with chronic arthritis aged 7–16 years, but only one child had significant evidence of depression. David et al[104] demonstrated a high frequency of depression among adults with juvenile-onset polyarticular arthritis, and this increased with the degree of disability. However, McAnarney et al[111] discovered that, in childhood, those patients with no disability had more emotional problems than disabled patients or controls. Having a child with chronic arthritis affects the whole family,[112,113] and family functioning also has effects on the outcome of arthritis.[113] Resistance factors within the family setting that predict better psychologic outcome include positive family support systems and family cohesion. Maternal depression, external stresses and lower family financial and educational status correlate with poorer psychosocial outcome, and should be indications for early psychosocial intervention and support. Wirrell et al[108] studied 61 young adults with juvenile-onset arthritis (mean age 23.4 years; range 18–31 years) using the RAND 36-Item Health Survey quality of life questionnaire. Scores were lower than average for physical functioning, but normal for emotional well-being, pain, energy and general health. Perceived social functioning scores, however, were more than one standard deviation below the mean but did not correlate with degree of physical disability or arthritis subtype. The authors stress the importance of addressing issues of self-esteem and coping skills in patients with all degrees of disability.

There are few studies that have looked specifically at sexual issues in juvenile-onset arthritis, which are covered in more detail in Chapter 15. Hill et al[107] surveyed 58 adults aged 19–37 years, at an average of 14.5 years after onset of arthritis. Fifty-two were interviewed by a sexual counsellor. Twenty-four were married or in long-term common-law relationships, all of whom were having sex regularly, although 16 reported limitation by pain, position or fatigue. Thirty-one were single, but over half (17) were having regular sexual intercourse, although 8 reported the same limitations. Severity of disease was a factor, with limitation of sexual activity being more common in those in Steinbrocker functional class III or IV. Thirty-eight per cent of those surveyed indicated a wish for further sexual counselling.

This underlines the importance of appropriate, sensitive and timely discussion of sexual issues. Teenagers, although often concerned about sex and relationships, may find it extremely difficult to initiate appropriate discussion, especially in a formal clinic setting and when accompanied by their parents. In the UK, Arthritis Care produce booklets entitled *Our Relationships, Our Sexuality* and *The Ruff Guide to Life for Young People with Arthritis*, which should be freely available in clinics where adolescents with chronic arthritis are seen. These are written for and by young people with arthritis, and explore many of the relevant issues. Young Arthritis Care also organizes local groups around the UK for mutual support and information sharing.

CONCLUSIONS

Arthritis in adolescence is a challenge for the entire multidisciplinary team. The disease itself may be particularly aggressive when it starts in adolescence. Chronic disease, with its origin in earlier childhood, may present new management problems in adolescence, of medical as well as psychological origin. To achieve the best possible outcome in the adolescent with arthritis, a holistic approach to management is essential. As well as concentrating on minimizing the impairments and disability with which our patients enter adult life, we also need to pay attention to broader quality-of-life issues by means of appropriate training, counselling and support for affected individuals and their families.

REFERENCES

1. Symmons P, Jones M, Osborne J, Sills J, Southwood T, Woo P. Pediatric rheumatology in the United Kingdom: data from the British Pediatric Rheumatology Group National Diagnostic Register. *Br J Rheumatol* 1996; **23**:1975–80.
2. White P, Shear E. Transition/job readiness for adolescents with juvenile arthritis and other chronic illness. *J Rheumatol* 1992; **19**(suppl 33):23–7.
3. Zirinsky L. The psychological impact of illness in adolescence. In: *The Practice of Medicine in Adolescence* (Brook C, ed). Edward Arnold: London, 1993:25–34.
4. White P. Paediatric rheumatology. Editorial: Future expectations: adolescents with rheumatic diseases and their transition into adulthood. *Br J Rheumatol* 1996; **35**:80–3.
5. Wood P. Nomenclature and classification of arthritis in children. In: *The Care of Rheumatic Children* (Munthe E, ed). EULAR: Basle, 1978:47–50.
6. Brewer E, Bass J, Baum J. Current proposed revision of JRA criteria. *Arthritis Rheum* 1977; **20**:S195–9.
7. Petty R. Classification of childhood arthritis: 1897–1997. *Rev Rhum (Engl Ed)* 1997; **64**: S161–2.
8. Smiley W. The eye in juvenile rheumatoid arthritis. *Trans Ophthal Soc UK* 1974; **94**:817–28.
9. Evans-Jones G, Fielder A, Jones R, Markham R, Stewart-Brown S. *Ophthalmic Services for Children*. The Royal College of Ophthalmologists and the British Paediatric Association: London, 1994.
10. Burgos-Vargas R, Pacheco-Tena C, Vazquez-Mellado J. Juvenile-onset spondyloarthropathies. *Rheum Dis Clin North Am* 1997; **23**:569–98.
11. Goodman J, McGrath P. The epidemiology of pain in children and adolescents. *Pain* 1991; **46**:247–64.
12. Gedalia A, Press J. Articular symptoms in hypermobile schoolchildren: a prospective study. *J Pediatr* 1991; **119**:944–6.
13. Southwood T, Sills J. Non-arthritic locomotor disorders in childhood. In: *Practical Problems, Series 2, No. 24, Reports on Rheumatic Diseases*, Arthritis and Rheumatism Council: Chesterfield, 1993.
14. Southwood T. Recent developments in the understanding of paediatric musculoskeletal pain syndromes. *Ann Rheum Dis* 1993; **52**: 490–2.
15. Brazier D, Venning H. Conversion disorders in adolescents: a practical approach to rehabilitation. *Br J Rheumatol* 1997; **36**:594–8.
16. Yunus M, Masi A. Juvenile primary fibromyalgia syndrome: a clinical study of thirty-three patients and matched normal controls. *Arthritis Rheum* 1985; **28**:138–44.

17. Schaller J. Arthritis as a presenting manifestation of malignancy in children. *J Pediatr* 1972; **81**:793–7.

18. Hughes R, Tempos K, Ansell B. A review of the diagnoses of hip pain presentation in the adolescent. *Br J Rheumatol* 1988; **27**:450–3.

19. Tertti M, Salminen J, Paajanen H, Terho PH, Kormono MJ. Low back pain and disk degeneration in children: a case control MR imaging study. *Radiology* 1991; **180**:503–7.

20. Fairbank J, Pynsent P, Van Poortvliet J, Phillips H. Influence of anthropometric factors and joint laxity in the incidence of adolescent back pain. *Spine* 1984; **9**:461–4.

21. Peterson L, Mason T, Nelson A, O'Fallon W, Gabriel S. Juvenile rheumatoid arthritis in Rochester, Minnesota 1960–1993. Is the epidemiology changing? *Arthritis Rheum* 1996; **39**:1385–90.

22. Oen K, Fast M, Postl B. Epidemiology of juvenile rheumatoid arthritis in Manitoba, Canada, 1975–92: cycles in incidence. *J Rheumatol* 1995; **22**:745–50.

23. Prieur A, Stavropoulos-Giokas C, Germinis A et al. Juvenile chronic arthritis (JCA): 12th International Histocompatibility Workshop study. In: *Proceedings of the Twelfth International Histocompatibility Workshop and Conference* (Charron D, ed). EDK: Paris, 1997:398–407.

24. Donn R, Ollier W. Juvenile chronic arthritis – a time for change? *Eur J Immunogenet* 1996; **23**:245–60.

25. Paul C, Schoenwald U, Truckenbrodt H et al. HLA-DP/DR interaction in early onset pauciarticular juvenile chronic arthritis. *Immunogenetics* 1993; **37**:442–8.

26. Miller LC, Lynch EA, Isa S, Logan JW, Dinarello CA, Steere AC. Balance of synovial fluid IL-1b and IL-1ra and recovery from Lyme arthritis. *Lancet* 1993; **341**:146–8.

27. McDowell T, Symons J, Ploski R, Forre O, Duff G. A genetic association between juvenile rheumatoid arthritis and a novel interleukin-1α polymorphism. *Arthritis Rheum* 1995; **38**:221–8.

28. Life P, Hassell A, Williams K et al. Responses to Gram-negative enteric bacterial antigens by synovial T cell from patients with juvenile chronic arthritis: recognition of heat shock protein HSP60. *J Rheumatol* 1993; **20**:1388–96.

29. de Graeff-Meeder ER, van Eden W, Rijkers GT et al. Juvenile chronic arthritis: T cell reactivity to human HSP60 in patients with a favorable course of arthritis. *J Clin Invest* 1995; **95**:934–40.

30. Lovell D, Giannini E, Brewer E. Time course of response to nonsteroidal anti-inflammatory drugs in patients with juvenile rheumatoid arthritis. *Arthritis Rheum* 1984; **27**:1433–7.

31. Lindsley C. Uses of nonsteroidal anti-inflammatory drugs in pediatrics. *Am J Dis Child* 1993; **147**:229–36.

32. Levy M, Barron K, Eichenfield A, Honig P. Naproxen-induced pseudoporphyria: a distinctive photodermatitis. *J Pediatr* 1990; **117**:660–4.

33. Allen R, Rogers M, Humphrey I. Naproxen induced pseudoporphyria in juvenile chronic arthritis. *J Rheumatol* 1991; **18**:893–6.

34. Allen R, Gross K, Laxer R, Malleson P, Beauchamp R, Petty R. Intra-articular triamcinolone hexacetonide in the management of chronic arthritis in children. *Arthritis Rheum* 1986; **29**:997–1001.

35. Schaller J. Drug therapy in adolescents with rheumatic diseases. *Rev Rhum (Engl Ed)* 1997; **64**:S194–5.

36. Markham A, Bryson H. Deflazacort: a review of its pharmacological properties and therapeutic efficacy. *Drugs* 1995; **50**:317–33.

37. Loftus J, Allen R, Hesp R et al. Randomized, double-blind trial of deflazacort versus prednisolone in juvenile chronic (or rheumatoid) arthritis: a relatively bone-sparing effect of deflazacort. *Pediatrics* 1991; **88**:428–36.

38. Miller J. Prolonged use of large intravenous steroid pulses in the rheumatic diseases of children. *Pediatrics* 1980; **65**:989–94.

39. Klein-Gitelman M, Pachman L. IV pulse corticosteroids (CS): adverse reactions are more variable than expected in children. *Arthritis Rheum* 1995; **38**:S338.

40. Wallace C, Levinson J. Juvenile rheumatoid arthritis: outcome and treatment for the 1990s. *Rheumatic Dis Clin North Am* 1991; **17**:891–905.

41. Harel L. Wagner-Weiner L, Poznanski A, Spencer C, Ekwo E, Magilavy D. Effects of methotrexate on radiologic progression in juvenile rheumatoid arthritis. *Arthritis Rheum* 1993; **10**:1370–4.

42. Giannini EH, Brewer EJ, Kuzmina N et al. Methotrexate in resistant juvenile rheumatoid arthritis. Results of the USA–USSR double-blind, placebo-controlled trial. The Pediatric Rheumatology Collaborative Study Group and the Cooperative Children's Study Group. *N Engl J Med* 1992; **326**:1043–9.

43. Woo P, Wilkes H, Southwood T, Prieur A-M. Low dose methotrexate is effective in extended oligoarticular arthritis but not in systemic arthritis of children. *Arthritis Rheum* 1997; **40**:S47.

44. Wallace C, Bleyer W, Sherry D, Salmonson K. Toxicity and serum levels of methotrexate in children with juvenile rheumatoid arthritis. *Arthritis Rheum* 1989; **32**:677–81.

45. Jundt J, Browne B, Fiocco G, Steele A, Mock D. A comparison of low dose methotrexate bioavailability: oral solution, oral tablet, subcutaneous and intramuscular dosing. *J Rheumatol* 1993; **20**:1845–9.

46. Wallace C, Sherry D. A practical approach to avoidance of methotrexate toxicity. *J Rheumatol* 1995; **22**:1009–12.

47. Brooks P, Spruil W, Parish R, Birchmore D. Pharmacokinetics of methotrexate administered by intramuscular and subcutaneous injections in patients with rheumatoid arthritis. *Arthritis Rheum* 1990; **33**:91–4.

48. Giannini E, Cassidy J. Methotrexate in juvenile rheumatoid arthritis – do the benefits outweigh the risks? *Drug Safety* 1993; **9**:325–39.

49. Graham L, Myones B, Rivas-Chacon R, Pachman L. Morbidity associated with long-term methotrexate therapy in juvenile rheumatoid arthritis. *J Pediatr* 1992; **120**:468–73.

50. Muzaffer M, Schneider R, Cameron B, Silverman E, Laxer R. Accelerated nodulosis during methotrexate therapy for juvenile rheumatoid arthritis. *J Pediatr* 1996; **128**:698–700.

51. Dupuis L, Koren G, Shore A, Silverman E, Laxer R. Methotrexate–nonsteroidal anti-inflammatory drug interaction in children with arthritis. *J Rheumatol* 1990; **17**:1469–73.

52. Wallace C, Smith A, Sherry D. Pilot investigation of naproxen/methotrexate interaction in patients with juvenile rheumatoid arthritis. *J Rheumatol* 1993; **20**:1764–8.

53. Ravelli A, Viola S, Ramenghi B, Aramini L, Ruperto N, Martini A. Frequency of relapse after discontinuation of methotrexate therapy for clinical remission in juvenile rheumatoid arthritis. *J Rheumatol* 1995; **22**:1574–6.

54. Van Rossum M, Fiselier T, Franssen M et al. Sulfasalazine in the treatment of juvenile chronic arthritis. *Rev Rhum (Engl Ed)* 1997; **64**:S247.

55. Dougados M, Van der Linden S, Leirisalo-Repo M et al. Sulfasalazine in the treatment of spondyloarthropathy: a randomized, double-blind, placebo-controlled study. *Arthritis Rheum* 1995; **38**:618–27.

56. Ansell B, Hall M, Loftus J et al. A multicentre pilot study of sulphasalazine in juvenile chronic arthritis. *Clin Exp Rheumatol* 1991; **9**:201–3.

57. Hertzberger-ten Cate R, Cats A. Toxicity of sulphasalazine in juvenile chronic arthritis. *Clin Exp Rheumatol* 1991; **9**:85–8.

58. Riley S, Lecarpentier J, Mani V, Goodman M, Mandal B, Turnberg L. Sulphasalazine induced seminal abnormalities in ulcerative colitis: results of mesalazine substitution. *Gut* 1987; **28**:1008–12.

59. Brewer E, Giannini E, Kuzmina N et al. Penicillamine and hydroxychloroquine in the treatment of severe juvenile rheumatoid arthritis. Results of the USA/USSR double-blind placebo-controlled trial. *N Engl J Med* 1986; **314**:1269–76.

60. Silman A, Shipley M. Ophthalmological monitoring for hydroxychloroquine toxicity: a scientific review of available data. *Br J Rheumatol* 1997; **36**:599–601.

61. Giannini E, Cassidy J, Brewer E, Shaikov A, Maximov A, Kuzmina N. Comparative efficacy and safety of advanced drug therapy in children with juvenile rheumatoid arthritis. *Semin Arthritis Rheum* 1993; **23**:34–46.

62. Giannini E, Brewer EJ, Kuzmina N. Auranofin in the treatment of juvenile rheumatoid arthritis. *Arthritis Rheum* 1990; **33**:466–76.

63. Ostensen M, Hoyeraal H, Kass E. Tolerance of cyclosporine A in children with refractory juvenile rheumatoid arthritis. *J Rheumatol* 1988; **15**:1536–38.

64. Pistoia V, Buoncompagni A, Scribanis R et al. Cyclosporin A in the treatment of juvenile chronic arthritis and childhood polymyositis. Results of a preliminary study. *Clin Exp Rheumatol* 1993; **11**:203–8.

65. Stephan J, Zeller J, Hubert P, Herbelin C, Dayer J, Prieur A. Macrophage activation syndrome and rheumatic disease in childhood: a report of four new cases. *Clin Exp Rheumatol* 1993; **11**:451–6.

66. Shaikov A, Maximov A, Speransky A, Lovell D, Giannini E, Solovyev S. Repetitive use of pulse therapy with methylprednisolone and cyclophosphamide in addition to oral methotrexate in children with systemic juvenile rheumatoid arthritis – preliminary results of a long term study. *J Rheumatol* 1992; **19**:612–16.

67. Silverman ED, Cawkwell GD, Lovell DJ et al. Intravenous immunoglobulin in the treatment of systemic onset juvenile rheumatoid arthritis: a randomized placebo controlled trial. *J Rheumatol* 1994; **21**:2353–8.

68. Elliot M, Woo P, Charles P, Long-Fox A, Woody J, Maini R. Treatment of systemic onset juvenile chronic arthritis (JCA) with monoclonal anti-TNFα.

Temporary control of systemic but not articular features of disease. *Arthritis Rheum* 1994; **37**:S276.

69. Bacon M, White P, Raiten D et al. Nutritional status and growth in juvenile rheumatoid arthritis. *Semin Arthritis Rheum* 1990; **20**:97–106.

70. Fraser P, Hoch S, Erlandson D, Partridge R, Jackson J. The timing of menarche in juvenile rheumatoid arthritis. *J Adolesc Health Care* 1988; **9**:483–7.

71. Stanhope R. Endocrinology. In: *The Practice of Medicine in Adolescence* (Brook C, ed). Edward Arnold: London, 1993:120–46.

72. Davies U, Rooney M, Preece M, Ansell B, Woo P. Treatment of growth retardation in juvenile chronic arthritis with recombinant growth hormone. *J Rheumatol* 1994; **21**:153–8.

73. Cassidy J, Hillman L. Abnormalities in skeletal growth in children with juvenile rheumatoid arthritis. *Rheum Dis Clin North Am* 1997; **23**:499–522.

74. Sambrook P, Kelly P, White C et al. Genetic determinants of bone mass. In: *Osteoporosis* (Marcus R, Feldman D, Kelsey J, eds). Academic Press: New York, 1996:477–82.

75. Lloyd T, Andon M, Rollings N et al. Calcium supplementation and bone mineral density in adolescent girls. *JAMA* 1993; **270**:841–4.

76. Cadogan J, Eastell R, Jones N, Barker M. Milk intake and bone mineral acquisition in adolescent girls: randomised, controlled intervention trial. *Br Med J* 1997; **315**:1255–60.

77. Welten D, Kemper H, Post G. Weight-bearing activity during youth is a more important factor for peak bone mass than calcium intake. *J Bone Miner Res* 1994; **9**:1089–96.

78. Hopp R, Degan J, Gallagher J, Cassidy J. Estimation of bone mineral density in children with juvenile rheumatoid arthritis. *J Rheumatol* 1991; **18**:1235–9.

79. Pepmueller P, Cassidy J, Allen S, Hillman L. Bone mineralization and bone mineral metabolism in children with juvenile rheumatoid arthritis. *Arthritis Rheum* 1996; **39**:746–57.

80. Reed A, Haugen M, Pachman L, Langman C. Abnormalities in serum osteocalcin values in children with chronic rheumatic diseases. *J Pediatr* 1990; **116**:574–80.

81. Reed A, Haugen M, Pachman L, Langman C. Repair of osteopenia in children with juvenile rheumatoid arthritis. *J Pediatr* 1993; **122**:693–6.

82. Abrams S, Lipnick R, Vieira N, Stuff J, Yergey A. Calcium absorption and metabolism in children with juvenile rheumatoid arthritis assessed using stable isotopes. *J Rheumatol* 1993; **20**:1196–200.

83. Bianchi ML, Bardare M, Caraceni MP et al. Bone metabolism in juvenile rheumatoid arthritis. *Bone Miner* 1990; **9**:153–62.

84. Warady B, Lindsley C, Robinson R, Luhert B. Effects of nutritional supplementation on bone mineral status of children with rheumatic diseases receiving corticosteroid therapy. *J Rheumatol* 1994; **21**:530–5.

85. Fantini F, Beltrametti P, Gallazzi M et al. Evaluation by dual-photon absorptiometry of bone mineral loss in rheumatic children on long-term treatment with corticosteroids. *Clin Exp Rheumatol* 1991; **9**:21–38.

86. Lepore L, Pennesi M, Barbi E, Pozzi R. Treatment and prevention of osteoporosis in juvenile chronic arthritis with disodium clodronate. *Clin Exp Rheumatol* 1991; **9**:33–5.

87. Falcini F, Bardare M, Zulian F et al. Alendronate improves bone mass in children with connective tissue diseases: preliminary results of a multicenter study. *Arthritis Rheum* 1997; **40**:S240.

88. Woo P. AA amyloidosis. In: *Topical Reviews, Series 3, No. 8, Reports on Rheumatic Diseases*, Arthritis and Rheumatism Council: Chesterfield, 1996.

89. Stoeber E. Prognosis in juvenile chronic arthritis: follow-up of 433 chronic rheumatic children. *Eur J Pediatr* 1981; **135**:225–8.

90. Schnitzer T, Ansell B. Amyloidosis in juvenile chronic polyarthritis. *Arthritis Rheum* 1977; **20**:245–52.

91. Filipowicz-Sosnowska A, Restropowiicz-Denisfewicz K, Rosenthal C, Baum J. The amyloidosis of juvenile rheumatoid arthritis. Comparative studies in Polish and American children. *Arthritis Rheum* 1978; **21**:699–703.

92. Savolainen H, Ylijoki H. Declining prevalence of secondary amyloidosis in JCA. *Clin Exp Rheumatol* 1995; **13**:551.

93. Woo P, O'Brien J, Robson M, Ansell B. A genetic marker for systemic amyloidosis in juvenile arthritis. *Lancet* 1987; **ii**:767–9.

94. David J, Vouyiouka O, Ansell B, Hall A, Woo P. Amyloidosis in juvenile chronic arthritis: a morbidity and mortality study. *Clin Exp Rheumatol* 1993; **11**:85–90.

95. Hawkins P. Diagnosis and monitoring of amyloidosis. *Baillières Clin Rheumatol* 1994; **8**:635–59.

96. Ostensen M. Problems related to pregnancy in

patients with juvenile chronic arthritis. *Rev Rhum (Engl Ed)* 1997; **64**:S196–7.

97. Pincus T, Summey J, Soraci SJ, Wallston K, Hummon N. Assessment of patient satisfaction in activities of daily living using a modified Stanford Health Assessment Questionnaire. *Arthritis Rheum* 1983; **26**:1346–53.

98. Miller J, Spitz P, Simpson U, Williams G. The social function of young adults who had arthritis in childhood. *J Pediatr* 1982; **100**:378–82.

99. Andersson Gare B, Fasth A. The natural history of juvenile chronic arthritis: a population based cohort study. II. Outcome. *J Rheumatol* 1995; **22**(2):308–19.

100. Peterson L, Mason T, Nelson A, O'Fallon W, Gabriel S. Psychosocial outcomes and health status of adults who have had juvenile rheumatoid arthritis: a controlled, population based study. *Arthritis Rheum* 1997; **40**:2235–40.

101. Ruperto N, Levinson J, Ravelli A et al. Long-term health outcomes and quality of life in American and Italian inception cohorts of patients with juvenile rheumatoid arthritis. I. Outcome status. *J Rheumatol* 1997; **24**:945–51.

102. Steinbrocker O, Traeger C, Batterman R. Therapeutic criteria in rheumatoid arthritis. *JAMA* 1949; **140**:659–62.

103. Laaksonen AI. A prognostic study of juvenile rheumatoid arthritis: analysis of 544 cases. *Acta Paediatr Scand* 1966; **166**:1–163.

104. David J, Cooper C, Hickey L et al. The functional and psychological outcomes of juvenile chronic arthritis in young adulthood. *Br J Rheumatol* 1994; **33**:876–81.

105. Cabral DA, Petty RE, Malleson PN, Ensworth S, McCormick AQ, Shroeder M-L. Visual prognosis in children with chronic anterior uveitis and arthritis. *J Rheumatol* 1994; **21**:2370–5.

106. Lovell D, Athreya B, Emery H et al. School attendance and patterns, special services and special needs in pediatric patients with rheumatic diseases. *Arthritis Care Res* 1990; **3**:196–203.

107. Hill R, Herstein A, Walters K. Juvenile rheumatoid arthritis: follow-up into adulthood – medical, sexual and social status. *Can Med Assoc J* 1976; **114**:790–6.

108. Wirrell E, Lang B, Camfield C. Social outcome in young adults with juvenile rheumatoid arthritis. *Arthritis Rheum* 1995; **38**:S184.

109. Shields C, Gaumond M, White P. Vocational maturity in adolescents with rheumatic diseases. *Arthritis Rheum* 1987; **30**:S210.

110. Baildam E, Holt P, Conway S, Morton M. The association between physical function and psychological problems in children with juvenile chronic arthritis. *Br J Rheumatol* 1995; **34**: 470–7.

111. McAnarney E, Pless I, Satterwhite B, Friedman S. Psychological problems of children with chronic juvenile arthritis. *Pediatrics* 1974; **53**:523–8.

112. Miller J. Psychosocial factors related to rheumatic diseases in childhood. *J Rheumatol* 1993; **20**:1–11.

113. McCormick M, Stemmler M, Athreya B. The impact of childhood rheumatic diseases on the family. *Arthritis Rheum* 1986; **29**:872–9.

6

Juvenile spondyloarthropathies and other causes of back pain

Janet McDonagh

INTRODUCTION

This chapter considers the spectrum of diseases seen in adolescence which affect the axial skeleton. Back pain in this transitional period from childhood to adulthood presents the rheumatologist with diagnostic challenges, particularly with respect to the interrelationships between the juvenile and adult presentations of similar conditions.

JUVENILE SPONDYLOARTHROPATHIES

Classification

Classification of idiopathic arthritis in childhood is still in a state of flux with the recent International League Against Rheumatism (ILAR) classification[1] having only recently been proposed and currently awaiting validation. Juvenile spondyloarthropathy usually presents in early adolescence and is often difficult to classify. Initial symptoms are often vague, with axial involvement and associated symptoms (e.g. associated inflammatory bowel disease (IBD)) often occurring many years after the onset of the peripheral arthritis. Presentation and/or diagnosis may therefore be delayed. Furthermore, the rate of misdiagnosis in this group has been reported to be 20%.[2,3]

Epidemiology

The incidence of juvenile spondyloarthropathies has been determined in Canadian children as 1.14 per 100 000 per year,[4] and a similar incidence has been reported by the British Paediatric Rheumatology Group National Diagnostic Register.[5] Juvenile spondyloarthropathy is the most common type of juvenile arthritis in North American Indian, Mexican and other non-Causcasian children.[6,7]

Clinical

There are two main subsets of spondyloarthropathies to be considered: the seronegative, enthesopathy and arthropathy (SEA) syndrome[8] and juvenile ankylosing spondylitis (JAS). The large 'undifferentiated' group of children will also be discussed. In these patients, enthesopathy is often a helpful distinguishing feature, only occasionally being seen in other juvenile arthritides and systemic lupus erythematosus (SLE),[9] and hence the new diagnostic grouping of 'enthesitis-related arthritides' (Table 6.1).[1] Enthesopathy is a more common feature in paediatric than in adult rheumatology practice, and is a cause of significant pain and disability.

The SEA syndrome
The SEA syndrome defines a group of children with enthesitis and arthralgia/arthritis and who are seronegative for both rheumatoid factor and antinuclear antibody.[8] Other features of this group include: a male preponderance, no axial involvement and compared to JAS, a lower

Table 6.1   Proposed ILAR classification of enthesitis-related arthritis[1]

1. Arthritis and enthesitis, or
2. Arthritis and at least two of the following:
    (i)   sacroiliac joint tenderness
    (ii)   inflammatory spinal pain
    (iii) HLA B27
    (iv)   positive family history (first- or second-
           degree relatives) of at least one of:
           (a) anterior uveitis with pain, redness or
                photophobia
           (b) spondyloarthropathy confirmed by a
                rheumatologist
           (c) inflammatory bowel disease
    (v)   anterior uveitis, which is usually associated
           with pain, redness or photophobia

Specific exclusions:
1. Excludes IBD related and reactive arthritis,
    juvenile psoriatic arthritis
2. Positive rheumatoid factor/antinuclear antibody

IBD, inflammatory bowel disease; HLA, human leucocyte antigen.

prevalence human leucocyte antigen (HLA) B27, a more frequent positive family history of arthritis (65% vs 25%, respectively), and a variable disease progression.[8,10–13]

When such children are followed-up into adulthood, the majority develop a spondyloarthropathy, although at varying rates.[10,11] Burgos-Vargas and Vazquez-Mellaod[14] reported that the highest risk factor for the development of JAS in such patients was severe persistent arthritis in five or more peripheral joints within the first year of illness.

Juvenile ankylosing spondylitis
The male preponderance in JAS becomes more obvious after puberty, raising the possibility of hormonal effects in disease pathogenesis. However, there may be a higher incidence of

JAS among females than previously thought.[15] The symptom pattern at onset is different from that in other juvenile arthritides (Table 6.2) and in adult ankylosing spondylitis (Table 6.3). Regardless of the occurrence of axial involvement, two distinct features distinguish JAS from other juvenile arthritides: enthesopathy (mainly involving the feet), and involvement of the tarsal joints.[14] Furthermore, isolated hip arthritis can be a presenting or early feature.[16] When there is upper-limb involvement, the small joints of the hand are least commonly affected.[14] In terms of juvenile versus adult forms, age at onset (and sex) appear to be the most important factor(s) influencing the clinical pattern of JAS.[17] Arthritis involving the tarsal and small joints of the feet is reported to be more frequent in the juvenile form of the disease.[17] However, involvement of the chest wall is seen less frequently in the latter.[18] Such differences help fuel debates about whether JAS and adult ankylosing spondylitis are the same, closely related, or JAS is indeed a distinct entity.

Axial involvement, both clinical and radiological, is the salient feature of adult onset ankylosing spondylitis but in JAS the opposite is true. Low back pain is unusual in JAS[14] and if sacroiliitis occurs, it is often late. Early signs may be subtle (e.g. loss of normal curve and/or hyperextension) and may be missed if not specifically looked for. In a study of Mexican patients, most children with JAS initially lacked significant axial involvement, with only 15% of patients affected within 1 year or less.[14] None had sole axial symptoms at onset, but all had developed axial disease within 10 years.[14] In JAS, pseudo-widening of the inferior synovial portion of the sacroiliac joints is seen on radiographs due to erosions prior to sclerosis and subsequent fusion. In contrast, sacroiliitis in other subgroups of juvenile arthritis is non-erosive, but involves similar loss of joint space and sclerosis. In JAS, the changes are initially unilateral and are seen only in the adolescent (over 12 years old).[11] The changes increase with disease duration, with 20% of patients exhibiting changes at 3 years compared to over 90% at 5 years.[11] Cervical spine involvement is infrequent

Table 6.2   Comparison of clinical features at disease onset between juvenile ankylosing spondylitis (JAS) and other types of juvenile chronic arthritis (JCA)[14]

	JAS	JCA	p
Total No. patients	35 (100%)	75 (100%)	
At 6 months:			
Pauciarticular involvement	19 (54.3%)	30.7	0.03
Enthesopathy	29 (82.9%)	0	< 0.0001
Tarsal involvement	25 (71.4%)	1.3	< 0.0001
Lumbosacral involvement	4 (11.4%)	0	0.02
At 12 months:			
Polyarticular involvement	28 (80%)	58 (77.3%)	NS
Enthesopathy	31 (88.6%)	3 (4%)	< 0.0001
Tarsal involvement	30 (85.7%)	8 (10.7%)	< 0.0001
Knee	35 (100%)	62 (82.7%)	0.04
Upper limb	13 (37.1%)	60 (80%)	< 0.0001
Lumbosacral involvement	5 (14.3%)	3 (4%)	NS

NS, not significant.

Table 6.3   Comparison of juvenile (JAS) and adult (AAS) forms of ankylosing spondylitis[17]

	JAS	AAS	p
Total No. patients	42 (100%)	15 (100%)	
Symptoms at onset:			
Peripheral arthritis	42 (89.4%)	15 (37.5%)	< 0.0001
Enthesopathy	30 (63.8%)	11 (27.5%)	0.001
Axial	11 (23.4%)	33 (82.5%)	< 0.0001
Peripheral arthritis (ever)	47 (100%)	23 (57.5%)	< 0.0001
Enthesopathy (ever)	37 (78.7%)	19 (47.5%)	0.005

and, when it occurs, follows lumbar spine involvement.[9] Atlantoaxial subluxation can occur, and neurological symptomatology and signs need to be borne in mind during follow-up of such patients.[9,19]

Extra-articular manifestations
Iritis appears to be less common than in the adult forms but is similarly acute, rarely preceding musculoskeletal manifestations and rarely causing residual deficit.[9]

The presence of diarrhoea and/or urethritis raises the possibility of IBD-associated arthritis or Reiter's disease (see below). Skin manifestations such as pyoderma gangrenosum, keratoderma blenorrhagicum and psoriasis similarly raise the possibility of alternative diagnoses.

Rare manifestations, including amyloidosis[20] and aortitis[21] have been reported.

Disease outcome

The outcome of the SEA syndrome has been discussed above. Peripheral joint disease tends to be more persistent than that seen in adults.[9] Reports of outcome are, however, variable.[22,23] Hip disease tends to be associated with poor outcome,[22] and may require a total hip replacement. Ectopic bone formation is seen more frequently after arthroplasty in such patients compared to other juvenile arthritides.[22] In view of the late axial involvement, follow-up of such patients must continue into adulthood.

Pathogenesis

There are two central foci of research into this group of diseases:

- Infective agents (enteric and/or genitourinary), which may be responsible for triggering and/or perpetuating juvenile spondyloarthropathy. At the present time there is evidence, but no proof, that this is true.
- A role for HLA B27 in this process. Some of the intriguing evidence reported to date is discussed below.

One theory is that juvenile spondyloarthropathies represent persistent reactive arthritides to enteric organisms. Supportive indirect evidence for this includes:

- The finding of inflammation at ileocolonoscopy, independent of non-steroidal anti-inflammatory drug (NSAID) usage, in 81% of patients with juvenile spondyloarthropathy.[24,25] HLA B27 may in turn be related to this inflammation (see below).[26]

- Reports of 7–20% of children with IBD developing arthritis[27–29] which responds to sulphasalazine (with a sulpha- antibiotic component).
- A dual binding capacity of mucosal lymphocytes to synovium and gut mucosa.[30]
- Demonstration of immune responses to enteric bacteria in the synovial compartment in juvenile spondyloarthropathies.[31]

The association with HLA B27 is well established, with HLA-B27-positive individuals 100 times more likely to develop arthritis after genitourinary or enteric infections.[32] Furthermore, 90% of B27-positive juvenile arthritis patients have synovial fluid lymphocyte populations that respond to enteric bacteria, compared with only 25% of B27-negative children.[31] HLA B27 may be directly involved in pathogenesis (e.g. the presentation of an arthritogenic peptide) or indirectly involved (e.g. linkage disequilibrium with another gene or reduced immune resistance to enteric bacteria at the level of antigen presentation).[33] The presence of HLA B27 cannot fully explain the development of ankylosing spondylitis. The majority of individuals with this antigen do not develop the disease, and B27-positive transgenic rats raised in sterile environments from birth did not develop arthritis.[34]

The link between infection and juvenile spondyloarthropathy may also involve molecular mimicry and cross-reactive immune responses (e.g. *Escherichia coli* heat shock protein 60 (hsp60); M Pugh, unpublished observations, 1996), although some reports dispute such hypotheses.[35] Research is ongoing in this area, and results are awaited with much interest.

OTHER JUVENILE ARTHRITIDES WITH AXIAL INVOLVEMENT

Juvenile psoriatic arthritis

Juvenile psoriatic arthritis is no longer considered as a juvenile spondyloarthropathy,[36] since it differs clinically, serologically and genetically from the latter as well as other arthritides in children. In contrast to juvenile spondyloarthropathy, juvenile psoriatic arthritis is more common in females, occurs in early childhood, exhibits a low frequency of enthesitis and lumbosacral involvement, and is often antinuclear antibody (ANA) positive.[37] In contrast to the association of adult psoriatic arthritis with HLA B27, several authors have found a normal frequency of HLA B27 in juvenile psoriatic arthritis,[36,37] although this has not been unanimous.[38]

IBD-associated arthritis

Of children with IBD, 7–21% develop arthritis, usually after diagnosis of the bowel disease.[27–29] Two patterns are seen.[9] The less common type is a HLA-B27-positive sacroiliitis and enthesitis with an oligoarticular lower limb arthritis and no relationship to bowel inflammatory activity. This form is the more likely to persist and progress despite control of the bowel disease and/or resection. The more common type is an oligo- or polyarticular arthritis with a predilection for the lower limbs.[9]

Reiter's disease

It is pertinent to include Reiter's disease in a book of adolescent rheumatology as one of the early descriptions was in a 16-year-old boy.[39] However, only a small minority of Reiter's disease cases is seen in the under 16 age group,[9] and only a third (35%) will have the classical triad of arthritis, urethritis and conjunctivitis.[40] The majority of patients are male (males/females 4 : 1)[41] and are mainly postdysenteric (*Shigella*, *Yersinia* or *Salmonella*), although sexually acquired reactive arthritis should be considered, particularly in this increasingly sexually active age group. Arthritis is seen in a quarter of patients, and is usually oligoarticular and asymmetrical, often with marked swelling affecting the lower limbs.[40] Enthesitis is seen in 58% and axial involvement in 23%, with 21% having radiological sacroiliitis.[40] HLA-B27-associated Reiter's disease (67%)[40] has been reported to be more protracted and systemic and to have a less favourable prognosis.[41] However 'juvenile Reiter's' generally has a good prognosis, with over half of patients going into

remission and the majority having no or minor disability at follow-up (mean duration of follow-up 28.6 months, range 2 months to 13.5 years).[40]

Other juvenile chronic arthritides

Arthritis involving the cervical spine is the main pattern of axial involvement in the remainder of the juvenile arthritides. However, vertebral fractures secondary to steroid-induced osteoporosis, growth retardation, and scoliosis secondary to unrecognized leg-length discrepancies need to be borne in mind.

The management of patients with juvenile spondyloarthropathy is given in Table 6.4.[9]

Finally, the following are important issues when considering inflammatory axial disease in adolescence as compared to adulthood:

- Measurement criteria for the axial joints, as used in adults, may not be directly comparable in childhood and adolescent disease (e.g. anterior spinal flexion[44] and chest expansion[18]).
- The differentiation of inflammatory and mechanical pain may be difficult in younger people, and may differ from that seen in adulthood.[45,46]
- Radiological criteria have a different impact on diagnosis (e.g. whereas radiological sacroiliitis is integral to the diagnosis of adult ankylosing spondylitis, it occurs much later after disease onset in children and adolescents, if at all[11]). Sacroiliac epiphyses do not fuse until age 21 years, and there is thus a potentially higher observer error in diagnosing sacroiliitis in adolescents in view of the normally wider joint space and indistinct subchondral margins during growth.[12]

NON-INFLAMMATORY BACK PAIN IN ADOLESCENCE

Epidemiology

There is a spectrum of opinion in the literature of back pain in childhood and adolescence which depends on the population studied. At one end

Table 6.4	Principles of management of juvenile spondyloarthropathies		

Drug therapy
- NSAID
- Sulphasalazine[42]
- Methotrexate[43]
- Steroids
  - intra-articular
  - injection of entheses
  - oral
  - topical (eye)

Disease education

Includes:
- Chronicity
- Possible complications
- Drug therapy
- Importance of exercise and physiotherapy
- Prognosis
- Importance of follow-up

Physiotherapy/occupational therapy/orthotics

Includes:
- Prevention of loss of range
- Maintenance of good posture
- Hydrotherapy
- Ultrasound
- Splints
- Insoles
- Heel raises/pads

Career advice

For example, avoidance of occupations stressful to the low back and lower limb joints

of the spectrum, authors of hospital-based studies recommend detailed assessment of all children with back pain because the experience was that it was an uncommon clinical presentation in this age group and serious underlying pathology was often found.[47–50] In contrast, large school-based surveys report a much higher prevalence (8–51%) of back pain among school children.[51–63] Interstudy variation in prevalence may be explained, at least in part, by study design. However, only a minority of young people (2–15%) seek medical help.[52,55,57,61,62]

Age and sex

The first episode of back pain usually occurs in the age range 13–14 years, tending to be earlier in males.[52] Thereafter, back pain is associated with increasing age,[51,54,55,52–63] as is recurrence of back pain.[62] There is a male predominance in prevalence, but no gender difference is observed in severity of pain.[62] However, sporting activities may be closely interrelated with gender differences (see below).

Family history

A positive family history is often seen but may be multifactorial (e.g. it may represent the presence of an underlying condition, such as spondylolisthesis,[64] disc herniation[65,66] or psychosocial factors.[55] A positive family history in parents and/or siblings may influence pain behaviour and coping strategies in a variety of ways. A significant association of child self-reported low back pain and parental back pain (treated) has been reported.[58,63] However, this is only significant in adolescents when both parents have low back pain.[63] and may indicate a more complex and precise understanding of pain in this age group.

Sports

Adolescence is often a period of increased (and often of new and/or varied) sporting activities (see also Chapter 12), and a corresponding increase in back pain has been reported.[61] However, it also appears to depend on what the activity is, the level of the athlete and their gender.

Sports involving twisting, hyperextension and bending (e.g. gymnastics, tennis, cycling and soccer[67–69]) are particularly associated with low back pain.

Balague et al[63] reported low back pain to be more common in competitive athletes (23.6%) compared with recreational athletes (15.8%). However, such pain is also increased at the other end of the activity spectrum (e.g. 'sport avoiders'[52] and 'less enthusiastic sportsmen'[62]).

The interrelationship of the gender difference with sporting activities has also been studied, and some authors have reported a positive link between sports and back pain only in boys,[55,62] in contrast to previous reports.[52,70]

Certain structural abnormalities (e.g. spondylolisthesis[69] and Scheuermann's disease[67]) have been reported to be more frequent in athletic teenagers. As well as finding more abnormalities on spinal radiographs of athletes compared to non-athletes,[67,69] different features have been reported in athletic individuals (e.g. Schmorl's nodes in athletes more frequently involved the anterior end-plate, possibly indicating a traumatic origin[67]).

In any study of athletic activity and back pain in adolescence it is important to remember the vulnerability of the growing spine with particular reference to the age of onset of athletic activity as well as any excess load on the spine and any direct trauma. The experience of pain in athletes may also differ from that of non-athletes, and may depend on individual susceptibility, level of motivation as well as the level of physical activity.

Anthropometric factors

Several studies have addressed the role of height, trunk length and weight in back pain in adolescents, with varying results.[52,56,71] Increased trunk length has been reported to be associated with low back pain.[52] The reported association of low back pain with time spent watching the television or time spent sitting[51,60] may be further supporting evidence for this hypothesis, and highlights possible areas for prevention (e.g. desk height and seating), particularly with regard to the increasing use of computers in this age group.

Other associations with low back pain in this age group include reduced spinal extension, reduced lower limb mobility,[52] reduced (back) muscle strength, particularly endurance strength,[56] and weak abdominal muscles.[58] However, association does not equal causality, and the possibility of a third unknown factor remains.

Relationship with back pain in adulthood

Although back pain in adolescence is common and recurrent, in general it does not deteriorate with time in the short term,[62] although some authors have reported a small subgroup of adolescents with more serious (long lasting or frequent) back pain.[72] However, the relationship with adult back pain remains unclear.[57,62,73] Harreby et al[73] used a prospective questionnaire based on a 25-year cohort study of 14 year olds (completion rate 83%). Eleven per cent of the cohort had a history of low back pain during adolescence; the lifetime prevalence of low back pain in these subjects as adults was 84%. Low back pain at age 14 years plus a positive family history of low back pain were highly associated with adult symptoms, with an 88% risk if both factors were present. Thirteen per cent of the total cohort had radiographic abnormalities (mainly of the Scheuermann's type), but these were not predictive of adult low back pain. An associated increased morbidity and reduced work capacity was observed in individuals with a history of low back pain during adolescence.[73]

This observation highlights the need for research into possible preventive measures in schools. Further prospective studies are needed, particularly in view of the high level of forgetfulness with regard to previous low back pain.[62]

DIFFERENTIAL DIAGNOSES OF BACK PAIN IN ADOLESCENCE

The differential diagnosis of back pain in adolescents differs from that in the very young child and in the adult (see below). A specific and/or serious cause has been reported to be found in 22–85% of children and adolescents.[74–77] Turner et al[74] reported that those with serious disease were usually over 12 years old and had clinical signs (e.g. neurological deficit, and reduced straight-leg raising). Urgent investigation is generally recommended in the very young, and in patients with persistent and/or increasing pain, associated weight loss, fever, radicular symptoms and sphincter disturbance. However, an underlying serious cause may present with only minor symptoms, and follow-up of patients in whom no cause can be identified is recommended. Further investigation is indicated if there is no response to appropriate therapy after 2 months.[78]

The main differential diagnoses fall into six categories:

- mechanical
- inflammatory
- infective
- neoplastic
- metabolic
- pain-amplification syndromes.

Mechanical causes of back pain

Spondylolysis and spondylolisthesis

These are the commonest identifiable causes of low back pain in adolescents.[79] The typical patient is an athletic, teenage boy. Reports of prevalence range from 2–7% in the general adolescent population, with a higher prevalence in certain athletic groups[67] (e.g. 11% in gymnasts[69]). Characteristically, spondylolysis

and spondylolisthesis occur after walking age, being uncommon in the under fives, with a peak at 20 years. It is more common in white populations,[77] and a familial pattern has been reported.[49,64]

Spondylolysis is a stress fracture of pars interarticularis and is seen on radiographs as a radiolucent defect, typically at L5.[80] A unilateral spondylolysis is not necessarily symptomatic and, if found in the presence of back pain, other causes of back pain should be considered. As unilateral spondsylolysis is not seen in non-ambulant patients,[81] it is thought to be acquired, particularly when lumbar lordosis is exaggerated, as occurs in vigorous training requiring repetitive flexion and extension (e.g. gymnastics, tennis and weight-lifting) and when more stress is placed on the pars. This is thought to lead to microfractures and subsequently to an overt fracture on one side (spondylolysis). However, a genetically weakened pars interarticularis has been proposed as a risk factor.[80] Spina bifida has been reported to be more frequent in these patients.[64,69,80]

The aims of the management of patients with spondylolysis are to reduce symptoms, prevent spondylolisthesis and facilitate return to premorbid activity. Advice regarding sporting activity (including avoidance) is vital. Conservative management includes analgesia and thoracolumbar bracing, but surgery (fusion) may be necessary (see below).

Once a spondylolysis has occurred, overloading of the intact side may occur subsequently and a bilateral spondylolysis may develop, and potentially a spondylolisthesis. The latter occurs in 50–60% of spondylolysis.[82] Neurological symptoms are uncommon due to the wide central canal in the young spine,[75] but patients may present with low back pain (characteristically exacerbated by hyperextension) and/or sciatica or tight hamstrings.[74,75] A degenerative L5/S1 disc has been reported in 25% of patients with a spondylolisthesis.[83] The former correlates with pain, which may indicate a discogenic rather than neuropathic origin.[83]

Unilateral spondylolysis may be missed on anteroposterior/lateral spine radiographs, and

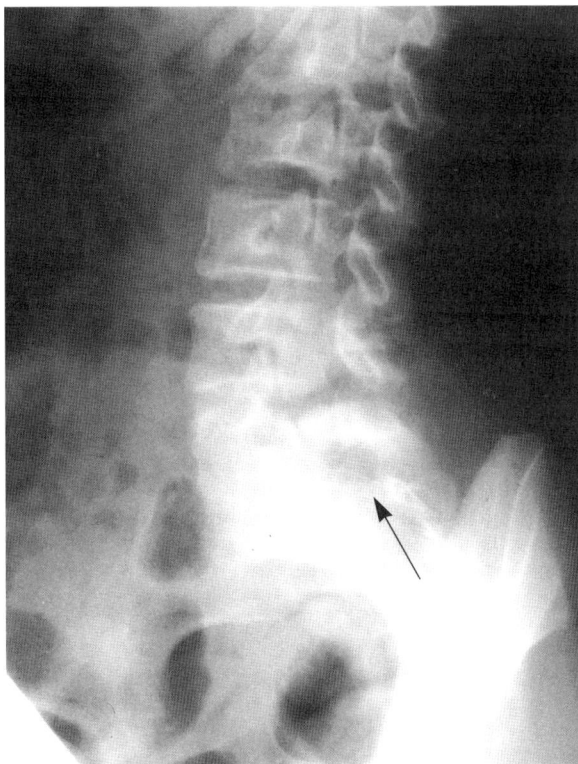

Figure 6.1 Oblique radiograph of the lumbar spine, showing L5 spondylolysis. The site of the missing collar of the 'Scottie dog' (i.e. the spondylolysis) is denoted by the arrow.

oblique views are the investigation of choice, when the famous 'Scottie dog' sign is seen (Figure 6.1). Flexion/extension views may be required to demonstrate any instability. If acute, the edges may look jagged and rough as compared with the elongated, sclerotic and smooth appearance of a chronic spondylolysis. The size of the gap depends on the degree of resorption and the presence or absence of a spondylolisthesis (see below). If the radiographs are normal and if symptoms have been present for less than 12 months, a bone scan will show increased uptake in the region of the metabolically active healing fracture. However, if the patient has been symptomatic for more than a year, a bone scan may be normal, and computed tomography (CT) or magnetic resonance imaging (MRI) are the investigations of choice.[84]

In general, spondylolisthesis in adolescence is benign, with a good prognosis.[80] In the absence of symptoms and a minimal slip, close monitoring (i.e. examination and radiographic investigation every 6 months during rapid growth periods) is all that is required. A spondylolisthesis of greater than 50% occurring before the growth spurt, progressive slip of greater than 30%, persistent pain, progressive scoliosis and/or neurological signs are indications for intervention.[79,83,85]

Scheuermann's disease

Scheuermann's disease is present in as many as 20–30% of the general population.[49] It is usually asymptomatic until the growth spurt and usually presents with back pain and/or deformity at age 11–15 years. It is more common in males and an increased prevalence has been reported in athletes.[67,82] It most commonly affects the thoracic spine (especially T7–10). The pain is characteristically worse at the end of the day and exacerbated by forward flexion and exercise and relieved by rest. The deformity is a fixed kyphosis, which increases on bending. Scheuermann's disease of the lumbar spine is less common, and is thought to be more painful[49] and more frequently associated with trauma.[67]

The diagnosis is both clinical and radiological (Figure 6.2), the latter being made according to the Bradford criteria:[86]

- one or more vertebrae with wedging of at least 5°
- irregular superior and inferior end-plates
- narrowing of disc spaces
- anterior vertebral wedging
- Schmorl's nodes (protrusion of disc material into adjacent vertebral body).

An associated spondylolysis has been reported in a third of cases.[87] It is important to note that any condition that decreases the mechanical properties of the end-plate or cancellous bone

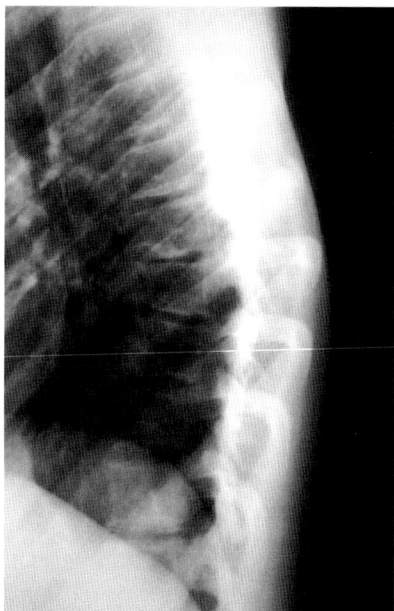

(a)

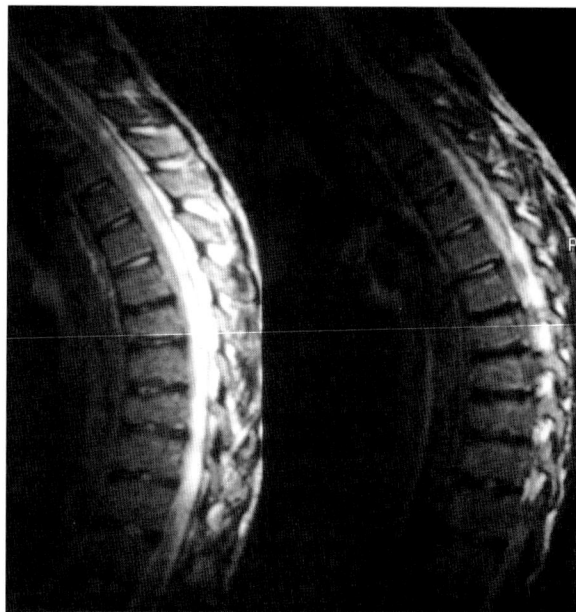

(b)

Figure 6.2 (a) Lateral radiograph showing thoracic Scheuermann's disease in a 14-year-old male. (b) MRI of the same patient showing vertebral changes of Scheuermann's disease with associated disc degeneration.

(e.g. osteoporosis, neoplasia, etc.) can cause intervertebral disc protrusions, and such conditions need to be considered in the differential diagnosis of such patients.[68]

However, the association of pain and radiologically confirmed Scheuermann's disease is not absolute, and other factors may be involved. Tertti et al[88] reported that, although there was no difference in prevalence of Scheuermann's disease in 15 years olds with low back pain compared to healthy controls, the former had more associated disc degeneration.

The exact cause of Scheuermann's disease is unknown, but possibilities include excessive and repetitive mechanical loading of the immature spine or an osteochondrosis.[9]

Management of Scheuermann's disease includes exercise, analgesia and/or splinting in a Milwaukee brace. Use of the latter has been reported to result in a rapid and significant return of disc height.[87] Back pain in later life is more common in patients with Scheuermann's disease, but is rarely severe.[89]

Slipped vertebral epiphysis

This occurs at the posterior rim of the inferior epiphysis, typically at L4 and usually with posterior displacement with the adjacent disc. The typical patient is an adolescent male with a history of heavy lifting. Diagnosis is made from a lateral radiograph and treatment is surgical.[90]

Disc degeneration

This is reported to occur in 6–16% of 10–19 year olds.[91,92] In a prospective study of 15–18 year olds, Salminen et al[93] reported a causal relationship between lower lumbar disc degeneration at age 15 and frequency of low back pain at age 18 (8%). However, in a case–control study comparing 15 year olds with and without back pain, Tertti et al[88] reported no significant difference in the frequency of disc degeneration (38% vs 26%, respectively). Disc degeneration was more often associated with either disc protrusion and/or Scheuermann's disease in the symptomatic teenagers.[88] The authors postulated that disc degeneration, which is associated with structural changes, may predispose to low-back disorders, and further follow-up of such patients is required. It remains unclear whether the disc degeneration is primary or secondary in such patients or if there is indeed a shared pathogenic mechanism (e.g. end-plate rupture).

Disc herniation

Up to 5.9% of all prolapsed intervertebral discs occur in adolescence.[47,65,66,71,94] It is slightly more common in males,[65,70] and the incidence increases with age.[66] Disc herniation is commonest at the L4/L5 and L5/S1 levels.[71] A positive family history is common.[64]

However, compared to adults, in adolescents disc herniation often presents with fewer findings[71] and diagnosis is often delayed. A third of patients have a history of trauma prior to onset.[94,95] Only two-thirds will present with back pain, and only a third with sciatica.[47] Abnormalities of straight-leg raising have been reported to be more prevalent and/or more dramatic in juvenile than in adult disc herniation.[47,71]

The natural history of juvenile disc herniation is that of slow resolution over 2 years.[95] Less than 2% of cases require surgical intervention, usually because of severe pain or persistent root pain. A good result with surgery is seen in the majority of cases.[95] Intradiscal chymopapain has also been used in the adolescent age group.[95]

Finally, studies of disc herniation in childhood and adolescents must include a consideration of possible false-positive MRI results.[88,96]

Facet joint abnormalities

Asymmetry of the facet joints has been reported in association with lumbar intervertebral disc herniation in children and adolescents,[97] and at greater frequency than in adults (41% vs 8%, respectively.[97,98] However, no relationship with location or side of disc herniation has been confirmed, and the hypothesis that the herniation is due to a mechanical imbalance remains unsubstantiated.[97,98]

Idiopathic scoliosis

In idiopathic scoliosis, the majority of spinal curve progression occurs in the age range 12–14 years. In the past, idiopathic scoliosis has not been included in causes of back pain, since it was thought to be always painless.[47] However, in a study of 2442 cases, 23% had back pain at presentation and 9% developed back pain during follow-up, with only 9% of patients with painful scoliosis having other underlying pathology.[99] Results from prospective controlled trials have shown that bracing for more than 20 h/day until completion of growth gives a better outcome than the natural history.[100] Pathogenesis appears to be multifactorial, including extraosseous and, possibly, osseous factors (e.g. significant osteopaenia has been reported, occurring before age 12 years and becoming significant in the age range 12–14 years[101]).

Inflammatory causes of back pain

Juvenile spondyloarthropathies
Axial disease often occurs late in this group of patients, and is rarely a presenting symptom (see above).

Juvenile intervertebral disc calcification
In contrast to the case in adults, juvenile intervertebral disc calcification is usually symptomatic, with acute pain and fever and an associated acute phase response. It affects the nucleus pulposus rather than the annulus fibrosis, and involves the cervical/thoracic spine rather than the lumbar spine as in adults.[102] It also spontaneously resolves, in contrast to the persistent calcification seen in adults. Older children tend to have more pain than younger ones. Symptomatic disc calcification tends to be cervical and to involve a single disc, rather than the multiple disc involvement seen in asymptomatic children. Intervertebral disc calcification is also seen in adolescents who have been treated for thalassaemia.[103]

Infective causes of back pain

Disciitis
As in adults, disciitis is rare in adolescents and more common in the younger age group (< 4

years old).[9] Disciitis most commonly occurs at the L4/L5 level.[9]

Organisms are difficult to isolate from the affected disc or peripheral blood and, if found, are usually *Staphylococcus aureus*. After 2–4 weeks changes are seen radiographically; the end-plate becomes poorly defined and there is loss of the joint space. A bone scan is more helpful, showing early increased uptake, but MRI is now the investigation of choice. Prognosis is good, although fusion of adjacent vertebrae may occur.

Vertebral osteomyelitis

In contrast to disciitis, vertebral osteomyelitis is more likely to affect the adolescent than the adult. It is usually staphylococcal in origin, although tuberculosis is an important possible cause to bear in mind.

Neoplastic causes of back pain

Tumours involving the adolescent spine are uncommon, but it is extremely important to keep them in mind. They are usually benign, although two-thirds of tumours in the lumbar spine are malignant. Common presentations include night-time and/or unremitting pain, a painful scoliosis, local tenderness, a palpable lump, bilateral sciatica, neurological signs and/or a disproportionate anaemia.

Benign tumours

The important benign bone tumours include osteoid osteoma and osteoblastoma, both of which affect the posterolateral elements. The osteoid osteoma is smaller (< 1 cm) than the osteoblastoma with a sclerotic rim and a radiolucent centre. Nocturnal pain that is relieved by NSAIDs is typical, although 50% of patients will have radicular pain.[104]

A fifth of aneurysmal bone cysts affect the spine; they primarily involve the posterior elements and usually present in adolescence.[105] Investigation may require scintigraphy, MRI and/or angiography. Treatment is by excision.

Eosinophilic granuloma can also present in adolescence with back pain, mainly thoracic. Neurological signs are rare. If more than one vertebra is involved, systemic histiocytosis should be considered.[104]

Malignant tumours

Ewing's sarcoma is the most common malignant tumour affecting the spine, and is associated with a fever, leucocytosis and a raised erythrocyte sedimentation rate (ESR). Other malignant tumours include lymphomas, leukaemia (presenting with compression fractures and/or involvement of the epidural space) and metastases (e.g. rhabdomyosarcomas and teratomas).

The majority of intraspinal tumours are benign (70%) and are usually slow growing.[106] The frequency of back pain varies from 40% to 77% of patients.[106,107] Other features include change in gait and/or a change in spinal movements or curvature. Loss of power and loss of sensation are late signs, with anal-sphincter disturbance occurring even later. The investigation of choice is MRI, although scintigraphy is usually abnormal, even when radiographs are normal. Treatment of tumours may also present further axial problems related to growth disturbance and increasing scoliosis.

Metabolic causes of back pain

The main metabolic bone disease that presents with back pain is osteoporosis, which is usually manifested by compression fractures. It is most commonly seen secondary to steroid therapy or due to an underlying disease process (e.g. osteogenesis imperfecta, diffuse marrow infiltration). It can also be primary (idiopathic juvenile osteoporosis). The latter presents late in childhood or at puberty, with arthralgia (ankles, knees) and back pain, and is characterized by the development of metaphyseal fractures resulting from the osteopaenia.[9,108] Biochemistry is normal except for the presence of hypercalciuria. The metabolic abnormalities disappear after completion of growth.[9]

Pain-amplification syndromes

A fifth of children exhibit musculoskeletal psychosomatic symptoms, and 17% of these have back pain.[109] The gender effect, as seen with headache, is less obvious with back pain.[57,59] Back pain is less of a feature in adolescent pain-amplification syndromes than in adults, and less lumbosacral tender points are present[110] (see Chapter 10).

Other causes of back pain

These are listed in Table 6.5.

SUMMARY

Adolescence is an interesting time for the axial skeleton, as it experiences the growth spurt as well as changes in both social and recreational activity. Important differences in the presentation of certain conditions, the clinical examination, radiological assessment and the differential diagnosis in this age group must be remembered by those caring for adolescents. Finally, further prospective studies of both inflammatory and non-inflammatory back pain are needed in order to define better the relationship between juvenile and adult conditions, particularly in view of the significant morbidity of back pain in today's society.

Table 6.5 Other causes of back pain in adolescence

- Congenital spinal anomalies:[47,49,50,68]
  - absence of a lumbar pedicle
  - spinal fusion with small neural foramen and/or spinal stenosis
- Microtrauma/overuse[47,48,82]
- Injury[47,48,50,104]
- Other infective causes:
  - epidural abscess[111]
  - iliopsoas abscess
  - hydatid bone lesion
- Sickle cell anaemia (e.g. bone infarction[49])
- Chronic recurrent multifocal osteomyelitis presenting with vertebral collapse[112]
- Fibrodysplasia ossificans[113]
- Juvenile dermatomyositis[114]
- Aortic dissection[115]
- Intra-abdominal disease
- Retroperitoneal disorder

REFERENCES

1. Fink CW. Proposal for the development of classification criteria for idiopathic arthritides of childhood. *J Rheumatol* 1995; **22**:1566–9.
2. Schaller JG, Ochs HD, Thomas ED et al. Histocompatibility antigens in childhood onset arthritis. *J Pediatr* 1976; **88**:926–30.
3. Rachelefsky GS, Steihm ER. Histocompatibility locus antigen W7 and the rheumatic diseases. *Pediatrics* 1975; **56**:498–500.
4. Malleson PN, Fung MY, Rosenberg AM et al. The incidence of paediatric rheumatic diseases: results from the Canadian Paediatric Rheumatology Association Disease Registry. *J Rheumatol* 1996; **23**:1981–7.
5. Symmons DPM, Jones M, Osborne J et al. Paediatric rheumatology in the United Kingdom: data from the British Paediatric Rheumatology Group National Diagnostic Register. *J Rheumatol* 1996; **23**:1975–80.
6. Goften JP, Chalmers A, Price GE et al. HLA-B27 and ankylosing spondylitis in BC Indians. *J Rheumatol* 1975; **2**:318–22.

7. Burgos-Vargas R, Lardizabal-Sanabria J, Katona G. Ankylosing spondylitis and related diseases in the Mexican Mestizo. *Spine* 1990; **4**:665–78.
8. Rosenberg AM, Petty RE. A syndrome of seronegative enthesopathy and arthropathy in children. *Arthritis Rheum* 1982; **25**:1041–7.
9. Cassidy JT, Petty RE (eds). *Textbook of Pediatric Rheumatology*, 3rd edn. WB Saunders: Philadelphia, 1995.
10. Cabral DA, Oen KG, Petty RE. SEA syndrome revisited: a long-term follow-up of children with a syndrome of seronegative enthesopathy and arthropathy. *J Rheumatol* 1992; **19**:1282–5.
11. Burgos-Vargas R, Clark P. Axial involvement in the seronegative enthesopathy and arthropathy syndrome and its progression to ankylosing spondylitis. *J Rheumatol* 1989; **16**:192–7.
12. Olivieri I, Foto M, Ruju GP et al. Low frequency of axial involvement in caucasian pediatric patients with seronegative enthesopathy and arthropathy syndrome after 5 years of disease. *J Rheumatol* 1992; **19**:469–75.

13. Sheerin KA, Giannini EH, Brewer EJ, Barron KS. HLA-B27 associated arthropathy in childhood: long-term clinical and diagnostic outcome. *Arthritis Rheum* 1988; **31**:1165–70.

14. Burgos-Vargas R, Vazquez-Mellaod J. The early clinical recognition of juvenile-onset ankylosing spondylitis and its differentiation from juvenile rheumatoid arthritis. *Arthritis Rheum* 1995; **38**:835–44.

15. Gomez KS, Raza K, Jones SD et al. Juvenile onset ankylosing spondylitis – more girls than we thought? *J Rheumatol* 1997; **24**:735–7.

16. Bowyer S. Hip contracture as the presenting sign in children with HLA-B27 arthritis. *J Rheumatol* 1995; **22**:165–7.

17. Burgos-Vargas R, Naranjo A, Castillo J, Katona G. Ankylosing spondylitis in the Mexican Mestizo: patterns of disease according to age at onset. *J Rheumatol* 1989; **16**:186–91.

18. Burgos-Vargas R, Castelazo-Duarte G, Orozco JA et al. Chest expansion in healthy adolescents and patients with the seronegative enthesopathy and arthropathy syndrome or juvenile ankylosing spondylitis. *J Rheumatol* 1993; **20**:1957–60.

19. Foster HE, Cairns RA, Burnell RH et al. Atlantoaxial subluxation in children with seronegative enthesopathy and arthropathy syndrome: 2 case reports and a review of the literature. *J Rheumatol* 1995; **22**:548–51.

20. Ansell BM. Juvenile spondylitis and related disorders. In: *Ankylosing Spondylitis* (Moll JMH ed). Churchill Livingstone: Edinburgh, 1980:120.

21. Stamato T, Laxer RM, de Freitas C et al. Prevalence of cardiac manifestations of juvenile ankylosing spondylitis. *Am J Cardiol* 1995; **75**:744–6.

22. Garcia-Morteo O, Maldonado-Cocco JA, Suarez-Almazor ME, Garay E. Ankylosing spondylitis of juvenile onset: comparison with adult onset disease. *Scand J Rheumatol* 1983; **12**:246–8.

23. Calin A, Elswood J. The natural history of juvenile-onset ankylosing spondylitis: a 24 year retrospective case-control study. *Br J Rheumatol* 1988; **27**:91–3.

24. Mielants H, Veys EM, Joos R et al. Late onset pauciarticular juvenile chronic arthritis: relation to gut inflammation. *J Rheumatol* 1987; **14**:459–65.

25. Mielants H, Veys EM, Goemare S et al. A prospective study of patients with spondyloarthropathy with special reference to HLA-B27 and to gut histology. *J Rheumatol* 1993; **20**:1353–8.

26. Mielants H, Veys EM, Joos R et al. HLA antigens in seronegative spondyloarthropathies. Reactive arthritis and arthritis in ankylosing spondylitis: relation to gut inflammation. *J Rheumatol* 1987; **14**:466–71.

27. Farmer RG, Michener WM. Prognosis of Crohn's disease with onset in childhood and adolescence. *Dig Dis Sci* 1979; **24**:752–7.

28. Hamilton JR, Bruce MD, Abdourhamam M et al. Inflammatory bowel disease in children and adolescents. *Adv Pediatr* 1979; **26**:311–22.

29. Lindsley C, Schaller J. Arthritis associated with inflammatory bowel disease in children. *J Paediatr* 1974; **84**:16–20.

30. Salmi M, Andrew DP, Butcher EC, Jalkanen S. Dual binding capacity of mucosal immunoblasts to mucosal and synovial endothelium in humans: dissection of the molecular mechanisms. *J Exp Med* 1995; **181**:137–49.

31. Life PF, Hassell A, Williams K et al. Responses to Gram-negative enteric bacterial antigens by synovial T cells from patients with juvenile chronic arthritis: recognition of heat shock protein HSP60. *J Rheumatol* 1993; **20**:1388–96.

32. Brewerton DA. Causes of arthritis. *Lancet* 1988; **ii**:1063–66.

33. Khare SD, Harvinder SL, David CS. Spontaneous inflammatory arthritis in HLA-B27 transgenic mice lacking β_2-microglobulin: a model of human spondyloarthropathies. *J Exp Med* 1995; **182**:1153–8.

34. Taurog JD, Richardson JA, Croft JT et al. The germ-free state prevents development of gut and joint inflammatory disease in HLA-B27 transgenic rats. *J Exp Med* 1994; **180**:2359–64.

35. Lahesmaa R, Skurnik M, Granfors K et al. Molecular mimicry in the pathogenesis of spondyloarthropathies. A critical appraisal of cross-reactivity between microbial antigens and HLA-B27. *Br J Rheumatol* 1992; **31**:221–9.

36. Roberton DM, Cabral DA, Malleson PN, Petty RE. Juvenile psoriatic arthritis: follow-up and evaluation of diagnostic criteria. *J Rheumatol* 1996; **23**:166–70.

37. Hamilton ML, Gladman DD, Shore A, Laxer R, Silverman ED. Juvenile psoriatic arthritis and HLA antigens. *Ann Rheum Dis* 1990; **49**:88–94.

38. Shore A, Ansell BM. Juvenile psoriatic arthritis – an analysis of 60 cases. *J Pediatr* 1982; **100**:529–35.

39. Reiter H. Uber eine bisher unerkannte Spirichaeteninfektion (Spirochaetosis arthritica). *Dtsch Med Wochenschr* 1916; **42**:1535–6.

40. Cuttica RJ, Scheines EJ, Garay SM et al. Juvenile onset Reiter's syndrome. A retrospective study of 26 patients. *Clin Exp Rheumatol* 1992; **10**:285–8.

41. Rosenberg AM, Petty RE. Reiter's disease in children. *Am J Dis Child* 1979; **133**:394–8.

42. Jobdeslandre C, Menkes CJ. Sufasalazine treatment in juvenile spondyloarthropathy. *Rev Rheumat* 1993; **60**:489–91.

43. Singsen BH, Goldbach-Mansky R. Methotrexate in the treatment of juvenile rheumatoid arthritis and other pediatric rheumatic and non-rheumatic disorders. *Rheum Dis Clin North Am* 1997; **23**:811–40.

44. Burgos-Vargas R, Lardizabal-Sanabria J, Katona G. Anterior spinal flexion in healthy Mexican children. *J Rheumatol* 1985; **12**:123–5.

45. Burgos-Vargas R, Vazquez-Mellado J, Cassis N et al. Genuine ankylosing spondylitis in children: a case–control study of patients with early definite disease according to adult onset criteria. *J Rheumatol* 1996; **23**:2140–7.

46. Calin A, Porta J, Fries JF, Schurman DJ. Clinical history as a screening test for ankylosing spondylitis. *JAMA* 1977; **237**:2613–5.

47. Bunnell WP. Back pain in children. *Orthop Clin North Am* 1982; **13**:587–604.

48. Smith MS. Psychosomatic symptoms in adolescence. *Med Clin North Am* 1990; **74**:1121–34.

49. Afshani E, Kuhn JP. Common causes of low back pain in children. *Radiographics* 1991; **11**:269–91.

50. King HA. Back pain in children. *Pediatr Clin North Am* 1984; **31**:1083–95.

51. Balague F, Dutoit G, Waldburger M. Low back pain in schoolchildren – an epidemiological study. *Scand J Rehab Med* 1988; **20**:175–9.

52. Fairbank JCT, Pynsent PB, van Poortvliet JA, Phillips H. Influence of anthropometric factors and joint laxity in the incidence of adolescent back pain. *Spine* 1984; **9**:461–4.

53. Kujala UM, Salminen JJ, Taimela S et al. Subject characteristics and low back pain in young athletes and non-athletes. *Med Sci Sports Exercise* 1992; **24**:627–32.

54. Mireau D, Cassidy JD, Yong-Hing K. Low-back pain and straight leg raising in children and adolescents. *Spine* 1989; **14**:526–8.

55. Balague F, Skovron M-L, Nordin M et al. Low back pain in school children. A study of familial and psychological factors. *Spine* 1995; **20**:1265–70.

56. Salminen JJ, Maki P, Oksanen A, Pentti J. Spinal mobility and trunk muscle strength in 15 year old schoolchildren with and without low-back pain. *Spine* 1992; **17**:405–11.

57. Olsen TL, Anderson RL, Dearwater SR et al. The epidemiology of low back pain in an adolescent population. *Am J Public Health* 1992; **82**:606–8.

58. Salminen JJ. The adolescent back. A field survey of 370 Finnish schoolchildren. *Acta Paediatr* 1984; **315**:8–122.

59. Kristjansdottir G. Prevalence of self-reported back pain in school children: a study of sociodemographic differences. *Eur J Pediatr* 1996; **155**:984–6.

60. Troussier B, Davoine P, de Gaudemaris R et al. Back pain in school children. A study among 1178 pupils. *Scand J Rehab Med* 1994; **26**:143–6.

61. Newcomer K, Sinaki M. Low back pain and its relationship to back strength and physical activity in children. *Acta Paediatr* 1996; **85**:1433–9.

62. Burton AK, Clarke RD, McClune TD, Tillotson KM. The natural history of low back pain in adolescents. *Spine* 1996; **21**:2323–8.

63. Balague F, Nordin M, Skovron ML et al. Non-specific low back pain among schoolchildren: a field survey with analysis of some associated factors. *J Spinal Disord* 1994; **7**:374–9.

64. Wynne-Davies R, Scott JHS. Inheritance and spondylolisthesis. A radiographic family survey. *J Bone Joint Surg* 1979; **61B**:301–5.

65. Varlotta GP, Brown MD, Kelsey JL, Golden AL. Familial predisposition for herniation of a lumbar disc in patients who are less than twenty-one years old. *J Bone Joint Surg (Am)* 1991; **73**:124–8.

66. Matsui H, Terahata N, Tsuji H et al. Familial predisposition and clustering for juvenile lumbar disc herniation. *Spine* 1992; **17**:1323–8.

67. Sward L, Hellstrom M, Jacobsson BO, Peterson L. Back pain and radiologic changes in the thoraco-lumbar spine of athletes. *Spine* 1990; **15**:124–9.

68. Balague F, Nordin M. Back pain in children and teenagers. *Clin Rheumatol* 1992; **6**:575–94.

69. Jackson DW, Wiltse LL, Cirincione RJ. Spondylolysis in the female gymnast. *Clin Orthop* 1976; **117**:68–73.

70. Salminen JJ, Erkintalo-Tertti, Paajanen HE. Magnetic resonance imaging findings of lumbar spine in the young: correlation with leisure time, physical activity, spinal mobility and trunk muscle strength in 15 year old pupils with or without low back pain. *J Spinal Disord* 1993; **6**:386–91.

71. Nelson CL, Janecki CJ, Gildenberg PL, Sava G. Disc protrusions in the young. *Clin Orthop Rel Res* 1972; **88**:142–50.

72. Taimela S, Kujala UM, Salminen JJ, Viljanen T. The prevalence of low back pain among children and adolescents. *Spine* 1997; **22**:1132–6.

73. Harreby M, Neergaard K, Hesselsoe G, Kjer J. Are radiologic changes in the thoracic and lumbar spine of adolescents risk factors for low back pain in adults? *Spine* 1995; **20**:2298–302.

74. Turner PG, Green JH, Galasko CSB. Back pain in childhood. *Spine* 1989; **14**:812–14.

75. Hensinger RN. Back pain in children. In: *The Paediatric Spine* (Bradford DS, Hensinger RN, eds). Thieme: New York, 1985:41–60.

76. Feldman DS, Wright JG, Hedden DM. Chronic back pain in children and adolescents. *Orthop Trans* 1995–6; **19**:592.

77. King HA. Back pain in children. *Paediatr Clin North Am* 1986; **33**:1489–93.

78. Sponseller PD. Back pain in children. *Curr Opin Pediatr* 1994; **6**:99–103.

79. Lindholm TS, Ragni P, Ylikoski M, Poussar M. Lumbar isthmic spondylolisthesis in children and adolescents – radiographic evaluation and result of operative treatment. *Spine* 1990; **15**:1350–5.

80. Danielson B, Frennered AK, Irstam LKH. Radiologic progression of isthmic lumbar spondylolisthesis in young patients. *Spine* 1991; **16**:422–5.

81. Rosenberg NJ, Bargar WL, Friedman B. The incidence of spondylolysis and spondylolisthesis in nonambulatory patients. *Spine* 1981; **6**:35–7.

82. Commandre FA, Gagnerie G, Zakarian M et al. The child, the spine and sport. *J Sports Med Phys Fitness* 1988; **28**:11–9.

83. Osterman K, Schlenzka D, Poussar M et al. Isthmic spondylolisthesis in symptomatic and asymptomatic subjects, epidemiology and natural history with special reference to disc abnormality and mode of treatment. *Clin Orthop* 1993; **297**:65–70.

84. Yamane T, Yoshida T, Mimatsu K. Early diagnosis of lumbar spondylolysis by MRI. *J Bone Joint Surg Br* 1993; **75**:764–8.

85. Muschik M, Zippel H, Perka C. Surgical management of severe spondylolisthesis in children and adolescents. *Spine* 1997; **22**:2036–43.

86. Bradford DS. Vertebral osteochondrosis. *Clin Orthop* 1981; **178**:83–90.

87. Greene TL, Hensinger RN, Huneter MD. Back pain and vertebral changes simulating Scheuermann's. *J Pediatr Orthop* 1985; **5**:1–7.

88. Tertti MO, Salminen JJ, Paajanen HEK et al. Low-back pain and disc degeneration in children: a case-control MR imaging study. *Radiology* 1991; **180**:503–7.

89. Murray PM, Wienstein SC, Spratt IF. The natural history and long-term follow-up of Scheuermann's kyphosis. *J Bone Joint Surg* 1993; **75**:236–48.

90. Handel SF, Twiford TW, Reigel JH, Kaufman HH. Posterior lumbar apophyseal fracture. *Radiology* 1979; **130**:629–33.

91. Powell MC, Wilson M, Szypryt P, Symonds EM. Prevalence of lumbar disc degeneration observed by magnetic resonance imaging in symptomless women. *Lancet* 1986; **ii**:1366–7.

92. Miller JAA, Schmatz C, Schultz AB. Lumbar disc degeneration: correlation with age, sex and spine level in 600 autopsy specimens. *Spine* 1988; **13**:173–8.

93. Salminen JJ, Erkintalo-Tertti M, Laine M. Pentti J. Low back pain in the young: a prospective three-year follow-up study of subjects with and without low back pain. *Spine* 1995; **20**:2101–7.

94. DeOrio JK, Bianco AJ. Lumbar disc excision in children and adolescents. *J Bone Joint Surg (Am)* 1982; **64**:991–6.

95. Bradbury N, Wilson LF, Mulholland RC. Adolescent disc protrusions. *Spine* 1996; **21**:372–7.

96. Gibson MJ, Szypryt EP, Buckley JH et al. Magnetic resonance imaging of adolescent disc herniation. *J Bone Joint Surg* 1987; **69B**:699–703.

97. Ishihara H, Matsui H, Osada R et al. Facet joint asymmetry as a radiologic feature of lumbar intervertebral disc herniation in children and adolescents. *Spine* 1997; **22**:2001–4.

98. Farfan HF, Sullivan JD. The relation of facet orientation to intervertebral disc failure. *Can J Surg* 1967; **10**:179–85.

99. Ramirez N, Johnston CE, Browne RH. The prevalence of back pain in children who have idiopathic scoliosis. *J Bone Joint Surg* 1997; **79A**:364–8.

100. Nachemson AL, Peterson LE, Bradford DS et al. Effectiveness of treatment with a brace in girls who have adolescent idiopathic scoliosis. A prospective, controlled study based on data from the brace study of the Scoliosis Research Society. *J Bone Joint Surg (Am)* 1995; **77A**:815–22.

101. Cheng JCY, Guo X, Osteopenia in adolescent idiopathic scoliosis. *Spine* 1997; **22**:1716–21.

102. Dias MS, Pang D. Juvenile intervertebral disc calcification: recognition, management and pathogenesis. *Neurosurgery* 1991; **28**:130–5.

103. Harkamp MJ, Babyn PS, Olivieri F. Spinal deformities in deferoxamine-treated homozygous β-thalassemia major patients. *Pediatr Radiol* 1993; **23**:525–8.

104. Hollingworth P. Back pain in children. *Br J Rheumatol* 1996; **35**:1022–8.

105. Cappana R, Albissini U, Picci P et al. Aneurysmal bone cysts of the spine. *J Bone Joint Surg* 1985; **67A**:527–31.

106. Cole GF. Intraspinal tumours. *Arch Dis Child* 1988; **63**:1007–9.

107. Parker APJ, Robinson RO, Bullock P. Difficulties in diagnosing intrinsic spinal cord tumours. *Arch Dis Child* 1996; **75**:204–7.

108. Smith R. Idiopathic juvenile osteoporosis: experience of 21 patients. *Br J Rheumatol* 1995; **34**:68–77.

109. Sherry DD, McGuire T, Mellins E, Salmonson K, Wallace CA, Nepom B. Psychosomatic musculoskeletal pain in childhood: clinical and psychological analyses of 100 children. *Pediatrics* 1991; **88**:1093–9.

110. Yunus MB, Masi AT. Juvenile primary fibromyalgia syndrome. *Arthritis Rheum* 1985; **28**:138–45.

111. McGee-Collett M, Johnston IH. Spinal epidural abscess: presentation and treatment. *Med J Aust* 1994; **155**:14–17.

112. Gamble JG, Rinsky LA. Chronic recurrent multifocal osteomyelitis: a distinct clinical entity. *J Paediatr Orthop* 1986; **6**:944–51.

113. Voynow JA, Charney EB. Fibrodysplasia ossificans progressiva presenting as osteomyelitis-like syndrome. *Clin Pediatr* 1986; **35**:373–5.

114. Fink CW, Cimaz RG. Back pain as the presenting symptom in juvenile dermato/polymyositis. *J Clin Rheumatol* 1995; **1**:90–2.

115. Griggs JR, Brisker JT, Mariscalco MM, Jefferson LS, Langston C. Back pain with cardiovascular collapse in a paediatric emergency department patient. *Pediatr Emerg Care* 1990; **6**:17–20.

7

Systemic lupus erythematosus

Clarissa Pilkington, Lori B Tucker and David A Isenberg

INTRODUCTION

Systemic lupus erythematosus (SLE) is a disease that has a multiplicity of presentations. In adolescence it may have an insidious onset, so that it can be months before a diagnosis can be made. The clinical picture can be complicated further by the difficulties of disentangling the psychological problems of normal adolescence from the effects of the disease process. Since SLE is not a common condition in childhood or adolescence, it is hardly surprising that it is often misdiagnosed, or diagnosed late, by general practitioners and paediatricians.

DEFINITION OF LUPUS

SLE is an autoimmune rheumatic disease that commonly affects the skin and musculoskeletal systems but can affect every organ, including the kidney, heart, lungs and the central nervous system. In children, the initial presenting symptom may be as subtle as school failure due to fatigue, or it can present in a more obvious way with a malar rash accompanied by fever, arthritis and serositis. In other cases, the kidney may be the first organ to be involved. This diversity in presentation and organ involvement can make the diagnosis and assessment of disease activity difficult. The American College of Rheumatology (ACR) published guidelines for disease classification in 1971 (revised 1982 and 1997).[1,2] These were proposed to ensure that research was based on comparable disease groups, but they have also been widely adopted for clinical diagnosis. In order to fulfil the criteria for lupus, a patient must meet 4 of the 11 criteria listed in Table 7.1.

Clinicians with little paediatric rheumatological experience may find it difficult to distinguish between arthritis occurring in childhood, dermatomyositis, scleroderma, the overlap syndromes and lupus. These diseases have some clinical and serological features in common, but there are clinical and laboratory clues that help to distinguish between the different rheumatological diseases. Patients with polyarticular juvenile idiopathic arthritis (see Chapter 4) can be positive for antinuclear antibody (ANA) and rheumatoid factor, but tend to have few systemic symptoms. However, a patient with polyarthritis, a high ANA titre and a positive rheumatoid factor needs to have the diagnosis of SLE considered. A full history must be taken to elicit subtle symptoms such as lethargy which is disproportionate to the arthritis, hair thinning, photosensitive rash or oral ulcers; and investigations including autoantibody profile, renal and haematological indices are strongly advised. Careful follow-up is required, as other features of lupus may develop over time. Gottren's papules tend to be associated with dermatomyositis rather than lupus. Scleroderma patients have skin lesions, but their skin is invariably 'tighter', and the face may have a 'pinched' look. Occasionally, a child may have clinical findings suggestive of several rheumatic conditions at disease onset, and a specific diagnosis may not emerge for months or even years.

Table 7.1 Revised criteria of the American Rheumatism Association for the classification of systemic lupus erythematosus (SLE)[1,2]

A person shall be said to have SLE if 4 or more of the 11 criteria are present, serially or simultaneously, during any interval of observation.

1. Malar rash
2. Discoid rash
3. Photosensitivity
4. Oral ulcers
5. Arthritis
6. Serositis:
   (a) pleuritis, or
   (b) pericarditis
7. Renal disorder:
   (a) proteinuria > 0.5 g/24 h or $\geqslant$ 3g persistently, or
   (b) cellular casts
8. Neurological disorder:
   (a) seizures, or
   (b) psychosis (having excluded other causes)
9. Haematological disorders:
   (a) haemolytic anaemia, or
   (b) leucopenia or < 4.0×10^9/l on two or more occasions
   (c) lymphopenia or < 1.5×10^9/l on two or more occasions
   (d) thrombocytopenia < 100×10^9/l
10. Immunological disorders:
    (a) raised antinative DNA antibody binding
    (b) anti-Sm antibody
    (c) positive finding of antiphospholipid antibodies based on:
        (i) abnormal serum level of IgG or IgM anticardiolipin levels, or
        (ii) positive test result for lupus anticoagulant or
        (iii) false-positive serological test for syphilis present for at least 6 months
11. Antinuclear antibody in raised titre

EPIDEMIOLOGY

The estimated incidence of lupus in children under the age of 15 years is 6 per 100 000.[3] As in adults, the incidence of lupus varies with racial origin. The reported racial mix differs depending on the geographical area from which the report originates. In the UK, a recent adult study from Birmingham showed a higher incidence in Afro-Caribbean women: 36.2 per 100 000 Caucasian, 90.6 per 100 000 Asian and 206 per 100 000 Afro-Caribbean women.[4] In Los Angeles, USA, the relative incidence in 10–18 year old females was reported to be 4.4 per 100 000 in whites, 19.86 per 100 000 in blacks, and 31.14 per 100 000 in Orientals.[5]

The sex ratio in childhood SLE is different from that in adults. In adults, lupus is very rare in males: it is 10–20 times more common in women.[6] The ratio in prepubertal children varies. In Boston it was reported as 1 : 5.5,[7] whereas in Israel it was reported as 1 : 2.8 (38 cases aged 7–16 years).[8] However, one report from India gives a sex ratio that is the same as in the adult population.[9]

The increased incidence of lupus in certain racial groups living within the same area suggests there is a genetic component to lupus. This is supported by reports of twin studies. In the largest study published to date, a concordance of 24% in monozygotic twins compared to 2% in dizygotic twins was noted.[10]

CLINICAL FEATURES

Adolescents can present with the classical photosensitive butterfly rash on the face (Figure 7.1). The rash can be urticarial, and in some cases is brought on by exposure to strip-lighting. Other skin presentations include vasculitic lesions of the hands and feet (Figure 7.2), which can be extremely painful, or Raynaud's phenomenon (Figure 7.3). Idiopathic Raynaud's phenomenon is fairly common in adolescents (especially girls), and patients who are ANA positive need to be kept under observation, as they may develop lupus, scleroderma or an overlap syndrome.

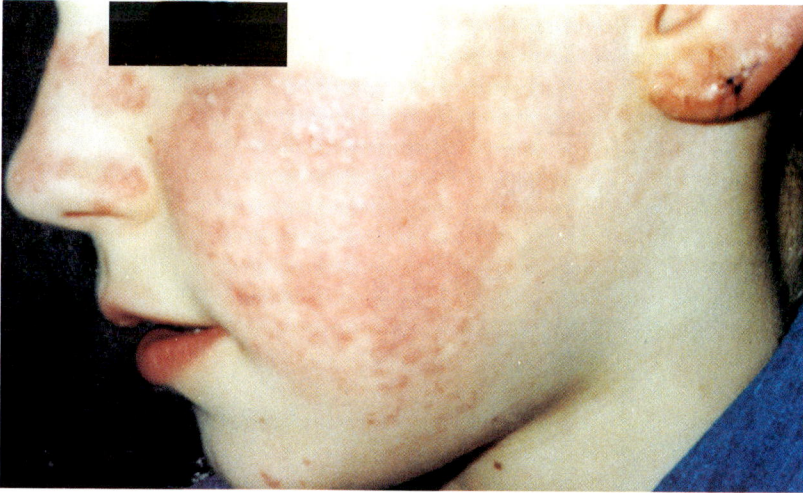

Figure 7.1 Butterfly rash.

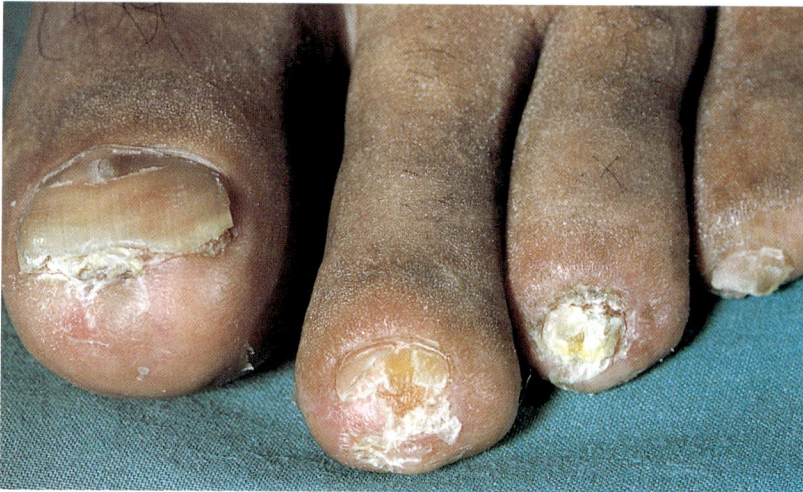

Figure 7.2 Vasculitis affecting the toes and toenails.

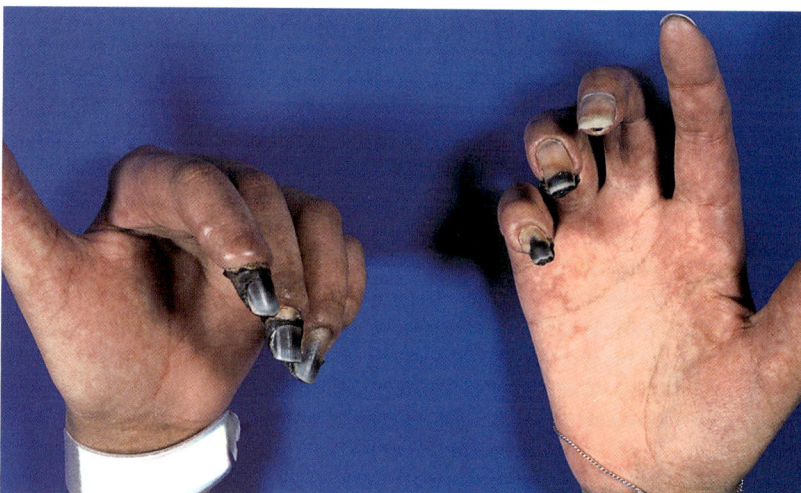

Figure 7.3 Severe vasculitis and Raynaud's phenomenon.

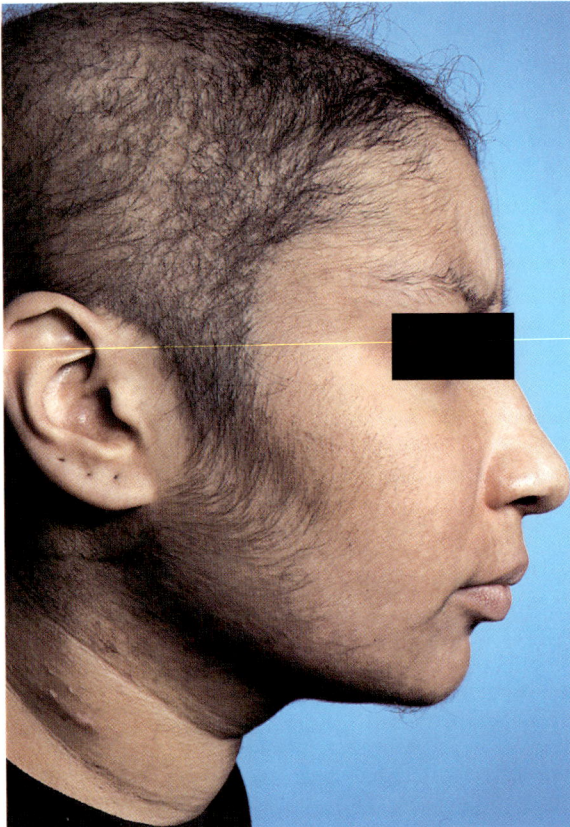

(a)

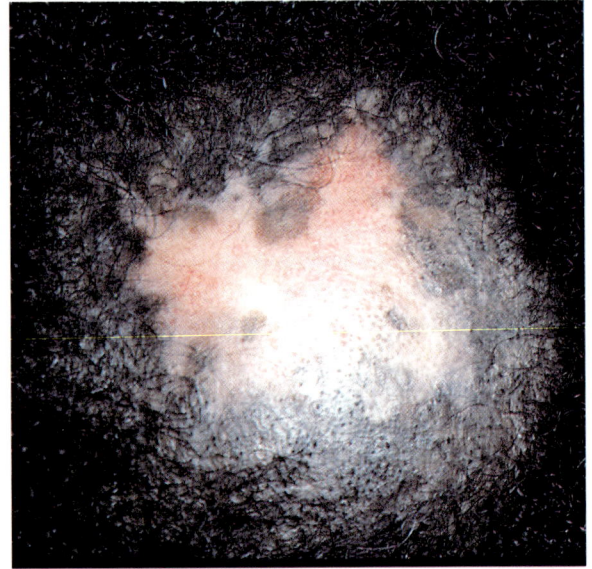

(b)

Figure 7.4 (a) Diffuse, non-scarring alopecia. (b) Alopecia which may become scarring.

Another presenting feature may be simply profound tiredness. This can be associated with arthralgia, or even arthritis. If there is an arthritis, there is usually tenosynovitis, and occasionally synovial effusions, but rarely erosive disease. The arthritis can cause an initial erroneous diagnosis of juvenile arthritis to be made. However, usually there are high titres of ANA present, and often the tiredness is out of proportion to the joint disease.

Direct questioning may reveal alopecia, which tends to be mild (Figure 7.4). Oral ulceration appears to be less common than in adults, but again has to be sought. Patients with severe lupus can present with pericarditis, pleuritis, pulmonary vasculitis or haemorrhage, which can be acute and fatal. Some patients present initially with renal involvement, in which case they are often referred to the renal paediatrician. Some of these cases do have preceding symptoms, but they have not been severe enough for medical advice to be sought.

Cerebral lupus can be difficult to diagnose in adolescents. Most reviews report that 9–45% of children have significant central nervous system (CNS) findings at disease onset. The ACR criteria for cerebral lupus are seizures and psychosis (see Table 7.1), having excluded causes such as drugs, infections and metabolic problems. However, a wide variety of other clinical features, from migraine headaches to aseptic meningitis, are recognized as CNS lupus manifestations. In a review of 108 patients with onset in childhood,[11] 25 had recorded neurological findings. The most frequent of these were headaches (16/25) and depression (9/25). Other findings included chorea, seizures, cerebrovascular accidents, cranial neuropathy and visual loss. Visual loss in lupus is most commonly due to retinal vessel thrombosis. Mononeuritis multiplex causes a peripheral neuropathy or, less commonly, a transverse myelitis can occur. In a study of 37 patients,[12] neuropsychiatric manifestations were reported, including organic brain syndrome, functional psychosis and personality disorder. In this study, headaches were also among the most frequently reported symptoms, as were behaviour disorders and memory alteration. However, a study of eight patients using neuropsychological assessments did not demonstrate significant behavioural or emotional distress.[13] This is discussed further later in this chapter.

Physical examination should be careful and thorough. Signs can be subtle, such as dilated capillaries in the nailbeds or vasculitic skin lesions. Patients may have lymphadenopathy, hepatosplenomegaly or evidence of a pleural or pericardial rub, even when they are not complaining of any symptoms.

DISEASE COURSE

As in adult-onset lupus, the disease course is highly variable, from patients with stable mild lupus to those who develop severe organ involvement. However, differences have been found between the disease patterns seen in adult- and childhood-onset lupus patients.[7] These are summarized in Table 7.2. Patients with childhood-onset lupus suffer more from major haematological disease and renal involvement, whereas those with adult-onset lupus suffer more from cardiopulmonary disease. There is little difference in the incidence of rash, joint or CNS involvement.

INVESTIGATIONS

Serological investigations may be divided into tests of end-organ dysfunction and immunological tests looking for the autoantibody profile of lupus. A full blood count is likely to show an anaemia of chronic disease, and, more specifically a lymphopaenia or a thrombocytopaenia. The erythrocyte sedimentation rate (ESR) is often raised, while the C-reactive protein (CRP)

Table 7.2 Cumulative features (as percentage of patients) in adult- and childhood-onset SLE[7]

	At 2 years		At 5 years	
	Adult	Paediatric	Adult	Paediatric
No. patients alive	163	37	113	28
No. patients dead	2	2	10	2
Rash	89	83	82	82
Arthritis	96	78	98	89
Cardiopulmonary disease	33	19	54	36
Renal disease	17	27	25	32
CNS disease	16	19	28	21
Major haematological disease	16	38*	20	39**

Statistically significant at: $*p < 0.001$; $**p < 0.025$.

level is normal. Renal function needs to be assessed, including plasma creatinine and urea. Hypocomplementaemia with a low C3 or C4 may be present. Levels of CH50 and complement activation products such as C3d and C4d can be helpful, but are not widely available. The complement levels, and the levels of double-stranded DNA antibodies (see below), are often a good reflection of disease activity.

ANAs are the most frequently found of the autoantibodies: in a recent review of 192 paediatric lupus patients,[14] over 97% were ANA positive. However, ANAs are not specific to lupus. In contrast, antibodies to double-stranded DNA of the immunoglobulin G (IgG) isotype are virtually diagnostic for lupus, and levels often reflect disease activity. However, a negative result does not exclude the diagnosis.

Antibodies which do not reflect disease activity, but are important for categorization, or for associated clinical problems, include antibodies to the extractable nuclear antigens (ENA), such as Ro, La, Sm, and RNP, as well as thyroid antibodies, anti-red-cell antibodies, antiplatelet antibodies, anti-IgG Fc antibodies (i.e. rheumatoid factor), anticomplement, and anticoagulation factors.[14]

Investigations to reveal haemolysis include a Coombs' test, although a positive result is not invariably associated with a haemolytic anaemia. Antiphospholipid antibodies are associated with fetal loss, thrombocytopaenia, thrombotic problems and coagulation abnormalities. A lupus anticoagulant is either an IgG or IgM antiphospholipid antibody that can interfere with phospholipid-dependent coagulation reactions and can cause a prolonged partial thromboplastin time. A lupus anticoagulant tends to be associated with thrombotic rather than haemorrhagic problems. Anticardiolipin antibodies are antiphospholipid antibodies of the IgG or IgM isotype. In adult lupus patients, anticardiolipin antibodies are associated with thrombosis, thrombocytopaenia, recurrent fetal abortions, pulmonary hypertension and cerebral disease.[6] The anticardiolipin syndrome may be the first manifestation of lupus, or it may occur as an isolated phenomenon (i.e. as a primary disease). In childhood-onset lupus, the reported incidence

of anticardiolipin antibodies has varied. In one study the incidence was found to be 50%,[15] and the anticardiolipin antibody levels were associated with anti-dsDNA antibody levels as well as neurological disease activity. In a more recent study, the incidence was found to be 79%, with an incidence of lupus anticoagulant of 42%.[16] In this study, the antibody levels did not correlate with disease activity, and the figures are much higher than for most reported series.

Neurological symptoms need to be investigated. Lumbar puncture, electroencephalography (EEG), magnetic resonance imaging (MRI) or computed tomography (CT) of the head may be useful in determining the cause of CNS symptoms. There are no specific investigations that will confirm cerebral lupus, although single photon emission CT (SPECT), if available, appears to be useful diagnostically.

On occasion, the diagnosis can be helped by skin biopsies demonstrating vasculitis and a positive lupus band test. This test identifies IgG or IgM linear deposition at the dermal–epidermal junction in non-light-exposed areas.

GENERAL TREATMENT

Important aspects of treatment include advice on lifestyle, such as taking adequate rest, the importance of contraception and sexual counselling, if needed. Advice about a low-salt, low-calorie diet is necessary for patients on steroid treatment. Skin protection is important: patients need to avoid exposure to sunlight as well as ultraviolet light from fluorescent lighting. Good-quality, high-factor sunblocks need to be prescribed and may need to be worn all year round. Sunblocks that are suitable for the patient's skin colour, and which are perceived as being trendy, will increase compliance. Fortunately, many teenagers are now very health conscious, and so are more likely to heed advice on avoiding exposure to sunlight.

DRUG TREATMENT

Patients with mild lupus affecting only the skin and joints can be treated successfully with non-steroidal anti-inflammatory drugs (NSAIDs) and hydroxychloroquine. Hydroxychloroquine is not only helpful in controlling the skin manifestations of lupus, but can also reduce the lethargy that afflicts many adolescents. Some patients respond slowly to hydroxychloroquine, and therefore it should be given on a 4–6 month trial basis before deciding whether or not it has been effective.

Corticosteroids

When the disease is more active with arthritis, pericarditis, pleuritis or serositis, corticosteroids are invariably the mainstay of treatment, either orally or intravenously. Maintenance treatment in the UK generally consists of oral enteric-coated prednisolone. Acute disease flares may be managed in part by either intravenous or intramuscular methylprednisolone. Due to their side-effects, steroids are reduced to a minimum at every available opportunity. However, the reduction in dose must be made with extreme caution, and over long periods of time. Careful attention has to be paid to disease control. Adolescents are frequently prescribed relatively high doses of steroids over prolonged periods of time in order to control their disease.

In adolescents, the most disastrous side-effect (from the patient's point of view) is that of altered appearance. They complain most bitterly about weight gain, and this can cause compliance problems. The problems with acne and striae seem to concern them less. The long-term problems of growth retardation and osteoporosis initially concern parents more than adolescents. However, it can become a real concern for adolescents who have required long-term steroid therapy when their peers start going into puberty and entering their pubertal growth spurt. It may be difficult to assess how much of the growth retardation and pubertal delay is due to disease activity and how much is due to steroid treatment. However, the combination of short stature and pubertal delay emphasizes the patient's differences from their friends and can cause psychological problems. If the pubertal delay is causing psychological problems, a

paediatric endocrinologist's advice can be useful in helping a teenager through puberty. As a teenager's final height may be reduced by long-term steroid therapy (as it reduces the length of growing time), the opinion of a paediatric endocrinologist is useful, and the adolescents often find the consultation helpful.

Osteoporosis

Osteoporosis is a side-effect of long-term steroid therapy, and the risk is increased by the low intake of calcium in most adolescents' diets. Calcium and vitamin D supplements need to be prescribed to prevent osteoporosis. On occasion, an adolescent will be convinced of the necessity of taking these by a bone density scan. Other side-effects of steroid therapy that need to be considered are steroid cataracts, and the problem of avascular necrosis, which seems to occur more often than in other paediatric autoimmune disorders requiring long-term steroid therapy.[17]

Atherosclerosis

A concern has been raised about the dangers of high lipid levels in patients on long-term steroid therapy, or with nephrotic renal disease. Steroid therapy may predispose to coronary atherosclerosis and it may be advisable to assess lipid levels, especially in patients with a strong family history of heart disease. The treatment of hypercholesterolaemia is controversial, but the use of cholesterol lowering agents should be considered.

Immunosuppressive agents

Immunosuppressive therapy is used in SLE, but which agent to use and when, are controversial topics. Azathioprine is an immunosuppressant widely used to help control disease activity, while keeping the steroid dose to a minimum. In cases of severe disease, especially lupus nephritis and cerebritis, cyclophosphamide is usually used. Its immunosuppressant effect is seen after several days, with the nadir of bone-marrow suppression around 10 days. Supportive treatment may be required, but if possible blood transfusions should be avoided, as most patients tend to develop antibodies over time and this may prejudice a later need for renal transplant. Many centres will give a monthly cyclophosphamide infusion for 6 months, followed by infusions every 2–3 months for up to 2 years,[18] depending on the disease activity and its response to the treatment. Obviously, in teenagers there is concern about the long-term effects of this drug, including its effect on female and male fertility. This issue needs to be addressed sensitively, as most adolescents find this a difficult area to cope with, even when they are well. If the patient is pubertal, then storage of sperm or eggs is a possibility. However, using the regime outlined above, Boumpas et al[18] showed that over 80% of those aged under 25 years will not develop infertility.

Plasmapheresis

Plasmapheresis has been used in lupus, often in conjunction with intravenous cyclophosphamide. Its role in the management of severe lupus has been controversial.[19] A recent multicentre trial comparing repeated plasmapheresis and intravenous cyclophosphamide with cyclophosphamide alone showed no additional clinical benefit and a greater number of side-effects with the combination treatment.[20] Therefore, there is no good evidence for plasmapheresis as a long-term treatment for lupus. However, in life-threatening situations it may help to 'buy time' while the immunosuppressants take effect.

Anticoagulation

The treatment of patients with antiphospholipid antibodies who are symptomatic consists either of low-dose aspirin or anticoagulation therapy. The use of anticoagulation after a single coagulation event requires evaluation: a single cerebral thrombotic event requires anticoagulation, but a single deep vein thrombosis may not. Care has to be taken in patients with recurrent spontaneous abortions: aspirin and low-dose heparin is recommended during pregnancy, with aspirin alone after pregnancy.[21] The treatment of patients who are asymptomatic is

controversial. It has been suggested that patients who are positive for both anticardiolipin antibodies and lupus anticoagulant may be more at risk of developing problems, and so should be treated with low-dose aspirin.[16]

IMMUNIZATIONS

Guidelines on immunizations need to be given to patients and their family doctors. In general, live vaccinations are contraindicated when on immunosuppressant drugs such as steroids, azathioprine or cyclophosphamide. Advice on exposure to chickenpox varies. Most adolescents are immune to varicella zoster, but this needs to be confirmed. Those who are not immune require zoster immune globulin if they come into contact with chickenpox and are on immunosuppressant drugs.

DIET

Many parents and adolescents seek advice on diet. There are many anecdotal reports of dietary restriction helping specific patients, with patients reporting that certain foods exacerbate their disease. There is little objective evidence published on dietary manipulation in lupus patients. An open study of lupus patients[22] showed a reduction in disease activity and a modest decrease in prednisolone after a year of a diet low in polyunsaturated fats. The only double-blind trial that has been published[23] looked at the effect of adding fish oil to a low-fat diet in 27 lupus patients with active disease. This showed that patients on a low-fat diet did significantly better when given a fish-oil supplement rather than a placebo.

OUTCOME ASSESSMENTS

As reviewed recently elsewhere,[6] it is evident that the outcome in patients with lupus depends upon the use of reliable, reproducible and valid disease activity, damage and patient health perception indices. Such indices have now been developed by adult rheumatologists. Among the activity indices the SLE Activity Measure (SLAM) and SLE Disease Activity Index (SLEDAI) offer useful global score assessments, whereas the British Isles Lupus Assessment Group (BILAG) system, which is based on the 'physician's intention to treat' principle, offers a more detailed 'at a glance' review of disease activity in eight organ systems. A damage index for lupus, the Systemic Lupus International Collaborative Clinics/American College of Rheumatology (SLICC/ACR) index[24] has been developed and widely accepted. Recent studies suggest that the SF-36 is a valuable health perception index to use in assessing patients with lupus.[25] The use of these assessments in adolescents is discussed further in Chapter 3.

PREGNANCY

Apart from patients with renal failure, fertility does not appear to be affected by lupus. Pregnancy is a time of enormous immunological change for healthy women. Despite this, pregnancy does not seem to adversely affect the mother with lupus. Although there are some reports to the contrary, the largest study of carefully matched pregnant and non-pregnant patients showed that pregnancy was not associated with an increased risk of SLE flare.[26] However, it is advisable to avoid pregnancy when the disease is active. Obviously lupus patients who are pregnant need careful monitoring, and disease flares may require corticosteroid treatment.

Pregnancy in any adolescent can be difficult to manage. The psychological effects of lupus on adolescents (discussed further below) are complicated enough, but if combined with pregnancy an 'explosive mixture' can be produced. Great care and sensitivity need to be used, especially as lupus can affect the fetus adversely.[6] There is a fetal mortality of around 20% due to spontaneous abortion and stillbirth. Premature delivery is common (up to 25%) due to maternal

ill-health or fetal distress. Babies born to mothers who are Ro and/or La positive may suffer from neonatal lupus. Neonatal lupus can cause a transient skin rash, or a permanent heart block requiring pacing.[17]

PSYCHOLOGICAL ISSUES

The diagnosis of lupus can be difficult at any age. However, the management of the disease in the adolescent years is particularly demanding and, ideally, requires the use of a team approach. Normal adolescent behaviour complicates even 'straightforward' chronic diseases. Active lupus appears to have a psychological effect on children and teenagers, even when they do not have overt signs of cerebral lupus. Our clinical psychologist, Shirley Corkhill, conducted a small pilot study of eight patients with lupus. This group included patients with mild disease who clinically appeared to be normal in their behaviour and attitudes. On psychological testing, even these patients responded in ways which were quite different from other children with other chronic disease, such as arthritis. In effect, their way of responding was more similar to children with psychiatric problems (S. Corkhill, personal communication). This suggests that in childhood lupus affects the CNS even when clinically there is no overt cerebral lupus.

In a study of mood and mood disorders in adult-onset lupus,[27] 39% of patients had clinical anxiety and 26% of the 80 patients were clinically depressed. Over 90% scored fatigue as one of the worst problems of their lupus, with 78% scoring depression as a problem. On neuropsychological testing, 15% were found to be cognitively impaired, although most of these had a preceding neurological problem (e.g. stroke, seizures or depression). However, this did not correlate with anxious or depressed moods. Nor did disease activity correlate with clinical anxiety, clinical depression, anxious mood or depressed mood.

There are few published studies on mood and psychological problems in childhood-onset lupus. A study of eight children aged 10–19

Table 7.3   Adolescent themes

- Control issues
- Separation from parents
- Sense of self
- Appearance
- Sexuality
- Cognitive development and planning for the future
- Vision of the future, self-concept

---

years with lupus looked at learning abilities as well as their behaviour and mood.[13] The children had globally lowered intellectual function, with the more complex functions of language processing and comprehension, as well as mathematical skills, most affected. Despite six of the patients being referred for altered mood or behaviour associated with their SLE, there was no significant behavioural or emotional distress, based on parental ratings and self-report ratings. However, adolescents with lupus often seem more 'difficult' than adolescents with other chronic diseases, and trying to distinguish psychological problems from disease activity can be very difficult. Often the clinician has to keep an open mind: symptoms that seem to be psychological may in fact turn out to be due to an unusual aspect of disease activity, or vice versa.

In dealing with adolescent lupus, there are several important adolescent themes that need to be considered (Table 7.3). These themes need to be considered in all the areas of an adolescent's life (school, social and family life).

In adolescence, the child is fighting the battle of emerging independence. It is a time of great turmoil for the individual, as well as their parents, who have to cope with their child's development as well as their own problems in trying to alter their role as a parent. In this context, the medical team has to treat the patient in their own right, but also has to support and gain the confidence of the family. Parents are used to caring for a child. Suddenly, the child is rebelling. On top of this, both the parents and their child are coming to terms with a chronic disease that is unpredictable and can affect all parts of the body. It is difficult for parents to let go and to have the confidence that the adolescent will make the right decisions. If some of these decisions affect health, it is difficult for parents to know when to step in and take control.

DRUG COMPLIANCE

One of the most frequent adolescent issues for the medical team is that of compliance. Many parents, quite rightly, will expect the medication to be taken unsupervised by their child. However, most adolescents are acutely aware of their bodies, and are very self-conscious. If they walk into a room, they are convinced that everyone is watching them and commenting on their appearance. They are having to come to terms with their own concept of self, as well as their sexuality. For example, from the adolescent's point of view the visible side-effects of steroids (increase in weight, especially the facial oedema, striae, hirsutism) far override the disease benefit. Therefore, many will either not take their steroids, or take them erratically. This leaves the physician in a quandary: are the symptoms due to undertreatment (in some cases to overtreatment) or to a lack of response to the medication? Sometimes parents will have an insight into what is going on, but often they have to be persuaded that their child is lying about compliance. At times this can only be done during a hospital admission where medication is closely supervised. Even in these cases, we have had teenagers who have managed to confound the nurses. Changing medication to syrup forms can help ensure that it is swallowed, but even so patients may have to be watched closely. Once the staff and parents are convinced that there is non-compliance, the team need to tackle the reasons for it. This usually requires the input of an experienced psychologist, who can take into account the adolescent's level of cognitive development.

METHODS OF COPING

In many ways, patients and their parents manage to cope with everyday life by a form of denial, which in adolescents has been referred to as a 'positive reappraisal' approach.[28] Lupus is often seen as a devastating disease by parents. Most teenagers, as well as their parents, are aware of the seriousness, unpredictability and chronicity of lupus. In spite of this, they manage to go to school, cope with family life and work. In order to get on with life, they have to positively reappraise their situation: they have to redefine their situation to see the positive side. In other words, passively accepting the pain, the fatigue and the despair that might be engendered by the reality of the disease is likely to be associated with adolescents who are less well-adjusted and have a lower sense of well-being.[28] The medical team (both nurses and doctors) must, to a certain extent, help in this denial or reappraisal process. Even when discussing disease possibilities, we tend to an optimistic view. As a team we feel the need to support the family in maintaining as 'ordinary' an existence as possible. The psychologist has an important role in allowing the parents and the patient to acknowledge the reality of their situation in a contained manner. It may be important to allow the adolescent time to express what they feel is different about them compared to their peers, and even compared to other patients on the ward. Teenagers have usually developed enough cognitive skills to hold a series of possibilities for the future, and they can think through the consequences of different actions. They also start to philosophize and become concerned with the 'unfairness' of having lupus. Helping the adolescent to move forward to a more positive reappraisal approach may lessen their distress.

SCHOOLING

Adolescents with lupus should be expected to attend school regularly. Adolescents with chronic disease tend to suffer from relapses and remissions. In lupus these tend to be unpredictable in their timing and severity. Patients miss school not only due to illness, but also for outpatient clinic visits, monitoring activities (e.g. blood tests) and treatment (e.g. physiotherapy). Even if these are done locally, time is lost from school, which not only affects academic achievement, but also makes it difficult for the adolescent to keep up with their peer group, both in emotional terms as well as socially. This is particularly true when the patient has long absences from school; even understanding mundane conversation can be difficult, as this is often based on recent common experience.

Patients with lupus often suffer from a lack of concentration, tiredness and lethargy. This can be due to disease activity (including cerebral lupus), drug treatment and, in some cases, an accompanying fibromyalgia. Adolescents with lupus may be able to manage the school day, but not the homework in the evenings. They may be expending all their energy in maintaining school, and maintaining their peer groups. These difficulties are increased if there are changes in physical appearance: many lupus patients suffer from rashes that come on very quickly and are very noticeable. Both girls and boys are acutely aware of patchy hair loss or vasculitic lesions on exposed areas. These changes in physical appearance, as well as those caused by the drug treatment, can be a cause of unpopularity at school. Thus, maintaining school can take a lot of physical as well as emotional energy. 'Whingeing' behaviour is often unpopular at school, and therefore adolescents with lupus may tend to express their distress or pain at home. This creates a problem in that parents may see an apparently different picture of how well their child is, from the picture seen by the school.

Parents may also see their child's level of achievement slipping due to fatigue and loss of concentration. They may find it difficult to persuade the school that extra help might be needed, or they may need to reassess what the realistic goals are for their child in view of their disease. These concerns can be very difficult to manage, as the adolescent years are important academically as well as from a career point of view.

FAMILY

The family of an adolescent with lupus encounters emotional demands and practical difficulties; they need to develop effective coping strategies. Many families do remarkably well. If difficulties arise, the family as a whole and how it functioned prior to the onset and diagnosis of lupus has to be considered. The team's role may be thought of as fostering the family's acquisition of relevant coping skills. This allows for greater independence and competence in dealing with stress within the family. Families who have good, open means of communication, and who work out problems together, often are more flexible in their routines and appear better 'adjusted'.[29] Parents will have increased levels of anxiety. They are faced with the issues of control and independence. During adolescence, parents have to decide what is and what is not safe for their child to do. With a chronic disease, different levels of control often have to be negotiated. On occasion, the teenager has to be helped to express which issues they would like to control, and which they would prefer to leave to others. This is followed by a negotiation over what is realistic. If this is done well, it can take an enormous amount of time with separate parent and child interviews. A busy outpatient clinic, with its lack of time and numerous interruptions, is unlikely to be a successful venue. In this respect, an experienced psychologist can be of great help.

Psychologists will incorporate time and privacy into their assessments. An experienced psychologist will often come up with an apparently simple solution to a problem, but it will have taken them time to achieve. They have to build up a relationship with the patient, and the adolescent has to believe that what they are saying is important to them as well as to the psychologist. Often, the psychologist will raise questions in order for the adolescent themself to find the answers, as opposed to doctors or nurses who are seen by patients as being the experts who provide all the answers and the advice. In the end, the key is in deciding which is the appropriate behavioural response in the context of the individual adolescent, and how to apply it.

Very little work has been done on fathers and their role in chronic disease. This needs to change, as many fathers are becoming more involved in their children's care. In research looking at mothers of children with chronic disease, it has been shown that potential isolation in giving up employment or careers can lead to anxiety and depression.[30] In the lower socio-economic groups, mothers cannot financially afford to give up their job, leading to the stress of juggling their job, a family and the burdens imposed by the disease. Whether or not a mother works outside the home, mothers do 'better' if they feel in control and are positively engaged in their child's disease management.[31] In fact, the mother's stress levels have been shown to be related to their perception of the child's disease severity, rather than to the child's, or doctor's perception.[32] Most parents perceive lupus as a much more menacing disease than many of the other rheumatological diseases.

Siblings of children with a chronic disease are an important part of the patient's family life. Siblings can feel neglected by their parents, and may have an increased burden of domestic chores and childcare-related activities within the family.[32] Siblings may be helped by an understanding of lupus, its unpredictability and how it can affect adolescents and alter their behaviour. However, differential treatment of a sick sibling still increases the likelihood of 'maladjustment' in a sibling,[33] and this may further increase the anxiety and stress within the family.

In childhood, as opposed to adolescence, children are highly dependent on parents. Therefore, attention has to be paid to the social environment in which coping strategies are developed. Parents can aid or hinder this. In adolescence, teenagers become more concerned with peer approval and their own status within their peer group.[32] They tend to use peer support for developing coping strategies. This is obviously difficult for adolescents with lupus, as their disease will be outside the experiences of their peer group.

Some psychologists talk about two different sorts of coping strategies: emotion focused and problem based. As they mature, children develop from using emotional strategies (such as wishful thinking or resignation) to problem-solving strategies. Illness can interfere with this development or cause the adolescent to regress in this respect. Unpredictable diseases such as lupus tend to encourage the use of emotion-focused coping strategies. Emotion-based coping strategies have been related to self-reports of depression, anxiety and substance abuse in adolescents, whereas when a problem-based approach is used mothers and children report fewer emotional and behaviour problems.[32] Therefore, each lupus patient needs to be assessed in order to ascertain their level of cognitive development: one cannot assume that older children, or children with a longer experience of lupus, will cope better.

Problem-solving skills are not the only area that needs to be assessed. Interpersonal skills and self-esteem are also important issues in adolescents with lupus. Chronic disease increases the likelihood of a teenager facing failure at school, either academically or at an interpersonal level. This is more often a problem in patients with lupus because of its effects on appearance, as well as its psychological effects, which may cause loss of self-esteem. This is at a time when many adolescents will be developing their ideas about themselves, their sexuality and their attitudes to smoking, alcohol and drug taking. It is a time when adolescents are developing a vision of what their future ambitions should be. In the context of an unpredictable disease, adolescents with lupus may need help in coming to terms with what their vision of the future can realistically be.

CONCLUSION

SLE is a disease that can affect any organ and the presentation of which can be acute or insidious. Once diagnosed, the disease course is variable and unpredictable. Careful follow-up is required. The management of adolescents with a chronic disease often benefits from a multidisciplinary team approach. This is especially true for the management of adolescents with lupus, where the effects of the disease are difficult to disentangle from 'normal' adolescent behaviour. The advice of a psychologist interested in adolescence can be very helpful. Adolescents, as well as their families, may need psychological help to come to terms with the illness, and to develop appropriate coping strategies.

REFERENCES

1. Tan EM, Cohen AS, Fries JF et al. The 1982 revised criteria for the classification of systemic lupus erythematosus. *Arthritis Rheum* 1982; **25**(11):1271–7.
2. Hochberg MC. Updating the American College of Rheumatology revised criteria for the classification of systemic lupus erythematosus. *Arthritis Rheum* 1997; **9**:1725.
3. Siegel M, Lee ML. The epidemiology of systemic lupus erythematosus. *Semin Arthritis Rheum* 1973; **3**:1–54.
4. Johnson AE, Gordon C, Palmer RG, Bacon PA. The prevalence and incidence of systemic lupus erythematosus in Birmingham, England. *Arthritis Rheum* 1995; **38**:551–8.
5. Lehman TJA. Systemic lupus erythematosus in children and adolescents. In: *The Clinical Management of Systemic Lupus Erythematosus* (Schur PH, ed), 2nd edn. Lippincott-Raven: Philadelphia, 1996:195–209.
6. Isenberg DA, Horsfall AC. Systemic lupus erythematosus in adults. In: *Oxford Textbook of Rheumatology* (Maddison PJ, Isenberg DA, Woo P, Glass DN, eds), 2nd edn. Oxford University Press: Oxford, 1998:1145–80.
7. Tucker LB, Menon S, Schaller JG, Isenberg DA. Adult- and childhood-onset systemic lupus erythematosus: a comparison of onset, clinical features, serology, and outcome. *Br J Rheum* 1995; **34**:866–72.
8. Brik R, Padeh S, Mukamel M et al. Systemic lupus erythematosus in children in Israel. *Harefuah* 1995; **129**:7–8.
9. Pande I, Sekharan NG, Kailash S et al. Analysis of clinical and laboratory profile in Indian systemic lupus erythematosus and its comparison with SLE in adults. *Lupus* 1993; **2**:83–7.
10. Deepen D, Escalante A, Weinrib L et al. A revised estimate of twin concordance in systemic lupus erythematosus. *Arthritis Rheum* 1992; **35**:311–18.

11. Parikh S, Swaiman KF, Kim Y. Neurologic characteristics of childhood lupus erythematosus. *Paediatr Neurol* 1995; **13**:198–201.

12. Yancey CL, Doughty RA, Athrea BH. Central nervous system involvement in childhood systemic lupus erythematosus. *Arthritis Rheum* 1981; **24**:1389–95.

13. Wyckoff PM, Miller LC, Tucker LB, Schaller JG. Neuropsychological assessment of children and adolescents with systemic lupus erythematosus. *Lupus* 1995; **4**:217–20.

14. Genth E, Mierau R. Autoantibodies in systemic rheumatic disorders, clinical and diagnostic relevance. *Rev Rhum (Engl Ed)* 1997; **10S**:149S–52S.

15. Shergy WJ, Kredich DW, Pisetsky DS. The relationship of anticardiolipin antibodies to disease manifestations in pediatric systemic lupus erythematosus. *J Rheum* 1988; **15**:1389–94.

16. Gattorno M, Buoncompagni A, Molinari AC et al. Antiphospholipid antibodies in paediatric systemic lupus erythematosus, juvenile chronic arthritis and overlap syndromes: SLE patients with both lupus anticoagulant and high-titre anticardiolipin antibodies are at risk for clinical manifestations related to the antiphospholipid syndrome. *Br J Rheum* 1995; **34**:873–81.

17. Silverman ED, Eddy AA. Systemic lupus erythematosus in children. In: *Oxford Textbook of Rheumatology* (Maddison PJ, Isenberg DA, Woo P, Glass DN, eds), 2nd edn. Oxford University Press: Oxford, 1998:1180–202.

18. Boumpas DT, Austin HA, Vaughan EM et al. Controlled trial of pulse methylprednisolone versus two regimens of pulse cyclophosphamide in severe lupus nephritis. *Lancet* 1992; **340**:741–5.

19. McClure C, Isenberg DA. Does plasma exchange have any part to play in the management of SLE? In: *Controversies in Rheumatology* (Isenberg DA, Tucker LB, eds). Martin Dunitz: London, 1997:75–85.

20. Schroeder JO, Schwab U, Zeuner R, Fastenrath S, Euler HH. Plasmapharesis and subsequent pulse cyclophosphamide in severe systemic lupus erythematosus. Preliminary results of the LPSG Trial. *Arthritis Rheum* 1997; **40S**:S325.

21. Rai R, Cohen H, Dave M, Regan L. Randomised controlled trial of aspirin and aspirin plus heparin in pregnant women with recurrent miscarriage associated with phospholipid antibodies. *Br Med J* 1997; **314**:253–7.

22. Thorner A, Walldius G, Nilsson B, Hadell K, Gullberg R. Beneficial effects of reduced intake of polyunsaturated fatty acids in the diet for one year in patients with systemic lupus erythematosus. *Ann Rheum Dis* 1990; **49**:134.

23. Walton AJE, Snaith ML, Locniskar M, Cumberland AG, Morrow WJW, Isenberg DA. Dietary fish oil and the severity of symptoms in patients with systemic lupus erythematosus. *Ann Rheum Dis* 1991; **50**:463–6.

24. Gladman DD, Ginzler E, Goldsmith C et al. The development and initial validation of the Systemic Lupus International Collaborating Clinics/American College of Rheumatology Damage Index for systemic lupus erythematosus. *Arthritis Rheum* 1996; **39**:363–9.

25. Stoll T, Gordon C, Seifert B et al. Consistency and validity of patient administered assessment of quality of life by the MOS SF-36; its association with disease activity and damage in patients with systemic lupus erythematosus. *J Rheum* 1997; **24**:1608–14.

26. Urowitz MB, Gladman DD, Farewell VT, Stewart J, McDonald J. Lupus and pregnancy studies. *Arthritis Rheum* 1993; **36**:1392–7.

27. Shortall E, Isenberg DA, Newman SP. Factors associated with mood and mood disorders in SLE. *Lupus* 1995; **4**:272–9.

28. Ebata AT, Moos RH. Coping and adjustment in distressed and healthy adolescents. *J Appl Dev Psychol* 1991; **12**:33–54.

29. Koocher GP, O'Malley JE. Implications for patient care. In: *The Damodes Syndrome: Psychological Consequences of Surviving Childhood Cancer* (Koocher GP, O'Malley JE, eds). New York: McGraw-Hill, 1981.

30. Wallander JL, Varni JW, Babani L, DeHeen CB, Wilcox KT, Banis HT. The social environment and the adaptation of mothers of physically handicapped children. *J Pediatr Psychol* 1989; **14**:371–88.

31. Obetz SW, Swenson WM, McCarthy CA, Gilchrist GS, Burgert EO. Children who survive malignant disease: emotional adaptation of the children and their families. In: *The Child with Cancer: Clinical Approaches to Psychosocial Care – Research in Psychosocial Aspects* (Schulman JL, Kupst MJ, eds). CC Thomas: Springfield, IL, 1980:194–210.

32. Eiser C. *Chronic Childhood Disease. An Introduction to Psychological Theory and Research.* Cambridge University Press: Cambridge, 1990.

33. Drotar D, Crawford P. Psychological adaptation of siblings of chronically ill children: research and practice implications. *Dev Behav Pediatr* 1985; **6**:355–62.

8

Myositis

Lauren M Pachman

INTRODUCTION

In children, inflammatory muscle disease includes an acute process, the aetiology of which is related to known viral or bacterial agents, and chronic myositis, encompassing juvenile dermatomyositis (JDM), juvenile polymyositis (JPM) and inflammatory myopathy associated with other autoimmune rheumatic disease or with parasitic infection. In the world at large, most of the inflammatory myopathies are a consequence of bacterial or parasitic infections, but in North America and Europe a viral aetiology is more common, and myopathy accompanying human T-cell lymphotropic virus-1 (HTLV-1) is now recognized.[1]

In the past few years, more attention has been focused on the paediatric inflammatory myopathies, providing increasing evidence (and controversy) concerning the similarities and differences between those illnesses that occur in childhood (aetiology, pathogenesis and response to therapy) and those that are found in the adult population. Specific validated information concerning the adolescent is much more scarce. In adults, over 50% of patients with myositis have specific clinical and epidemiological features and enter specific subsets of inflammatory myopathy;[2] however, these subsets are rare in children.[3] Recent evidence suggests that genetic[4] and infectious factors may play a part in disease susceptibility, as well as disease severity/chronicity. In this chapter the available clinical and laboratory evidence concerning JDM is discussed and areas in which new data have been accrued are identified.

The primary clinical feature of both JDM and JPM is chronic and progressive weakness of proximal muscles. In JDM the vasculopathy and distinctive skin manifestations are commonly associated with muscle involvement; in JPM, the skin is spared. A diagnosis of definite JDM is made if, in addition to the typical rash, three of the following four criteria are present:[5]

- elevated serum levels of muscle-derived enzymes
- electromyographic evidence of inflammatory myopathy
- positive muscle biopsy
- proximal muscle weakness.

A diagnosis of definite JPM is made if three of the four criteria are present.[5] Because myositis is often a part of other autoimmune rheumatic diseases, it is essential to exclude such conditions as systemic lupus erythematosus, mixed connective tissue disease,[6] chronic arthritis in children (especially of systemic onset),[7] the spondyloarthropathies and Sjögren's syndrome. Inclusion-body myositis, which often runs a steroid-resistant course, has also been described in children.[8] Furthermore, the inflammatory myopathy can be focal, such as in orbital myositis,[9] nodular or proliferative,[3] or involve an eosinophilic infiltration of the fascia.[10] Other types of musculoskeletal disorder that may present with muscle weakness and/elevated levels of serum-derived enzymes must also be excluded, the most common of which are the muscular dystrophies (see below).

EPIDEMIOLOGY

Demographic data

In childhood there is a bimodal age distribution for polymyositis/dermatomyositis (at 5–9 years of age, 3.7 cases/million/year; at 10–14 years of age, 4.3 cases/million/year) as well as a separate adult peak (at 45–64 years of age, 10 cases/million/year).[11] A study of 79 American patients with JDM of the age at disease onset confirmed the bimodal distribution in both boys and girls (Figure 8.1).[12] Children with disease onset under the age of 7 years may have a milder course.[13] In the USA, JDM is more frequently reported in Caucasians (male/female 2 : 1),[12] although children of African or Asian origin may be at increased risk for chronic myositis.[14] In the UK and Ireland, five times as many girls were diagnosed as boys, with an incidence of 1.9/million children under age 16 years.[15] A similar trend was found in China.[16] However, in Japan, the overall incidence was 1.3 males to 1 female; none had associated malignancy or interstitial lung disease.[17] In Singapore, for children below the age of 5 years with JDM the sex ratio was equal.[18] This is in contrast to data from our Chicago clinic population of 127 children with JDM, in which the female/male ratio was 1.7 (no significant change with age), or from the National New Onset JDM Registry (146 children) in which, overall, the female/male ratio was 2.17 (for children aged 5 years and below the ratio was 2.08). In children, JPM accounts for about 8% of the inflammatory myopathies,[19] as compared with adults in whom the frequency is estimated to be about 27%.[20] In contrast to reports of one-third mortality and one-third morbidity prior to the use of corticosteroids,[21] both of these adverse outcomes have decreased.[22,23] In Japan, during a 10-year period (1973–1983) there was a 2.9% mortality rate,[24] which is similar to estimates from USA data, although no long-term data are available. Association with malignancy is frequent in adults with dermatomyositis,[25] but not in children;[24] only sporadic cases of both an inflammatory myopathy and malignancy have been reported.[26] Furthermore, a population-based

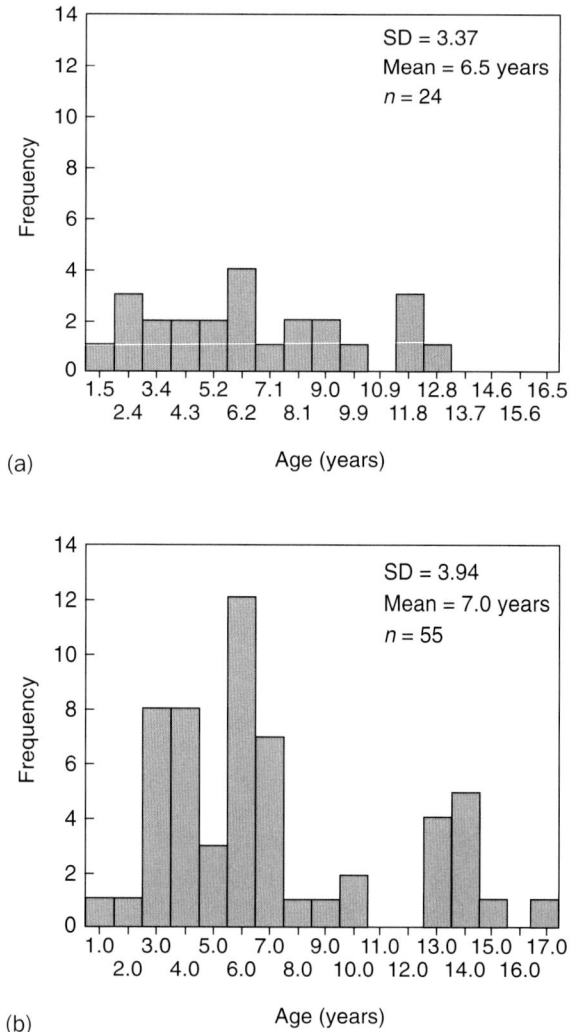

Figure 8.1 The age at diagnosis of JDM in (a) girls and (b)boys.

survey did not find malignancy in children aged 16 years or under.[27]

There is some controversy about the season of year of disease onset of juveniles with dermatomyositis and adults with polymyositis–dermatomyositis. The data appear to vary by geographical region and by year. In the north central region of the USA, children with definite JDM (diagnosed within 4 months of onset) were more likely to have their first symptoms in the months of January to June than at other periods of time in each of 7 years (1974–1980).[28] An investigation of 79 newly diagnosed JDM patients from all regions of the USA (1989–1992) identified an increased frequency of disease onset in the spring and summer of some years,[12] although another preliminary survey of JDM in the USA did not confirm this impression.[19] In Canada, clustering of new cases of JDM was observed as well, suggesting an environmental influence.[29] In the UK and Ireland, several clusters of disease onset were identified, the largest of which was in April and May in 1992; the timing of these clusters appeared to vary from year to year.[15] A case–control study of children in the USA validated the impression of a significant increase in antecedent symptoms in children with JDM in the 3 months prior to diagnosis.[30] It is not yet firmly established if the preference for season of onset is the same for both adults and children living in the same region, or if the peak onset of polymyositis is in the same time-frame as that of dermatomyositis in both age groups. A National Institutes of Health (NIH) sponsored National New Onset Registry has been established in the USA to determine more about the onset of dermatomyositis in children.[31]

Infectious agents and juvenile dermatomyositis

In addition to temporal, seasonal differences, there may be regional differences in agents associated with disease onset. Agents associated with the onset (and, on occasion, flare) of JDM are group A β-haemolytic streptococci,[19,32,33] hepatitis B[34] and the RNA picornaviruses.[30,35,36] Sera from newly diagnosed children (1974–1980) from the Chicago area had an increased frequency of antibody (both neutralizing (N) and complement fixing (CF)) to coxsackie B virus,[37] which were not reproduced by the same group of investigators in a study of 20 children with dermatomyositis from the same region with onset of disease in the years 1987–1992.[36] Enteroviral RNA was identified in the muscle of UK patients with polymyositis or

dermatomyositis,[35,38] but other investigators have not found viral RNA in cases from the USA, either in Jo-1 positive adults[39] or in magnetic resonance imaging (MRI) directed muscle biopsy of 20 newly diagnosed untreated children with active dermatomyositis.[36] Other infectious agents considered as triggers for JDM include *Toxoplasma gondii*,[40,41] and hepatitis B,[34] but antibody titres to these factors were not found to be increased, either in a regional study[28] or in a case–control national study of new-onset juvenile dermatomyositis spanning the years 1987–1992.[36,43] Although Theiler's murine encephalomyelitis virus (TMEV) was identified in adult polymyositis, none of the children with JDM were positive for this agent.[44] Taken together, the above data suggest that the aetiology of JDM is multifactorial, including a possible role of molecular mimicry. Supporting evidence for this hypothesis is found in a report of a sequence found in skeletal myosin (which has homology with the streptococcal type 5 M protein) stimulating lymphocytes from children with recurrent dermatomyositis following streptococcal infection.[32,33] Non-infectious exposures currently posited as causative agents in myositis include vaccines,[45] drugs,[46] growth

Table 8.1 Symptoms present in 79 newly diagnosed children with juvenile dermatomyositis

Symptom	n	
Rash	79	(100%)
Weakness	79	(100%)
Muscle pain	58	(73%)
Fever	51	(65%)
Dysphagia	35	(44%)
Hoarseness	34	(43%)
Abdominal pain	29	(37%)
Arthritis	28	(35%)
Calcifications	18	(23%)
Melena	10	(13%)

Table 8.2   First symptom (rash and/or weakness) of JDM and interval of time (median and range) before second symptom

	n	Rash First	Rash–weakness interval (months)	Weakness First	Weakness–rash interval (months)	Rash and weakness occurred at same time
Caucasian	59	30	2.0 (0.2–12.9)	15	2.0 (0.7–9.6)	14
Minority	20	12	3.5 (1.0–9.4)	4	6.0 (4.6–20.0)	4
All	79	42	2.0 (0.2–12.9)	19	3.2 (0.7–20.0)	18

hormone[47] and bone-marrow transplants, in which graft-versus-host myositis occurs as a component of immune activation.[48]

CLINICAL PRESENTATION

The most common physical findings in children with JDM at diagnosis are presented in Table 8.1. In addition, hepatosplenomegaly and generalized lymphadenopathy are present at onset in about 5% of children.

Cutaneous manifestations

In 53% of children with JDM the rash pre-dates the onset of symmetrical weakness in proximal muscles, while in 23% it is recognized at the same time as the weakness. In 24% of children, weakness is the first symptom. The distribution in minority and non-minority children and the interval between the first and second symptom is shown in Table 8.2. Sun exposure can precipitate exacerbation of symptoms (the children may sunburn more easily), either initially or once the disease has been diagnosed and treated; 41% of children with JDM had their first symptom during the summer months. Periorbital erythema and oedema, and/or eyelid telangiectasia (which may persist long after other signs and symptoms of disease activity have resolved) are seen in 50–90% of affected children. The rash has a violaceous or heliotrope hue, and is often most prominent on the eyelid (Figure 8.2a), where small infarctions may be seen. As in children with systemic lupus, the erythematous rash may cross the bridge of the nose. Other areas of erythema, involving the upper torso, the extensor surfaces of the arms and legs, the medial malleoli of the ankles and the buttocks, may occur in the absence of raised serum concentrations of muscle-derived enzymes. Partial baldness, which is particularly distressing to the adolescent, may result as a consequence of chronic scalp inflammation (Figure 8.2b).[49] The skin over the knuckles is often either hypertrophic or pale red (Gottron's sign), evolving into colourless bands of atrophic skin which, during active disease, may have a papular, 'alligator skin' like appearance (Gottron's papules) (Figure 8.2c). These hypertrophic, often erythematous, lesions (which fade as the disease resolves) occur primarily over the metacarpal phalangeal joints, the extensor aspect of the elbows or knees, or the medial canthus of the eyelid. Some recent data indicate that all children with the amyopathic form of JDM (rash only) will develop myositis (often with calcinosis) later in their disease course,[50] but this view is strongly contested.[51] Diffuse vasculopathy (nailbed telangiectasia (Figure 8.2d)), infarction of oral epithelium and skin folds, or digital ulceration) is clearly associated with more severe disease, and is correlated with the clinical course of the disease.[52] The progression

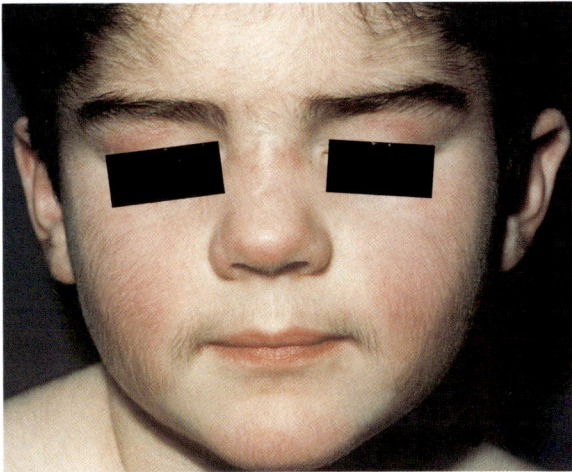
(a)

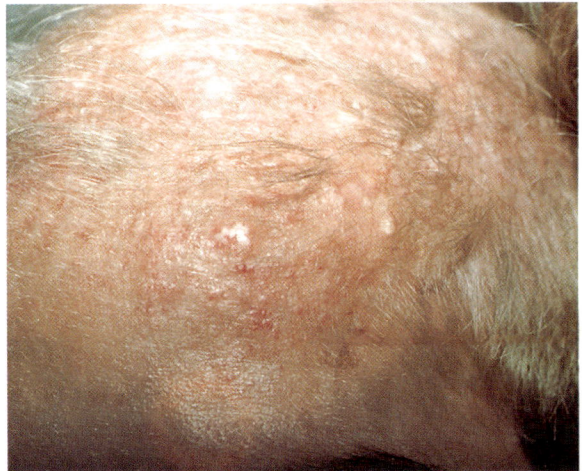
(b)

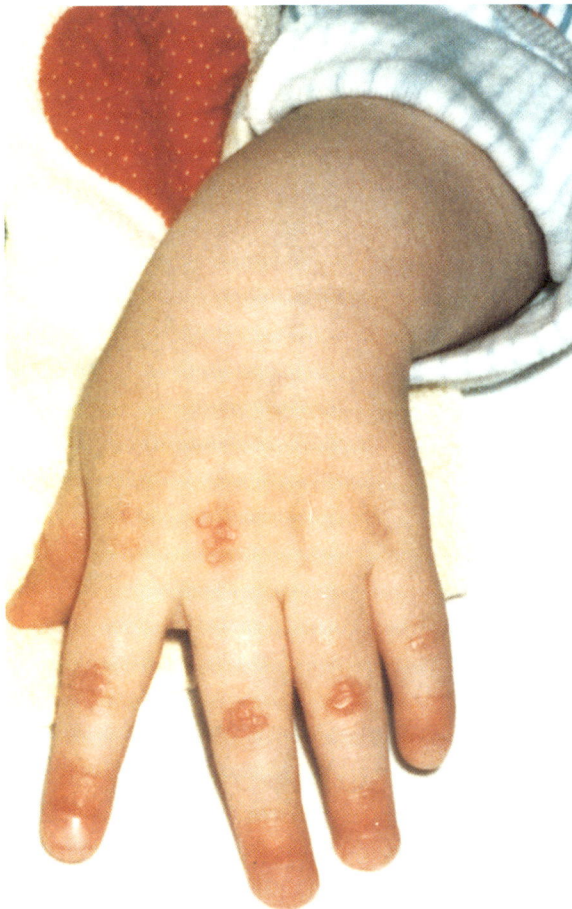
(c)

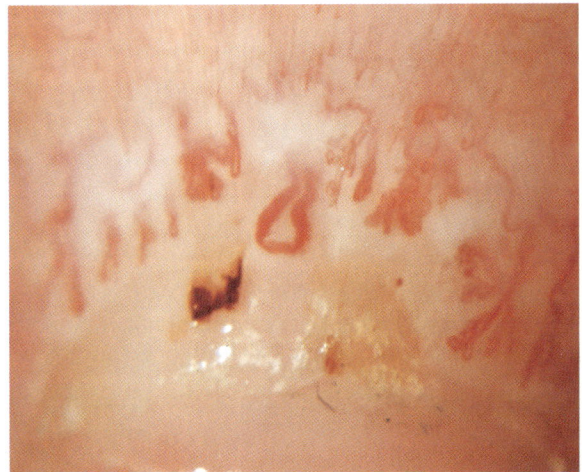
(d)

Figure 8.2 The cutaneous hallmarks of JDM. (a) The face of a child with JDM, showing eyelid capillary vessel dilatation and thrombosis, malar rash (which may cross the nasal bridge) and perioral pallor. (b) Alopecia in an adolescent: a consequence of chronic inflammation in the scalp. (c) The hand of a child with JDM, demonstrating erythematous Gottron's papules across the proximal interphalangeal and metacarpal phalangeal joints and evident periungual erythema. (d) Nailfold changes in chronic JDM, showing marked capillary dilatation and areas of capillary thrombosis.

(a)

(b)

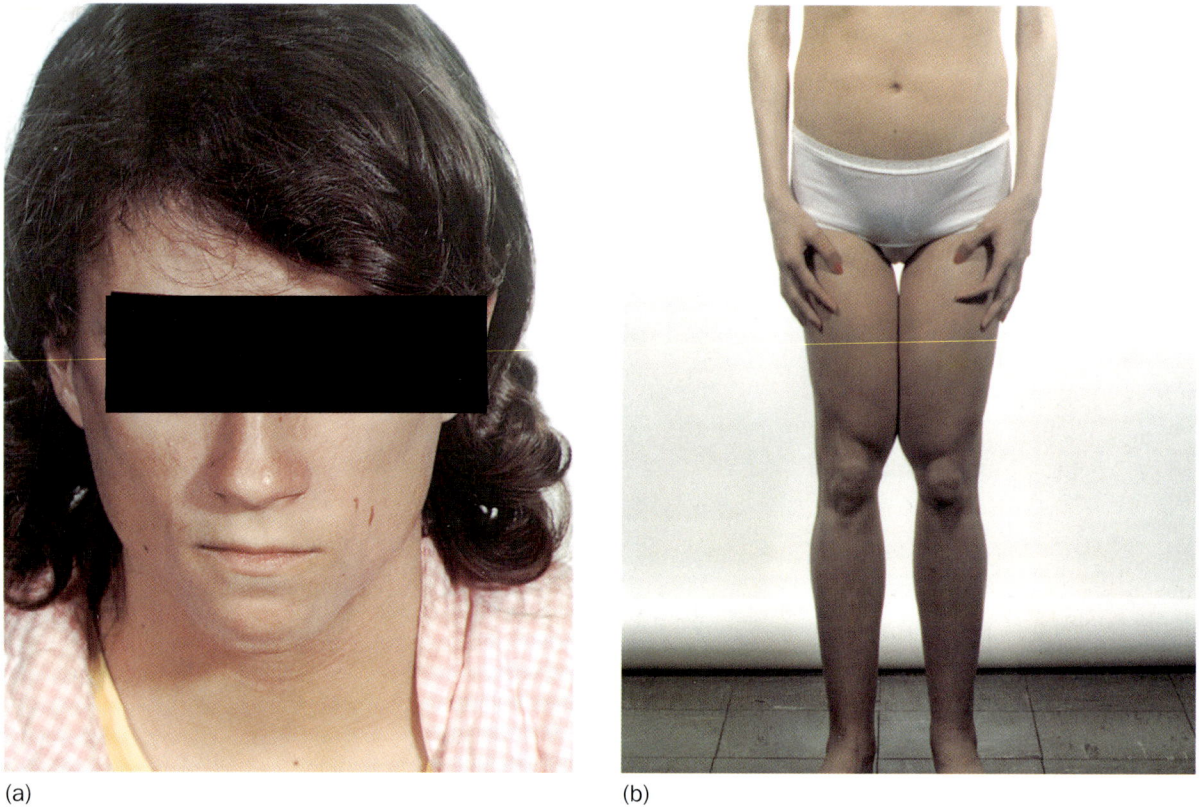

Figure 8.3   An adolescent in whom JDM was diagnosed at age 3 years, showing some of the characteristics of partial lipodystrophy. (a) Her face displays atrophy of the buccal fat pad. (b) The body habitus shows truncal obesity, with loss of fat from the limbs, and early 'potbelly'.

and regression of the vasculopathy can be quantitated using freeze-frame video microscopy.[53,54]

One of the major consequences of JDM seen in adolescents with chronic symptoms is partial lipoatrophy,[55,56] subcutaneous tissue loss which is pronounced in the buccal fat (Figure 8.3a) and in the extremities (Figure 8.3b). The areas are not tender, despite a lymphohistiocytic panniculitis.[57] Other clinical features of partial lipoatrophy include acanthosis nigricans, increased insulin levels, an abnormal glucose tolerance test (GGT) level associated with insulin-resistant diabetes, and virilization.[58,59] If the onset is before menarche in females, sterility may follow. A cross-sectional study of 34 children with JDM

confirmed[56] that children with chronic symptoms are more at risk (two had insulin resistance), again providing impetus for rapid disease control.[60]

Musculoskeletal symptoms

Although cutaneous findings are often the definitive sign of JDM, weakness can occur as the first symptom (see Table 8.2). Proximal muscle weakness, as evidenced by difficulty in climbing stairs, getting up from a chair, combing hair, or using the hands to push off from the body in an attempt to stand (Gower's sign), is common; weakness of the neck flexors is a particularly sensitive indicator of muscular impairment; but a young child (under the age of 4 years) will not be able to do a sit-up (clear the scapula), even when normal. This functional disability can be measured reliably by means of a questionnaire.[61] Over 60% of children complain of pain on muscle compression, but it is less severe than the muscle pain in the bacterial-related myopathies. Children with spinal muscular atrophy do not usually have muscle pain on compression. Fatigue is common, and is also exhibited by children with the dystrophies (most commonly those of Duchenne and Becker). Usually the child is more comfortable when the limbs are held in the flexed position, which promotes the development of flexion contractures. Active myositis can often be confirmed by electromyography or muscle biopsy, despite normal serum levels of muscle derived enzymes.[62] The use of MRI-directed biopsies minimizes error in sampling uninvolved area in this focal disease,[63] and can, under special circumstances, be an excellent means of monitoring a child's response to therapy.[64–66] The myositis as shown on MRI may normalize several months later than the muscle enzymes stabilize in their normal ranges.[67] Phosphorus-32 spin MRI has been in use for the past few years, and gives useful information about the child's muscle strength and performance.[68] Decreased bone density (associated with a depressed serum osteocalcin) is frequent in untreated juvenile dermatomyositis, which places the child at risk of bony fracture,[69,70] which is augmented further by steroid administration.

Cardiorespiratory abnormalities

The electrocardiogram is abnormal at disease onset in over half of children with definite JDM. Asymptomatic conduction abnormalities predominate, with an occasional complete block of the right bundle branch,[71] which usually resolves as disease activity decreases. Dilated cardiomyopathy can be a presenting complaint,[72] and tachycardia during the disease course reflects cardiac compromise. A decrease in ventilatory capacity, with a normal diffusion of carbon dioxide (DLCO) was found in 78% of JDM patients negative for antibody to the t-RNA synthetase, Jo-1.[71] This decrease in ventilatory capacity can be associated with diminished speech volume; several of our children have developed vocal-cord nodules, presumably as a result of the stress of trying to be heard. Pulmonary fibrosis is more commonly found in individuals who carry antibody to the t-RNA synthetases, of which anti-Jo-1 is the most common (see the section on pathophysiology below). For the adolescent who may want to smoke cigarettes, further impairment of lung function is a very serious issue, and merits straightforward discussion. Return to taxing competitive sports should only be permitted once there is evidence of normal cardiorespiratory function.

Gastrointestinal involvement

One of the most severe prognostic indicators is impairment of the flow of secretions, which is associated with decreased oesophageal motility (documented by radiographic contrast studies showing retained barium in a widened atonic, pyriform sinus).[73] The swallowing of liquids may also be impaired; oesophageal reflux may result in aspiration pneumonia, and appropriate precautions (e.g. using thickened foods, raising the bed head, and attention to clearing the respiratory tree) should be taken to prevent this.

Smooth-muscle dysfunction can also result in decreased lower gastrointestinal motility, making constipation an annoying symptom. Involvement of the masseter may result in difficulty in chewing. Vasculopathy affects any part of the gastrointestinal tract; in severe disease there is weight loss and mucosal ulceration, with melaena and the possibility of life-threatening perforation. In the young child, development of normal speech patterns can be disturbed; soft-palate involvement is often revealed by nasal, high-pitched speech (e.g. by saying the alphabet) and usually resolved with a decrease in the inflammatory component of the myositis.

Genitourinary function

Massive breakdown of muscle elements, as well as primary compromise of the renal parenchyma itself, may occur in children with an active myopathic process. This requires prompt hydration and monitoring of renal function. If unchecked, renal failure can occur. Necrosis of the ureter has been reported, involving the middle one-third (iliac) segment, because of the relatively sparse blood supply to this region compared with the upper (lumbar) or lower (pelvic) segments.[74] With respect to reproductive function, menses may cease during severe disease, but will resume once the active inflammation has been controlled. Anticardiolipin antibodies (ACAs) have been identified in JDM[75] (often with a negative lupus anticoagulant), and can be associated with increased fetal wastage.[76,77] Birth-control measures should take into account the possible presence of ACAs, to avoid the risk of increased intravascular thrombosis.

Ophthalmological findings

Infarctions of eye-related tissue most often occur over the medial canthus, which heals, leaving a depressed scar. In active disease, transient retinal exudates and 'cotton-wool' spots may occur after the occlusion of small vessels, leading to intraretinal oedema, with injury to retinal nerve fibres, optic atrophy and sustained visual loss. Neovascularization of the retina with spontaneous regression has also been reported.[78] Disease of conjunctival vessels can also lead to an avascular zone, with a potential for infarction. Children treated with steroids should be monitored for both glaucoma and for the development of sublenticular cataracts, which are related to the dose of corticosteroids given.[79] If there is a family history of red–green colour blindness, the use of hydroxychloroquine should be avoided. Orbital myositis can be documented by MRI, either as an isolated finding or as part of the spectrum of inflammatory myopathy, and responds to corticosteroid administration.[9]

Other disease manifestations

Vasculopathy involving the central nervous system may be associated with depression and/or wide mood swings, which may be exacerbated by steroid therapy (see below). It is not usual for a child with JDM to present with Raynaud's phenomenon; these symptoms are more frequently found as an isolated phenomenon, in overlap syndromes, or in those children who go on to develop scleroderma.

DIFFERENTIAL DIAGNOSIS

General

The differential diagnosis of this inflammatory myopathy includes many of the major neuromuscular disorders of infancy and childhood, as well as metabolic and infectious diseases that can be symptomatic at any age. Some of the most common potential candidates for consideration are listed in Table 8.3.

Cutaneous signs

Gottron's sign can be mimicked by psoriatic lesions, accompanied by healing foci of hypopigmentation found in areas usually unaffected in JDM, such as the pretibial region. These rashes may clear with sun exposure, rather than becoming more prominent. In contrast, as in systemic lupus erythematosus (SLE), sun exposure can precipitate symptoms.[80]

Muscle complaints

Other conditions associated with muscle cramps and contractures include hypothyroidism, uraemia and electrolyte imbalance such as hypokalaemia (either iatrogenic or in conjunction with familial periodic paralysis). Pretibial tenderness is seen with erythema nodosum, but is not a feature of JDM. Pain that awakens the child at night should be investigated for another cause such as malignancy, osteoid osteoma or osteomyelitis. Muscle weakness can be seen in adrenal dysfunction, or after long-term high-dose steroid administration. In addition, thyroid, pitu-

---

Table 8.3 Differential diagnosis of juvenile dermatomyositis and polymyositis

Juvenile dermatomyositis

- Autoimmune rheumatic diseases: systemic lupus erythematosus, overlap syndromes, systemic-onset juvenile rheumatoid arthritis, scleroderma
- Infectious myopathies: echovirus, parvovirus, toxoplasmosis, Lyme disease, hepatitis B, leishmaniasis
- Other autoimmune diseases: psoriasis, eczema, allergic reactions
- Drug- and toxin-induced myopathies: hydroxyurea, phenobarbital, photosensitizers, some antibiotics, non-steroidal anti-inflammatory drugs, diuretics, vaccines

Juvenile polymyositis

- Infectious myopathies: influenza, parainfluenza, hepatitis B, adenovirus, human T-cell leukaemia virus-1, HIV
- Pyomyositis: *Staphlococcus aureus*, group A streptococcus
- Drug- and toxin-induced myopathies: corticosteroids, hydroxychloroquine, penicillamine, penicillin, sulphonamides, ketoconazole, cimetidine, ranitidine, levostatin, azidothymidine, vaccines
- Dystrophies: Duchenne, Becker, facioscapulohumeral, myotonic, infantile
- Endocrine myopathies: thyroid, diabetes
- Mitochondrial myopathies

AZT, azidothymidine; FSH, follicle stimulating hormone; HIV, human immunodeficiency virus; sulpha, sulphur containing compounds.

itary and parathyroid dysfunction may be accompanied by skeletal complaints. Metabolic muscle diseases include defects of glycolysis (e.g. phosphofructokinase deficiency), and are associated with contractures, exercise intolerance, myoglobinuria and a positive ischaemic lactate test. The child may have defects in lipid metabolism, such as a carnitine deficiency state,[81] which may be exacerbated by non-steroidal anti-inflammatory drugs (NSAIDs), or may manifest a myalgia syndrome, which can be detected by a positive ischaemic ammonia test.

Acute infectious viral myositis in children, most frequently attributed to influenza A or B, is clinically differentiated from chronic myositis by its localization to the muscles of the calf, severe pain and rapid resolution in 1–4 weeks.[82] The agent of this acute myositis has been isolated from cultures of muscle biopsy, accompanied by a rise in complement-fixing antibody titres to influenza; the myopathy is characterized by myoglobinuria, electromyographic changes and elevated creatine kinase. As in adults infected

with the human immunodeficiency virus (HIV) or HTLV-1, children with these illnesses may also have muscle complaints.[1] In children and adolescents, other autoimmune rheumatic disorders may also be accompanied by inflammatory muscle disease. Children with systemic-onset arthritis, with spiking fevers and an evanescent rash, may have a positive MRI and increased concentrations of muscle enzymes.[7] Confusion may be created if a child has classical Gottron's papules, elevated muscle enzymes and muscle-biopsy evidence of perifascicular atrophy in the presence of antibody to RNP or PM/Scl. Such children with overlap syndrome are less likely to have resolution of their disease, and will require long-term therapy into adult life.

Electromyography

Evidence of an inflammatory myopathy on electromyography (EMG) is not specific to JDM. Selection of a site of active involvement is facilitated by using MRI to identify focally involved muscles (20% of EMGs are negative[12]). Once the location of the electrodes has been chosen (not the site of a future biopsy), insertional irritability, followed by spontaneous electrical activity at rest is often observed. This pattern can be also seen in the muscular dystrophies and in early acute myositis. Abnormal, early, full recruitment of muscle fibres with moderate effort occurs in about 45% of patients with JDM, and bizarre, high-frequency discharges occur in 15–20% of patients tested. Reduced motor-unit activity is seen in Duchenne's muscular dystrophy as well as in JDM. Myasthenia gravis can coexist with an inflammatory myopathy, resulting in a greater degree of instability of motor-unit potential than is found in the uncomplicated inflammatory myopathies.

PATHOPHYSIOLOGY

Histopathology

In JDM, even in the presence of normal serum levels of muscle-derived enzymes, the MRI-directed muscle biopsy can reveal active foci of inflammation;[83] these children may also have elevated levels of von Willebrand-factor antigen and neopterin, or an elevated percentage of circulating cluster determinant (CD) 19+ B cells. The vasculopathy of this disease may occur in the absence of a prominent inflammatory component.[84,85] In JDM damage to capillaries and arterioles with loss of the capillary network results in structural change in the nailfold capillary bed as well as in muscle, with a subsequent decrease in the capillary/fibre ratio. The muscle pathology in JDM reflects vascular compromise and capillary dropout, with perifasicular atrophy of both type I and type II fibres (Figure 8.4). Multiple satellite cells are frequently seen in atrophic fibres; focal repair takes place concomitantly with fibre atrophy.[86] Low-grade ischaemia may also be related to expression of class I and class II major histocompatibility complex (MHC) gene products, which again have been found

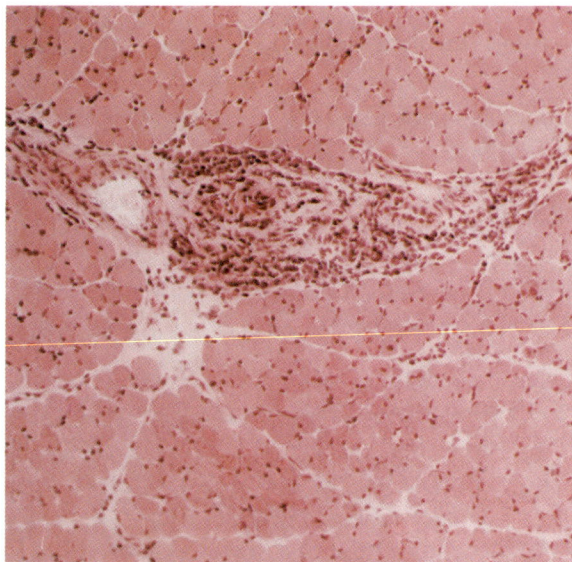

Figure 8.4   A muscle biopsy (haematoxylin and eosin stain) showing the typical changes seen in JDM: occlusion of capillaries, perifascicular atrophy and round-cell infiltrate, which is primarily composed of lymphocytes and macrophages.

primarily in the perifascicular area.[87] In contrast, in polymyositis there appears to be less primary involvement of vessels – they may be normal in number and structure. In new-onset, untreated JDM, there is a marked increase in the number of CD8+ T cells that localize in the muscle, compared with the decreased number of CD8+ T cells in the peripheral blood.[88] There is some evidence of oligoclonality of these muscle-associated lymphocytes, suggesting an antigen-driven process.[89] CD14+ macrophages on biopsy are associated with serum levels of neopterin; they both decrease in response to therapy.[90] Neopterin, a member of the pteridine family, is derived from guanosine triphosphate (GTP) via guanosinetriphosphate cyclohydrolase and released from macrophages as a consequence of T-cell-dependent interactions[91] involving interferon-γ (IFN-γ). Neopterin levels correlate with the clinical disease activity score in over 65% of cases.[92] The results of these studies[93] have been confirmed,[94] but no association was found with lymphocyte secretion of IFN-γ in vitro.[95] In dermatomyositis, there appears to be close relationship between CD4+ T cells and B cells, as well as macrophages, suggesting a cytotoxic mechanism, perhaps directed against immune-complex-modified endothelial cells.[96] Examination of biopsies from adults with dermatomyositis has shown increased synthesis of interleukin-10, -6 and -8 (IL-10, IL-6, IL-8).[97]

In the interpretation of the histopathology, it is helpful to have access to a description of the patients with respect to myositis-specific antibodies, duration of inflammatory disease, previous therapy at the time of biopsy, and verification that the site biopsied was appropriate (e.g. positive on MRI or ultrasound scanning). A consistent scoring of the various tissue and vascular components at biopsy before institution of therapy will permit a more reasoned evaluation of the child's response to therapy.[83,98]

Calcification in soft tissues

Calcium deposits are reported in 23–28% of JDM patients at diagnosis.[12,13] The aetiology of the calcinosis must be determined and clearly differentiated from other syndromes in which calcinosis occurs, such as heterotopic calcinosis or following trauma. In JDM, calcinosis may be a correlate of disease severity and duration, a delay in diagnosis and/or insufficient therapy.[12] There is increased urinary excretion of γ-carboxyglutamic acid (GLA), a component of the vitamin-K-dependent coagulation pathway.[99] The calcifications may resolve spontaneously, draining as a white cheesy or serosanguinous exudate, and leave dry, pitted scars. In persistent, active myositis, the calcifications may progress to become a sheath, impairing flexion and function, and breaking the barrier of the skin to form a site of entry of infection. Sepsis is not uncommon in this event, and contributes to morbidity and mortality from this disease. The calcifications are not correlated with antinuclear antibody, immune complexes or class II human leucocyte antigen (HLA).[100]

Immunological, genetic and haematological data

Humoral immunity

Humoral immunity may be abnormal in a minority of patients: in early disease, immunoglobulin M (IgM)[71] or IgG[88] may be elevated, or IgA deficiency may be present.[71] Antinuclear antibody (ANA) was found to be present in sera from 60–70% of 89 newly diagnosed children compared with 105 age- and sex-matched controls ($p < 0.005$, $p < 0.001$, respectively); no other autoantibodies were identified using an array of tissue and organ substrates[100] and standard tests for rheumatological disease.[75] The ANA is speckled and cytoskeletal in pattern in 60–70% of children (often in high titres), but is Jo-1 negative.[100,101] An antibody specificity for heat shock protein 60 (hsp60) in the juvenile dermatomyositis sera has been noted,[102] as has antibody to a 56-kDa nuclear protein[103] identified as annexin XI, which is seen in a wide spectrum of connective-tissue diseases, including JDM.[104] Unlike the adult population with inflammatory myopathies, in children myositis-specific antibodies have been described,[105] but these are rare.[106] In general, the few children with Jo-1 who have been identified recently are similar to adults with antisynthetase antibodies, and are characterized by dyspnoea on exertion, a pulmonary perfusion deficit with evidence of pulmonary fibrosis on both histologic and radiographic examination, and disease flares on reduction of therapy.[107] Most have severe arthritis; some have 'mechanic's hands',[107] but this is much more common in adults, being rare in children.

Complement activation has been implicated in several studies that included children with JDM: the C5b-9 membrane-attack complex was localized to the intramuscular microvasculature in 10 of 12 patients,[108] and was correlated with the duration of the clinical disease.[109] Immune complexes appear to participate in the pathophysiology of this disease, with complement activation (despite normal levels of total haemolytic complement, C3 and C4) accompanied by increased levels of fibrinopeptide A and von Willebrand factor antigen (vWF:Ag).[110]

Cellular immunity

Children with active untreated JDM are lymphopenic.[88] Despite this lymphopenia, there is a relative increase in the percentage of B cells (defined by anti-CD19 monoclonal antibody), which is positively correlated with a clinical disease activity score. In contrast, the percentages of CD4, CD8 and CD25 cells are not correlated with disease activity.[111] This increased percentage of B cells may reflect response to medical therapy, by returning to normal ranges later than other serological indicators.[112] The CD4/CD8 T-cell ratio is increased, suggesting that there is a decrease in circulating CD8+ T cells in the periphery.[88] Clonal expansion of T cells in the muscle of new-onset, untreated children with JDM has demonstrated a specific increase in T-cell receptor (TCR) variable gene expression (Vβ) as determined by polymerase chain reaction and sequencing of the CDR3 region in six children positive for the HLA antigen DQA1*0501.[89]

Genetic data

Records of JDM in more than one family member are sporadic, but the disease has been reported in monozygotic twins who developed muscle related abnormalities 2 weeks after an upper respiratory tract infection.[113] The association of the supratype A1, Cw7, B8, DR3 suggests that there might be a genetic component to disease susceptibility or expression: and HLA-DQA1*0501 was identified. The frequency of the C4a null allele was observed on the basis of linkage disequilibrium in 30 Caucasian patients with JDM compared with regional controls matched for HLA DR3.[114] This observation was sustained when other racial groups in the USA were studied,[115] as well as analysis of family studies, which have confirmed the increased association of DAQ1*0501 in children with JDM.[116] However, this association does not appear to be true for Czech children with this disease.[117]

Haematological data

In JDM, the usual indicators of an acute-phase reaction are often within normal limits, although children with acute severe disease or infected sites of calcinosis may have elevated values.

Lymphopenia is not commonly accompanied by an abnormal platelet count, although a mild microcytic anaemia may be present. A sensitive indicator of inflammatory disease is an elevated vWF:Ag,[118,119] which may precede a disease flare (when muscle enzyme data are normal), or remain elevated once the enzyme levels have normalized.[110] In over 50% of children, levels of vWF:Ag correlate with a clinical score of disease activity; analysis of the multimers confirms that it is endothelial in origin, this reflecting endothelial cell damage.[120,121]

These clues to disease activity (MRI, neopterin and vWF:Ag levels, and the percentage of B cells) are still imperfect guides to therapy,[122] but may be of substantial use in characterizing the severity of the immunologically mediated inflammatory process.[112]

DISEASE COURSE AND THERAPY

Disease course

The outcome of JDM has greatly improved since the 1960s, when one-third of the children died, one-third were crippled and one-third recovered.[21] Several types of disease course have been described – monocyclic, recurrent and continuous[123] – but the course may be altered by early diagnosis and aggressive therapy. The frequency of calcinosis (which was associated with loss of mobility) has decreased from over 60% of cases[124] to about 23% at diagnosis (see Table 8.1). Late disease recurrence after years of apparent inactivity has been reported,[125] suggesting the need for periodic monitoring using more sensitive indicators of disease activity. It is difficult to predict outcome at the onset of illness, although the magnitude of the initial serum levels of creatine kinase appears to be a direct correlate of disease severity.[126] Several groups have found that prognosis is directly related to the degree of vascular involvement.[124,127]

Therapy

There is continuing controversy over the type, duration and route of medication to be instituted.[128] Recommendations are limited because of lack of long-term outcome data. A comprehensive review of the current status of medical therapy has recently been published.[3] For uncomplicated JDM, oral prednisone 1–2 mg/kg is commonly used.[3] Linear growth may be temporarily arrested if the oral dosage of steroids used exceeds 4 mg/m^2. This, combined with increased weight secondary to both the therapy regimen and lack of exercise, proves a challenge for the body-image-conscious teenager. Return to high-impact sports activities can be considered once an improvement in bone density has occurred due to disease control. For the adolescent with increased weight gain, oral prednisone may pose problems with compliance, which is circumvented by documented intravenous administration of medication.

In the last two decades several investigators have observed the utility of high-dose, intravenous, intermittent (pulse) methylprednisolone (IVMP) for the treatment of JDM.[66,129,130] Children treated with an intravenous course (30 mg/kg, 1 g maximum dose) plus low-dose daily prednisone (0.5 mg/kg/day) had a shorter disease course with respect to persistence of rash (1.5 vs 3.9 years) and weakness (1.5 vs 2.7 years) than children on the standard treatment of oral prednisolone, and they did not have calcinosis, spine compression fracture or growth retardation, although the frequency of cataracts was the same in both groups.[131] Limited treatment with IVMP alone was not effective.[132] When a subset of JDM patients who sustained a monocyclic disease course was subjected to a cost analysis, the intravenous-treated group had 2 years disease-free, but their bill was about US$10 000 higher than those given PO therapy.[133] This cost was equalized when there was increased use of day hospital and out-patient facilities for the intravenous-treated group at diagnosis; the first series of patients treated with IVMP had been cared for in an in-patient setting.[134]

Adequate hydration lessens the possibility of renal damage. If there is evidence of dysphagia or difficulty in handling secretions, the immediate use of weekly intravenous methotrexate at a starting dose of 15 mg/m^2 to be administered in conjunction with high-dose IVMP (30 mg/kg/day) is suggested. The frequency of the IVMP steroid administration is determined by the muscle biopsy findings, and the rate of the child's response, using those parameters that are useful for the particular patient. Low-dose oral steroids 0.5 mg/kg/day are given in the morning on the days that IVMP is not infused. The protocol for each child is individualized. In general, an intensive course of IVMP is used until there is normalization of the laboratory data, with gradual reduction in therapy. The use of high-dose IVMP is not without adverse reactions. Analysis of a prospective log kept over a 5 year period of 213 children with various types of serious rheumatic disease given over 2622 doses, 22% ($n = 46$) experienced an adverse reaction of which 21 (47%) had behavioural changes ranging from euphoria to emotional lability. There was one case of anaphylaxis.[135] Adverse reactions to IVMP were closely associated with a record of previous accounts of cutaneous allergic eruptions to antibiotics.[136]

With severe skin involvement, hydroxychloroquine (7 mg/kg/day) is given if there is no family history of red–green colour blindness. With milder involvement, the cutaneous symptoms often resolve within several weeks, making the use of this drug less necessary. Topical agents to lessen dryness help the occasional pruritis, as do topical steroids, which should be used sparingly.[137] For breaks in the integument, a 'skin substitute' (e.g. 'second skin' or duoderm) should be considered. Sepsis secondary to infected calcinosis (e.g. staphylococcal or streptococcal infection) must be treated aggressively.

For the past two decades, children who have severe onset of disease, or who do not respond to steroids, have been treated with methotrexate.[138] More recently, earlier use of this modality at doses of 15 mg/m^2/week has reduced the morbidity of the disease[139] and permitted the use of lower doses of steroids. In active disease, intravenous or subcutaneous administration of methotrexate ensures drug absorption; as the disease becomes quiescent, oral administration is tolerated. Complaints of nausea can be circumvented by dividing the dose but giving the full amount in a 24-hour period. The function of the liver and bone marrow must be monitored. It is particularly important to inform the adolescent with JDM who is treated with methotrexate to avoid sun exposure (due to increased sunburn and vitiligo) and alcohol ingestion (liver toxicity).

If the child remains severely ill (sometimes despite normalization of muscle enzymes), evaluation of the immune system may help to guide therapy (e.g. the percentage of B cells remains elevated[140]). Intravenous cyclophosphamide therapy, starting at 500 mg/m^2 every 3 weeks (following adequate hydration), with mesna for bladder protection, can be considered. Serum levels of IgG must be checked on a periodic basis to ensure that they are adequate; if not, replacement therapy (4 g/kg every 3–4 weeks) is needed to prevent recurrent infections. Pneumocystis has been reported in immunosuppressed myositis patients.[141]

In the adolescent, steroid therapy may exacerbate the age-related predisposition to acne. Administration of tetracycline, which is commonly used to treat acne, may lower the available levels of methotrexate, contributing to disease flare.

When considering therapies other than steroids, high-dose (not replacement) intravenous gammaglobulin may initially help the rash,[142,143] especially if given early in the disease course.[144] A summary of case reports of the response of 27 JDM patients to intravenous gammaglobulin suggests that, while it may be a good adjunct to other medical therapy, prolonged control of disease activity may not be achieved with this drug alone. Plasmapheresis alone does not appear to be effective in adults,[145] and no data are available on children. A total of 23 children with JDM treated with cyclosporin A (CYA) have been reported, and the results appear encouraging;[3] evaluation of the efficacy of CYA has been proposed,[146] but has been hampered by coexisting therapies.[147] FK506 has been found useful in the treatment of adults with Jo-1 myopathy.[148]

At the moment there is no successful therapy for long-standing calcinosis in children with inactive disease. MRI may reveal inflammation associated with calcinosis, permitting more aggressive medical therapy, which may result in regression (and, occasionally, radiologic resolution) of the calcinosis. Once the myositis has been controlled, some of the calcific sites can be carefully appraised and, if not too extensive, excised while the child is covered by methotrexate, without recurrence in the wound site, which is common.

Previous studies have documented a decrease in bone density and osteocalcin (an indicator of bone mineral metabolism) in untreated active JDM.[70] In adolescents, who often decrease their intake of calcium-containing foods, administration of vitamin D and increasing the calcium intake may aid in calcium absorption from the gastrointestinal tract in the face of steroid therapy (which inhibits calcium absorption). This approach may decrease the occurrence of one of the most serious consequences of steroid therapy, osteopenia, which can progress to spinal cord compression fractures.[79]

Combined medical therapy (to suppress inflammation) and physiotherapy (gentle, passive stretching) is required in the early phase of the disease, and more intensive, graded physiotherapy is effective at later stages of the disease, once the inflammation has abated. Prevention of sunburn, both by avoidance of the sun and by use of barriers (clothing UVA/UVB parabenzoic acid (PABA)-free sunblocks over sun protection factor (SPF) 30) helps keep inflammation in both muscle and skin in remission.

Recognition of the psychological factors that dominate the adolescent's response to chronic illness is very important in achieving a good outcome. The mood swings that occur both as a result of the level of maturation and the administration of corticosteroids can be devastating if not recognized and treated appropriately. It is particularly important to allow the adolescent to participate in decisions affecting therapy and to encourage age-appropriate independence, to establish an identity and to master the tools needed for financial independence.[149]

Overall, the outcome of JDM has improved, with a reduction in morbidity and mortality; but few data are available concerning long-term follow-up. The limited available evidence suggests that children do well in adulthood on socio-economic and functional assessment, but no prospective data are currently available concerning the consequences of more recent aggressive interventions.

In summary, the aetiology and pathogenesis of juvenile dermatomyositis, an immunologically mediated vasculopathy, is under intense investigation. This is an exciting time, because knowledge of the specific factors that play a role in both disease susceptibility and disease severity will lead to more effective and targeted therapies. This information should be of some interest to both the adolescent with an inflammatory myopathy and those who provide them with care.

REFERENCES

1. Smadja D, Bellance R, Cabre P, Arfi S, Vernant JC. Clinical characteristics of HTLV-1 associated dermato-polymyositis. Seven cases from Martinique. *Acta Neurol Scand* 1995; **92**:206–12.
2. Pachman LM, Miller FW. Inflammatory myopathies: dermatomyositis, polymyositis and related disorders in the child and adult. In: *Samter's Immunological Disease* (Frank M, Austin F, Claman H, Unanuae E, eds). Little, Brown: Boston, 1994:791–803.
3. Rider LG, Miller FW. Classification and treatment of the juvenile idiopathic inflammatory myopathies. *Rheum Dis Clin North Am* 1997; **23**:619–55.
4. Friedman JM, Rachman LM, Maryjowski ML et al. Immunogenetic studies of juvenile dermatomyositis: HLA-DR antigen frequencies. *Arthritis Rheum* 1983; **26**:214–6..
5. Bohan A, Peter JB. Polymyositis and dermatomyositis. Parts 1 and 2. *N Engl J Med* 1975; **292**:344–347, 403–7.
6. Citera G, Espada G, Maldonado Cocco JA. Sequential development of two connective tissue diseases in juvenile patients. *J Rheumatol* 1993; **20**:2149–52.
7. Miller ML, Levinson L, Pachman LM, Poznanski AK. Abnormal muscle MRI in a patient with systemic juvenile rheumatoid arthritis. *Pediatr Radiol* 1995; **25**:S107–8.
8. Serratrice G, Schiano A, Pellissier JF, Desnuelle C. Les expressions anatomocliniques des pollymyosites chez l'enfant. *Ann Pediatr (Paris)* 1989; **36**:237–43.
9. Pollard ZF. Acute rectus muscle palsy in children as a result of orbital myositis. *J Pediatr* 1996; **128**:230–3.
10. Huang KW, Chen XH. Pathology of eosinophilic fascitis and relation to polymyositis. *Can J Neurol Sci* 1987; **4**:632–7.
11. Medsger TA Jr, Dawson WN, Masi AT. The epidemiology of polymyositis. *Am J Med* 1970; **48**:715–23.
12. Pachman LM, Hayford JR, Chung A et al. Juvenile dermatomyositis at diagnosis: clinical characteristics of 79 children. *J Rheumatol* 1998; **25**:1998–204.
13. Rider LG, Okada S, Sherry DD et al. Presentations and disease courses of juvenile idiopathic inflammatory myopathy (JIIM). *Arthritis Rheum* 1995; **38**:S362.
14. Benbassat J, Geffel D, Zlotnick A. Epidemiology of polymyositis–dermatomyositis in Israel. *Isr J Med Sci* 1980; **16**:197–200.
15. Symmons DPM, Sills JA, Davis SM. The incidence of juvenile dermatomyositis: results from a nation-wide study. *Br J Rheumatol* 1995; **43**:732–6.
16. Wang Y-J, Lii Y-P, Lan J-L, Chi C-S, Mak S-C, Scian W-J. Juvenile and adult dermatomyositis among the Chinese: a comparative study. *Chin Med J (Taipei)* 1993; **52**:285–92.
17. Hiketa T, Matsumoto Y, Ohashi M, Sakaki R. Juvenile dermatomyositis: a statistical study of 114 patients with dermatomyositis. *J Dermatol* 1992; **19**:470–6.
18. See Y, Giam YC, Chng HH. A retrospective study of 13 oriental children with juvenile dermatomyositis. *Ann Acad Med, Singapore* 1997; **26**:210–14.
19. Rider LG, Okada S, Sherry DD et al. Epidemiologic features and environmental exposure associated with illness onset in juvenile idiopathic inflammatory myopathy (JIIM). *Arthritis Rheum* 1995; **38**:S362.
20. Love LA, Leff RL, Fraser DD et al. A new approach to the classification of idiopathic inflammatory myopathy: myositis-specific autoantibodies define useful homogeneous patient groups. *Medicine (Baltimore)* 1991; **70**:360–74.

21. Bitnum C, Daeschner CW, Travis LB et al. Dermatomyositis. *J Pediatr* 1964; **64**:101–31.

22. Ansell BA, Miller JJ III, Pachman LM, Sullivan DB. Controversies in juvenile dermatomyositis. *J Rheumatol* 1990; **17**(suppl 22):1–6.

23. Hochberg MC. Epidemiology of polymyositis/dermatomyositis. *Mt Sinai J Med* 1988; **55**:447–52.

24. Hidano A, Keneka K, Arai Y. Survey of the prognosis for dermatomyositis with special reference to its associated malignancy and pulmonary fibrosis. *J Dermatol* 1986; **13**:233–41.

25. Masi AT, Hochberg MC. Temporal association of polymyositis–dermatomyositis with malignancy: methodologic and clinical considerations. *Mt Sinai J Med* 1988; **55**:471–8.

26. Sherry DD, Haas JE, Milstein JM. Childhood polymyositis as a paraneoplastic phenomenon. *Pediatr Neurol* 1993; **9**:155–6.

27. Sigurgeirsson B, Lindelöf B, Edhag O, Allander E. Risk of cancer in patients with dermatomyositis or polymyositis; a population-based study. *N Engl J Med* 1992; **326**:363–7.

28. Christensen ML, Pachman LM, Maryjowski ML. Antibody to coxsackie-B virus: increased incidence in sera from children with recently diagnosed juvenile dermatomyositis. *Arthritis Rheum* 1983; **26**:S24.

29. Rosenberg AM. Geographical clustering of childhood dermatomyositis in Saskatchewan. *Arthritis Rheum* 1994; **37**:S402.

30. Pachman LM, Hayford JR, Hochberg MC et al. New-onset juvenile dermatomyositis: comparisons with a healthy cohort and children with juvenile rheumatoid arthritis. *Arthritis Rheum* 1997; **40**:1526–33.

31. Pachman LM, Mendez E, Chiu Y-I et al. New onset juvenile dermatomyositis (JDM): increased time to diagnosis and therapy in minority children by physician report. *Arthritis Rheum* 1997; **40**:S333.

32. Martini A, Ravelli A, Albani S et al. Recurrent juvenile dermatomyositis and cutaneous necrotizing arteritis with molecular mimicry between streptococcal type 5M protein and human skeletal myosin. *J Pediatr* 1992; **121**:739–42.

33. Albani S, Costouros N, Massa M, Liotta M, Pachman LM, Martini A. Identification of cross-reactive epitopes on human skeletal myosin and streptococcal M5 protein in patients with juvenile dermatomyositis (JDM). *Arthritis Rheum* 1997; **40**:S140.

34. Mihas AA, Kirby JD, Kent SP. Hepatitis B antigen and polymyositis. *J Am Med Wom Assoc* 1978; **239**:221–2.

35. Bowles NE, Dubowitz V, Sewry CA, Archard LC. Dermatomyositis, polymyositis, and coxsackie-B-virus infection. *Lancet* 1987; **i**:1004–7.

36. Pachman LM, Litt DL, Rowley AH et al. Lack of detection of enteroviral RNA or bacterial DNA in MRI directed muscle biopsies from twenty children with active untreated juvenile dermatomyositis. *Arthritis Rheum* 1995; **38**:1513–18.

37. Christensen ML, Pachman LM, Schneiderman R, Patel DC, Friedman JM. Prevalence of coxsackie B virus antibodies in patients with juvenile dermatomyositis. *Arthritis Rheum* 1986; **29**:1365–70.

38. Yousef GE, Isenberg DA, Mowbray JF. Detection of enterovirus specific RNA sequences in muscle biopsy specimens from patients with adult onset myositis. *Ann Rheum Dis* 1990; **49**:310–5.

39. Leff RL, Miller FW, Greenberg SJ, Klein EA, Dalakas MC, Plotz PH. Viruses in idiopathic inflammatory myopathies: absence of candidate viral genomes in muscle. *Lancet* 1992; **339**:1192–5.

40. Lapetina F. Toxoplasmosis and dermatomyositis: a causal or casual relationship. *Pediatr Med Chir* 1989; **11**:197–3.

41. Schroter HM, Sarnet HB, Matheson DS, Seland TP. Juvenile dermatomyositis induced by toxoplasmosis. *J Child Neurol* 1987; **2**:101–4.

42. Pachman LM, Hayford JR, Hochberg M et al. New onset juvenile dermatomyositis: comparisons with children with JRA and healthy children. *Arthritis Rheum* 1997; **40**:1526–33.

43. Pachman LM, Hayford JR, Hochberg MC et al. Seasonal onset in juvenile dermatomyositis (JDMS): an epidemiological study. *Arthritis Rheum* 1992; **35**:S88.

44. Rosenberg NL, Rotbart HA, Abzug MJ, Ringel SP, Levin MJ. Evidence for a novel picornavirus in human dermatomyositis. *Ann Neurol* 1989; **26**:204–9.

45. Cotterill JA, Shapiro H. Dermatomyositis after immunization. *Lancet* 1978; **ii**:1158–9.

46. Swartz MO, Silver RM. D-Penicillamine induced polymyositis in juvenile chronic arthritis: report of a case. *J Rheumatol* 1984; **11**:251–2.

47. Yordam N, Kandemir N, Topaloglu H et al. Myositis associated with growth hormone therapy. *J Pediatr* 1994; **125**:671.

48. Adams C, August CS, Maguire H et al. Neuromuscular complications of bone marrow transplantation. *Pediatr Neurol* 1995; **12**:58–61.

49. Kasteler JS, Callen JP. Scalp involvement in dermatomyositis. Often overlooked or misdiagnosed. *JAMA* 1994; **272**:1939–41.

50. Eisenstein D, Paller A, Pachman LM. Juvenile dermatomyositis presenting with rash alone. *Pediatrics* 1997; **100**:391–2.

51. Cosnes A, Amaudric F, Gherardi R et al. Dermatomyositis without muscle weakness. Long-term follow-up of 12 patients without systemic corticosteroids. *Arch Dermatol* 1995; **131**:1381–85. Comments, *Arch Dermatol* 1995; **131**:1458–9.

52. Silver RM, Maricq HR. Childhood dermatomyositis: serial microvascular studies. *Pediatrics* 1989; **83**:278–83.

53. Pachman LM, Sundberg J, Kinder J, Maduzia L, Daugherty C. Nailfold capillary studies in children with pediatric connective tissue diseases: systemic lupus erythematosus (SLE), juvenile dermatomyositis (JDMS), Raynaud's phenomenon (RP) – comparison with data from normal children. *Arthritis Rheum* 1996; **39**:R14.

54. Pachman LM, Sundberg J, Maduzia L, Daugherty C, Litt D. Sequential studies of nailfold capillary vessels (NFC) in 10 children with juvenile dermatomyositis (JDMS): correlation with disease activity score (DAS) but not von Willebrand factor antigen (vWF:Ag). *Arthritis Rheum* 1995; **38**:S361.

55. Tucker LB, Sadegi-Neged A, Schaller JG. The association of acquired lipodystrophy with juvenile dermatomyositis. *Arthritis Rheum* 1990; **33**:S1496.

56. Kitson H, Malleson PN, Sanderson S, Cabral DA, Petty RE. Lipodystrophy in juvenile dermatomyositis patients: evaluation of clinical and metabolic abnormalities. *Arthritis Rheum* 1997; **40**:S140.

57. Commens C, O'Neill P, Walker G. Dermatomyositis associated with multifocal atrophy. *J Am Acad Dermatol* 1990; **22**:966–9.

58. Huang JL. Juvenile dermatomyositis associated with partial lipodystrophy. *Br J Clin Pract* 1996; **50**:112–13.

59. Quecedo E, Febrer I, Serrano G, Martinez-Aparicio A, Aliaga A. Partial lipodystrophy associated with juvenile dermatomyositis: report of two cases. *Pediatr Dermatol* 1996; **13**:477–82.

60. Klein-Gitelman MS, Daaboul J, Oren PP, Kinder J, Pachman LM. Acquired lipodystrophy in juvenile dermatomyositis (JDM): who is at risk? *J Invest Med* 1997; **45**:342A.

61. Feldman BM, Ayling-Campos A, Luy L, Stevens D, Silverman ED, Laxer RM. Measuring disability in juvenile dermatomyositis: validity of the childhood health assessment questionnaire. *J Rheumat* 1995; **22**:326–31.

62. Miller LC, Michael AF, Kim Y. Childhood dermatomyositis. *Clin Pediatr* 1987; **26**:561–8.

63. Pitt AM, Fleckenstein JL, Greenlee RG Jr et al. MRI-guided biopsy in inflammatory myopathy: initial results. *Magn Reson Imaging* 1993; **11**:1093–9.

64. Keim DR, Hernandez RJ, Sullivan DB. Serial magnetic resonance imaging in juvenile dermatomyositis. *Arthritis Rheum* 1991; **34**:1580–4.

65. Hernandez RJ, Sullivan DB, Chenevert TL. MR imaging in children with dermatomyositis: musculoskeletal findings and correlation with clinical and laboratory findings. *Am J Roentgenol* 1993; **161**:359–66.

66. Yanagisawa T, Sueishi M, Nawata Y et al. Methylprednisolone pulse therapy in dermatomyositis. *Dermatologica* 1983; **167**:47–51.

67. Huppertz HI, Kaiser WA. Serial magnetic resonance imaging in juvenile dermatomyositis – delayed normalization. *Rheumatol Intl* 1994; **4**:127–9.

68. Park JH, Vital TL, Ryder NM et al. Magnetic resonance imaging and P-31 magnetic resonance spectroscopy provide unique quantitative data useful in the longitudinal management of patients with dermatomyositis. *Arthritis Rheum* 1994; **37**:736–46.

69. Perez MD, Abrams SA, Koenning G, Stuff JE, O'Brien KO, Ellis KJ. Mineral metabolism in children with dermatomyositis. *J Rheumat* 1994; **21**:2364–9.

70. Reed AM, Haugen M, Pachman LM, Langman CB. Abnormalities in serum osteocalcin values in children with chronic rheumatic diseases. *J Pediatr* 1990; **116**:574–80.

71. Pachman LM, Cooke N. Juvenile dermatomyositis: a clinical and immunologic study. *J Pediatr* 1980; **96**:226–34.

72. Cuny C, Eicher JC, Collet E et al. Cardiomyopathie dilatee relevant une dermatopolymyosite attitude therapeutique. *Ann Cardiol Angeiol* 1993; **42**:155–8.

73. Pachman LM. Juvenile dermatomyositis. *Pediatr Clin North Am* 1986; **33**:1097–117.

74. Borrelli MP, Cordeiro MJ, Wroclawski P et al. Uretal necrosis in dermatomyositis. *J Urol* 1988; **139**:1275–7.

75. Montecucco C, Ravelli A, Caporali R et al. Autoantibodies in juvenile dermatomyositis. *Clin Exp Rheumatol* 1990; **8**:193–6.

76. Harris A, Webley M, Usherwood M, Burge S. Dermatomyositis presenting in pregnancy. *Br J Dermatol* 1995; **133**:783–5.

77. Ohno T, Imai A, Tamaya T. Successful outcomes of pregnancy complicated with dermatomyositis. Case reports. *Gynecol Obstet Invest* 1992; **33**:187–9.

78. Fong LP, Yeung J. Spontaneous regression of retinal neovascularization in juvenile dermatomyositis. *Aust NZ J Ophthalmol* 1990; **18**:107–8.

79. Callen AM, Pachman LM, Hayford JR, Chung A, Ramsey-Goldman R. Intermittent high-dose intravenous methylprednisolone (IV pulse) therapy prevents calcinosis and shortens disease course in juvenile dermatomyositis (JDMS). *Arthritis Rheum* 1994; **37**:R10.

80. Drake LA, Dinehart SM, Farmer ER et al. Guidelines for care of dermatomyositis. *J Am Acad Dermatol* 1996; **34**:824–9.

81. Breningstall GN. Carnitine deficiency syndromes. *Pediatr Neurol* 1990; **6**:75–81.

82. Mejlszenkier JD, Safran AE, Healy JJ. The myositis of influenza. *Arch Neurol* 1973; **29**:441–3.

83. Pachman LM, Crawford S, Morello F, Maduzia L, Caliendo J, Heller S. MRI directed needle biopsy for the assessment of juvenile dermatomyositis (JDMS) response to therapy: comparison of initial and follow-up biopsies using a histological rating scale evaluating disease severity/chronicity. *Arthritis Rheum* 1996; **39**:R14.

84. Banker BQ, Victor M. Dermatomyositis (systemic angiopathy) of childhood. *Medicine* 1966; **45**:261–89.

85. Emslie-Smith AM, Engel AG. Microvascular changes in early and advanced dermatomyositis: a quantitative study. *Ann Neurol* 1990; **27**:343–56.

86. Woo M, Chung SJ, Nonaka I. Perifascicular atrophic fibers in childhood dermatomyositis with particular reference to mitochrondrial changes. *J Neurol Sci* 1988; **88**:133–43.

87. Karpati G, Pouliot Y, Carpenter S. Expression of immunoreactive major histocompatibility complex products in human skeletal muscles. *Ann Neurol* 1988; **23**:64–72.

88. O'Gorman MRG, Corrochano V, Roleck J, Donovan M, Pachman LM. Flow cytometric analysis of the lymphocyte subsets in peripheral blood of children with untreated active juvenile dermatomyositis. *Clin Diag Lab Immunol* 1995; **2**:205–8.

89. Pachman LM, O'Gorman MRG, Lawton TP et al. Evidence of a TCR Vβ8 motif and increased CD56⁺ NK cells in muscle biopsies (Mbx) from DQAI*0501 positive untreated children with juvenile dermatomyositis (JDM) very early in their disease course. *Ped Res* 1998; **43**:338A

90. Pachman LM, Maduzia L, Liotta M, Schlis K, Crawford S. Serum neopterin (NEO) correlates with increased macrophages (CD14+) in MRI directed muscle biopsies in active juvenile dermatomyositis (JDMS). *Arthritis Rheum* 1996; **39**:S191.

91. Barak M, Merzback D, Gruener N. The effect of immunomodulators on PHA or IFN-γ induced release of neopterin from purified macrophages and peripheral blood mononuclear cells. *Immunol Lett* 1989; **21**:317–22.

92. Pachman LM, Maduzia L, Chung A, Donovan M, Ramsey-Goldman R. Juvenile dermatomyositis (JDMS): disease activity scores are correlated with levels of neopterin in serum. *Arthritis Rheum* 1995; **38**:R16.

93. Myones BL, Luckey JP, Hayford JR, Pachman LM. Increased neopterin levels in juvenile dermatomyositis correlate with disease activity and are indicative of macrophage activation. *Arthritis Rheum* 1989; **52**:S83.

94. DeBenedetti F, DeAmici M, Aramini L, Ruperto N, Martini A. Correlations of serum neopterin concentrations with disease activity in juvenile dermatomyositis. *Arch Dis Child* 1993; **69**:232–35.

95. Chung D, Liotta M, Daugherty C, O'Gorman MRG, Pachman LM. In vitro synthesis of IFN-γ by peripheral blood mononuclear cells (PBMCs) in active juvenile dermatomyositis (JDMS): lack of association with serum levels of neoptin (NEO). *Invest Med* 1996; **44**:368A.

96. Engel AG, Arahata K. Mononuclear cells in myopathies: quantitation of functionally distinct subsets, recognition of antigen-specific cell-mediated cytotoxicity in some diseases, and implications for the pathogenesis of the different inflammatory myopathies. *Hum Pathol* 1986; **17**:704–21.

97. Hagiwara E, Adams EM, Plotz PH, Klinman DM. Abnormal numbers of cytokine producing cells in patients with polymyositis and dermatomyositis. *Clin Exp Rheum* 1996; **14**:485–91.

98. Pachman LM, Crawford S, Morello F et al. MRI directed muscle biopsy (Bx) for assessment of juvenile dermatomyositis (JDMS) response to therapy; comparison of initial and follow-up biopsies using a histological rating scale evaluating disease severity/chronicity. *Arthritis Rheum* 1996; **39**:S191.

99. Lian JB, Pachman LM, Gundberg CM, Partridge

REH, Maryjowski ML. γ-Carboxyglutamate excretion and calcinosis in juvenile dermatomyositis. *Arthritis Rheum* 1982; **25**:1094–100.

100. Pachman LM, Friedman JM, Maryjowski MC et al. Immunogenetic studies in juvenile dermatomyositis III: study of antibody to organ-specific and nuclear antigens. *Arthritis Rheum* 1985; **28**:151–7.

101. Pachman LM, Hardin JA, Cobb MA, Arroyave CM. The antinuclear antibody (ANA) in juvenile dermatomyositis (JDMS) is not Jo-1, suggesting that JDMS and polymyositis (PM) are different diseases. *Arthritis Rheum* 1984; **27**:S45.

102. Patterson BK, Lee C, Lane WC et al. Antinuclear antibody (ANA) positive sera from juvenile dermatomyositis (JDMS) has specificity for heat shock protein 60 (HSP-60). *Pediatr Res* 1993; **33**:157A.

103. Cambridge G, Ovadia E, Isenberg DA, Dubowitz V, Sperling J, Sperling R. Juvenile dermatomyositis: serial studies of circulating autoantibodies to a 56 kDa nuclear protein. *Clin Exp Rheumatol* 1994; **12**:451–7.

104. Misaki Y, van Venrooij WJ, Priijn GJ. Prevalence and characteristics of anti-56K/annex XI autoantibodies in systemic autoimmune disease. *J Rheumatol* 1995; **22**:97–192.

105. Rider LG, Miller FW, Targoff IN et al. A broadened spectrum of juvenile myositis: myositis-specific autoantibodies in children. *Arthritis Rheum* 1994; **37**:1534–8.

106. Feldman BM, Reichlin M, Laxer RM, Targoff IN, Stein LD, Silverman ED. Clinical significance of specific autoantibodies in juvenile dermatomyositis. *J Rheumatol* 1996; **23**:1794–7.

107. Rider LG, Targoff IN, Taylor-Albert ES et al. Anti-Jo-1 autoantibodies define a clinically homogenous subset of childhood idiopathic inflammatory myopathy (IIM). *Arthritis Rheum* 1995; **38**:S62.

108. Kissel JT, Mendell JR, Rammohan KW. Microvascular deposition of complement membrane attack complex in dermatomyositis. *N Engl J Med* 1986; **314**:329–334.

109. Kissel JT, Halterman RK, Rammohan KW, Mendell JR. The relationship of complement-mediated microvasculopathy to the histologic features and clinical duration of disease in dermatomyositis. *Arch Neurol* 1991; **48**:26–30.

110. Scott JP, Arroyave C. Activation of complement and coagulation in juvenile dermatomyositis. *Arthritis Rheum* 1987; **30**:572–6.

111. Eisenstein DM, O'Gorman MRG, Donovan M, Pachman LM. Percentage of B cells in peripheral blood of patients with JDMS. *Arthritis Rheum* 1995; **38**:R15.

112. Pachman LM. Juvenile dermatomyositis (JDMS): new clues to diagnosis and pathogenesis. *Clin Exp Rheumatol* 1994; **12**:S69–73.

113. Harati Y, Niakan E, Bergman EW. Childhood dermatomyositis in monozygotic twins. *Neurology* 1986; **36**:721–3.

114. Reed AM, Pachman LM, Ober C. Molecular genetic studies of major histocompatibility complex genes in children with juvenile dermatomyositis: increased risk associated with HLA-DQA1*0501. *Hum Immunol* 1991; **32**:235–40.

115. Reed AM, Stirling J, Rivas R, Kredich D. The HLA-DAQ1*0501 allele in JDMS is seen in multiple racial groups. *Arthritis Rheum* 1992; **29**:S52.

116. Reed AM, Pachman LM, Hayford JR, Ober C. Immunogenetic studies in families of children with juvenile dermatomyositis (JDMS). *J Rheumatol* 1998; **25**:1000–2.

117. Vavrincova P, Havelka S, Cerna M, Stastny P. HLA class II alleles in juvenile dermatomyositis. *J Rheumatol* 1993; **20**(suppl 37):17–18.

118. Guzman J, Petty RE, Malleson PN. Monitoring disease activity in juvenile dermatomyositis: the role of von Willebrand factor and muscle enzymes. *J Rheumatol* 1994; **21**:739–43.

119. Bowyer SL, Ragsdale CG, Sullivan DB. Factor VIII related antigen and childhood rheumatic diseases. *J Rheumatol* 1989; **16**:1093–7.

120. Bloom BI, Tucker LB, Miller LC, Schaller JG. Von Willebrand factor in juvenile dermatomyositis. *J Rheumatol* 1995; **22**:320–5.

121. Miller CH, Donovan JM, Maduzia L, Chung A, Pachman LM. Relationship of von Willebrand factor antigen to disease activity in juvenile dermatomyositis. *Arthritis Rheum* 1995; **39**:R13.

122. Pachman LM. Imperfect indications of disease activity in juvenile dermatomyositis. *J Rheumatol* 1995; **2**:193–7.

123. Spencer CH, Hanson V, Singsen BH, Bernstein BH, Kornreich HK, King KK. Course of treated juvenile dermatomyositis. *J Pediatr* 1984; **105**:399–8.

124. Bowyer SL, Blane CE, Sullivan DB. Childhood dermatomyositis: factors predicting functional outcome and development of dystrophic calcification. *J Pediatr* 1983; **103**:882–8.

125. Lovell HB, Lindsley CB. Late recurrence of childhood dermatomyositis. *J Rheumatol* 1986; **13**:821–2.

126. Van Rossum MAJ, Hiemstra I, Prieur AM, Rijkers GT, Kuis W. Juvenile dermato/polymyositis: a retrospective analysis of 33 cases with special focus on initial CPK levels. *Clin Exp Rheumatol* 1994; **12**:339–42.

127. Crowe WE, Love KE, Levinson JE, Hilton PK. Clinical and pathogenetic implications of histopathology in childhood polydermatomyositis. *Arthritis Rheum* 1982; **25**:126–39.

128. Malleson PN. Controversies in juvenile dermatomyositis. *J Rheumatol* 1990; **17**:731–2.

129. Laxer RM, Stein LD, Petty RE. Intravenous pulse methylprednisolone treatment of juvenile dermatomyositis. *Arthritis Rheum* 1987; **30**:328–34.

130. Miller JJ III. Prolonged use of large intravenous steroid pulses in the rheumatic diseases of children. *Pediatrics* 1980; **65**:989–94.

131. Pachman LM, Callen AM, Hayford JR, Chung A, Sinacore J, Ramsey-Goldman R. Juvenile dermatomyositis (JDMS): decreased calcinosis (Ca^{2+}) with intermittent high-dose intravenous methylprednisolone (IV pulse) therapy. *Arthritis Rheum* 1994; **37**:S429.

132. Lang BA, Dooley J. Failure of pulse intravenous methylprednisolone treatment in juvenile dermatomyositis. *J Pediatr* 1996; **128**:429–32.

133. Klein-Gitelman MS, Waters T, Pachman LM. A comparison of the cost effectiveness of IV and PO corticosteroids in the treatment of juvenile dermatomyositis (JDMS). *Arthritis Rheum* 1996; **39**:R13.

134. Klein-Gitelman MS. Outpatient pulse IV cyclophosphamide (PIVCYP) is cost effective and safe. Personal communication.

135. Klein-Gitelman MS, Pachman LM. IV pulse corticosteroids (CS): adverse reactions are more variable than expected in children. *Arthritis Rheum* 1995; **38**:S338.

136. Klein-Gitelman MS, Pachman LM. Intravenous pulse corticosteroids (CS): adverse reactions are more variable than expected in children. *J Rheum* 1998, in press.

137. Stonecipher MR, Callen JP, Jorizzo JL. The red face: dermatomyositis. *Clin Dermatol* 1993; **11**:261–73.

138. Jacobs JC. Methotrexate and azathioprine treatment of childhood dermatomyositis. *Pediatrics* 1977; **59**:212–18.

139. Miller LC, Sisson BA, Tucker LB, DeNardo BA, Schaller JG. Methotrexate treatment of recalcitrant childhood dermatomyositis. *Arthritis Rheum* 1992; **35**:1143–9.

140. Eisenstein DM, O'Gorman MRG, Pachman LM. Peripheral blood lymphocyte (PBLn) subsets in patients with juvenile dermatomyositis (JDMS). *Arthritis Rheum* 1995; **38**:S361.

141. Bachelez H, Schremmer B, Cadranel J et al. Fulminant pneumocystis carinii pneumonia in 4 patients with dermatomyositis. *Arch Intern Med* 1997; **157**:1501–3.

142. Roifman CM, Schaffer FM, Wachsmuth SE, Murphy G, Gelfand EW. Reversal of chronic polymyositis following intravenous immune serum globulin therapy. *JAMA* 1987; **258**:513–15.

143. Lang BA, Laxer RM, Murphy G, Silverman ED, Roifman CM. Treatment of dermatomyositis with intravenous gammaglobulin. *Am J Med* 1991; **91**:169–72.

144. Basta M, Dalakas MC. High-dose intravenous immunoglobulin exerts its beneficial effect in patients with dermatomyositis by blocking endomysial deposition of activated complement fragments. *J Clin Invest* 1994; **95**:1729–35.

145. Miller FW, Leitman SF, Cronin ME et al. Controlled trial of plasma exchange and leukapheresis in polymyositis and dermatomyositis. *N Engl J Med* 1992; **326**:1380–4.

146. Heckmatt JZ, Hasson N, Saunders CE et al. Effectiveness of cyclosporin for dermatomyositis. *Lancet* 1989; **i**:1063–6.

147. Pistoia V, Buoncompagni A, Scribanis R et al. Cyclosporin A in the treatment of juvenile chronic arthritis and childhood polymyositis–dermatomyositis. Results of a preliminary study. *Clin Exp Rheumatol* 1993; **11**:203–8.

148. Oddis CV, Carroll P, Abu-Elmgd K, McCauley J, Fung JJ, Starzl TE. FK506 in the treatment of polymyositis. *Arthritis Rheum* 1994; **37**:S286.

149. White PH. Success on the road to adulthood: issues and hurdles for adolescents with disabilities. *Rheum Dis Clin North Am* 1997; **23**:697–707.

9

Scleroderma in children and adolescents

Ronald M Laxer

INTRODUCTION

The scleroderma group of disorders is marked clinically by the presence of hard skin and pathologically by the deposition of excessive amounts of collagen in various organ systems. Although the systemic variety of scleroderma is one of the least common of the classic 'autoimmune rheumatic diseases' in a paediatric rheumatology clinic, the multisystem involvement, morbidity, mortality and absence of disease-remitting agents make it challenging to care for. Annual costs for scleroderma patients in the USA have been estimated at $1.5 billion, mostly due to indirect costs resulting from the severe morbidity and loss of productivity in the workforce.[1] In children and adolescents, these disorders make up only a very small percentage of patients in a general rheumatology clinic, and the frequency of the various subtypes is very different from that in the adult population. Therefore, most of the information on systemic sclerosis in adolescents is derived from adult studies, with reports in children being limited to small case series and no therapeutic trials.[2–10] In contrast, localized forms of scleroderma are much more common than the systemic type in paediatrics, and form the focus of most of the paediatric scleroderma literature (Table 9.1).

SYSTEMIC SCLEROSIS

The last decade has witnessed a sense of optimism in some quarters surrounding the systemic sclerosis group of disorders. Advances

---

Table 9.1   Classification of scleroderma

- Systemic sclerosis:
  - diffuse (formerly known as progressive systemic sclerosis)
  - limited (formerly known as CREST* syndrome)
  - overlap syndromes with scleroderma
- Localized scleroderma:
  - morphea
  - linear scleroderma
    - (a) on an extremity
    - (b) on the face (*en coup de sabre*)
  - generalized fasciitis
- Eosinophilic morphea
- Secondary forms:
  - drug induced
  - chemical induced
- Pseudoscleroderma

*Calcinosis, Raynauld's phenomena, oesophageal dysmotility, sclerodactyly, telangiectasiae

---

in cell biology, immunology and inflammation, immunogenetics and connective-tissue biology have resulted in an understanding of some of the pathogenetic events that may be involved. New supportive therapies for the systemic manifestations have reduced the morbidity and mortality. New methods of monitoring the disease (clinical and laboratory) have led to a renewed interest in clinical trials of these disorders. It is hoped that some of these advances will also lead to further understanding of the types of scleroderma that are more common in the paediatric and adolescent age groups.

Incidence and epidemiology

In recent adult studies, the incidence of systemic sclerosis has been found to range from 3.7 per million to 19 per million population, with a prevalence rate ranging from 31 per million to 240 per million.[11] The prevalence is influenced by genetic, ethnic and environmental backgrounds. The systemic disease peaks in the 30–50 year old age group; paediatric patients make up less than 10% of all patients. In adults, females outnumber males by anywhere from 3 : 1 to 14 : 1,[12] but this ratio is lower in younger children. The disease is more common in blacks, who also have worse disease. In the most recent survey of the American Pediatric Rheumatology disease registry (SL

Bowyer, personal communication, 1998), patients with systemic sclerosis made up only 0.17% of all cases. To put this in perspective, in three recent paediatric rheumatology registries, the ratio of patients with systemic sclerosis to patients with systemic lupus erythematosus (SLE) ranged from 1 : 5 to 1 : 17.[13–15] Although there is no distinct immunogenetic profile associated with scleroderma in general, linkages are seen when the disease is put into subsets by autoantibody profile, disease severity and course.[16] These linkages include several human leucocyte antigen (HLA) DR and DQ associations. Rarely, familial cases may occur.[17]

Pathogenesis

The pathogenesis of scleroderma is not fully understood, but to determine a model it must be assessed from the perspective of the endothelial cell, the immune system and the fibroblast[18–20] (Figure 9.1). Central to any hypothesis is that

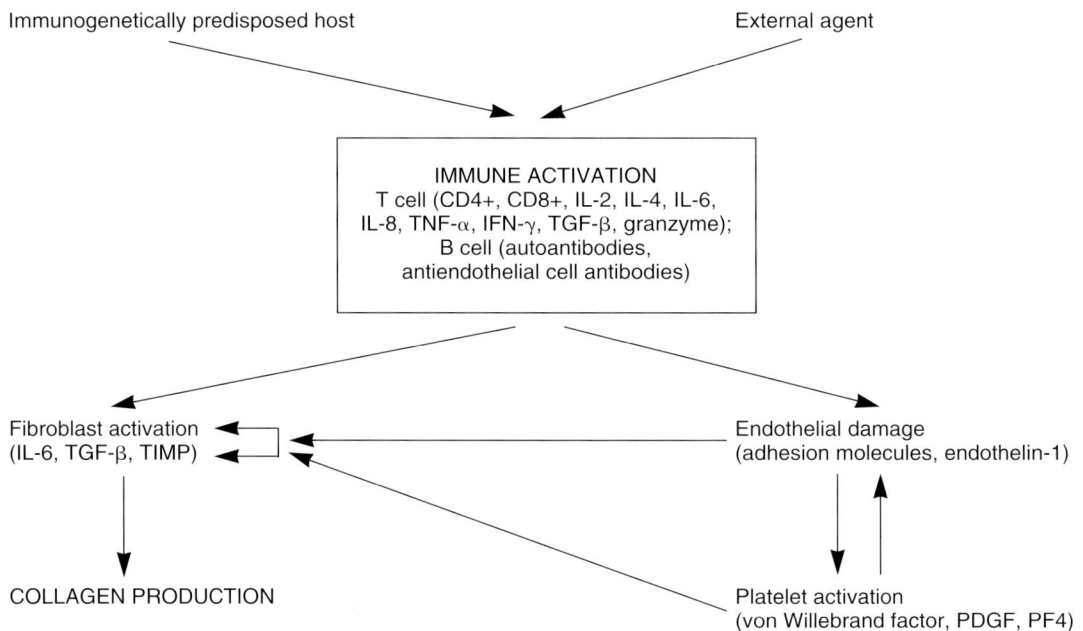

Figure 9.1 Hypothetical model for the pathogenesis of scleroderma (see text).

immune activation leads to a cascade of events, which ultimately results in excessive deposition of collagen. The immunogenetic associations in systemic sclerosis[16] and the production of scleroderma-like syndromes with various toxins and drugs suggest that environmental stimuli act upon the immune system of a genetically predisposed host to activate the immune system. There is evidence of both T cell[19–21] (cluster determinant 4+ (CD4+) cells in early skin lesions, CD8+ T cells in bronchoalveolar lavage (BAL) fluid, and altered cytokine expression) and B cell[22] (autoantibodies and antiendothelial-cell antibodies) activation. T-cell effector mechanisms activate fibroblasts to increase collagen production.[23] Endothelial-cell activation and damage by both T- and B-cell mechanisms further activates the immune system and, with the expression of endothelial cell adhesion molecules,[24] attracts inflammatory cells to the local lesions, which further act upon fibroblasts to increase the production of collagen.[25] In addition, the release of endothelin leads to potent vasoconstriction. Platelet activation (increased von Willebrand factor, platelet factor 4 (PF4) and platelet-derived growth factor (PDGF)) results from endothelial cell damage. This leads to platelet aggregation and microthrombi, vascular permeability with egress of inflammatory and immunostimulatory cells to the extravascular space, and further stimulation of fibroblasts to produce collagen. The fibroblast also produces mediators, which act in an autocrine fashion to perpetuate collagen production,[26] as well as tissue inhibitors of metalloproteinases (TIMP), which prevent the breakdown of newly formed collagen. Mast cells[27] and eosinophils,[28] which are found near to the lesions, may also play important roles in the fibrosis. The similarity of the scleroderma lesions to those of chronic graft-versus-host disease (GVHD) have led to the hypothesis that fetal cells may cross the placenta into the maternal circulation and provide donor lymphocytes that recognize disparate lymphocyte antigens, resulting in a reaction similar to chronic GVHD. Subsequent activation of these cells by environmental stimuli may result in disease development.[29]

Table 9.2   Criteria for the diagnosis of systemic sclerosis[30]

Major criterion
- Scleroderma proximal to the metacarpophalangeal joints

Minor criteria
- Sclerodactyly
- Digital pitting scars of fingertips or loss of substance of the distal finger pad
- Bilateral basilar pulmonary fibrosis

Clinical manifestations

The American Rheumatism Association/ American College of Rheumatology (ARA/ ACR) classification criteria (Table 9.2) have a sensitivity of 97% and a specificity of 98% for definite systemic sclerosis compared to patients with SLE, polymyositis/dermatomyositis and Raynaud's phenomenon.[30]

Skin

The hallmark of scleroderma is the development of tight, hard skin. The distribution of involvement, rapidity of evolution, disease severity and outcome vary by subtype. Diffuse disease (formerly known as progressive systemic sclerosis), associated with the presence of anti-Scl 70 antibodies, evolves rapidly over the first 1–3 years of disease and involves the proximal extremities (above the knee and elbow) in addition to the trunk, whereas skin involvement in limited systemic sclerosis (formerly known as CREST (calcinosis, Raynaud's phenomenon, oesophageal involvement, sclerodactyly, and telangiectasiae) syndrome), associated with the presence of anticentromere antibodies, progresses much more slowly, is generally limited to the skin of the distal extremities and face, and spares the trunk.

The earliest cutaneous feature is peripheral oedema, particularly of the hands. This oedema is not pitting, is painless, and limits motion

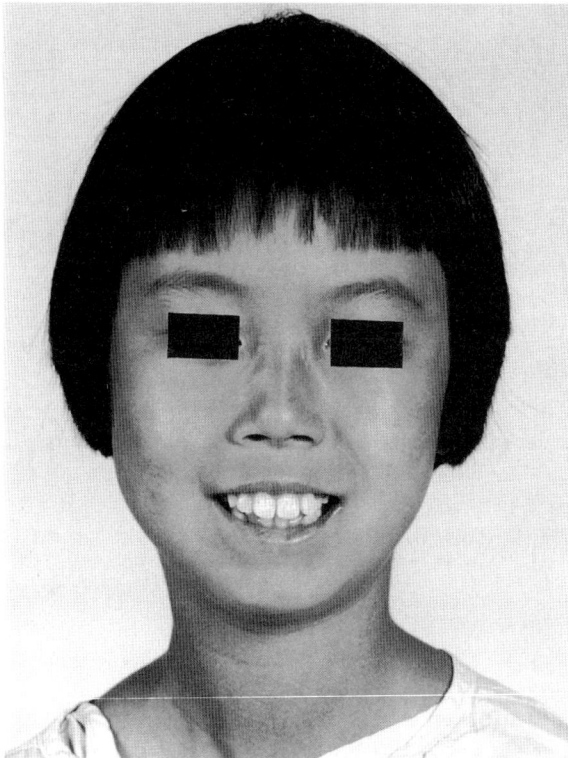

Figure 9.2 The face of a 10-year-old girl with a 2-year history of diffuse systemic sclerosis shows a 'pinched' appearance.

Pigmentary changes occur frequently. Both hyperpigmentation[31] and hypopigmentation can occur, and can result in a 'salt and pepper' appearance, with hyperpigmentation over the hair follicles with surrounding hypopigmentation. Cutaneous telangiectasia are especially prominent in the limited variant of systemic sclerosis, particularly over the finger pads, oral mucosa and neck. Ulcerations may develop over thin skin that has been traumatized, and may also occur in more distal areas as a result of ischaemia (see below). Characteristic 'ice-pick' scars of the finger pads (Figure 9.3) and loss of finger pulp space may result from Raynaud's phenomenon, and in fact, this is one of the minor diagnostic criteria. Subcutaneous calcinosis occurs in both varieties, but much more commonly in limited systemic sclerosis. Prominent areas of involvement include the fingers, knees, elbows and buttocks. Large calcific deposits may impair joint function and require surgical removal. These areas may also become superinfected. Skin nodules may develop over flexor tendons. The 'neck sign' (ridging and tightening of the skin of the neck on extending the head) is present in 90% of patients with systemic sclerosis.[32]

The cutaneous histopathology in the early phase reveals oedema, endothelial-cell swelling

(resulting in stiffness). There is a firm feel on palpation. This early oedematous phase is associated with inflammatory changes in the subcutaneous tissue, which becomes progressively thicker and tighter. In the extremities, this results in stiffness and loss of motion; and in the face, a 'pinched' appearance, with a loss of facial creases develops (Figure 9.2). As the skin thickens and tightens, there is also loss of skin appendages. As the skin tightens over the extremities, joint contractures develop. The skin is susceptible to minor trauma, particularly over bony prominences. In addition to the feeling of tightness, early symptoms may include dryness and pruritus. Paradoxically, over time, there is progressive softening of the skin, regardless of treatment.

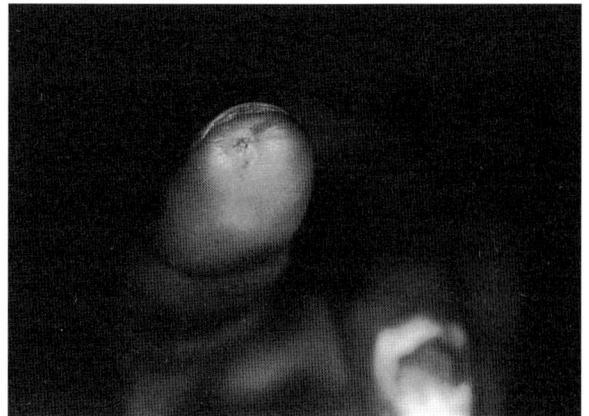

Figure 9.3 Digital pitting scar in a 5-year-old girl with scleroderma–myositis overlap syndrome.

and a perivascular infiltrate of mononuclear cells.[33] With progression of the lesion, other cells, including macrophages, eosinophils, mast cells and plasma cells, appear. With time, there is excessive deposition of sheets of collagen throughout the dermis and subcutaneous tissue, with loss of rete pegs and replacement of skin appendages. There is no evidence of vasculitis. While systemic effects of vascular changes, inflammatory cells and growth factors are thought to account for these changes, a report of clinically normal skin becoming sclerodermatous when transplanted into a sclerodermatous area suggests that local factors are important as well.[34]

Over the last several years, several methods of quantifying skin involvement have been developed.[35] Skin scores are based upon dividing the body into several areas and measuring the degree of skin thickening in each area,[36] and have been shown to be reliable predictors of prognosis.[37] Close correlations have been found between skin thickening and the weight of skin-core biopsies (after careful removal of all subcutaneous fatty tissue).[38] They can be used to monitor the course of disease as well as of treatment in individual patients, and serve as reliable markers for the response to therapy in drug trials. High-frequency ultrasound has recently been proposed as another way of monitoring skin thickness in scleroderma, but this requires the use of specialized equipment.[39,40] Several new methods of assessing skin involvement[41,42] may be more objective than the skin score and deserve further study. These techniques, if validated, may also be useful in evaluating localized scleroderma.

Raynaud's phenomenon
Raynaud's phenomenon is such an important symptom of systemic sclerosis, occurring in over 90% of patients, that the diagnosis of systemic sclerosis should be questioned if it is not present. In fact, it is the presenting symptom in 70% of patients, and may antedate the development of other stigmata of systemic sclerosis by years, especially in the limited variant of the disease.

The manifestations of Raynaud's phenome-

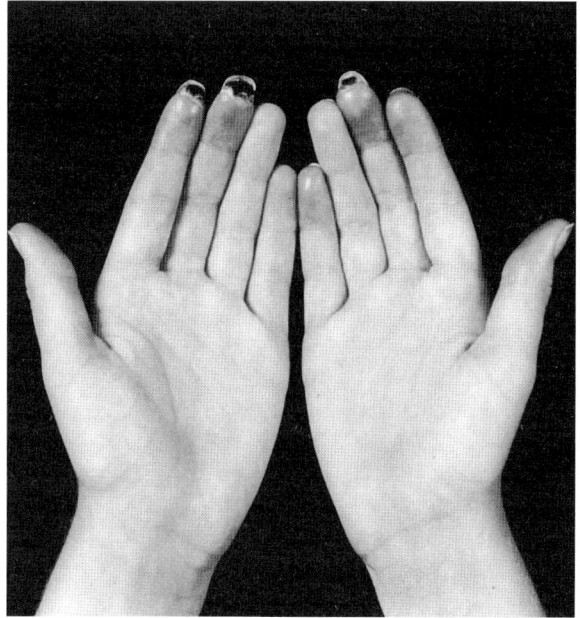

Figure 9.4 Dry gangrene of three digits secondary to Raynaud's phenomenon.

non result from vasospasm, usually in response to environment stimuli. The most common triggers are cold and stress: the cold provocation may be minimal. Typically, Raynaud's phenomenon occurs in three phases: the ischaemic phase, resulting in cutaneous pallor; the hypoxic phase, resulting in cyanotic colour change; and the reperfusion phase (hyperaemia), resulting in redness. In the fingers and toes, there is a well-demarcated area of involvement, and clear demarcation should be sought carefully in the history. Symptoms of Raynaud's phenomenon vary from none, to peripheral numbness and tingling, to severe pain if the ischaemic phase is prolonged. Recurrent severe attacks may result in tissue loss (flattening of pulp spaces) and tiny pitted scars on the fingertips (see Figure 9.3). Occasionally, the vasospasm may be so severe that gangrenous changes can develop (Figure 9.4). These may be superficial or extend to bone, resulting in auto-amputation. Other acral areas, including the ear lobes and tip of the nose, may

Table 9.3   Raynaud's phenomenon: differential diagnosis

- Primary
- Disorder of blood vessel:
  - connective tissue disease
  - vibration
  - cold injury
- Drug
- External pressure/compression:
  - anatomic (e.g. thoracic outlet syndrome)
- Abnormal blood viscosity:
  - cryoglobulinaemia, cryofibrinogenaemia, hyperviscosity syndromes

Musculoskeletal system

Articular involvement may be the first manifestation of systemic sclerosis and, if the skin manifestations are subtle, this may result in a mistaken diagnosis of juvenile idiopathic arthritis. Eventually, almost all patients will develop joint involvement. Joint involvement may be secondary to synovial inflammation,[44] which is not common; more commonly, it results from fibrosis of the joint capsule and tightness of the overlying skin.[45] While the predominantly involved joints are the small joints of the hands, wrists and ankles, many other joints can be affected. Erosions are extremely uncommon unless the systemic sclerosis is part of an overlap syndrome. Progressive joint dysfunction, however, results from the tightness of the skin and fibrosis of the joint capsule.

Bony abnormalities occur and are thought to result form ischaemia. Acro-osteolysis occurs with severe Raynaud's but, in and of itself, is of little consequence.[46] Mandibular resorption is a characteristic musculoskeletal feature that may result from several external effects, including facial tightness, decreased oral aperture and atrophy of the masticatory muscles.[47]

Muscle involvement occurs in up to 80% of patients,[48] and can be associated with both the diffuse and limited forms of disease.[49] It can take one of two forms.[50] An indolent myopathy with minimal to mild weakness, mildly raised enzymes, and minimal inflammation on biopsy is the more common type, and does not necessarily require treatment (or only low-dose corticosteroids). A more inflammatory process as part of an overlap syndrome may also occur, and can resemble the myopathy of either polymyositis or dermatomyositis, especially if myositis-associated antibodies are present. Adult patients with muscle involvement may also be at higher risk for myocardial dysfunction, and thus detection of myopathy in scleroderma patients should prompt a search for cardiac disease.[51]

Tendon friction rubs are a characteristic feature, occurring most commonly in diffuse disease. They may be palpable or audible and represent fibrotic changes of the tenosynovium.[45]

occasionally be involved.

It is extremely important to differentiate the Raynaud's phenomenon of systemic sclerosis from other causes (Table 9.3). Features suggestive of primary Raynaud's phenomenon include a positive family history, absence of scarring, ulcers and other trophic changes, a negative antinuclear antibody (ANA) test and normal nailfold capillaries. The two most important indicators that a patient with Raynaud's phenomenon is destined to develop systemic sclerosis (or another connective-tissue disease) are a positive ANA and abnormal nailfold capillaries.[43] In the clinic, use of an ophthalmoscope at + 40 diopters with immersion oil placed on the nailbed magnifies vessels for examination. Normally, an unbroken 'picket-fence' pattern of hair-pin vessels is observed. In the systemic sclerosis group of disorders, areas of capillary enlargement, dropout and bushy dilatation may be seen, which likely reflect changes in the vascular beds in other organs.

The course of Raynaud's phenomenon is monitored primarily by history and physical examination. Measurement of finger temperature, systolic pressure and Doppler wave studies are primarily research tools.

These are most common over the wrist, ankle and knee. The presence of one or more tendon friction rubs early in the course of systemic sclerosis was one of the best predictors of both evolution to diffuse scleroderma and reduced survival.[52]

Pleuropulmonary disease

Pleuropulmonary disease is present in the vast majority of patients, but its evolution differs in diffuse and limited systemic sclerosis. Both pulmonary hypertension and interstitial fibrosis occur. Pulmonary hypertension occurs as an isolated phenomenon in the limited disease variant, whereas interstitial fibrosis occurs early in diffuse systemic sclerosis. Anticentromere antibodies can be associated with a lower risk of interstitial lung disease.[53] With time, interstitial fibrosis may lead to cor pulmonale and subsequent pulmonary hypertension.[54] Pulmonary abnormalities in childhood systemic sclerosis have been reported to be similar to those in the adult disease.[55]

Pulmonary involvement should be suspected and searched for in every patient with systemic sclerosis, as there is some suggestion that early treatment can reverse inflammatory changes.[56] The onset of pulmonary disease is usually insidious. Clinically, the symptoms are shortness of breath on exertion, dry cough, fatigue and reduced energy. Physical findings include dry basilar rales, reduced chest expansion, occasional pleural effusions and, with time, signs of right-sided heart failure. Clubbing is rare, perhaps due to poor perfusion and tight skin over the fingers. Aspiration pneumonia may develop in patients with gastro-oesophageal reflux.

Plain radiographs show changes of basilar pulmonary fibrosis (Figure 9.5a), and honeycomb lung in the advanced stages. However, chest radiograph changes occur late and do not correlate well with pulmonary function. Nuclear medicine studies[57,58] can document inflammatory disease prior to its clinical or radiographic appearance. BAL can also be used to study the local production of inflammatory cells and cytokines. Neutrophilic alveolitis can be found in 50–60% of patients, and suggests a poor

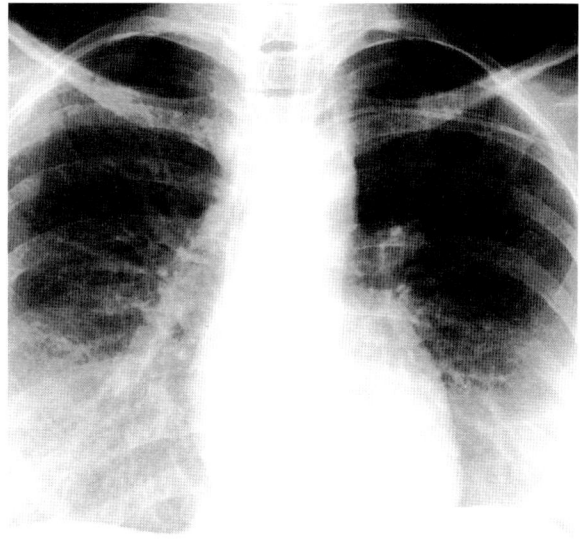

(a)

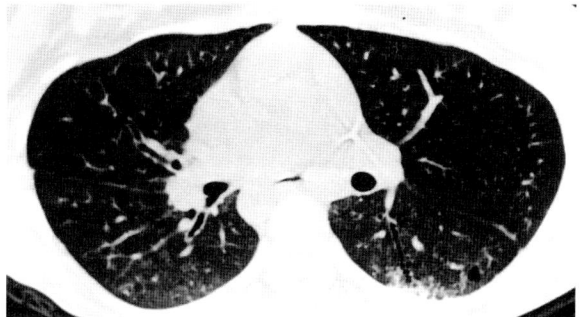

(b)

Figure 9.5 (a) Frontal view of the chest of an 18-year-old girl with a 4-year history of scleroderma overlap, demonstrating a fine and subtle diffuse interstitial process. (b) High-resolution CT scan of the chest, demonstrating a mixed interstitial pattern of peripheral linear densities, some of which represent interlobular septal thickening, combined with small 'cysts', suggesting a pattern of early honeycombing as seen in cases of interstitial fibrosis.

outcome.[59] The presence of the fibrogenic cytokines platelet-derived growth factor-1 (PDGF-1) and transforming growth factor β (TGF-β) may explain the pulmonary fibrosis.[60]

The recent advent of high-resolution computed tomography (CT) has been important in the early detection of lung disease, and should be used to monitor the course of disease.[61,62] Small, ill-defined signals in the posterior segments of the lower lobe followed by a reticulonodular appearance in a subpleural distribution correlate with early scleroderma lung disease (Figure 9.5b).

Pulmonary function tests are a simple way to detect and follow the course of lung disease. Fibrosis causes restrictive lung disease, and this is documented by a reduction in the total lung capacity (TLC) and forced vital capacity (FVC). The most sensitive indicator of early interstitial lung disease is a reduction in the diffusing capacity of carbon monoxide (DLCO), which reflects impaired gas exchange. A reduced DLCO is also associated with the development of pulmonary hypertension in cases of limited systemic sclerosis, and correlates closely with the findings of fibrosing alveolitis on CT scans.[63]

Asymptomatic pleural effusions are common. There is an increased incidence of carcinoma of the lung in patients with systemic sclerosis.[64] The dangers of smoking cannot be overemphasized to adolescents, who are so strongly influenced by their peer group.

Gastrointestinal manifestations
Gastrointestinal (GI) involvement is common and any point along the GI tract can be affected. In order of decreasing incidence, the oesophagus, anorectal area, small bowel and colon can be involved.[65,66] Morbidity from GI involvement is one of the most important components of systemic sclerosis. Fortunately, development of new agents has improved the plight of these patients.

Oral findings include xerostomia, which results from an overlap with Sjögren's syndrome but more commonly from fibrosis of the salivary glands. Dental loosening results from involvement of the periodontal membrane and mandibular resorption. Tongue atrophy leads to impaired taste and further anorexia. Most important, progressive tightening of the skin of the face leads to an inability to open the mouth. The interincisor distance (normally ≥ 4 mm) can be used to monitor the tightening of the skin of the face.

Oesophageal disease is the GI hallmark of systemic sclerosis and occurs in almost all children and adolescents with the disease.[67] Both abnormalities of the lower oesophageal sphincter (LES) and fibrosis of the lower two-thirds of the oesophagus are common. The result leads to very poor propulsive activity and 'lower dysphagia'. The reduced sphincter pressure allows for reflux of gastric contents, the acid content of which leads to oesophagitis. This may lead to stricture formation and a further reduction in oesophageal motility. Symptoms of reflux include burning chest pain and water-brash. Severe reflux can result in aspiration pneumonia. Barrett's metaplasia may occur and may be associated with the development of oesophageal carcinoma.[68]

The diagnosis is made by history, but is often delayed. Oesophageal cineradiography may demonstrate abnormal peristalsis. Manometry can determine sphincter pressure and can document motility abnormalities, and shows abnormalities much earlier than standard barium studies. The presence of reflux can be documented using a pH probe, but this is a painful test. Radionuclide oesophageal scanning for the presence of reflux has not been applied in paediatrics.

Involvement of the stomach is common and results in delayed gastric emptying. Severe atony can give rise to the 'watermelon stomach'.[69] Small bowel disease results from similar events as in the rest of the GI tract, with smooth muscle fibre atrophy and fibrosis predicting the clinical picture. Reduced motility of the small intestine results in pseudo-obstruction, with symptoms of bloating and cramping.[70] More importantly, this reduced motility can lead to bacterial overgrowth, with malabsorption and diarrhoea. Radiologically, dilatation of the duodenum and jejunum are common, and a prolonged transit time and intestinal sacculations are observed. Large bowel disease is often asymptomatic and can only be defined radiologically by loss of colonic haustra and pseudo-diverticula. Occasionally, constipation may be so severe as to require colectomy.

Cardiovascular system

As with other organ systems, involvement of the cardiovascular system can begin in an indolent fashion. Asymptomatic cardiac disease is common and can be detected by routine electrocardiography (ECG), echocardiography and thallium scanning.[71–73] With time, progressive fibrosis of both the myocardium and conducting tissue leads to significant morbidity. The characteristic cardiac abnormality results from very small vessel obliterative disease, leading to small areas of ischaemia and reperfusion; the pathological correlate is 'contraction band necrosis'. Progressive myocardial fibrosis can result in a restrictive cardiomyopathy and congestive heart failure. Myocarditis is rare, and is associated with polymyositis and significant morbidity and mortality.[51] Significant lung disease with pulmonary hypertension can also lead to cor pulmonale. Symptoms of involvement include fatigue (as a result of reduced myocardial function or myocarditis), dyspnoea from pulmonary hypertension, congestive heart failure, and palpitations from arrhythmias. A cardiac score, derived from routine ECG and echocardiographic studies, can be used to predict survival from scleroderma.[74] Thallium perfusion defects are predictive of increased risk of developing subsequent cardiac disease or death.[75]

Renal system

Prior to the development of angiotensin converting enzyme (ACE) inhibitors, renal disease was the major cause of mortality in scleroderma. Renal involvement occurs as a result of intimal thickening of small arteries and endothelial cells. These changes occur early, and almost only with diffuse disease. This vasculopathy results in a reduced cortical blood flow and multiple small cortical infarcts. Any reduction in blood flow (e.g. hypovolaemia) can lead to critical reduction in renal cortical flow and rapid and sustained activation of the renin–angiotensin systems, with malignant hypertension.[76,77] This formerly fatal event is now treatable with the use of ACE inhibitors.[78]

The earliest sign of renal disease is mild proteinuria. With time, there may be an increase in proteinuria and a mild decrease in creatinine clearance. Hypertension occurs in up to 50% of adult patients, and is usually associated with proteinuria. The development of hypertension or reduction in the creatinine clearance should be an indication to treat with an ACE inhibitor. The development of malignant hypertension, which occurs in 10–20% of cases, is frequently accompanied, and occasionally preceded, by microangiopathic haemolytic anaemia.

Other organ involvement

Other organ systems can occasionally be involved. Central nervous system disease is rare, but neuropathies, reflecting fibrotic impingement, can occur, particularly trigeminal neuropathy.[79,80] Sicca symptoms are more likely to result from glandular fibrosis than lymphocytic infiltration. Hypothyroidism, while rare, results from similar mechanisms.[81]

Disease course and mortality

The course of systemic sclerosis is determined by the subtype. Diffuse disease is associated with rapidly progressive skin involvement and vital organ disease, while limited disease may be stable for many years before the development of pulmonary hypertension. The appearance of renal, cardiac or pulmonary disease within the first year of disease onset is associated with a poor outcome. The standardized mortality rate in a cohort of 237 patients was 4.69, compared to an age- and sex-matched control group,[82] with overall 3-, 6-, and 9-year survival rates of 86%, 76% and 61%, respectively.[83] A more recent series, documented a 7-year survival rate of 76.5%, broken down to 81% for limited disease and 72% for diffuse disease.[84] It is likely that the recent advances in the treatment of renal and pulmonary disease will result in improved survival rates. Death in childhood cases has resulted from cardiac, renal or pulmonary failure. While in the past, childhood systemic sclerosis was considered to have a very poor prognosis and quality of life, a recent international survey suggested better outcomes.[85] In this group of 120 patients reported from 32 centres, the mean age of disease onset was 8.7 years, with a mean disease duration at last follow-up of 4.9 years. The 1-year survival was 100%, 2 year-survival 97% and 4-year survival 95%. The outcome was classified as 'excellent' in 9%, 'satisfactory' in 69% and 'poor' in 17%. There were six deaths (5%); the causes of death were heart failure in four, renal failure in one and sepsis in one patient. These preliminary data are much more encouraging than the published data on adults, and may suggest a better outcome for children and adolescents with systemic sclerosis.

Laboratory features

In contrast to most other autoimmune rheumatic disorders, there is no significant elevation of the erythrocyte sedimentation rate (ESR) in scleroderma, unless it is part of an overlap syndrome. In fact, elevation of the ESR may indicate a poor prognosis, and should suggest a search for other disorders. Anaemia can result from several causes, including GI blood loss (oesophagitis), malabsorption, poor nutrition and chronic disease. The white blood cell count and differential are normal.

ANAs are present in 90% of patients; the antibody specificity differs by disease subtype and disease course (Table 9.4).[22] The production of these autoantibodies seems to be genetically determined.[86] Indirect immunofluorescence staining on human cells gives either nuclear or nucleolar patterns, depending on the specificity of the autoantibody. The major antibody systems are antitopoisomerase-1 (also called Scl-70), anticentromere and antinucleolar proteins.

Table 9.4   Autoantibodies in scleroderma*

Autoantigen	Location	Sclerosis subset	Associated organ involvement
Topoisomerase-1 (Scl-70)	Nucleus, nucleoplasm	Diffuse cutaneous	Pulmonary fibrosis, vasculopathy
RNA polymerase I, II, III	Nucleus, nucleoplasm	Diffuse cutaneous	Renal, less frequently pulmonary
Centromere proteins	Nucleus, nucleoplasm	Limited cutaneous	Calcinosis, telangiectasiae
Fibrillarin	Nucleolus	None	Pulmonary hypertension
Th/To	Nucleolus	Limited cutaneous	Puffy fingers, small bowel disease, hypothyroidism, arthropathy
Pm-Scl	Nucleolus	Overlap syndrome	Limited skin thickening, myopathy, arthropathy

*Adapted from Okano.[22]

Antibodies to topoisomerase-1 occur in 20–40% of patients with systemic sclerosis, but in up to 60% with diffuse disease. As such, the presence of these antibodies is associated with a poor outcome. Topoisomerase-1 is a non-histone basic protein that catalyses the uncoiling of DNA. Antibodies to RNA polymerases I, II and III are also associated with diffuse disease and occur in 3–33% of systemic sclerosis patients. Antibodies to centromere occur in 15–30% of patients overall, and in 70–80% of patients with limited disease. These antibodies are markers for milder disease in general, except for the late development of pulmonary hypertension. The role of these autoantibodies is unclear, but the consistent association with disease subsets suggests that they play some role in disease pathogenesis. The sequence homology between topoiso-merase-1 and a retrovirus suggests that molecular mimicry may play a role in the production of some of the autoantibodies.[19] Other autoantibodies that are fairly unique to scleroderma include antifibrillarin and PM-Scl.[22]

The significance of anticardiolipin antibodies, which are found in approximately one-third of patients, is uncertain.[87,88] Antihistone antibodies are also found in one-third of patients and correlate with diffuse disease.[89]

Management

The management of the patient with systemic sclerosis (Table 9.5) requires close and careful observation, protective measures and the care of a supportive multidisciplinary health-care team.

Table 9.5 Management of scleroderma by organ system

Vascular
Keep warm, vasodilators/calcium channel blockers, prostaglandin E1, prostacyclin, tissue plasminogen activator, sympathectomy, local vascular microsurgery

Renal
Maintain good perfusion (avoid volume reduction), angiotensin-converting agents, antihypertensives

Heart
Calcium-channel blockers, antiarrhythmic agents, transplantation, corticosteroids

Lungs
Corticosteroids, cyclophosphamide, calcium-channel blockers, vasodilators, D-penicillamine

Skin
Lubricants, topical corticosteroid, diltiazem

Gastrointestinal system
Prokinetic agents, proton-pump inhibitors, intermittent antibiotics, stool softeners, total parenteral nutrition

Disease-modifying agents
D-Penicillamine, cyclosporine, methotrexate, γ-interferon, vitamin D, PUVA, bone-marrow transplantation

PUVA, psoralens + UVA radiation.

The major advances in treating systemic sclerosis over the last decade have been in the treatment of end-organ disease. The ACR guidelines for the conduct of clinical trials in system sclerosis[90,91] should lead to important new information on management. The results of randomized controlled trials of disease-modifying drugs in scleroderma have been disappointing to date, with the majority of the reported studies being negative.[92]

Systemic therapy is directed at the underlying process(es) implicated in the pathogenesis of the fibrosis. D-penicillamine[93–95] may improve skin and lung disease if started early; it requires prolonged treatment and has significant potential side-effects, including haematological, renal and autoimmune effects. Doses used are 10–15 mg/kg/day. In a placebo-controlled trial, methotrexate has been reported to reduce skin scores.[96] Cyclosporine A improved skin scores, but may be associated with hypertension and other renal toxicity.[97,98] Relaxin decreases collagen synthesis by cultured human scleroderma fibroblasts,[99] and has shown promise in an early study.[100] It is administered by continuous subcutaneous infusion, and is therefore not very practical. Studies are currently in progress to determine the role of relaxin in the various forms of scleroderma. The use of extracorporeal photochemotherapy, in which the patient's leucocytes are treated with a photosensitizing compound, removed by leucapheresis, exposed to UVA irradiation and re-infused, has been reported with variable results, and is currently not recommended.[101,102] UVA treatment with psoralens[103] and vitamin D_3[104] have been reported to be successful in open-labelled studies.

α-Interferon was not very effective in musculoskeletal or visceral disease in the one study reported.[105] γ-Interferon has been shown to reduce collagen production, and therefore might be considered useful in treating systemic sclerosis. Several studies have been reported, with variable results and toxicity; it deserves further study.[106–109]

The failure to control the rapidly progressive disease and the poor outcomes have led to a new protocol for allogeneic bone-marrow transplantation.[110] One child with systemic sclerosis has been successfully transplanted with autologous peripheral stem cells.[111] Whether this becomes an accepted form of therapy requires further experience, given a 5–10% mortality from the procedure alone.

In patients with newly diagnosed systemic sclerosis the present author recommends systemic treatment with either D-penicillamine (10–15 mg/kg/day) or methotrexate (10–15 mg/m^2 per week).

Raynaud's phenomenon

Protective measures are most important and must be re-emphasized at each visit. This is particularly true in adolescents (e.g. wear warm clothing, do not smoke). Avoidance of cold exposure as much as possible, use of warm clothing, and mittens (with 'hot packs') instead of gloves are the keys to preventing or ameliorating attacks of Raynaud's phenomenon. Calcium channel blocking agents have also proved to be very effective in managing patients.[112] Long-acting nifedipine is the agent of choice, and the dose should be titrated to prevent attacks and also side-effects.[113] If this is inadequate and patients are having severe recurrent attacks, use of intravenous prostaglandin E1[114] or prostacyclin[115] have been shown to be effective in some series; they are also effective for ulcers that are refractile to treatment.[116] The role of ketansirin (a serotonin antagonist), antiplatelet agents, anticoagulants, antifibrinolytics and pentoxyphilline have not been proven. Biofeedback may be helpful in selected patients.[117] Microsurgery (digital sympathectomy) is occasionally attempted, with variable success.[118]

In the present author's experience, most patients with Raynaud's phenomenon can be managed with careful attention to symptomatic measures together with nifedipine. The dose should be based on the weight of the child, generally starting at 10–20 mg/day long-acting nifedipine. This dose can be increased as tolerated, depending on side-effects (primarily headache and postural hypotension). If these measures are not effective, I have tried topical nitroglycerine, with occasional benefit. Short-term impressive improvements in patients with impending tissue loss or non-healing ulcers have been seen with intravenous prostacyclin.

Skin and musculoskeletal system

The skin of patients with systemic sclerosis often feels very dry and may be pruritic; emollients are often most helpful. In case reports diltiazem has been reported to be effective in improving calcinosis.[119] Physical therapy, including active and passive exercises and splinting, is usually adequate treatment for joint disease. Non-steroidal anti-inflammatory drugs (NSAIDs) are occasionally necessary. For severe myopathy, high-dose corticosteroids should be used.

Gastrointestinal manifestations

As patients are prone to disorders of motility and reflux, supportive measures are important. Patients should have small frequent meals rather than large meals, and should reduce their fatty food intake. They should remain upright for at least 2 hours after a meal. Omeprazole has been very effective in the treatment of reflux oesophagitis.[120] Oesophageal motility and LES dysfunction may be improved with prokinetic agents such as cisapride and erythromycin.[70,121] Intestinal motility may be improved by these agents or octrerotide.[122] If there is suggestion of malabsorption, treatment with broad-spectrum antibiotics should be instituted. Supportive treatment for pseudo-obstruction should include intravenous hydration, nutrition and nasogastric suction. Severe constipation may require the use of enemas or, rarely, the excision of affected bowel.

Pulmonary disease

Once pulmonary fibrosis has developed, the process appears to be irreversible. Therefore early detection of inflammatory changes (see above) is critical to attempt to reverse the process. Early use of D-penicillamine may reduce or delay the development of lung disease.[94] Recently, treatment with cortico-steroid and cyclophosphamide has shown some potential in reducing the pulmonary fibrosis

that follows alveolitis.[56] Vasodilator agents have not been effective in treating pulmonary hypertension. If pulmonary fibrosis is severe, lung transplantation may be attempted; survival appears to be similar to that of other patients with lung transplantation.[123]

LOCALIZED SCLERODERMA

The localized scleroderma group of disorders make up the majority of cases of scleroderma in the paediatric and adolescent age groups, in fact outnumbering cases of systemic sclerosis significantly in these age groups. As the term suggests, localized scleroderma is not associated with the degree of systemic involvement as is systemic sclerosis, although there occasionally may be involvement in organ systems other than the skin and subcutaneous tissue.[124] An important issue for all patients is whether the disease should be classified as part of the spectrum of generalized scleroderma, as localized lesions occasionally may be seen in cases of systemic sclerosis or in fact other connective-tissue diseases.[125] Only occasionally does localized scleroderma evolve into systemic sclerosis or another connective-tissue disease.[126–128] It has been suggested that patients with scleroderma nailfold abnormalities may go on to develop systemic disease.[129] Evolution to systemic disease is so unusual that in our clinic we attempt to explain to families that these are essentially different processes and use the term 'morphea' rather than 'scleroderma'. However, other paediatric rheumatologists feel that children with morphea do frequently progress to systemic sclerosis, and therefore the issue remains controversial.

Epidemiology

In the most thorough epidemiologic study reported to date (the Rochester Epidemiology Project), the overall incidence was 2.7 per 100 000 of the entire population. Twenty-eight per cent of the cases reviewed in the period 1960–1993 occurred in patients aged less than 18 years. Of these, 40% had linear scleroderma and the remainder had various forms of morphea. The linear form was the only variety more common in the paediatric/adolescent age group than in adults. Interestingly, the age- and sex-specific incidence rates increased over the three decades of study.[130] In most series, females outnumber males by 3–4 : 1,[131–135] but this incidence ratio may vary by subtype.

Classification

Several classification schemes have been proposed.[135,136] Subgroups include morphea and linear scleroderma. When there are multiple patches of morphea (more than 3 or 4), the disorder may be called *generalized morphea*. When localized scleroderma involves the face and/or scalp, it is known as *scleroderma en coup de sabre*. In most series, linear lesions are the most common, followed by morphea and generalized morphea.[126,131–135] Clinically, there is significant overlap with other dermatological conditions, including lichen sclerosis et atrophicus, atrophederma of Pasini and Pierini, and lipoatrophy,[137] although some feel that these should all be classified in the morphea group of disorders.[135] *Pan-sclerotic morphea* is another variant with coalescent areas of morphea that extend deep to bone.[138] *Parry–Romberg syndrome* is another variant with atrophy of subcutaneous tissue and fat of the skin of the face occurring below the forehead. There is little, if any, sclerosis of the skin and subcutaneous tissue, although there may be overlap of Parry–Romberg and morphea variants of the disease.[139] Despite the many variants of localized scleroderma, several may occur together in the same patient, suggesting that the division may be somewhat arbitrary.

Clinical features

The diagnosis is based on clinical features, and a skin biopsy is rarely necessary. When done it shows the same pathology as that of generalized scleroderma: bland sheets of collagen with replacement of rete pegs and loss of dermal appendages. There is very little inflammation on the skin biopsy. As the clinical presentation is usually an indolent one, the date of onset is rarely determined. This makes determination of

aetiology particularly difficult. While some authors have postulated trauma as an inciting feature, this is extremely difficult to prove without a case–control study.[140,141] An intriguing association has been seen with spina bifida occulta.[126] The reason for the association is unclear, but it may suggest a neurologic role. An association with *Borrelia* infection has been proposed. This may vary by geographic area; it seems to be more consistently associated in Europe (but not in all studies) and Japan[142,143] than in North America.[144] Radiation may also lead to localized scleroderma.[145]

Morphea lesions most commonly occur on the trunk, abdomen or proximal extremity (Figure 9.6). Typically, the lesions present as ivory

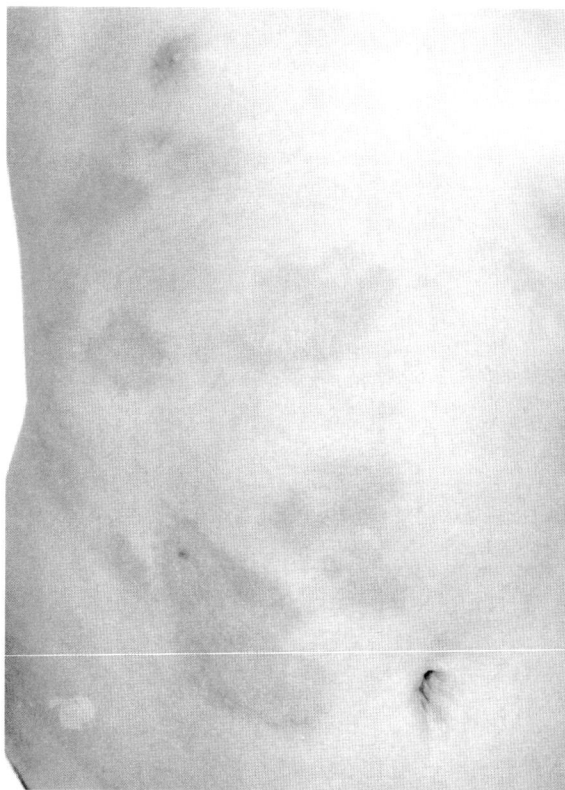

Figure 9.6 Multiple hyperpigmented plaques of morphea.

coloured, oval to circular patches of 0.5 cm to many centimetres of thickened skin. When surrounded by a lilac-coloured halo, the process is considered to be active. The lesions may be warm to the touch. They usually remain active for a period of 3–5 years, regardless of treatment, and subsequently resolve with skin softening, often becoming hyperpigmented as they do so. Symptoms of morphea are unusual, but occasionally there may be tingling, burning or itching of the lesion.

Linear lesions are of a much more important concern, and the duration of activity may be longer than that of morphea lesions. The patient or their parent may note a band of discolouration that feels firm to touch, in a linear distribution, over an extremity or on the forehead and scalp. These lesions do not follow a dermatomal pattern. There may be associated erythema or warmth, signs that suggest disease activity. With time, there may be thinning of the extremity or the forehead, and reduced motion if the band crosses the joint. These lesions are more common in the lower than in the upper extremity. Growth changes may be significant. When involving an extremity, there may be shortening. Over the face, there may be significant atrophy of facial structures. A lesion that crosses the chest wall can be associated with underdevelopment of breast tissue (Figures 9.7–9.9).

Although considered a localized process and not truly a part of generalized systemic sclerosis,

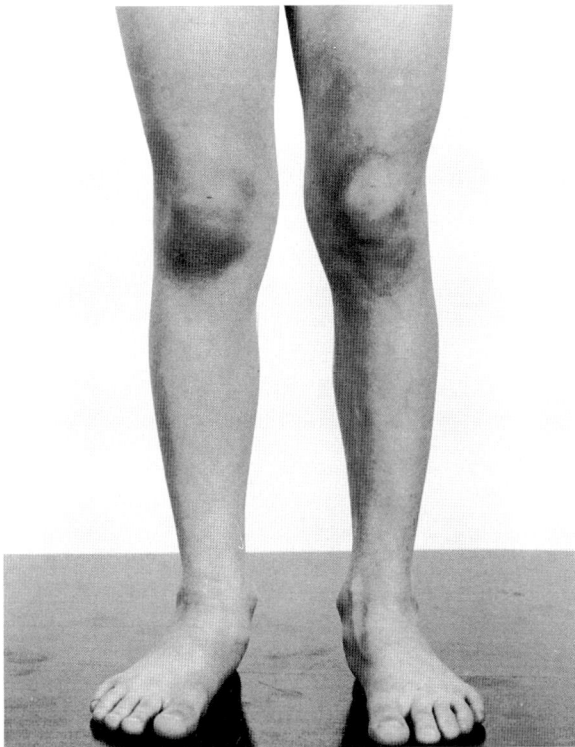
(a)

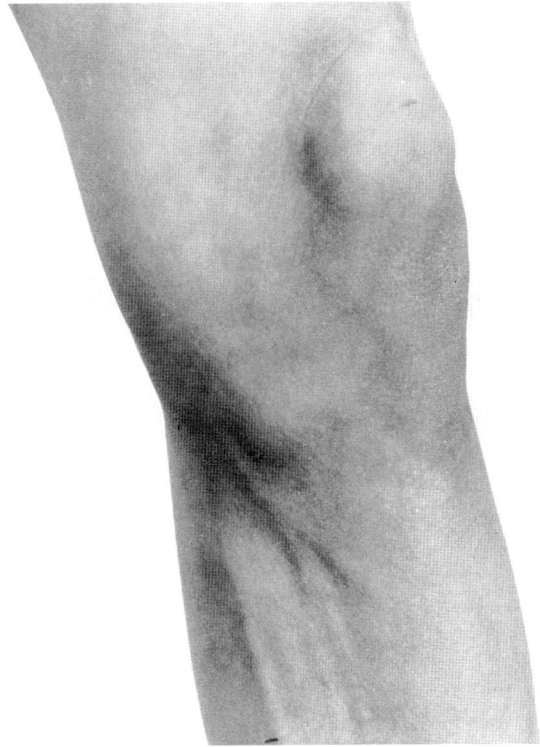
(b)

Figure 9.7 Localized linear scleroderma of the left leg. Note asymmetry of the musculature (a), hyperpigmentation and atrophy of the soft tissue (b).

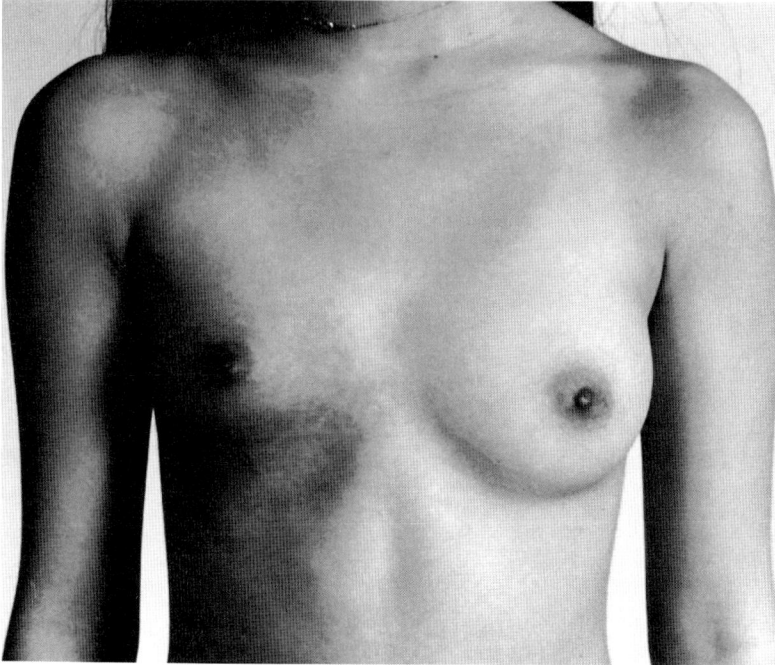

Figure 9.8 A 15-year-old girl with a 4-year history of morphea over the right chest wall, with marked underdevelopment of the right breast.

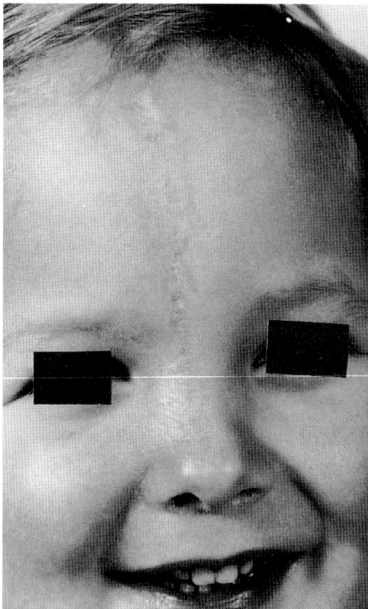

(a)

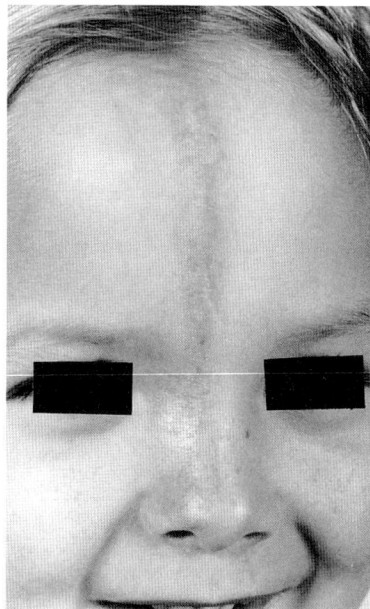

(b)

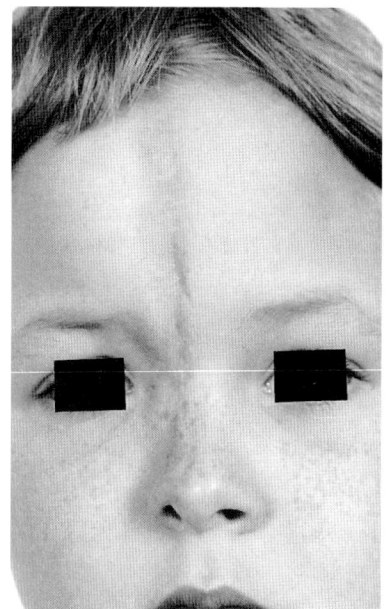

(c)

Figure 9.9 Progressive changes over a 5-year period of linear scleroderma *en coup de sabre*. The band has become deeper, hyperpigmented and has extended almost to the tip of the nose. No treatment was administered.

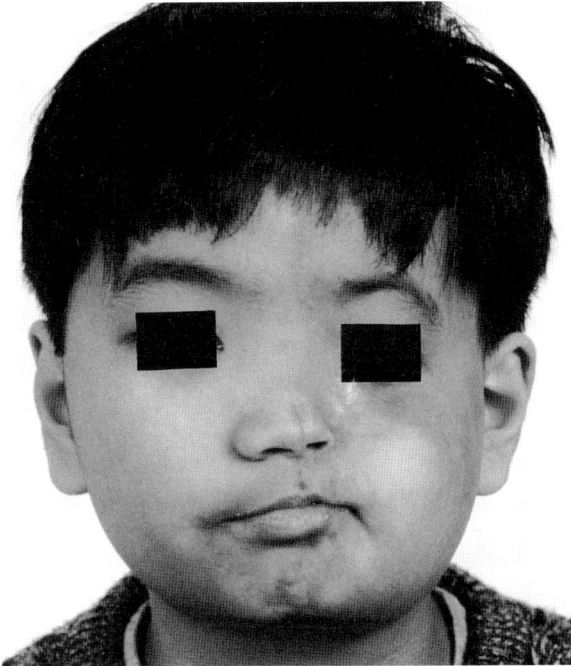

(a)

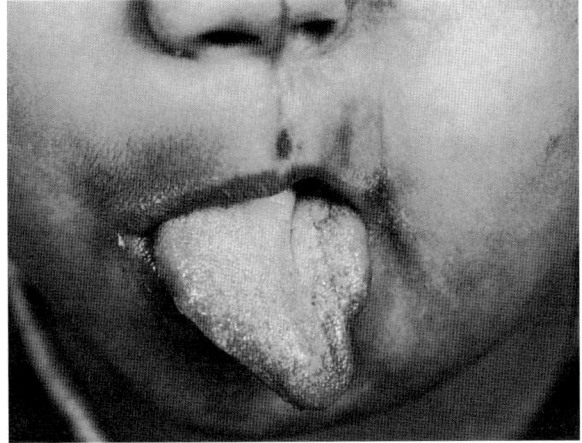

(b)

Figure 9.10 A 13-year-old boy with combined linear scleroderma *en coup de sabre* and Parry–Romberg syndrome. Note the tightening around the mouth (a), with atrophy of the tongue (b).

other systems can be involved as well. Polyarthralgia occurs in 10–25% of cases, and actual synovitis of the small and medium-sized joints in a fewer number. Extensive linear lesions that cross joint lines will lead to significant muscle atrophy, limb shortening and joint contracture. These effects may occasionally be so severe as to require amputation for functional activity. Myopathy has been rarely reported.[146]

Internal organ involvement other than mentioned above is rare,[124] and probably reflects another associated disease. Oesophageal disturbance has been reported, but is asymptomatic.[124,147] A very recent study examined 43 children with localized scleroderma and determined frequent cardiac abnormalities.[148] Until these results are confirmed by other authors, we do not recommend anything other than a thorough history and physical examination with careful follow-up.

En coup de sabre lesions may be associated with alopecia, ptosis, uveitis, cataract and keratopathy.[149] Seizures have been noted occasionally, and are thought to result from invasion of the sclerodermatous plaque to the brain causing an irritant focus.[147,150] Intracerebral calcifications and white-matter lesions have been noted on CT and MRI scans, but the significance of these is not clear.[150,151] Parry–Romberg syndrome has been reported with some neurological defects as well.[152,153] Atrophy of the pinna and tongue with deviation to the involved side may also occur (Figure 9.10).

Laboratory features

Laboratory abnormalities are common but non-specific, and generally do not predict either subtype or disease activity. Some authors have suggested that hypergammaglobulinaemia and eosinophilia may represent active disease.[154] Rheumatoid factor occurs in 10–30% and ANA in 20–80% of cases.[131,135,155,156] The autoantibody specificities seen in systemic sclerosis do not usually occur in localized scleroderma.[157]

Autoantibody specificities in localized scleroderma include antidenatured DNA, antibodies to histones and antibodies to high mobility group proteins.[155,156,158,159] The similarities and differences of antibody associations between localized scleroderma and systemic sclerosis could be used to support or refute the argument that there are similar immunopathogenetic mechanisms; alternatively, there may be no role of these antibodies in the aetiopathogenesis of these diseases, and they may only be epiphenomenon in disorders in which skin involvement occurs. Additional autoantibody studies have shown antimitochondrial antibodies in older patients with localized scleroderma, but their significance in adolescents is unclear.[160] Similarly, certain anti-heat shock protein antibodies have been found in adults with localized scleroderma.[161] The role is unknown in the paediatric population, but they may relate to an as yet unidentified infectious trigger.

In addition to autoantibody formation, there are other immunological abnormalities in localized scleroderma. A role for TGF-β and connective-tissue growth factor, while not as extensively studied as in systemic sclerosis, has been suggested in localized scleroderma.[162] Immune activation has also been suggested by the presence of soluble interleukin-2 (IL-2) receptors which, in a retrospective study, correlated with disease activity, suggesting the importance of T-cell activation, although these results have not been consistent in all studies.[141,163,164] Further evidence of T-cell activation includes the findings of elevated levels of soluble CD4 and CD8 in patients with generalized morphea,[165] as well as elevated levels of circulating IL-2, IL-4 and IL-6 compared to controls.[166] Elevated levels of soluble CD23 indicate B-cell activation.[167] In addition, in another study, increased levels of circulating intercellular adhesion molecule-1 (ICAM-1) correlated with the number of lesions and the number of involved areas.[168] There has also been a recent suggestion of abnormalities in vascular activation with a subclinical coagulopathy.[141] These studies suggest an important role of the immune system in the pathogenesis of these disorders.

Management

The pharmacological management of localized scleroderma is limited by a lack of understanding of the aetiology and pathogenesis, absence of specific clinical or laboratory markers of disease activity, and potential toxicity of systemic therapy in a disease the natural history of which is to improve with time. A major challenge is to be able to predict those patients who will have a prolonged course, with disability or cosmetic change. Most reports of successful treatment are anecdotal; no controlled trials have been undertaken. It is vital that outcome measures be developed, as they have been for systemic sclerosis.

For isolated morphea lesions, nothing more than simple follow-up may be necessary. Many practitioners recommend a topical fluorinated corticosteroid cream administered three times daily, or intralesional steroids. Some authors have advocated massage as a way of softening the skin.

For generalized lesions, linear lesions that cross joints, or facial lesions that are cosmetically disfiguring, systemic therapy may be indicated. Reports of successful treatment have included the use of prednisone,[169] phenytoin,[170] cyclophenyl,[171] D-penicillamine,[172,173] calcitriol,[174,175] cyclosporin[176] and, more recently, methotrexate[177] and ultraviolet-A (UVA) light with or without psoralens.[178–180] One must weigh the known risks of these agents against the potential benefits, and inform families appropriately. Ideally, multicentre protocols should be developed to address this important problem. In early lesions in which systemic treatment may be beneficial, corticosteroids are used for 3 months (either oral, dose to be tapered; or three monthly pulses of 3 days of intravenous methylprednisolone 1 g/kg) and subcutaneous methotrexate up to 1 mg/kg/week; for lesions that appear active but are not new, we use methotrexate, but not corticosteroids.

Supportive management is mandatory. The family's concern that localized scleroderma will progress to systemic sclerosis must be addressed sensitively. When lesions cross joint lines, aggressive physiotherapy must be instituted early to reduce or prevent joint contracture, which can be debilitating. In addition, muscle strengthening and gait training are important to consider. The use of splints and custom-moulded foot orthoses to keep joints stretched and well aligned is important. Occasionally, surgery with lengthening of the Achilles tendon may be considered, and has been performed success-fully.[181,182] The skin has healed well in previously reported cases. Skin grafts will take and remain normal if the disease remains inactive.

En coup de sabre lesions (Parry–Romberg syndrome) can be disfiguring. A supportive family and health-care team is vital to maintain self-esteem. Consideration to rebuilding tissue may be given once the process has become inac-tive.[183] Specific treatment will be directed to other systems if they are involved.

SCLERODERMA-LIKE DISORDERS

Eosinophilic fasciitis

Eosinophilic fasciitis may be localized or gener-alized. According to its early descriptions, eosinophilic fasciitis followed trauma or physi-cal exertion. Clinically, involvement of one or several extremities is accompanied by pain, swelling and brawny oedema. The classic triad of laboratory abnormalities is a raised ESR, increased immunoglobulin G and peripheral eosinophilia. Rarely, ANA and rheumatoid factor may be present. The diagnosis is confirmed by a full-thickness skin and muscle biopsy which shows diffuse thickening of the fascia. There is also a mononuclear cell infiltrate, and, although eosinophilic infiltration is charac-teristic, it is not universal; it is more common early in the disease. There is usually a rapid improvement with systemic corticosteroid ther-apy, with clinical resolution of the oedema and laboratory resolution of the eosinophilia and other inflammatory parameters; however, there may be long-term sclerodermatous changes and persistence of flexion contractures.[184,185] In fact, in one review, two-thirds of children developed cutaneous fibrosis without internal organ involvement. Early onset (age $\leq$ 7 years) and extensive disease (3 or 4 extremities involved) each seemed to predict the progression to fibro-sis.[185] There is also a frequent overlap with morphea lesions,[186] suggesting that eosinophilic fasciitis and localized scleroderma are part of the same spectrum of disorders. In adults, there is the risk of the later development of aplastic anaemia.[187]

Eosinophilia–myalgia syndrome

The eosinophilia–myalgia syndrome, reported in the late 1980s, has been traced to the ingestion of L-tryptophan that had been contaminated during the preparation process.[188] It is a multi-system illness with scleroderma-like features including oedema and thickening of the skin, myalgias, neuropathies and erythematous macules. Unlike systemic sclerosis, the face and acral portions of the body are usually spared and Raynaud's phenomenon is uncommon. Like the toxic-oil syndrome, in which contamination of rape-seed oil in Spain led to 300 deaths in approximately 20 000 affected cases of a sclero-derma-like disease,[189,190] it reminds us to search for environmental triggers in cases of sclero-derma or scleroderma-like disorders.

The controversy over the association of sili-cone breast implants and the subsequent devel-opment of scleroderma seems to have been settled by some recent meta-analyses which indicate that there is no evidence of a link.[191,192] A report of oesophageal motility disturbances in newborns breast-fed by mothers who had sili-cone implants, and also of scleroderma-like disorders in males with testicular silicone implants is intriguing.[193,194]

Chronic guest-versus-host disease

Chronic GVHD occurs more than 100 days following an allogeneic bone-marrow transplan-tation and can lead to fibrotic changes in the skin, fascia and internal organs that together resemble scleroderma. Cyclosporine has led to an improvement in the long-term prognosis of this potentially disabling condition.[195]

Scleredema adultorum of Buschke

This is an uncommon disorder characterized by thickening of the dermis of the neck, head and upper trunk and proximal extremities. However, in contrast to scleroderma, it does not involve the hands or feet and spares internal organs. It resolves over several months, and has been associated with the recent onset of a streptococcal infection.[196]

Drug/chemical-induced disease

Several drugs, including pentazocine[197] and bleomycin,[198] may result in skin and/or pulmonary fibrosis. Similarly, occupational exposure to chemicals such as silica[199] has been associated with a scleroderma-like illness.

Pseudoscleroderma

Pseudoscleroderma occurs when scleroderma-like skin fibrosis is not associated with other 'connective-tissue' disease manifestations, and includes endocrine and metabolic causes (e.g. diabetes, scleromyxoedema and phenylketonuria).

BIRTH CONTROL AND PREGNANCY

The issue of pregnancy will be on the mind of most adolescents diagnosed with scleroderma. The fertility rate appears to be similar to that of healthy controls, but there is a higher rate of premature and low-birth-weight births. Patients with severe renal, cardiac or pulmonary disease

may be best advised to avoid pregnancy until the disease stabilizes. Care must be taken to avoid potentially teratogenic medications during pregnancy.[200]

SUMMARY

The sclerodermatous disorders represent a wide spectrum of disorders, ranging from isolated skin lesions to severe multisystem involvement with significant morbidity and mortality. Patients with systemic sclerosis require careful attention in order to detect early end-organ involvement, as supportive management is crucial and can lead to a significant improvement in the quality of life of the patient. A supportive health-care team is essential in working with adolescents and their families. The localized forms of scleroderma are much more common than the systemic varieties and, while not commonly associated with internal organ involvement, they can have serious local complications. No treatment has been shown to be effective in randomized, placebo-controlled trials. Current research efforts are aimed at attempting to understand the role of the fibroblast, endothelial cell and immune system in these disorders, and will hopefully lead to the discovery of specific defects that are central to scleroderma. This knowledge should allow for the design of new agents aimed at correcting the abnormalities. Well-designed, collaborative multicentre trials will be critical in proving the effectiveness of therapeutic agents in this fascinating group of diseases.

REFERENCES

1. Wilson L. Cost-of-illness of scleroderma: the case for rare diseases. *Semin Arthritis Rheum* 1997; **27**:73–84.
2. Cassidy JT, Sullivan DB, Dabich L, Petty RE. Scleroderma in children. *Arthritis Rheum* 1977; **20**:351–4.
3. Kornreich HK, King KK, Bernstein BH, Singsen BH, Hanson V. Scleroderma in childhood. *Arthritis Rheum* 1977; **20**:343–50.
4. Goel KM, Shanks RA. Scleroderma in childhood. *Arch Dis Child* 1974; **49**:861–6.
5. Bernstein RM, Pereira RS, Holden AJ, Black CM, Howard A, Ansell BM. Autoantibodies in childhood scleroderma. *Ann Rheum Dis* 1985; **44**:503–6.
6. Lababidi HM, Nasr FW, Khatib Z. Juvenile progressive systemic sclerosis: report of five cases. *J Rheumatol* 1991; **18**:885–8.

7. Martinez-Cordero E, Fonseca MC, Aquilar Leon DE, Padilla A. Juvenile systemic sclerosis. *J Rheumatol* 1993; **20**:405–7.

8. Fujita Y, Yamamori H, Hiyoshi K, Inamo Y, Harada K, Fujikawa S. Systemic sclerosis in children: a national retrospective survey in Japan. *Acta Paediatr Jpn* 1997; **39**:263–7.

9. Ansell BM, Nasseh GA, Bywaters EG. Scleroderma in childhood. *Ann Rheum Dis* 1976; **35**:189–97.

10. Dabich L, Sullivan DB, Cassidy JT. Scleroderma in the child. *J Pediatr* 1974; **85**:770–5.

11. Mayes MD, Epidemiology of systemic sclerosis and related diseases. *Curr Opin Rheumatol* 1997; **9**:557–61.

12. Mayes MD. Scleroderma epidemiology. *Rheum Dis Clin North Am* 1996; **22**:751–64.

13. Bowyer S, Roettcher P. Pediatric rheumatology clinic populations in the United States: results of a 3 year survey. Pediatric Rheumatology Database Research Group. *J Rheumatol* 1996; **23**:1968–74.

14. Malleson PN, Fung MY, Rosenberg AM. The incidence of pediatric rheumatic diseases: results from the Canadian Pediatric Rheumatology Association Disease Registry. *J Rheumatol* 1996; **23**:1981–7.

15. Symmons DP, Jones M, Osborne J, Sills J, Southwood TR, Woo P. Pediatric rheumatology in the United Kingdom: data from the British Pediatric Rheumatology Group National Diagnostic Register. *J Rheumatol* 1996; **23**:1975–80.

16. Reveille JD. Molecular genetics of systemic sclerosis. *Curr Opin Rheum* 1995; **7**:522–8.

17. Stephens CO, Briggs DC, Whyte J et al. Familial scleroderma – evidence for environmental versus genetic trigger. *Br J Rheumatol* 1994; **33**:1131–5.

18. Furst DE, Clements PJ. Hypothesis for the pathogenesis of systemic sclerosis. *J Rheumatol* 1997; **48**(suppl):53–7.

19. White B. Immunopathogenesis of systemic sclerosis. *Rheum Dis Clin North Am* 1996; **22**:695–708.

20. Sollberg S, Kreig T. New aspects in scleroderma research. *Int Arch Allergy Immunol* 1996; **111**:330–6.

21. Needleman BW, Wigley FM, Stair RW. Interleukin-1, interleukin-2, interleukin-4, interleukin-6, tumor necrosis factor alpha, and interferon-gamma levels in sera from patients with scleroderma. *Arthritis Rheum* 1992; **35**:67–72.

22. Okano Y. Antinuclear antibody in systemic sclerosis (scleroderma). *Rheum Dis Clin North Am* 1996; **22**:709–35.

23. Jimenez SA, Hitraya E, Varga J. Pathogenesis of scleroderma. *Rheum Dis Clin North Am* 1996; **22**:647–764.

24. Denton CP, Xu S, Black CM, Pearson JD. Scleroderma fibroblasts show increased responsiveness to endothelial cell-derived IL-1 and bFGF. *J Invest Dermatol* 1997; **108**:269–74.

25. Postlethwaite AE. Connective tissue metabolism including cytokines in scleroderma. *Curr Opin Rheum* 1994; **6**:616–20.

26. Kawakami T, Ihn H, Xu W, Smith E, LeRoy C, Trojanowska M. Increased expression of TGF-β receptors by scleroderma fibroblasts: evidence for contribution of autocrine TGF-β signaling to scleroderma phenotype. *J Invest Dermatol* 1998; **110**:47–51.

27. Gruber BL. Mast cells: accessory cells which potentiate fibrosis. *Int Rev Immunol* 1995; **12**:259–79.

28. Cox D, Earle L, Jimenez SA, Leiferman KM, Gleich GJ, Varga J. Elevated levels of eosinophil major basic protein in the sera of patients with systemic sclerosis. *Arthritis Rheum* 1995; **38**:939–45.

29. Artlett CM, Welsh KI, Black CM, Jimenez SA. Fetal–maternal HLA compatibility confers susceptibility to systemic sclerosis. *Immunogenetics* 1998; **47**:17–22.

30. Subcommittee for Scleroderma Criteria of the American Rheumatism Association Diagnostic and Therapeutic Criteria Committee. Preliminary criteria for the classification of systemic sclerosis (scleroderma). *Arthritis Rheum* 1980; **23**:581–90.

31. Pope JE, Shum DT, Gottschalk R, Stevens A, McManus R. Increased pigmentation in scleroderma. *J Rheumatol* 1996; **23**:1912–6.

32. Barnett AJ. The 'neck sign' in scleroderma. *Arthritis Rheum* 1989; **32**:209–11.

33. Kraling BM, Maul GG, Jimenez SA. Mononuclear cellular infiltrates in clinically involved skin from patients with systemic sclerosis of recent onset predominantly consist of monocytes/macrophages. *Pathobiology* 1995; **63**:48–56.

34. Herrick AL, Marcuson R, Freemont AJ, Jayson MI. Clinically normal skin becomes sclerodermatous when transplanted into a sclerodermatous area. *Br J Rheumatol* 1992; **31**:707–9.

35. Aghassi D, Monoson T, Braverman I. Reproducible measurements to quantify cutaneous involvement in scleroderma. *Arch Dermatol* 1995; **131**:1160–6.

36. Clements P, Lachenbruch P, Siebold J et al. Inter and intraobserver variability of total skin thick-

ness score (modified Rodnan TSS) in systemic sclerosis. *J Rheumatol* 1995; **22**:1281–5.

37. Clements PJ, Lachenbruch PA, Ng SC, Simmons M, Sterz M, Furst D. Skin score. A semiquantitative measure of cutaneous involvement that improves prediction of prognosis in systemic sclerosis. *Arthritis Rheum* 1990; **33**:1256–63.

38. Rodnan GP, Lipinski E, Luksick J. Skin thickness and collagen content in progressive systemic sclerosis and localized scleroderma. *Arthritis Rheum* 1979; **22**:130–40.

39. Scheja A, Akesson A. Comparison of high frequency (20 MHz) ultrasound and palpation for the assessment of skin involvement in systemic sclerosis (scleroderma). *Clin Exp Rheumatol* 1997; **15**:283–8.

40. Ihn H, Shimozuma M, Fujimoto M et al. Ultrasound measurement of skin thickness in systemic sclerosis. *Br J Rheumatol* 1995; **34**:535–8.

41. Enomoto DN, Mekkes JR, Bossuyt PM, Hoekzema R, Bos JD. Quantification of cutaneous sclerosis with a skin elasticity meter in patients with generalized scleroderma. *J Am Acad Dermatol* 1996; **35**:381–7.

42. Ishikawa T, Tamura T. Measurement of skin elastic properties with a new suction device (II): systemic sclerosis. *J Dermatol* 1996; **23**:165–8.

43. Duffy CM, Laxer RM, Lee P, Ramsay C, Fritzler M, Silverman ED. Raynaud syndrome in childhood. *J Pediatr* 1989; **114**:73–8.

44. Misra R, Darton K, Jewkes RF, Black CM, Maini RN. Arthritis in scleroderma. *Br J Rheumatol* 1995; **34**:831–7.

45. Schumacher HR. Joint involvement in progressive systemic sclerosis. *Am J Clin Pathol* 1973; **60**:593–600.

46. Bassett LW, Blocka KL, Furst DE, Clements PJ, Gold RH. Skeletal findings in progressive systemic sclerosis (scleroderma). *Am J Roentgenol* 1981; **136**:1121–6.

47. Ryall KS, Hopper FE, Cotterill TA. Mandibular resorption on systemic sclerosis. *Br J Dermatol* 1982; **107**:711–4.

48. Blocka KL, Bassett LW, Furst DE, Clements PJ, Paulus HE. The arthropathy of advanced progressive systemic sclerosis. A radiographic survey. *Arthritis Rheum* 1981; **24**:874–84.

49. Hietaharju A, Jaaskelainen S, Kalimo H, Hietarinta M. Peripheral neuromuscular manifestations in systemic sclerosis (scleroderma). *Muscle Nerve* 1993; **16**:1204–12.

50. Clements PJ, Furst DE, Campion DS et al. Muscle disease in progressive systemic sclerosis: diagnostic and therapeutic considerations. *Arthritis Rheum* 1978; **21**:62–71.

51. Follansbee WP, Zerbe TR, Medsger TA Jr. Cardiac and skeletal muscle disease in systemic sclerosis (scleroderma): a high risk association. *Am Heart J* 1993; **125**:194–203.

52. Steen VD, Medsger TA Jr. The palpable tendon friction rub: an important physical examination finding in patients with systemic sclerosis. *Arthritis Rheum* 1997; **40**:1146–51.

53. Kane GC, Varga J, Conant EF, Spirn PW, Jimenez S, Fish JE. Lung involvement in systemic sclerosis (scleroderma): relation to classification based on extent of skin involvement or autoantibody status. *Respir Med* 1996; **90**:223–30.

54. Koh ET, Lee P, Gladman DD, Abu-Shakra M. Pulmonary hypertension in systemic sclerosis: an analysis of 17 patients. *Br J Rheumatol* 1996; **35**:989–93.

55. Garty BZ, Athreya BH, Wilmott R, Scarpa N, Doughty R, Douglas SD. Pulmonary functions in children with progressive systemic sclerosis. *Pediatrics* 1991; **88**:1161–7.

56. Vallance DK, Lynch JP III, McCune WJ. Immunosuppressive treatment of the pulmonary manifestations of progressive systemic sclerosis. *Curr Opin Rheumatol* 1995; **7**:174–82.

57. Fanti S, De Fabritiis A, Aloisi D et al. Early pulmonary involvement in systemic sclerosis assessed by technetium-^{99}m-DTPA clearance rate. *J Nucl Med* 1994; **35**:1933–6.

58. Falcini F, Pignone A, Matucci-Cerinic M et al. Clinical utility of non-invasive methods in the evaluation of scleroderma lung in pediatric age. *Scand J Rheumatol* 1992; **21**:82–4.

59. Silver RM. Clinical problems. The lungs. *Clin Rheumatol Dis* 1996; **22**:825–40.

60. Bolster MB, Ludwicka A, Sutherland SE, Strange C, Silver RM. Cytokine concentrations in bronchoalveolar lavage fluid of patients with systemic sclerosis. *Arthritis Rheum* 1997; **40**:743–51.

61. Remy-Jardin M, Remy J, Wallaert B, Bataille D, Hatron PY. Pulmonary involvement in progressive systemic sclerosis: sequential evaluation with CT, pulmonary function tests, and bronchoalveolar lavage. *Radiology* 1993; **188**:499–506.

62. Seely JM, Effmann EL, Muller NL. High-resolution CT of pediatric lung disease: imaging findings. *Am J Roentgenol* 1997; **168**:1269–75.

63. Wells AU, Hansell DM, Rubens MB et al. Fibrosing alveolitis in systemic sclerosis: indices of lung function in relation to extent of disease on

computed tomography. *Arthritis Rheum* 1997; **40**:1229–36.

64. Abu-Shakra M, Guillemin F, Lee P. Cancer in systemic sclerosis. *Arthritis Rheum* 1993; **36**:460–4.

65. Young MA, Rose S, Reynolds JC. Gastrointestinal manifestations of scleroderma. *Rheum Dis Clin North Am* 1996; **22**:797–823.

66. Lock G, Holstege A, Lang B, Scholmerich J. Gastrointestinal manifestations of progressive systemic sclerosis. *Am J Gastroenterol* 1997; **92**:763–71.

67. Flick JA, Boyle JT, Tuchman DN et al. Esophageal motor abnormalities in children and adolescents with scleroderma and mixed connective tissue disease. *Pediatrics* 1988; **82**:107–11.

68. Katzka DA, Reynolds JC, Saul SH et al. Barrett's metaplasia and adenocarcinoma of the esophagus in scleroderma. *Am J Med* 1987; **82**:46–52.

69. Marie I, Cailleux N, Levesque H. Watermelon stomach and systemic sclerosis: localization of digestive system involvement? *Arthritis Rheum* 1996; **39**:1439.

70. Sjogren RW. Gastrointestinal motility disorders in scleroderma. *Arthritis Rheum* 1994; **37**:1265–82.

71. Follansbee WP, Curtiss EI, Medsger TA Jr et al. Physiologic abnormalities of cardiac function in progressive systemic sclerosis with diffuse scleroderma. *N Engl J Med* 1984; **310**:142–8.

72. Byers RJ, Marshall DAS, Freemont AJ. Pericardial involvement in systemic sclerosis. *Ann Rheumatol Dis* 1997; **56**:393–4.

73. Janosik DL, Osborn TG, Moore TL, Shah DG, Kenney RG, Zuckner J. Heart disease in systemic sclerosis. *Semin Arthritis Rheum* 1989; **19**:191–200.

74. Clements PJ, Lachenbruch PA, Furst DE, Paulus HE, Sturz MJ. Cardiac score. A semiquantitative measure of cardiac involvement that improves prediction of prognosis in systemic sclerosis. *Arthritis Rheum* 1991; **34**:1371–80.

75. Steen VD, Follansbee WP, Conte CG, Medsger TA Jr. Thallium perfusion defects predict subsequent cardiac dysfunction in patients with systemic sclerosis. *Arthritis Rheum* 1996; **39**:677–81.

76. Steen VD, Medsger TA Jr, Osial TA Jr, Ziegler GL, Shapiro AP, Rodnan GP. Factors predicting development of renal involvement in progressive systemic sclerosis. *Am J Med* 1984; **76**:779–86.

77. Clements PJ, Lachenbruch PA, Furst DE, Maxwell M, Danovitch G, Paulus HE. Abnormalities of renal physiology in systemic sclerosis. A prospective study with 10-year followup. *Arthritis Rheum* 1994; **37**:67–74.

78. Zawada ET Jr, Clements PJ, Furst DA, Bloomer HA, Paulus HE, Maxwell MH. Clinical course of patients with scleroderma renal crisis treated with captopril. *Nephron* 1981; **27**:74–8.

79. Cerinic MM, Generini S, Pignone A, Casale R. The nervous system in systemic sclerosis (scleroderma). Clinical features and pathogenetic mechanisms. *Rheum Dis Clin North Am* 1996; **22**:879–92.

80. Langevitz P, Buskila D, Lee P. Ilioinguinal nerve entrapment in a patient with systemic sclerosis. *Clin Rheum* 1993; **12**:540–1.

81. De Keyser L, Narhi DC, Furst DE et al. Thyroid dysfunction in a prospectively followed series of patients with progressive systemic sclerosis. *J Endocrinol Invest* 1990; **13**:161–9.

82. Abu-Shakra M, Lee P. Mortality in systemic sclerosis: a comparison with the general population. *J Rheumatol* 1995; **22**:2100–2.

83. Lee P, Langevitz P, Alderdice CA et al. Mortality in systemic sclerosis (scleroderma). *Q J Med* 1992; **82**:139–48.

84. Silman AJ. Scleroderma – demographics and survival. *J Rheum* 1997; **48**(suppl):58–61.

85. Foeldvari I, Zhavania M, Birdi N et al. A favorable outcome in 120 children with progressive systemic sclerosis (PSS): results of a multinational questionnaire. *Arthritis Rheum* 1997; **40** (suppl):S101.

86. Reveille JD, Durban E, Goldstein R, Moreda R, Arnett FC. Racial differences in the frequencies of scleroderma-related autoantibodies. *Arthritis Rheum* 1992; **35**:216–8.

87. Picillo U, Migliaresi S, Marcialis MR, Ferruzzi AM, Tirri G. Clinical setting of patients with systemic sclerosis by serum autoantibodies. *Clin Rheum* 1997; **16**:378–83.

88. Katayama I, Otoyama K, Kondo S, Nishioka K, Nisiyama S. Clinical manifestations in anticardiolipin antibody-positive patients with progressive systemic sclerosis. *J Am Acad Dermatol* 1990; **23**:198–201.

89. Sato S, Ihn H, Kikuchi K, Takehara K. Antihistone antibodies in systemic sclerosis. Association with pulmonary fibrosis. *Arthritis Rheum* 1994; **37**:391–4.

90. White B, Bauer EA, Goldsmith LA et al. Guidelines for clinical trials in systemic sclerosis (scleroderma). I. Disease-modifying interventions. The American College of Rheumatology Committee on Design and Outcomes in Clinical

Trials in Systemic Sclerosis. *Arthritis Rheum* 1995; **38**:351–60.

91. Pope JE, Bellamy N. Outcome measurement in scleroderma clinical trials. *Semin Arthritis Rheum* 1993; **23**:22–33.

92. Pope JE. Treatment of systemic sclerosis. *Clin Rheumatol Dis* 1996; **22**:893–907

93. Steen VD, Medsger TA Jr, Rodnan GP. D-Penicillamine therapy in progressive systemic sclerosis (scleroderma): a retrospective analysis. *Ann Intern Med* 1982; **97**:652–9.

94. Steen VD, Owens GR, Redmond C, Rodnan GP, Medsger TA Jr. The effect of D-penicillamine on pulmonary findings in systemic sclerosis. *Arthritis Rheum* 1985; **28**:882–8.

95. Jimenez SA, Sigal SH. A 15-year prospective study of treatment of rapidly progressive systemic sclerosis with D-penicillamine. *J Rheumatol* 1991; **18**:1496–503.

96. van den Hoogen FH, Boerbooms AM, Swaak AJ, Rasker JJ, van Lier HJ, van de Putte LB. Comparison of methotrexate with placebo in the treatment of systemic sclerosis: a 24 week randomized double-blind trial, followed by a 24 week observational trial. *Br J Rheumatol* 1996; **35**:364–72.

97. Clements PJ, Lachenbruch PA, Sterz M et al. Cyclosporine in systemic sclerosis. Results of a forty-eight-week open safety study in ten patients. *Arthritis Rheum* 1993; **36**:75–83.

98. Al-Mayouf S, Silverman ED, Feldman B, Thorner P, Laxer RM. Cyclosporine in the treatment of an unusual case of juvenile systemic scleroderma. *J Rheumatol* 1998; **25**:791–3.

99. Unemori EN, Bauer EA, Amento EP. Relaxin alone and in conjunction with interferon-γ decreases collagen synthesis by cultured human scleroderma fibroblasts. *J Invest Dermatol* 1992; **99**:337–42.

100. Seibold JR, Korn J, Simms R et al. Controlled trial of recombinant human relaxin (rhRlxn) in diffuse scleroderma (DS). *Arthritis Rheum* 1997; **40**(suppl):S123.

101. Rook AH, Freundlich B, Jegasothy BV et al. Treatment of systemic sclerosis with extracorporeal photochemotherapy. Results of a multicenter trial. *Arch Dermatol* 1992; **128**:337–46.

102. Cribier B, Faradji T, Le Coz C, Oberling F, Grosshans E. Extracorporeal photochemotherapy in systemic sclerosis and severe morphea. *Dermatology* 1995; **191**:25–31.

103. Kenakura T, Fukumaru S, Matsushita S, Terasaki K, Mizoguchi S, Kanzak T. Successful treatment of scleroderma with PUVA therapy. *J Dermatol* 1996; **23**:455–4.

104. Humbert P, Dupond JL, Agache P et al. Treatment of scleroderma with oral 1,25-dihydroxyvitamin D_3: evaluation of skin involvement using non-invasive techniques. Results of an open prospective trial. *Acta Dermatol Venereol* 1993; **73**:449–51.

105. Stevens W, Vancheeswaran R, Black CM. α-Interferon-2a (Roferon-A) in the treatment of diffuse cutaneous systemic sclerosis: a pilot study. UK Systemic Sclerosis Study Group. *Br J Rheumatol* 1992; **31**:683–9.

106. Freundlich B, Jimenez SA, Steen VD, Medsger TA Jr, Szkolnicki M, Jaffe HS. Treatment of systemic sclerosis with recombinant interferon-γ. A phase I/II clinical trial. *Arthritis Rheum* 1992; **35**:1134–42.

107. Vlachoyiannopoulos PG, Tsifetaki N, Dimitriou I, Galaris D, Papiris SA, Moutsopoulos HM. Safety and efficacy of recombinant γ-interferon in the treatment of systemic sclerosis. *Ann Rheum Dis* 1996; **55**:761–8.

108. Polisson RP, Gilkeson GS, Pyun EH, Pisetsky DS, Smith EA, Simon LS. A multicenter trial of recombinant human interferon-γ in patients with systemic sclerosis: effects on cutaneous fibrosis and interleukin-2 receptor levels. *Rheumatology* 1996; **23**:654–8.

109. Hunzelmann N, Anders S, Fierlbeck G et al. Systemic scleroderma. Multicenter trial of 1 year of treatment with recombinant interferon-γ. *Arch Dermatol* 1997; **13**:609–13.

110. Nash RA, McSweeney PA, Storb R et al. Development of a protocol for allogeneic marrow transplantation for severe systemic sclerosis: paradigm for autoimmune disease. *J Rheumatol* 1997; **24**(suppl 48):72–8.

111. Martini A, Maccario R, Ravelli A et al. Marked and sustained improvement one year after autologous peripheral stem cell transplant in a girl with severe progressive systemic sclerosis. *Arthritis Rheum* 1997; **40**(suppl):S139.

112. Smith CD, McKendry RJ. Controlled trial of nifedipine in the treatment of Raynaud's phenomenon. *Lancet* 1982; **ii**:1299–301.

113. Wigley FM, Flavahan NA. Raynaud's phenomenon. *Clin Rheum Dis* 1996; **22**:765–81.

114. Langevitz P, Buskila D, Lee P, Urowitz MB. Treatment of refractory ischemic skin ulcers in patients with Raynaud's phenomenon with PGE1 infusions. *J Rheumatol* 1989; **16**:1433–5.

115. Wigley FM, Wise RA, Seibold JR et al. Intravenous iloprost infusion in patients with Raynaud phenomenon secondary to systemic sclerosis. A multicenter, placebo-controlled, double-blind study. *Ann Intern Med* 1994; **120**:199–206.

116. Zachariae H, Halkier-Sorensen L, Bjerring P, Heickendorff L. Treatment of ischaemic digital ulcers and prevention of gangrene with intravenous iloprost in systemic sclerosis. *Acta Dermatol Venereol* 1996; **76**:236–8.

117. Freedman RR, Keegan D, Migaly P, Galloway MP, Mayes M. Plasma catecholamines during behavioral treatments for Raynaud's disease. *Psychosom Med* 1991; **5**:433–9.

118. Koman LA, Smith BP, Pollock FE Jr, Smith TL, Pollock D, Russell GB. The microcirculatory effects of peripheral sympathectomy. *J Hand Surg (Am)* 1995; **20**:709–17.

119. Dolan AL, Kassimos D, Gibson T, Kingsley GH. Diltiazem induces remission of calcinosis in scleroderma. *Br J Rheumatol* 1995; **34**:576–8.

120. Shoenut JP, Wieler JA, Micflikier AB. The extent and pattern of gastro-oesophageal reflux in patients with scleroderma oesophagus: the effect of low-dose omeprazole. *Aliment Pharmacol Ther* 1993; **7**:509–13.

121. Kahan A, Chaussade S, Gaudric M et al. The effect of cisapride on gastro-oesophageal dysfunction in systemic sclerosis: a controlled monometric study. *Br J Clin Pharmacol* 1991; **31**:683–7.

122. Verne GN, Eaker EY, Hardy E, Sninsky CA. Effect of octreotide and erythromycin on idiopathic and scleroderma-associated intestinal pseudoobstruction. *Dig Dis Sci* 1995; **40**:1892–901.

123. Levine SM, Anzueto A, Peters JI, Calhoon JH, Jenkinson SG, Bryan CL. Single lung transplantation in patients with systemic disease. *Chest* 1994; **105**:837–41.

124. Dehen L, Roujeau JC, Cosnes A, Revuz J. Internal involvement in localized scleroderma. *Medicine* 1994; **73**:241–5.

125. Soma Y, Tamaki T, Kikuchi K et al. Coexistence of morphea and systemic sclerosis. *Dermatology* 1993; **186**:103–5.

126. Christianson HB, Dorsey CS, O'Leary PA, Kierland RR. Localized scleroderma. A clinical study of 235 cases. *Am Med Assoc Arch Dermatol* 1956; **74**:629–39.

127. Goldenstein-Schainberg C, Pereira RMR, Cossermelli W. Linear scleroderma and systemic

lupus erythematosus. *J Rheumatol* 1990; **17**:1427–8.

128. Birdi N, Laxer RM, Thorner P, Fritzler MJ, Silverman ED. Localized scleroderma progressing to systemic disease. (Case report and review of literature). *Arthritis Rheum* 1993; **36**:410–15.

129. Maricq HR. Capillary abnormalities, Raynaud's phenomenon, and systemic sclerosis in patients with localized scleroderma. *J Am Acad Dermatol* 1985; **12**:844–51.

130. Peterson LS, Nelson AM, Su WP, Mason T, O'Fallon WM, Gabriel SE. The epidemiology of morphea (localized scleroderma) in Olmsted County 1960–1993. *J Rheumatol* 1997; **24**:73–80.

131. Uziel Y, Krafchik BR, Silverman ED, Thorner PS, Laxer RM. Localized scleroderma in childhood: a report of 30 cases. *Semin Arthritis Rheum* 1994; **23**:328–40.

132. Falanga V, Medsger TA Jr, Reichlin M, Rodnan GP. Linear scleroderma. Clinical spectrum, prognosis, and laboratory abnormalities. *Ann Intern Med* 1986; **104**:849–57.

133. Silman A, Jannini S, Symmons D, Bacon P. An epidemiological study of scleroderma in the West Midlands. *Br J Rheumatol* 1988; **27**:286–90.

134. Torok E, Ablonczy E. Morphoea in children. *Clin Exp Dermatol* 1986; **11**:607–12.

135. Peterson LS, Nelson AM, Su WP. Classification of morphea. *Mayo Clin Proc* 1995; **70**:1068–76.

136. Tuffanelli DL, Winkelmann RK. Systemic scleroderma. *Arch Dermatol* 1961; **84**:359–71.

137. Connelly MG, Winkelmann RK. Coexistence of lichen sclerosus, morphea, and lichen planus. Report of four cases and review of the literature. *J Am Acad Dermatol* 1985; **12**:844–51.

138. Diaz-Perez JL, Connolly SM, Winkelmann RK. Disabling pansclerotic morphea of children. *Arch Dermatol* 1980; **116**:169–73.

139. Lehman TJA. The Parry–Romberg syndrome of progressive facial hemiatrophy and linear scleroderma *en coup de sabre*. Mistaken diagnosis or overlapping conditions? *J Rheumatol* 1992; **19**:844–5.

140. Littman BH. Linear scleroderma: a response to neurologic injury? Report and literature review. *J Rheumatol* 1989; **16**:1135–40.

141. Vancheeswaran R, Black CM, David J et al. Childhood-onset scleroderma: is it different from adult-onset disease? *Arthritis Rheum* 1996; **39**:1041–9.

142. Alonso-Llamazares J, Persing DH, Anda P, Gibson LE, Rutledge BJ, Iglesias L. No evidence

for *Borrelia burgdorferi* infection in lesions of morphea and lichen sclerosus et atrophicus in Spain. A prospective study and literature review. *Acta Dermatol Venereol* 1997; **77**:299–304.

143. Fujiwara H, Fujiwara K, Hashimoto K et al. Detection of *Borrelia burgdorferi* Dna (*B. garinii* or *B. afzelii*) in morphea and lichen sclerosus et atrophicus tissues of German and Japanese but not of US patients. *Arch Dermatol* 1997; **133**:41–4.

144. Dillon WI, Saed GM, Fivenson DP. *Borrelia burgdorferi* DNA is undetectable by polymerase chain reaction in skin lesions of morphea, scleroderma, or lichen sclerosus et atrophicus of patients from North America. *J Am Acad Dermatol* 1995; **33**:617–20.

145. Davis DA, Cohen PR, McNeese MD, Duvic M. Localized scleroderma in breast cancer patients treated with supervoltage external beam radiation: radiation port scleroderma. *J Am Acad Dermatol* 1996; **35**:923–7.

146. Dunne JW, Heye N, Edis RH, Kakulas BA. Necrotizing inflammatory myopathy associated with localized scleroderma. *Muscle Nerve* 1996; **19**:1040–2.

147. Kornreich HK, King KK, Bernstein BH, Singsen BH, Hanson V. Scleroderma in childhood. *Arthritis Rheum* 1977; **20**(suppl 2):343–50.

148. Rokicki W, Dukalska M, Rubisz-Brzezinska J, Gasior Z. Circulatory system in children with localized scleroderma. *Pediatr Cardiol* 1997; **18**:213–17.

149. Goldenstein-Schainberg C, Pereira RMR, Gusukuma MC, Messina WC, Cossermelli W. Childhood linear scleroderma 'en coup de sabre' with uveitis. *J Pediatr* 1990; **117**:581–4.

150. Fry JA, Alvarellos A, Fink CW, Blaw ME, Roach ES. Intracranial findings in progressive facial hemiatrophy. *J Rheumatol* 1992; **19**:956–8l.

151. Liu P, Uziel Y, Chuang S, Silverman E, Krafchik B, Laxer R. Localized scleroderma: imaging features. *Pediatr Radiol* 1994; **24**:207–9.

152. Leao M, da Silva ML. Progressive hemifacial atrophy with agenesis of the head of the caudate nucleus. *J Med Genet* 1994; **31**:969–71.

153. Menni S, Marzano AV, Passoni E. Neurologic abnormalities in two patients with facial hemiatrophy and sclerosis coexisting with morphea. *Pediatr Dermatol* 1997; **14**:113–6.

154. Falanga V, Medsger TA Jr. Frequency, levels, and significance of blood eosinophilia in systemic sclerosis, localized scleroderma, and eosinophilic fasciitis. *J Am Acad Dermatol* 1987; **17**:648–56.

155. Takehara K, Moroi Y, Nakabayashi Y, Ishibashi Y. Antinuclear antibodies in localized scleroderma. *Arthritis Rheum* 1983; **26**:612–6.

156. Rosenberg AM, Uziel Y, Krafchick BR et al. Antinuclear antibodies in children with localized forms of cutaneous scleroderma. *J Rheumatol* 1995; **22**:2337–43.

157. Ruffatti A, Peserico A, Glorioso S et al. Anticentromere antibody in localized scleroderma. *J Am Acad Dermatol* 1986; **15**:637–42.

158. Sato S, Ihn H, Soma Y et al. Antihistone antibodies in patients with localized scleroderma. *Arthritis Rheum* 1993; **36**:1137–41.

159. Sato S, Fujimoto M, Ihn H, Kikuchi K, Takehara K. Clinical characteristics associated with antihistone antibodies in patients with localized scleroderma. *J Am Acad Dermatol* 1994; **31**:567–71.

160. Fujimoto M, Sato S, Ihn H et al. Autoantibodies to mitochondrial 2-oxo-acid dehydrogenase complexes in localized scleroderma. *Clin Exp Immunol* 1996; **105**:297–301.

161. Fujimoto M, Sato S, Ihn H, Takehara K. Autoantibodies to the heat-shock protein hsp73 in localized scleroderma. *Arch Dermatol Res* 1995; **287**:581–5.

162. Takehara K, Connective tissue growth factor gene expression in tissue sections from localized scleroderma, keloid, and other fibrotic skin disorders. *J Invest Dermatol* 1996; **106**:729–33.

163. Uziel Y, Krafchik BR, Feldman B, Silverman ED, Rubin LA, Laxer RM. Serum soluble interleukin-2-receptor levels: a marker of disease activity in localized scleroderma. *Arthritis Rheum* 1994; **37**:898–901.

164. Ihn H, Sato S, Fujimoto M, Kikuchi K, Takehara K. Clinical significance of serum levels of soluble interleukin-2 receptor in patients with localized scleroderma. *Br J Dermatol* 1996; **134**:843–7.

165. Sato S, Fujimoto M, Kikuchi K, Ihn H, Tamaki K, Takehara K. Soluble CD4 and CD8 in serum from patients with localized scleroderma. *Arch Dermatol Res* 1996; **288**:358–62.

166. Ihn H, Sato S, Fujimoto M, Kikuchi K, Takehara K. Demonstration of interleukin-2, interleukin-4 and interleukin-6 in sera from patients with localized scleroderma. *Arch Dermatol Res* 1995; **287**:193–7.

167. Sato S, Fujimoto M, Kikuchi K, Ihn H, Tamaki K, Takehara K. Elevated soluble CD23 levels in the sera from patients with localized scleroderma. *Arch Dermatol Res* 1996; **288**:74–8.

168. Ihn H, Fujimoto M, Sato S et al. Increased levels of circulating intercellular adhesion molecule-1

in patients with localized scleroderma. *J Am Acad Dermatol* 1994; **31**:591–5.

169. Ansell BM, Falcini F, Woo P. Scleroderma in childhood. *Clin Dermatol* 1994; **12**:299–307.

170. Neldner KH. Treatment of localized linear scleroderma with phenytoin. *Cutis* 1978; **22**:569–72.

171. Pachor ML, Nicolis F, Lunardi C et al. Morphea: treatment of two clinical cases with cyclophenyl. *Clin Exp Rheumatol* 1987; **5**:293–4.

172. Curley RK, Macfarlane AW, Evans S, Woodrow JC. The treatment of linear morphoea with D-penicillamine. *Clin Exp Dermatol* 1987; **12**:56–7.

173. Falanga V, Medsger TA Jr. D-Penicillamine in the treatment of localized scleroderma. *Arch Dermatol* 1990; **126**:609–12.

174. Hulshof MM, Pavel S, Breedveld FC, Dijkmans BA, Vermeer BJ. Oral calcitriol as a new therapeutic modality for generalized morphea. *Arch Dermatol* 1994; **130**:1290–3.

175. Humbert P, Aubin F, Dupond JL, Delaporte E. Oral calcitriol as a new therapeutic agent in localized and systemic scleroderma. *Arch Dermatol* 1995; **131**:850–1.

176. Peter RU, Ruzicka T, Eckert F. Low-dose cyclosporine A in the treatment of disabling morphea. *Arch Dermatol* 1991; **127**:1420–1.

177. Lehman TJA. Systemic and localized scleroderma in children. *Curr Opin Rheumatol* 1996; **8**:576–9.

178. Kerscher M, Dirschka T, Volkenandt M. Treatment of localised scleroderma by UVA1 phototherapy. *Lancet* 1995; **346**:1166.

179. Stege H, Berneburg M, Humke S et al. High-dose UVA1 radiation therapy for localized scleroderma. *J Am Acad Dermatol* 1997; **36**:938–44.

180. Gruss C, Stucker M, Kobyletzki G, Schreiber D, Altmeyer P, Kerscher M. Low dose UVA1 phototherapy in disabling pansclerotic morphoea of childhood. *Br J Dermatol* 1997; **136**:293–4.

181. Uziel Y, Krafchik BR, Silverman ED, Liu P, Laxer RM. Orthopedic manifestations of localized scleroderma in children. *J Orthoped Rheumatol* 1994; **7**:224–7.

182. Buckley SL, Skinner S, James P, Ashley RK. Focal scleroderma in children: an orthopaedic perspective. *J Pediatr Orthop* 1993; **13**:784–90.

183. Ousterhout DK. Correction of enophthalmos in progressive hemifacial atrophy: a case report. *Ophthal Plast Reconstr Surg* 1996; **12**:240–4.

184. Grisanti MW, Moore TL, Osborn TG, Haber PL. Eosinophilic fasciitis in children. *Semin Arthritis Rheum* 1989; **19**:151–7.

185. Farrington ML, Haas JE, Nazar-Stewart V, Mellins ED. Eosinophilic fasciitis in children frequently progresses to scleroderma-like cutaneous fibrosis. *J Rheumatol* 1993; **20**:128–32.

186. Miller JJ III. The fasciitis–morphea complex in children. *Am J Dis Child* 1992; **146**:733–6.

187. Littlejohn GO, Keystone EC. Eosinophilic fasciitis and aplastic anaemia. *J Rheumatol* 1980; **7**:730–2.

188. Kilbourne EM, Philen RM, Kamb ML, Falk H. Tryptophan produced by Showa Denko and epidemic eosinophilia–myalgia syndrome. *J Rheumatol* 1996; **46**(suppl):81–8.

189. Alonso-Ruiz A, Calabozo M, Perez-Ruiz F, Mancebo L. Toxic oil syndrome. A long-term follow-up of a cohort of 332 patients. *Medicine* 1993; **72**:285–95.

190. Izquierdo M, Mateo I, Rodrigo M et al. Chronic juvenile toxic epidemic syndrome. *Ann Rheum Dis* 1985; **44**:98–103.

191. Spiera H, Spiera RF. Silicone breast implants and connective tissue disease: an overview. *Mt Sinai J Med* 1997; **64**:363–71.

192. Blackburn WD Jr, Everson MP. Silicone-associated rheumatic disease: an unsupported myth. *Plast Reconstr Surg* 1997; **99**:1362–7.

193. Levine JJ, Ilowite NT. Sclerodermalike esophageal disease in children breast-fed by mothers with silicone breast implants. *JAMA* 1994; **271**:213–6.

194. Jacobs JC, Imundo LF. Silicone implants and autoimmune disease. *Lancet* 1994; **343**:354–5.

195. Siadak M, Sullivan KM. The management of chronic graft-versus-host disease. *Blood Rev* 1994; **8**:154–60.

196. Cron RQ, Swetter SM. Scleredema revisited. A poststreptococcal complication. *Clin Pediatr* 1994; **33**:606–10.

197. Palestine RF, Millns JL, Spigel GT, Schroeter AL. Skin manifestations of pentazocine abuse. *J Am Acad Dermatol* 1980; **2**:47–55.

198. Cohen I, Mosher M, O'Keefe EJ, Klaus SN, De Conti RC. Cutaneous toxicity of bleomycin therapy. *Arch Dermatol* 1972; **107**:553–5.

199. Sanchez-Roman J, Wichmann I, Salaberri J, Varela JM, Nunez-Rolden A. Multiple clinical and biological autoimmune manifestations in 30 workers after occupational exposure to silica. *Ann Rheum Dis* 1993; **52**:534–8.

200. Steen VD, Scleroderma and pregnancy. *Clin Rheum Dis* 1997; **23**:133–47.

10

Systemic vasculitis

Bianca A Lang

INTRODUCTION

Systemic vasculitis can present in adolescents with a wide variety of signs and symptoms, since blood vessels of any size and in any organ may be affected. A number of clinical features that suggest the presence of vasculitis are listed in Table 10.1. It is essential to diagnose the specific type of vasculitis because certain previously fatal forms can now be effectively treated with rapid initiation of steroid and immunosuppressive therapy. In addition, it is important to avoid potentially toxic therapy in the teenager with self-limited cutaneous leucocytoclastic vasculitis or Henoch–Schönlein purpura. This chapter will help the clinician to distinguish between the main primary forms of vasculitis that can affect adolescents, and briefly mentions a few of the secondary causes.

DEFINITION AND CLASSIFICATION

Inflammation and necrosis of blood-vessel walls is common to all forms of vasculitis. In secondary forms the cause of inflammation is known, while in primary forms the cause is unknown. Because we do not know the causative agents or specific pathogenesis of the various forms of primary systemic vasculitis, our attempts at classification remain unsatisfactory. The first classification of vasculitis was proposed by Zeek[1] in the 1950s. Since then there have been many attempts to classify systemic vasculitis.[2–5] Recently, the American College of Rheumatology (ACR) has developed a classification system based on data derived from patients with well-established classic diseases.[2] Although this is useful for making comparisons between defined groups of patients for study purposes, these criteria were not designed for the diagnosis of individual patients or to help the clinician distinguish a primary vasculitis from various illnesses that mimic vasculitis. In 1994, the Chapel Hill Consensus Conference (CHCC) on the Nomenclature of Systemic Vasculitis agreed on terminology and definitions for the most common forms of non-infectious systemic

---

Table 10.1   Clinical features that suggest a systemic vasculitis*

- Palpable purpura, chronic urticaria
- Gangrene
- Unexplained fever
- Unexplained arthralgias/arthritis
- Unexplained myalgias/myositis
- Mononeuritis multiplex
- Unexplained pulmonary or cardiovascular disease
- Unexplained renal disease
- Unexplained central nervous system disease
- Unexplained hypertension
- Absent pulses; bruits

*A combination of constitutional symptoms with two or more organ systems involved increases the suspicion of a systemic vasculitis.

Table 10.2 A classification of primary systemic vasculitis in children

- Leucocytoclastic vasculitis:
  - Henoch–Schönlein purpura
  - hypersensitivity vasculitis
  - mixed cryoglobulinemia
- Polyarteritis:
  - polyarteritis nodosa
  - microscopic polyarteritis
  - cutaneous polyarteritis
  - Kawasaki disease
- Granulomatous vasculitis:
  - Wegener's granulomatosis
  - allergic granulomatosis (Churg–Strauss syndrome)
  - primary angiitis of the central nervous system
- Giant cell arteritis:
  - Takayasu's arteritis
  - temporal arteritis
- Other vasculitides:
  - Behçet's disease
  - Cogan's syndrome

vasculitis[3] and categorized them on the basis of vessel size. The main problem with this classification system is that many of the primary vasculitides involve vessels of various sizes. A modification of the classification system proposed by Zeek is presented in Table 10.2 and provides a useful framework within which to consider the various causes of systemic vasculitis that affect children and adolescents.

LEUCOCYTOCLASTIC VASCULITIS

Leucocytoclastic vasculitis is a term often used to encompass a wide group of conditions where there is prominent vasculitis of small blood vessels, including arterioles, capillaries and venules. The term 'hypersensitivity vasculitis' is sometimes used interchangeably with leucocytoclastic vasculitis, because in many patients the inflammatory process appears to follow exposure to a precipitating antigen such as a drug, foreign protein or infectious agent. In other patients, similar histological findings are seen in association with cryoglobulinaemia, or they may occur without a defined trigger, such as in Henoch–Schönlein purpura. Leucocytoclastic vasculitis may also be seen as part of other systemic illnesses, including autoimmune rheumatic diseases, certain malignancies and other primary forms of systemic vasculitis. In some cases, leucocytoclastic vasculitis may be idiopathic and limited to the skin.[3,6]

The characteristic histopathology of leucocytoclastic vasculitis is necrotizing inflammation of small blood vessels, in particular the postcapillary venules. Typically, vessel walls and perivascular tissues are infiltrated by neutrophils and there is fragmentation of nuclei.[6] In some patients with small-vessel vasculitis the inflammatory infiltrates consist predominantly of mononuclear cells. This may represent a late stage of leucocytoclastic vasculitis or a different mode or degree of response to injury.[7]

The clinical hallmarks of leucocytoclastic vasculitis are palpable petechiae and purpura, and less commonly chronic or recurrent urticaria. Other rashes may also occur. When leucocytoclastic vasculitis is limited to the skin, it usually resolves spontaneously within several weeks or a few months.[6] In some patients, systemic disease can follow skin manifestations by months to years. Because of the association with systemic illnesses, in all patients with leucocytoclastic vasculitis where the history and examination have not led to a specific diagnosis, a number of investigations should be considered as outlined in Table 10.3. Certain clinical features and a few specific investigations often suggest the diagnosis of one of the more important causes of small-vessel vasculitis in adolescents, including Henoch–Schönlein purpura, hypersensitivity vasculitis and cryoglobulinaemic vasculitis.

Table 10.3 Investigations in a patient with leucocytoclastic vasculitis

CBC	C-reactive protein
ESR	Rheumatoid factor
AST	Cryoglobulins
BUN	Serum protein electrophoresis
Creatinine	ANCAs
C_3, C_4, CH50	HBs Ag
ANA, anti-DNA	Urinalysis
IgG, IgA, IgM	Chest radiograph

CBC, complete blood cell count; AST, aspartate aminotransferase; BUN, blood urea nitrogen.

Henoch–Schönlein purpura

Henoch–Schönlein purpura (HSP) is a form of leucocytoclastic vasculitis characterized by predominant involvement of the skin, joints, gastrointestinal tract and kidneys. It is one of the most common forms of systemic vasculitis in childhood, occurring most often in children aged 2–10 years, with a peak incidence at age 5 years.[8] In adolescents, HSP is quite common under the age of 16 years,[9] but occurs less frequently in older adolescents. In the ACR study to determine classification criteria for HSP, 85 patients with HSP were studied.[8] Sixty-four per cent were younger than age 16; however, only 7% were aged 16–20 years. HSP is frequently preceded by an upper respiratory tract infection and, in some cases, group A streptococcal infection; however, no specific organism has been implicated in its causation.[9] It is important to make a diagnosis of HSP correctly because the course is usually self-limited and specific treatment is not usually required. Because HSP is less common in adolescents than in younger children, a more serious form of systemic vasculitis must be excluded, particularly if the presentation is atypical.

Clinical features
Most patients with HSP present with a purpuric rash, abdominal pain and joint pain which develop over several days or weeks. Palpable petechiae and purpura at different stages of development are typically seen on the buttocks and lower extremities. In some cases the rash may begin as erythematous macules or urticaria which later become purpuric, and if skin lesions are severe they may ulcerate. Subcutaneous oedema is much less common in adolescents than in younger children. Most patients have colicky abdominal pain at the time of onset of the purpura, and they may have vomiting or occult blood in their stools.[10–12] Melena, haematemesis, intussusception and acute perforation are uncommon. Even rarer complications include haemorrhagic pancreatitis, ulcerative colitis and other enteropathy.[12,13] Arthritis or arthralgias occur in over 50% of patients with HSP, most often affecting the knees and ankles, but less commonly other joints, including the small joints of the fingers. Swelling is most often periarticular and usually resolves within a week. Renal involvement has been reported in 20–50% of children with HSP; however, chronic renal failure is very uncommon.[9,14,15] Data vary from series to series, with earlier studies based in paediatric referral centres suggesting that chronic renal disease developed in up to 5–10% of patients. A more recent study of unselected children in Belfast who developed HSP found that 20% had renal involvement at diagnosis and less than 1% of patients developed persistent renal disease.[15] The spectrum of renal disease varies from microscopic haematuria and mild proteinuria to a nephritic/nephrotic syndrome, hypertension or renal failure. Most patients with renal disease will manifest it within the first 3 months; however, rarely, nephritis occurs many months or rarely years later.[9]

Unusual manifestations of HSP include central nervous system (CNS) vasculitis, peripheral neuropathy and pulmonary haemorrhage.[16,17] If an adolescent with suspected HSP develops one of these manifestations a careful work-up for a more serious systemic vasculitis is essential.

Laboratory investigations
There are no diagnostic laboratory abnormalities in HSP. Complement levels are usually normal.

An elevated serum immunoglobulin A (IgA) level is present in up to 50% of patients,[18] and circulating IgA containing immune complexes and cryoglobulins may be present.[19] In the adolescent with possible HSP, laboratory tests should be performed to exclude other diseases such as systemic lupus erythematosus (SLE), another systemic vasculitis, disseminated intravascular coagulation, septicaemia, haemolytic uraemic syndrome, post-streptococcal glomerulonephritis and others, depending on the clinical presentation. A positive antineutrophil cytoplasmic antibody (ANCA) should suggest a more serious small- to medium-vessel vasculitis and prompt further investigations. In questionable cases, a diagnosis of HSP should be confirmed by the pathological findings of IgA deposition in the walls of affected dermal vessels as well as in the glomerular mesangium.[20,21]

Treatment and prognosis
The overall prognosis in HSP is excellent and most patients require only supportive care. The illness usually resolves within 4 weeks, although recurrences are common.[22] Severe gastrointestinal complications, particularly severe gastrointestinal bleeding, may warrant the use of corticosteroids for 2–3 weeks, although their use remains controversial.[11]

Corticosteroids are generally not indicated to treat the renal disease;[9,23] however, their use together with immunosuppressives may have a role in cases of rapidly progressive glomerulonephritis.[24,25] End-stage renal disease is very uncommon in children with HSP; however, adolescents with nephritic or nephrotic syndrome at presentation may be at higher risk.[22,26] Transplantation has been successful, although recurrences in the graft have rarely been reported.

Hypersensitivity vasculitis

Hypersensitivity vasculitis is believed to be a relatively common cause of leucocytoclastic vasculitis in adolescents, although incidence figures are not available.[24] It is most often seen following drug treatment, usually occurring 7–10 days after onset of treatment, but occasionally beginning earlier or up to 3 weeks after the onset of treatment. Drugs known to cause a small-vessel vasculitis include penicillin, sulphonamides, cefaclor, thiazides, iodides, antithyroid drugs, retinoids, hydantoins and occasionally others.[27] Other antigens, including infectious agents,[28] may also trigger hypersensitivity vasculitis and, historically, the administration of homologous antiserum to treat such conditions as tetanus or diphtheria was an important trigger of so-called 'serum sickness'. More recently, foreign proteins such as monoclonal antibodies and cytokines have caused an immune-complex-mediated vasculitis.[29]

Clinically, symptoms may be limited to the skin, with petechiae and purpura, which are usually all at a similar stage of development. Urticaria, erythema multiforme and other skin lesions may also be seen. Systemic symptoms are relatively common, including fever, myalgias, arthralgias, lymphadenopathy and, occasionally, arthritis. Rarely, other organ systems may be involved, including kidneys, nervous system, heart and lungs.[9] The illness is usually short lived, resolving within a few weeks of removing the trigger. Occasionally corticosteroids are necessary for severe or prolonged cases.

Cryoglobulinaemic vasculitis

Cryoglobulinaemia is a very rare cause of leucocytoclastic vasculitis in children and adolescents.[30] Hepatitis B antigen has occasionally been associated with this disorder in the past.[31] However, more recently, hepatitis C has been implicated as a possible aetiologic factor.[32,33] With intravenous drug use the most common cause of hepatitis C infection, and with 72% of intravenous drug abusers less than 24 years of age found to be infected in one recent study,[33,34] there is reason for concern that in some areas this form of vasculitis may be seen more commonly in the older adolescent population. The typical presentation is with periodic crops of petechiae or purpura on the distal lower extremities precipitated by exposure to cold or prolonged standing.[31] Arthralgias and weakness are also common, and Raynaud's phenomenon, nephritis and, rarely, peripheral neuropathy or pulmonary disease may be seen.[30,31,35] A diagnosis is made by detecting mixed cryoglobulins in the blood. These are usually composed of one or more classes of polyclonal immunoglobulins (IgG and IgM) and possess rheumatoid factor activity.[6] A very low C_4 level with normal C_3 levels supports the diagnosis. Treatment is often limited to non-steroidal anti-inflammatory drugs (NSAIDs) for arthralgias and painful skin lesions, although corticosteroids with or without immunosuppressive drugs may be required to treat glomerulonephritis which is the main cause of long-term morbidity.[33] Preliminary reports suggest a possible role for interferon-α and plasmapheresis in the treatment of patients with associated hepatitis C infection.

POLYARTERITIS GROUP

Polyarteritis nodosa (macroscopic)

The classic form of polyarteritis nodosa (PAN) was first described by Küssmaul and Maier in 1866.[36] It is a condition characterized by inflammation and necrosis of medium-sized arteries, which may lead to the development of aneurysms and the infarction of affected organs. Classic PAN is rare but does occur in children and adolescents.[4,37–42] No reports of PAN specifically in adolescents have been published. However, in the large series of 130 patients reported by Frohnert and Sheps,[42] 7% (9/130) were between 10 and 19 years old. Boys and girls are affected almost equally.[38,42] The aetiology of PAN is unknown; however, immune-complex deposition is believed to play a role in the vessel-wall destruction.[5]

Clinical features
Most adolescents with classic PAN present with fever, malaise and weight loss in association with one or more of the following features: abdominal pain, arthralgia/arthritis, myalgia, skin rash, hypertension, haematuria, or peripheral or CNS disease.[4,38,40,41] Adolescents are often misdiagnosed as having an infectious illness, an autoimmune

rheumatic disease, or malignancy before the correct diagnosis of PAN is established.

Polyarthralgias are very common; however, if present, arthritis is usually transient and affects only a few joints. Myalgias are common and weakness may occur, but diffuse myositis is uncommon. Abdominal pain is a common presenting symptom and is often non-specific. The patient may present with a surgical abdomen due to small bowel infarction or perforation, gastrointestinal haemorrhage, visceral rupture, infarctive cholecystitis or necrotizing pancreatitis.[43,44] SLE and inflammatory bowel disease must be considered in the differential diagnosis. Renal involvement is common, and typically results in loin pain due to infarcts secondary to vasculitis of the arcuate artery system.[6] Urinary sediment abnormalities are typically mild, which helps differentiate classic PAN from microscopic PAN. The latter is almost always characterized by severe crescentic glomerulonephritis with significant haematuria, proteinuria and, often, oliguria or anuria.[45] In classic PAN, neurological involvement may present as seizures, focal deficits, unilateral visual loss, organic psychoses or mononeuritis multiplex. The latter results from vasculitis affecting the vasovasorum of several peripheral sensory and motor nerves leading to a sensorimotor peripheral neuropathy. Paraesthesias followed by weakness typically occur, with foot drop a common finding in older patients. Skin lesions of classic PAN, resulting from vasculitis of small and medium sized arteries in the panniculus and muscle, include subcutaneous nodules, ulcerative lesions, livedo reticularis and, occasionally, gangrene of a digit.[6,46] Petechiae, purpura and erythema multiforme have also been described and, although some would argue that this is more suggestive of microscopic PAN,[3] most would agree that these can also be seen with classic PAN.[2] Other organ system disease is seen less commonly, including cardiac, respiratory and testicular involvement.

Pathology
The typical pathology of PAN is a necrotizing arteritis affecting the entire thickness of predominantly medium-sized muscular arteries. The inflammatory cells are predominantly neutrophils.

The lesions are spotty in distribution and, in contrast to hypersensitivity vasculitis, acute and chronic lesions will often be seen on the same biopsy.[6] Aneurysm formation is typical and thrombosis may be present. In one study which compared the pathology in children and adolescents with PAN with the pathology in adults with the same disease, no differences were found.[4]

Laboratory and radiological investigations
Most adolescents with PAN have anaemia, leucocytosis, thrombocytosis, an elevated erythrocyte sedimentation rate (ESR) and C-reactive protein (CRP), and hypergammaglobulinaemia. However, these do not help make a specific diagnosis.[9,38,40] Antinuclear antibodies (ANAs) and rheumatoid factor (RF) are only occasionally detected. Factor VIII related antigen may be increased,[47] and circulating immune complexes may be present. Serum complement levels are usually normal or increased, but C_3 and C_4 may be decreased. ANCAs, described in detail later in this chapter, are usually negative in classic PAN.[24,48] In the small number of patients with classic PAN in whom ANCAs have been reported, more had p-ANCA, with specificity for myeloperoxidase, than c-ANCA.[24,49] EMG and nerve conduction studies may be valuable in confirming nerve and muscle involvement, and may suggest the need for a muscle biopsy. Skin biopsies should be full thickness, including subcutaneous tissue. Abdominal angiography with selective visualization of the renal, hepatic, splenic and mesenteric arteries may demonstrate multiple aneurysms at the bifurcations of medium sized arteries.[50] Stenoses or tortuosity are less common findings. It must be kept in mind that aneurysms are not specific for PAN and may be seen with Wegener's granulomatosis, SLE, infection and other causes. Magnetic subtraction angiography may have a role in demonstrating aneurysms in the future. Renal scans may show patchy areas of decreased uptake associated with renal vasculitis. Renal biopsy is less helpful in diagnosing classic PAN than microscopic PAN, but may demonstrate small or medium vessel vasculitis in some patients. Glomerular changes do not help make a specific diagnosis, but aggressive glomerulonephritis is more suggestive of microscopic PAN or another disease.

Treatment and prognosis
Standard initial therapy for PAN includes daily prednisone 1–2 mg/kg/day up to 60–80 mg/day in divided doses for about 4 weeks, followed by a slow taper.[9,51] This regime of high-dose corticosteroids is invariably associated with toxicity. It is essential to discuss the treatment plan with the adolescent and explain the potential side-effects of corticosteroids. Most adolescents are extremely self-conscious about their appearance; the cushingoid facies, weight gain and acne associated with prednisone will undoubtedly be disturbing. Non-compliance and alteration of the dosage of prednisone by the adolescent is best avoided by education and repeated discussions at each return visit. Adolescents often will not express their concerns unless they are directly questioned by their physicians. Look for evidence of acne and, if it is present, take the initiative to address it and commence treatment. This will be appreciated by the embarrassed adolescent who otherwise may have resorted to over-the-counter preparations which could have aggravated the problem.

In patients with severe major organ involvement or with progressive disease despite corticosteroids, cyclophosphamide could be added.[52] Both daily oral cyclophosphamide 2 mg/kg/day and intravenous pulse cyclophosphamide[52] have been used. Plasmapheresis has been used in life-threatening cases,[24] but is not always effective.[53] Adjunctive treatment with anti-platelet drugs may be useful.[24]

The prognosis reported for PAN in children and adolescents has been variable, and reflects differences in disease severity and probably differences in classification of patients in different series. Prior to the use of steroids, the 5-year survival rate was close to 10%.[42] This improved to 50% with the use of steroids,[42] and the addition of immunosuppressive therapy in selected patients has further improved outcome.[51] Despite improved survival, mortality can still be as high as 20–30%.[24] Severe visceral or CNS disease is associated with a poorer prognosis.

Microscopic polyarteritis (polyangiitis)

Microscopic polyarteritis (MPA) was a term first used by Davson et al in 1948 to classify a subgroup of patients with PAN who had significant segmental necrotizing glomerulonephritis.[5] Since then, MPA has been defined as a necrotizing small-vessel vasculitis associated with glomerulonephritis but without granulomatous inflammation.[54] MPA is not recognized as a separate entity in the ACR classification criteria of systemic vasculitis.[2] In contrast, MPA is probably overemphasized in the CHCC nomenclature, where it is diagnosed histologically in any patient with necrotizing small-vessel vasculitis in the absence of immune deposits or granulomatous inflammation; even in the presence of medium-sized vessel vasculitis.[3] Although there are no data on its incidence, MPA does occur in adolescents. Children and adolescents have been included within large series of adult patients, but no specific information on the disease in adolescents is available.[48] Nevertheless, MPA is an important diagnostic consideration in the teenager who presents with severe glomerulonephritis or pulmonary–renal syndrome.

Clinical features

MPA has many clinical similarities to classic PAN, including constitutional symptoms, cutaneous manifestations, musculoskeletal and gastrointestinal involvement, and peripheral neuropathy. It can usually be clinically differentiated from PAN by the type and degree of renal and pulmonary involvement. Microscopic PAN is almost always accompanied by crescentic rapidly progressive glomerulonephritis.[48,54] An adolescent with MPA usually has significant haematuria, proteinuria, and often rapidly develops acute renal failure. Hypertension is associated with severe nephritis rather than with vasculitis of the renal arteries.[45] Pulmonary involvement is common and MPA is one of the most common causes of the pulmonary–renal syndrome.[49] Although specific data in adolescents are lacking, 20–30% of patients in several adult series with MPA had pulmonary haemorrhage.[48] Haemoptysis usually starts within 1 month of presentation and may be mild or severe. It is associated with significant morbidity and mortality. MPA must be differentiated from Wegener's granulomatosis, Goodpasture's syndrome, SLE and other causes of pulmonary–renal syndrome. Ear, nose and throat, as well as ocular manifestations, are more common in MPA than in classic PAN; however, they are less prominent than in Wegener's granulomatosis.[48]

Pathology

Pathology in MPA is characterized by necrotizing vasculitis affecting predominantly small vessels (capillaries, arterioles and venules) without granuloma formation. Necrotizing crescentic glomerulonephritis without immunoglobulin or complement deposition is characteristic, and pulmonary capillaritis is common. Necrotizing vasculitis of small and medium-sized arteries may also occur.[48]

Laboratory measures

Differentiating laboratory features of MPA include a high frequency of ANCAs, this being reported in 50–80% of patients.[54–56] In most cases, this is anti-p-ANCA (antimyeloperoxidase), although c-ANCA (anti-PR3) has been detected in some patients. In contrast to classic PAN, visceral angiography is usually normal and aneurysms are absent.[48]

Treatment and prognosis

There are no data on treatment of MPA specifically in adolescents and children, and there are few data in adults, because MPA has only recently been defined as a specific disease entity. The similarities in renal histology and the association with ANCA in MPA and Wegener's granulomatosis, as well as available data to date, suggest that MPA may be similar to Wegener's in response to treatment. Current recommended treatment is a combination of high-dose daily steroids with daily cyclophosphamide if there is glomerulonephritis or other major organ disease. Intravenous pulse steroids and pulse cyclophosphamide have also been used.[48] Plasmapheresis should be considered in life-threatening disease, particularly with lung haemorrhage. The prognosis for fulminating MPA is guarded, with the 5-year survival in one adult series being reported as 65%. Two-thirds of deaths in this series were due to active vasculitis complicated by renal failure and lung haemorrhage or to treatment side-effects. Relapses are frequent and occur in approximately one-third of patients within 2 years.[48] Further study of this subcategory of vasculitis in adolescents is needed.

Cutaneous polyarteritis

Cutaneous polyarteritis should be differentiated from classic PAN and MPA in adolescents because the prognosis is generally excellent. Symptoms often begin following a sore throat or otitis, and in a number of patients a preceding streptococcal infection has been documented.[57–60] Painful nodules, often on the medial side of the foot, are the most common skin lesions, but livedo reticularis, purpura and ulceration also may occur. Myalgias, arthralgias and arthritis are common, and oedema of the extremities may be seen. Peripheral neuropathy and abdominal pain are less common. The outcome is generally excellent. However, relapses are common and may occur in association with streptococcal or other infections, with tapering of steroids, or at any time.[24] Treatment usually includes penicillin, NSAIDs and corticosteroids.[24] Because of the association with streptococcal infection, penicillin prophylaxis should be considered.[4] A few children have been reported to develop classic PAN, and in these patients and patients with major systemic disease immunosuppressive therapy may be needed.[24]

Hepatitis B associated PAN

In adults, PAN may develop after infection with hepatitis B virus, usually within 6 months of infection. Most paediatric series of PAN have not shown an association with hepatitis B.[38,40] However, ages are not always specified in the predominantly adult series of PAN with hepatitis B, and these may have included a few adolescents.

The hepatitis may be silent and patients may present with symptoms and signs typical of PAN. Certain clinical features are more typical of hepatitis B associated PAN, including malignant hypertension, renal infarction and orchiepididymitis. Although the disease may initially be severe, with appropriate treatment the outcome is very good. Antiviral agents and plasmapheresis, rather than immunosuppressive treatment, are now generally recommended. Hepatitis C is not a common cause of PAN.[49]

Kawasaki disease

Kawasaki disease is a necrotizing vasculitis affecting small and medium-sized arteries. The cause remains unknown, although an infectious basis is still suspected. The diagnostic criteria for Kawasaki disease are listed in Table 10.4. Kawasaki disease is the most common vasculitis of childhood.[62,63] It usually affects infants and children under 5 years of age. It is uncommon in adolescents, and is thus only briefly reviewed here.

The major clinical features of this disease are outlined in Table 10.4 and include fever persisting for at least 5 days, bilateral non-suppurative conjunctivitis, acute cervical lymphadenopathy, rash, typical peripheral extremity changes, and typical changes of the lips and oral cavity. Coronary artery aneurysms occur in 20–30% of patients without treatment, and other cardiac complications, including pericarditis, myocarditis, myocardial infarction and cardiac failure, may occur. Other organ systems may be involved, and patients may have arthritis, gastrointestinal disturbances (including hydrops of the gallbladder), sterile pyuria and proteinuria, cough, seizures and aseptic meningitis.[9] Leucocytosis in the acute phase and thrombocytosis in the subacute phase, as well as non-specific findings of inflammation, are typical. Current treatment includes high-dose aspirin and intravenous immunoglobulin (IVIG) as a single dose of 2 g/kg in the acute phase,[63] followed by low-dose aspirin for at least 8 weeks, or longer if there are coronary artery abnormalities. Dipyridamole is occasionally

Table 10.4 Kawasaki disease: frequency and characteristics of diagnostic criteria*

Criterion	Frequency (%)	Characteristics
Fever	100	Duration of 5 days or more
Conjunctivitis	85	Bilateral, bulbar, non-suppurative
Lymph-node enlargement	70	Cervical, acute, non-purulent, > 1.5 cm
Rash	80	Polymorphous, no vesicles or crusts
Changes of lips or oral mucosa	90	Dry, red, vertically fissured lips, 'strawberry' tongue Diffuse erythema of oropharynx
Changes of extremities	70	Initial stage: erythema of palms or soles, indurative oedema of hands or feet. subacute stage: desquamation from fingertips

*From Cassidy and Petty.[9]

used, and if giant aneurysms are present, anti-coagulation should be considered. The use of steroids has been controversial, although together with low-dose aspirin they may have a role in patients refractory to IVIG. The overall prognosis is good, although there may be some increased risk of stenotic arterial lesions later in life.[64]

GRANULOMATOUS VASCULITIS GROUP

Wegener's granulomatosis

Wegener's granulomatosis (WG) is a necrotizing granulomatous vasculitis characterized by upper and lower respiratory tract disease, glomerulonephritis, and a systemic small-vessel vasculitis.[65] A limited form of the disease has also been recognized where renal disease is absent.[65] Although it is a rare disease, it is well described in adolescents.[65–69] In a large series reported by the National Institutes of Health (NIH), 15% (23/158) of cases occurred in patients under 19 years of age.[70] In this series, most aspects of the disease were found to be similar in adolescents and children compared with adults, with the exception of an increased frequency of subglotic stenosis and saddle nose deformity at younger ages. The onset of WG in all age groups may be insidious or fulminant. Fever, malaise and weight loss are common. Upper respiratory tract disease is the most common presenting feature of WG, occurring in > 70% of patients.[65,70] Sinusitis, nasal mucosal ulceration, epistaxis, nasal septal perforation, otitis media and hearing loss are all common. Saddle nose deformities were found to be twice as common in patients less than 19 years of age compared with adults (48% vs 25%).[69] Subglottic stenosis secondary to granulomatous laryngo-tracheal inflammation is also more common in adolescents, reported in 48%, compared with 10% of adults.[69,71] This may result in stridor or, in some cases, life-threatening airway obstruction. It is best assessed by direct laryngoscopy, which may reveal signs of inflammation or chronic scarring. Oral ulcers and parotitis have been reported less commonly.

Although a few patients have only upper airway disease, most also have lower airway disease, and almost half of patients present with pulmonary symptoms.[65,69,70] Cough, haemoptysis and pleuritis are common. Asymptomatic pulmonary nodules and fleeting infiltrates also occur frequently. Diffuse pulmonary haemorrhage due to alveolar capillaritis is less common, but has a high mortality and requires urgent immunosuppressive therapy. Unlike Churg–Strauss syndrome (CSS), lung disease is not associated with asthma or peripheral blood eosinophilia.

Less than 30% of patients with WG have nephritis at presentation; however, approximately 80% will develop glomerulonephritis during their disease course. Microscopic haematuria is common, but hypertension is uncommon. A rapidly progressive crescentic glomerulonephritis may be seen in almost half of patients who develop renal failure.[65]

Ocular involvement is often seen during the course of WG, and inflammation of any component may occur. Proptosis (often unilateral) due to retro-orbital granulomatous inflammation, is the most characteristic eye finding in WG.[65]

Neurological manifestations include peripheral neuropathies as well as CNS involvement. If present, computed tomography (CT) or magnetic resonance imaging (MRI) should be used to assess for infarction, haemorrhage, mass lesions and meningeal enhancement. Angiography is not usually helpful because of the small size of the vessels involved.

Other fairly non-specific manifestations of WG include arthralgias and arthritis, pericarditis and coronary vasculitis. Cutaneous lesions, including palpable purpura, ulcers and subcutaneous nodules, may be seen, and usually reflect active systemic disease. Gastrointestinal and genitourinary involvement are very uncommon.[65]

Pathology

The pathology of the upper and lower respiratory tract typically includes necrosis, granulomas and vasculitis. Because of the small amount of tissue obtained from most nasal and sinus biopsies, it is uncommon for all these features to be detected, making it difficult to confirm the diagnosis histologically.[65] Capillaritis is a common but non-specific finding on lung biopsy. Kidney biopsies show a focal segmental proliferative glomerulonephritis, often with crescent formation and with absent or minimal immunoglobulin deposition. This does not differ from the glomerular changes seen with microscopic PAN, CSS, or an idiopathic disease limited to the kidneys. Vasculitis of medium-sized renal arteries and granulomatous changes are rarely seen in the kidney.

Laboratory

Leucocytosis without eosinophilia is common and the ESR is usually markedly elevated. RF is positive in about 50% of adult patients. Most patients have circulating antineutrophil cytoplasmic antibodies (ANCAs) present in their serum which on immunofluorescent studies show a characteristic granular cytoplasmic distribution (c-ANCA).[72] The value of ANCA in the systemic vasculitides is discussed briefly at the end of this section on WG.

Treatment and prognosis

Current standard treatment for WG consists of a combination of high-dose steroids and daily oral cyclophosphamide (2 mg/kg/day).[65,70,73] Data strongly suggest that steroids alone are inadequate to treat active major organ involvement in WG, and glomerulonephritis in particular. The use of daily oral cyclophosphamide together with steroids has been shown to result in improvement in 91% of patients with WG, with complete remission achieved in 75% of patients.[70] Intermittent intravenous cyclophosphamide has been advocated by some; however, its use in WG remains controversial.[74,75] The high incidence of morbidity related to drug toxicity in WG has led to the evaluation of less-toxic therapy. Recent studies suggest that methotrexate may be an effective and less-toxic alternative to cyclophosphamide for patients who do not have life-threatening disease or who have had cyclophosphamide-related toxicity.[74,76] Methotrexate may also have a role in maintenance therapy. Alternative immunosuppressives to daily cyclophosphamide or weekly methotrexate should only be used if patients are intolerant or unresponsive to these treatments.

Trimethoprim–sulphamethoxazole is not appropriate for treating major organ involvement, but may be useful in preventing upper airway relapses and treating isolated upper airway disease.[77] In addition, aggressive treatment of infection, particularly sinusitis, is very important, because such intercurrent infections can simulate increased disease activity, but infection should not be treated with increased immunosuppression. Plasmapheresis may be considered in life-threatening situations.

Appropriate treatment of subglottic stenosis is particularly important in adolescents because of the high incidence of this complication in this age group. In some cases, subglottic stenosis may not respond to systemic immunosuppressive therapy, but may improve with intratracheal dilatation and injection with a long-acting corticosteroid.[78]

Wegener's granulomatosis was almost always fatal before the use of current immunosuppressive therapy. In contrast, recent figures from the NIH study which included adults and children indicate a 20% mortality rate over 8 years.[70,73] Similarly, a 15% mortality rate has been reported for patients treated at the Hospital for Sick Children (Great Ormond Street) in London.[24] Despite improved mortality, approximately 50% of patients have at least one relapse within 5 years, which usually requires reinstitution of induction therapy.[70] Morbidity is significant, and in the prospective NIH study of 23 children with Wegener's granulomatosis 86% had permanent morbidity. This figure for overall morbidity was similar to that found for adults. However, treatment-related morbidity was less common in children (22%) compared with adults (45%), and no paediatric patients developed cyclophosphamide-related malignancies compared with 11% of adults.[69] Nevertheless, it is essential to discuss openly the potential side-effects of cyclophosphamide, including alopecia, haemorrhagic cystitis, bone-marrow suppression, infectious complications, sterility and the increased risk of malignancy. Adolescents should be encouraged to ask questions and express their concerns about the disease and the treatment plan. Adolescents diagnosed with WG are likely to experience significant anger and may reject the recommended treatment options. Such patients may be persuaded to accept the necessary treatment if the physician does not give up, but provides explanations and counselling in an empathetic way. It is essential that the physician maintains optimism for the adolescent's improvement. Once patients are stable and improving, they should be encouraged to participate in reasonable and rewarding activities. This will allow the adolescents to rebuild a sense of peer acceptance which will be a critical resource in helping them to cope.

Dealing with contraception in sexually active patients and addressing issues related to future fertility are critical in adolescents who require treatment with cyclophosphamide. Injectable contraception with Depo-Provera and depot medoxyprogesterone acetate (DMPA) may be preferred to oral contraceptives in some patients to improve compliance. However, the finding of decreased bone density in patients using this form of contraception needs further study,[79] particularly as adolescents with WG require corticosteroid treatment in addition to immunosuppressives. Future fertility is of great concern to many adolescents with WG who require daily cyclophosphamide. Consideration should be given to storing eggs and/or sperm when an adolescent is about to be treated with cyclophosphamide, just as it is considered in patients starting chemotherapy for a malignant disease.

Antineutrophil cytoplasmic antibodies

ANCAS AND THEIR MEASUREMENT
Antineutrophil cytoplasmic antibodies (ANCAs) are antibodies directed against specific enzymes contained within the granules of polymorphonuclear granulocytes (PMNs) and monocytes. These enzymes include myeloperoxidase and several serine proteases, including proteinase-3, neutrophil elastase, and cathepsin G. ANCAs can be detected by indirect immunofluorescence microscopy using ethanol-fixed PMNs as the substrate.[72] Two main staining patterns on immunofluorescence have been seen; the cytoplasmic ANCA (c-ANCA) pattern

and the perinuclear ANCA (pANCA) pattern. The c-ANCA pattern is characterized by diffuse fine granular staining of the PMN cytoplasm. The main antigen associated with the cANCA pattern is proteinase-3 (PR3). The pANCA pattern is characterized by a perinuclear or nuclear staining pattern. The main antigen associated with pANCA is myeloperoxidase (MPO). The perinuclear staining pattern occurs because MPO, which originates from the same granules as PR3, redistributes to the nucleus when the PMN is fixed in ethanol.[80] ANAs also show a nuclear staining pattern on ethanol-fixed cells, and must be differentiated using Hep-2 cells. Antibodies directed against other PMN enzymes (e.g. elastase and cathepsin G) may also give a perinuclear or other staining pattern. Specific enzyme-linked immunosorbent assays (ELISAs) are now available to determine if ANCAs are directed against PR3 or MPO.

ROLE OF ANCAS IN THE DIAGNOSIS OF SYSTEMIC VASCULITIS

A role for ANCAs in the diagnosis of Wegener's granulomatosis was first suggested by Van der Woude et al in 1985.[72] Since then, ANCAs have been found to be associated with three major categories of vasculitis: Wegener's granulomatosis, microscopic polyarteritis and CSS, as well as with idiopathic rapidly progressive glomerulonephritis.[80–82] Although either cANCA or pANCA may occur in a patient with any of these disorders, most patients with WG have cANCA (PR3), and patients with MPA are more likely to have pANCA. cANCA and pANCA are both commonly seen with idiopathic rapidly progressive glomerulonephritis, and either may be seen in CSS. Combining the results of immunofluorescence tests with the results of ELISAs increases the sensitivity and specificity of these tests. cANCAs (by immunofluorescence and ELISA) are present in 80–90% of patients with active generalized WG.[57,72,83,84] However, they are detected in only about half of patients with active limited WG. The specificity is generally 95%, but may vary with different laboratories. pANCAs, usually with MPO specificity, have been reported in 50–80% of patients with

MPA.[54,56,57] ANCA results in patients with CSS have been variable and data are limited. Although it has been reported that up to 70% of patients with CSS may be ANCA positive, in one study only 5 of 25 patients with CSS were ANCA positive (all cANCA),[85] and in another study 8 of 12 patients with CSS were ANCA positive (four cANCA; four pANCA).[86] pANCAs and/or atypical staining patterns have also been variably reported in patients with inflammatory bowel disease, primary sclerosing cholangitis, rheumatoid arthritis, as well as in patients with vasculitis associated with drugs, infection and malignancy.[56,57] In summary, cANCAs have a role in the diagnosis of generalized WG, but other ANCA results should be interpreted with caution.

ROLE OF ANCAS IN THE TREATMENT OF SYSTEMIC VASCULITIS

Several small studies have suggested that a rise in ANCA titre is predictive of disease relapse in patients with WG. Although ANCA titres may vary with disease activity in some patients, discordance also occurs, and disease flares are not necessarily predicted by a rise in cANCA titre. Data are still limited, and adjustment of immunosuppressive therapy on the basis of cANCA levels alone is not recommended.[70,81,87]

ROLE OF ANCAS IN DISEASE PATHOGENESIS

The role of ANCAs in disease pathogenesis has not yet been determined. In vitro studies have shown that ANCAs may have a role in the activation and degranulation of PMNs and monocytes, resulting in release of toxic oxygen metabolites, which may contribute to vascular injury.[88,89] Evidence against a primary pathogenic role for ANCAs is the observation that not all patients with WG are ANCA positive, particularly those with limited disease, and ANCAs are found even less consistently in MPA or CSS. In addition, many patients with WG who are in remission continue to have high cANCA titres for many years.[90,91]

Churg–Strauss syndrome

Churg–Strauss syndrome, also known as allergic granulomatosis, is extremely rare in children and adolescents. No features have been identified that distinguish adolescents with CSS from adults with the disease. However, the literature is limited to occasional case reports and a few patients within larger series of adult patients.[92–95] Of interest, the original description of CSS included four female adolescents whose asthma began at 17–18 years of age and who died with systemic vasculitis within 4–10 years.[92] A history of asthma and allergic rhinitis preceding the onset of symptoms and signs of a systemic vasculitis, along with peripheral blood eosinophilia ($> 1500/mm^3$), allow the condition to be distinguished from PAN and other vasculitides.[92,95,96] The asthma typically precedes the onset of vasculitis by 2–5 years, although this is variable.[92] Lung involvement is almost always present in CSS, with transient patchy infiltrates often seen on chest radiographs.[94,97] Skin lesions are common, and include palpable purpura as well as tender subcutaneous nodules, often found on the scalp or extremities. The pathology of these nodules reveals granulomatous inflammation with a predominantly eosinophilic infiltrate. Coronary arteritis and myocarditis are the main causes of morbidity and mortality, and may be silent at presentation.[49] Renal disease is less common or severe compared with PAN and WG.[98] Peripheral neuropathy is quite common, occurring in 60–70% of patients,[54,99] and gastrointestinal involvement with eosinophilic infiltration may also occur.[92] The diagnosis of CSS is confirmed by the characteristic pathology, which includes necrotizing vasculitis with eosinophilic infiltrates and extravascular granulomata.[92] Leucocytosis with eosinophilia accounting for up to 80% of the increase is common. Patients may be ANCA positive, but the frequency and patterns detected have been variable and the data limited to small numbers.[85,86] High-dose corticosteroids alone are usually adequate for initial therapy. If there is life-threatening disease with vasculitis of the gastrointestinal tract or heart, or severe glomerulonephritis, or if the course of the disease is refractory or relapsing, the addition of cyclophosphamide should be considered.[54,95,100] Plasmapheresis has not been shown to be beneficial.[53]

Primary angiitis of the central nervous system

Isolated vasculitis of the CNS is a very rare disorder characterized by necrotizing granulomatous inflammation of small and medium-sized vessels of the brain and spinal cord.[101] Clinical presentation includes headaches, nonspecific mental changes, and focal neurologic deficits, including hemiparesis.[102] Associated systemic symptoms are usually absent. CT or MRI may show evidence of cerebral infarction, cerebral angiography may demonstrate multifocal areas of stenosis and ectasia, and spinal fluid examination usually shows increased cells and protein due to meningeal vessel involvement. CNS biopsy may be needed to make a definitive diagnosis. Primary angiitis of the CNS is extremely rare and other disorders must always be excluded. Other diagnoses to consider include infection, drug use (especially amphetamines and cocaine), malignancy, vasospastic disorders and other systemic vasculitides.

GIANT CELL ARTERITIS

Takayasu's arteritis

Takayasu's arteritis is a large-vessel vasculitis that typically causes stenosis and aneurysms of the aorta, its major branches and, less commonly, the pulmonary arteries. It is most commonly diagnosed in young females aged 20–30 years; however, it is also relatively common in adolescents.[103,104] World-wide, Takayasu's arteritis is the third most common primary systemic vasculitis in childhood, after Henoch–Schönlein purpura and Kawasaki disease.[24,103] Paediatric cases of Takayasu's arteritis often occur in adolescents, and in Japan almost 20% of cases of Takayasu's arteritis occur between the ages of 10 and 19 years.[9] In Mexico, 77% of a large series of 107 patients with

Takayasu's arteritis had onset of their disease between ages 10 and 20 years.[104] In a recent study of North American patients with Takayasu's arteritis performed at the NIH, the median age at diagnosis was 25 years, and 19 patients (32%) were less than 20 years old.[105] A concerning finding of this study was a median delay in diagnosis in adolescents and children of 19 months from what, in retrospect, were significant signs or symptoms of large-vessel disease. This delay in diagnosis was almost four times that of adults, and emphasizes the fact that the diagnosis will be missed unless the clinician keeps this disorder in mind and looks for its main clinical features.[105,106]

Clinical features

The clinical presentation of Takayasu's arteritis has traditionally been described as occurring in two distinct phases: the early phase, characterized by symptoms and signs of systemic inflammation; and the later 'pulseless' phase, characterized by symptoms and signs related to occlusive arterial disease.[104,107] Although this pattern of presentation does occur in some patients, and has led to the misdiagnosis of acute rheumatic fever and juvenile arthritis in patients later diagnosed with Takayasu's arteritis,[108,109] this clinical presentation is not seen in all patients. It has been emphasized recently that the presentation and course of Takayasu's arteritis can be extremely variable, and this must be taken into account if an early diagnosis of this disease is to be made in adolescents.[106]

A number of patients will present with systemic symptoms, including fever, malaise, weight loss, night sweats, myalgias and/or arthralgias. Arthritis and erythema-nodosum-like lesions have also been reported;[105,107,110,111] however, the frequency of these symptoms at disease onset is quite variable. A study of 26 children aged 3–15 years in Mexico found that 65% presented with constitutional symptoms and/or arthritis.[111] In contrast, the recent NIH study, which included 19 patients less than 20 years of age, found that only one-third of patients had constitutional symptoms at disease onset.[105] This study also found that almost 60% of patients

never had constitutional symptoms, and in some patients constitutional symptoms occurred primarily late in the disease course.

Another important clinical pattern of presentation of Takayasu's arteritis in children and young adolescents is with symptoms and signs of hypertension and congestive heart failure.[104,111,112] Common presenting symptoms include, dyspnoea, palpitations, headaches and generalized weakness. In a study of Korean children, five of eight presented with hypertensive encephalopathy,[112] and in the series of paediatric patients from Mexico mentioned previously, two-thirds presented with congestive heart failure.[111] Patients with Takayasu's arteritis may also present with other symptoms or signs of large-vessel inflammation and/or occlusion, including the presence of bruits, absent or diminished peripheral pulses, asymmetric blood pressures, or symptoms or signs of CNS ischaemia, including dizziness, syncope, seizures, stroke or visual changes.[104,105,107,111,112] Claudication and paraesthesias are often reported in adults; however, claudication was found to be less common in patients under 20 years of age in the recent NIH study (11% vs 46% in adults).[105] Signs of severe ischaemia such as necrosis and gangrene are uncommon in adolescents and adults because of collateral circulation. Arteriovenous anastomoses in and around the optic disc with preretinal haemorrhages are the classic eye findings associated with this disease. These were present in the child originally reported by Takayasu; however, they are extremely rare.[113] Pulmonary hypertension due to pulmonary artery stenosis is also uncommon.[105] It appears that the presenting features of Takayasu's arteritis vary in different races, geographic areas and age groups, and further documentation of the clinical features of this disease in adolescents in North America and Europe is needed.

Pathology

Typical pathology in Takayasu's arteritis consists of segmental giant cell granulomatous inflammation and fibrosis affecting all three layers of the vessel wall.[6] There is characteristic destruction of the elastic lamina and extensive fibrosis of the media. Giant cells may surround these areas of destruction; however, in some cases few giant cells are seen. Intimal thickening and secondary thrombosis are common. In some cases, histologically active disease may be seen in asymptomatic patients, as was the case in four of nine patients in the NIH study who had active vasculitis documented on studied biopsy specimens.[105]

Investigations

Most laboratory tests are non-specific in Takayasu's arteritis, and although the ESR may be elevated, it may be normal despite other evidence of active disease.[105] An elevated factor VIII related antigen may be helpful in indicating active disease in some patients.[47] A positive tuberculin test is common in certain parts of the world, but this is not the case in North America.[107] Occasionally the diagnosis of Takayasu's arteritis is suggested by widening or calcification of the aorta seen on plain films of the chest or abdomen. More commonly, the diagnosis of Takayasu's arteritis is made on angiography of the aorta and its major branches, which demonstrates vessel narrowing and post-stenotic fusiform aneurysmal dilatations.[114] Involvement of the descending thoracic and abdominal aorta are particularly common in adolescents and children,[9,103] whereas the aortic arch is most commonly involved in adults. MRI and Doppler ultrasound are less invasive techniques which, with refinement, may play a role in the diagnosis and follow-up of this disease in the future.[111,115,116] Other diseases affecting the aorta should be excluded in adolescents with suspected Takayasu's arteritis, including Kawasaki disease, Behçet's disease, Cogan's syndrome, sarcoidosis, and infectious causes and disorders of connective tissue such as Ehlers–Danlos or Marfan's syndromes.

Treatment and prognosis

High-dose corticosteroids are the main treatment of Takayasu's arteritis and appear to be most effective early in the course of the disease. They usually decrease systemic symptoms, and in some cases help to reverse arterial stenoses.[111,117,118] However, not all patients respond to steroids. Some patients who do not improve with steroids will respond to the addition of immunosuppressive treatment such as cyclophosphamide or methotrexate.[105,118,119] Other patients are refractory to all treatment. In the NIH study, 23% of patients never achieved remission.[105] Additional aspects of treatment in Takayasu's arteritis include control of renal hypertension and antiplatelet therapy.[24,120] In adolescents and adults with inactive disease, reconstructive surgery and transluminal angioplasty have been used.[118]

Prognosis is variable. In the series of children with Takayasu's arteritis reported from Mexico, the mortality rate was 35% over a 5-year period.[111] Infection likely played a significant role in this immunosuppressed population. In contrast, the 5-year survival rates from the two large North American series from the Mayo Clinic and the NIH were 94% and 97%, respectively.[105,107] Despite these encouraging mortality statistics in North America, morbidity remains significant. Almost half of all patients who achieved remission in the NIH study had at least one relapse, and approximately half of all patients were occupationally disabled.[105]

Giant cell (temporal) arteritis

Temporal arteritis is a localized form of giant cell arteritis which occurs mainly in adults aged over 55 years in association with polymyalgia rheumatica.[121] It is very rare in adolescents, but one case has been reported as an overlap picture with another systemic vasculitis.[122] Typical presentation includes localized pain and tenderness over the temporal artery associated with a persistent headache. There may be intermittent jaw claudication as well as tender nodules along the temporal artery. Retinal artery inflammation may lead to optic ischaemia and sudden blindness. Therefore early diagnosis and treatment is essential. Polymyalgia rheumatica, characterized by pain and diffuse stiffness of the proximal arms and legs with or without fever, occurs in about 50% of adult patients with temporal arteritis. Diagnosis is made on temporal artery biopsy, and treatment consists of corticosteroids. An entity termed 'juvenile temporal arteritis' has been described in adolescents and children which should be differentiated from giant cell temporal arteritis. This rare, localized, benign process usually presents with painless temporal artery nodules, although occasionally the nodules may be tender.[123] Unlike in older adults, there is no associated visual disturbance, no myalgias, no elevation of the ESR, and the temporal artery biopsy shows an eosinophilic panarteritis without granulomatous inflammation or giant cells. No specific treatment is required.

OTHER VASCULITIDES

Behçet's disease

Behçet's disease is rare, but may occur in adolescents.[124–126] A recent study from Turkey reported that in 95 of 1784 (5.3%) patients with Behçet's disease, onset of illness was before age 16 years (51 males/44 females).[126] Most of these patients presented between ages 10 and 16 years. Behçet's disease is characterized by the triad of aphthous stomatitis, genital ulceration and uveitis. Anterior and posterior uveitis may be severe and may lead to blindness. In the recent study from Turkey,[126] 27% of patients with juvenile Behçet's had ocular involvement and developed blindness. Skin manifestations are common in Behçet's disease and include erythema nodosum, ulceration and other rashes. Meningoencephalitis is the most common CNS manifestation.[127] Polyarthritis is common, and an association with sacroiliitis has been reported but remains unclear.[128] Gastrointestinal disease may be indistinguishable from ulcerative colitis or Crohn's disease. Any part of the gastrointestinal tract may be affected, including the oesophagus. Vascular involvement includes arteritis, aneurysm formation, as well as venous thrombosis. The high frequency of Behçet's disease in older males, as well as the high incidence of venous disease, helps distinguish it from Takayasu's arteritis. Steroids are effective in some, but not all, patients with Behçet's disease. Other treatment options have included colchicine, levamisol, thalidomide, cyclosporin A and chlorambucil.[24,129,130] Azathioprine and cyclophosphamide have been used to treat severe disease with variable efficacy. The disease is usually prolonged with a relapsing course.

Cogan's syndrome

Cogan's syndrome is characterized by interstitial keratitis with vestibuloauditory dysfunction.[131] It occurs most commonly in young adults, but has also been reported in adolescents and children.[132] Patients may present with photophobia, hearing loss, vertigo or symptoms or signs secondary to aortitis or, less commonly, widespread systemic vasculitis. Steroids are the mainstay of treatment; however, hearing loss may be permanent.[9] The use of cyclosporin A in cases of severe disease, especially with aortitis, has been advocated and appeared effective in a 19 year old with Cogan's syndrome who had aortic valve involvement.[133]

Other causes

There are other rare causes of primary vasculitis which are beyond the scope of this chapter. In addition, there are many important secondary causes of vasculitis in adolescents,[7,9] only a few

---

Table 10.5   Secondary causes of vasculitis

- Infection
- Malignancy
- Autoimmune rheumatic disease
- Drug reactions
- Substance abuse
- Radiation vasculitis
- Transplant vasculitis
- Inflammatory bowel disease
- Retroperitoneal fibrosis
- Sarcoidosis

Table 10.6 Mimics of systemic vasculitis

- Familial Mediterranean fever
- Stevens–Johnson syndrome
- Sweet's syndrome
- Goodpasture's syndrome
- Relapsing polychondritis
- Weber–Christian disease
- Left atrial myxoma
- Antiphospholipid syndrome
- Vasospastic disorders
- Haemolytic uraemic syndrome
- Thrombotic thrombocytopenia purpura
- Ergot poisoning
- Neurofibromatosis
- Moya moya disease

vasculitis, usually involving small vessels. The important secondary causes of vasculitis that must be considered in adolescents are outlined in Table 10.5. Certain other disorders may mimic vasculitis,[7] and must also be considered in the differential diagnosis of the adolescent with possible vasculitis (Table 10.6).

CONCLUSION

The adolescent who presents with suspected vasculitis often poses a challenge to the physician. After recognizing that vasculitis is present, secondary causes such as an underlying infection, connective-tissue disease, malignancy or other disorder must always be excluded, and mimics of vasculitis must also be considered. If the adolescent appears to have a primary systemic vasculitis, careful consideration of the patient's clinical features, the laboratory and radiological investigations, and the pathological findings, should allow the clinician to make a specific diagnosis in most cases. This will ensure that patients with self-limited disease are not overtreated, and that adolescents with an aggressive form of primary systemic vasculitis receive early appropriate treatment, which can dramatically improve outcome.

of which have been reviewed briefly here. Autoimmune rheumatic diseases, including SLE, juvenile dermatomyositis, scleroderma and juvenile arthritis, particularly the RF-positive and systemic forms, can all be associated with a

REFERENCES

1. Zeek PM. Periarteritis nodosa and other forms of necrotizing angiitis. *N Engl J Med* 1953; **248**:764–72.
2. Hunder GG, Arend WP, Block DA et al. 1990 criteria for the classification of vasculitis. *Arthritis Rheum* 1990; **33**:1065–7.
3. Jennette JC, Falk RJ, Andrassy K et al. Nomenclature of systemic vasculitides: proposal of an international consensus conference. *Arthritis Rheum* 1994; **37**:187–92.
4. Fink CW. Polyarteritis and other diseases with necrotizing vasculitis in childhood. *Arthritis Rheum* 1977; **20**(suppl):378–84.
5. Davson J, Ball J, Platt R. The kidney in periarteritis nodosa. *Q J Med* 1948; **17**:175–202.
6. Fan PT, Davis JA, Somer T, Kaplan L, Bluestone R. A clinical approach to systemic vasculitis. *Semin Arthritis Rheum* 1980; **9**:248–304.
7. Churg J, Churg A. Idiopathic and secondary vasculitis: a review. *Mod Pathol* 1989; **2**:144–60.
8. Mills JA, Michel BA, Bloch DA et al. 1990 criteria for the classification of Henoch–Schönlein purpura. *Arthritis Rheum* 1990; **33**:1114–21.
9. Cassidy JT, Petty RE. Vasculitis. In: *Textbook of Pediatric Rheumatology*, 3rd edn. WB Saunders: Philadelphia, 1995:365–422.
10. Allen DM, Diamond LK, Howell DA. Anaphylactoid purpura in children (Schönlein–Henoch syndrome): review with a follow-up of the renal complications. *Am J Dis Child* 1960; **99**:833–54.
11. Winter HS. Steroid effects on the course of abdominal pain in children with Henoch–Schönlein purpura. *Pediatrics* 1987; **79**:1018–21.
12. Feldt R, Stickler GB. The gastrointestinal manifestations of anaphylactoid purpura in children. *Mayo Clin Proc* 1962; **37**:465–73.

13. Garner JAM. Acute pancreatitis as a complication of anaphylactoid (Henoch–Schönlein) purpura. *Arch Dis Child* 1977; **52**:971–2.

14. Koskimies O, Rapola J, Savilahi E et al. Renal involvement in Schönlein–Henoch purpura. *Acta Pediatr Scand* 1974; **63**:357–63.

15. Stewart M, Savage JM, Bell B et al. Long term renal prognosis of Henoch–Schönlein purpura in an unselected childhood population. *Eur J Pediatr* 1988; **147**:113–5.

16. Wright WK, Krous HF, Griswold WR et al. Pulmonary vasculitis with hemorrhage in anaphylactoid purpura. *Pediatr Pulmonary* 1994; **17**:269–71.

17. Belman AL, Leicher CR, Moshe SL, Mezey AP. Neurologic manifestations of Schönlein–Henoch purpura: a report of three cases and review of the literature. *Pediatrics* 1985; **75**:687–92.

18. Trygstad CW, Stiehm ER. Elevated serum IgA globulin in anaphylactoid purpura. *Pediatrics* 1971; **47**:1023–8.

19. Levinsky RJ, Barratt TM. IgA immune complexes in Henoch–Schönlein purpura. *Lancet* 1979; **ii**:1100–3.

20. Giangiacomo J, Tsai CC. Dermal and glomerular deposition of IgA in anaphylactoid purpura. *Am J Dis Child* 1977; **131**:981–3.

21. Baart de La Faille-Kuyper EH, Kater L, Kooiker CJ, Dorhout Mees EJ. IgA-deposits in cutaneous blood vessel walls and mesangium in Henoch–Schönlein syndrome. *Lancet* 1973; **21**:892–3.

22. Counahan R, Winterborn MH, White RHR et al. Prognosis of Henoch–Schönlein nephritis in children. *Br Med J* 1977; **2**:11–14.

23. Habib R, Cameron JS. Schönlein–Henoch purpura. In: *The Kidney and Rheumatic Diseases* (Bacon PA, Hadler NM, eds). Butterworth: London, 1982:178–201.

24. Dillon MJ, Ansell BM. Vasculitis in children and adolescents. *Rheum Dis Clin North Am* 1995; **21**:1115–36.

25. Bergstein J, Leiser J, Andreoli S. Response of crescentic Henoch–Schönlein purpura nephritis (HSP GN) to corticosteroid and azathioprine (AZA) therapy. *J Am Soc Nephrol* 1996; **7**:328.

26. Goldstein AR, White RHR, Akuse R, Chantler C. Long-term follow-up of childhood Henoch–Schönlein nephritis. *Lancet* 1992; **339**:280–2.

27. Wolkenstein P, Revuz I. Drug-induced severe skin reactions: incidence, management and prevention. *Drug Safety* 1995; **13**:56–68.

28. Kunnamo I, Kallio P, Pelkonen P et al. Serum-sickness-like disease is a common cause of acute arthritis in children. *Acta Paediatr Scand* 1986; **75**:964–9.

29. Lantin JP, Gattesco S, Duclos A et al. Anaphylactoid purpura like vasculitis following fibrinolytic therapy: role of the immune response to streptokinase. *Clin Exp Rheumatol* 1994; **12**:429–33.

30. Weinberger A, Berliner S, Pinkhas J. Articular manifestations of essential cryoglobulinemia. *Semin Arthritis Rheum* 1981; **10**:224–9.

31. Levo Y, Gorevic PD, Kassab HJ et al. Association between hepatitis B virus and essential mixed cryoglobulinemia. *N Engl J Med* 1977; **296**:1501–4.

32. Agnello V, Chung RT, Kaplan LM. A role for hepatitis C virus infection in type II cryoglobulinemia. *N Engl J Med* 1992; **327**:1490–95.

33. Agnello V, Romain PL. Mixed cryoglobulinemia secondary to hepatitis C virus infection. *Rheum Dis Clin North Am* 1996; **22**:1–21.

34. Kelen GD, Green GB, Purcell RH et al. Hepatitis B and hepatitis C in emergency department patients. *N Engl J Med* 1992; **326**:1399–404.

35. Gorevic PD, Kassab HJ, Levo Y et al. Mixed cryoglobulinemia: clinical aspects and long-term follow-up of 40 patients. *Am J Med* 1980; **69**:287–308.

36. Küssmaul A, Maier R. Über eine bisher nicht beschriebene eigenthümliche Arterienerkrankung (periarteritis nodosa), die mit Morbus Brightii und rapid fortschreitender allgemeiner Muskellähmung einhergeht. *Dtsch Arch Klin Med* 1866; **1**:484–517.

37. Reimold EW, Weinberg AG, Fink CW et al. Polyarteritis in children. *Am J Dis Child* 1976; **130**:534–41.

38. Blau EB, Morris RF, Yunis EJ. Polyarteritis nodosa in older children. *Pediatrics* 1977; **60**:227–34.

39. Petty RE, Magilavy DB, Cassidy JT et al. Polyarteritis in childhood. A clinical description of eight cases. *Arthritis Rheum* 1977; **20**(suppl):392–4.

40. Magilavy DB, Petty RE, Cassidy JT et al. A syndrome of childhood polyarteritis. *J Pediatr* 1977; **91**:25–30.

41. Ettlinger RE, Nelson AM, Burke EC et al. Polyarteritis nodosa in childhood. A clinical pathologic study. *Arthritis Rheum* 1979; **22**:820–5.

42. Frohnert PP, Sheps SG. Long-term follow-up study of periarteritis nodosa. *Am J Med* 1967; **43**:8–14.

43. Cabal E, Holtz S. Polyarteritis as a cause of intestinal hemorrhage. *Gastroenterology* 1971; **61**:99–105.
44. Ostrum BJ, Soder PD. Periarteritis nodosa complicated by spontaneous perinephritic hematoma: roentgenographic findings in three cases and a review of a literature. *Am J Roentgenol* 1960; **84**:849–60.
45. Coward RA, Hamdy NAT, Shortland JS et al. Renal micro polyarteritis: a treatable condition. *Nephrol Dialysis Transplant* 1986; **1**:31–7.
46. Diaz-Perez JL, Winkelmann RK. Cutaneous periarteritis nodosa. *Arch Dermatol* 1974; **110**:407–14.
47. Woolf AD, Wakerley G, Wallington TB et al. Factor VIII related antigen in the assessment of vasculitis. *Ann Rheum Dis* 1987; **46**:441–7.
48. Lhote F, Guillevin L. Polyarteritis nodosa, microscopic polyangiitis, and Churg-Strauss syndrome. *Rheum Dis Clin North Am* 1995; **21**:911–47.
49. Niles JL, Bottinger EP, Saurina GR et al. The syndrome of lung hemorrhage and nephritis is usually an ANCA-associated condition. *Arch Intern Med* 1996; **156**:440–5.
50. McLain LG, Bookstein JJ, Kelsch RC. Polyarteritis nodosa diagnosed by renal arteriography. *J Pediatr* 1972; **80**:1032–5.
51. Sack M, Cassidy JT, Bole GG. Prognostic factors in polyarteritis. *J Rheumatol* 1976; **2**:411–20.
52. Fauci AS, Katz P, Haynes BF et al. Cyclophosphamide therapy of severe necrotizing vasculitis. *N Engl J Med* 1979; **301**:235–8.
53. Guillevin L, Fain O, Lhote F et al. Lack of superiority of steroids plus plasma exchange to steroids alone in the treatment of polyarteritis nodosa and Churg–Strauss syndrome. A prospective randomized trial in 78 patients. *Arthritis Rheum* 1992; **35**:208–15.
54. Jennette JC, Falk RJ. Small-vessel vasculitis. *N Engl J Med* 1997; **337**:1512–23.
55. Jennette JC, Falk RJ. Diagnostic classification of antineutrophil cytoplasmic autoantibody-associated vasculitides. *Am J Kidney Dis* 1991; **18**:184–7.
56. Nolle B, Specks U, Ludemann J, Rohrbach MS, DeRemee DA, Gross WL. Anticytoplasmic autoantibodies: their immunodiagnostic value in Wegener's granulomatosis. *Ann Intern Med* 1989; **111**:28–40.
57. David J, Ansell BM, Woo P. Polyarteritis nodosa associated with *Streptococcus*. *Arch Dis Child* 1993; **69**:685–8.
58. Diaz-Perez JL, Winklemann RK. Cutaneous periarteritis nodosa: a study of 33 cases. In: *Vasculitis* (Winklemann RK, Woolf K, eds). Lloyd-Luke: London, 1980:273.
59. Kumar L, Thapa BR, Sarkar B, Walia BNS. Benign cutaneous polyarteritis nodosa in children below 10 years of age – a clinical experience. *Ann Rheum Dis* 1995; **54**:134–6.
60. Fink CW. The role of *Streptococcus* in post-streptococcal reactive arthritis and childhood polyarteritis nodosa. *J Rheumatol* 1991; **18**(suppl 29):14–20.
61. Yanagawa H, Kawasaki T, Shigematsu I. Nationwide survey on Kawasaki disease in Japan. *Pediatrics* 1987; **80**:58–62.
62. Schackelford PG, Strauss AW. Kawasaki syndrome. *N Engl J Med* 1991; **324**:1664–6.
63. Newburger JW, Takahashi M, Beiser AS et al. A single intravenous infusion of gammaglobulin as compared with four infusions in the treatment of acute Kawasaki syndrome. *N Engl J Med* 1991; **324**:1633–9.
64. Brecker SJD, Gray HH, Obedershaw PJ. Coronary artery aneurysms and myocardial infarction: adult sequelae of Kawasaki disease. *Br Heart J* 1988; **59**:509–12.
65. Duna GF, Galperin C, Hoffman GS. Wegener's granulomatosis. *Rheum Dis Clin North Am* 1995; **21**:949–86.
66. Moorthy AV, Chesney RW, Segar WE et al. Wegener granulomatosis in childhood: prolonged survival following cytotoxic therapy. *J Pediatr* 1977; **91**:616–8.
67. Orlowski JP, Clough JD, Dyment PG. Wegener's granulomatosis in the pediatric age group. *Pediatrics* 1978; **61**:83–90.
68. Hall SL, Miller LC, Duggan E et al. Wegener granulomatosis in pediatric patients. *J Pediatr* 1985; **1–6**:739–44.
69. Rottem M, Fauci AS, Hallahan DW et al. Wegener granulomatosis in children and adolescents: clinical presentation and outcome. *J Pediatr* 1993; **122**:26–31.
70. Hoffman GS, Kerr GS, Leavitt RY et al. Wegener's granulomatosis: an analysis of 158 patients. *Ann Intern Med* 1992; **116**:488–98.
71. Lebovics RS, Hoffman GS, Leavitt RY et al. The management of subglottic stenosis in patients with Wegener's granulomatosis. *Laryngoscope* 1992; **102**:1341–5.
72. van der Woude FJ, Lobatto S, Permin H, vanderGiessen M, Rasmussen N, Wiik A.

Autoantibodies against neutrophils and monocytes: tool for diagnosis and marker of disease activity in Wegener's granulomatosis. *Lancet* 1985; **i**:425–9.

73. Fauci AS, Haynes BF, Katz P et al. Wegener's granulomatosis: prospective clinical and therapeutic experience with 85 patients for 21 years. *Ann Intern Med* 1983; **98**:76–85.

74. Hoffman GS. Treatment of Wegener's granulomatosis: time to change the standard of care? *Arthritis Rheum* 1997; **40**:2099–104.

75. Guillevin L, Cordier JF, Lhote F et al. A prospective, multicenter, randomized trial comparing steroids and pulse cyclophosphamide versus steroids and oral cyclophosphamide in the treatment of generalized Wegener's granulomatosis. *Arthritis Rheum* 1997; **40**:2187–98.

76. Hoffman GS, Leavitt RY, Kerr GS et al. The treatment of Wegener's granulomatosis with glucocorticosteroids and methotrexate. *Arthritis Rheum* 1992; **35**:1322–9.

77. Leavitt RY, Hoffman GS, Fauci AS. Response: the role of trimethoprim/sulfamethoxazole in the treatment of Wegener's granulomatosis. *Arthritis Rheum* 1988; **31**:1073–4.

78. Langford CA, Sneller MC. New developments in the treatment of Wegener's granulomatosis, polyarteritis nodosa, microscopic polyangiitis, and Churg–Strauss syndrome. *Curr Opin Rheum* 1997; **9**:26–30.

79. Cromer BA, Blair JM, Mahan J et al. A prospective comparison of bone density in adolescent girls on depot medroxyprogesterone acetate (Depo-Provera), levonorgestrel (Norplant), or oral contraceptives. *J Pediatr* 1996; **129**:671–76.

80. Hagen EC, Ballieux BEPB, Daha MR, Van Es LA, van der Woude FJ. Fundamental and clinical aspects of antineutrophil cytoplasmic antibodies. *Autoimmunity* 1992; **11**:199–207.

81. Wong SN, Shah V, Dillon MJ. Anti-neutrophil cytoplasmic antibodies (ANCA) in childhood systemic vasculitis. *Eur J Pediatr* 1995; **154**:43–45.

82. Jennette JC, Falk RJ. Anti-neutrophil cytoplasmic autoantibodies: discovery, specificity, disease associations and pathogenic potential. *Adv Pathol Lab Med* 1995; **8**:363–72.

83. Cohen-Tervaert JW, van der Woude FJ, Fauci AS et al. Association between active Wegener's granulomatosis and anticytoplasmic antibodies. *Arch Intern Med* 1989; **149**:2461–5.

84. Specks U, Wheatley CL, McDonald TJ, Rohrbach MS, DeRemee DA. Anticytoplasmic autoantibodies in the diagnosis of Wegener's granulomatosis. *Mayo Clin Proc* 1989; **64**:28–36.

85. Hauschild S, Schmitt WH, Csernok E et al. ANCA in systemic vasculitides, collagen vascular disorders and inflammatory bowel diseases. In: *ANCA-associated Vasculitis* (Gross WL, ed). Plenum: New York, 1993:245–51.

86. Guillevin L, Visser H, Noël LH et al. Antineutrophil cytoplasm antibodies in systemic polyarteritis nodosa with and without hepatitis B virus infection and Churg–Strauss syndrome: 62 patients. *J Rheumatol* 1993; **20**:1345–9.

87. Pettersson E, Heigl Z. Antineutrophil cytoplasmic antibody (c-ANCA and p-ANCA) titers in relation to disease activity in patients with necrotizing vasculitis: a longitudinal study. *Clin Nephrol* 1992; **37**:219–28.

88. Jennette JC, Ewert B, Falk RJ. Do antineutrophil cytoplasmic autoantibodies cause Wegener's granulomatosis and other forms of necrotizing vasculitis? *Rheum Dis Clin North Am* 1993; **19**:1–14.

89. Falk RJ, Terrell RS, Charles LA et al. Antineutrophil cytoplasmic autoantibodies induce neutrophils to degranulate and produce oxygen radicals in vitro. *Proc Natl Acad Sci USA* 1990; **87**:4115–9.

90. Kerr GS, Fleisher TA, Hallahan CW, Leavitt RY, Fauci AS, Hoffman GS. Limited prognostic value of changes in antineutrophil cytoplasmic antibody titer in patients with Wegener's granulomatosis. *Arthritis Rheum* 1993; **36**:365–71.

91. Sneller, MC. Wegener's granulomatosis. *JAMA* 1995; **273**(16):1288–91.

92. Churg J, Strauss L. Allergic granulomatosis, allergic angiitis, and periarteritis nodosa. *Am J Pathol* 1951; **27**:277–94.

93. Frayha RA. Churg–Strauss syndrome in a child. *J Rheumatol* 1982; **9**:807–9.

94. Treitman P, Herskowitz JL, Bass HN. Churg–Strauss syndrome in a 14 year old boy diagnosed by transbronchial lung biopsy. *Clin Pediatr* 1991; **30**:502–5.

95. Chumbley LC, Harrison EG, DeRemee RA. Allergic granulomatosis and angiitis (Churg–Strauss syndrome). Report and analysis of 30 cases. *Mayo Clin Proc* 1977; **52**:477–84.

96. Haas C, Geneau C, Odinot JM et al. Allergic angiitis with granulomatosis: Churg–Strauss syndrome. *Ann Intern Med* 1991; **142**:335–42.

97. Orriols R, Roman A, Bosch J et al. Churg–Strauss syndrome: eight cases in the last 10 years. *Med Clin (Barcelona)* 1989; **92**:241–4.

98. Clutterbuck EJ, Evans DJ, Pusey C. Renal involvement in Churg–Strauss syndrome. *Nephrol Dialysis Transplant* 1990; **5**:161–7.

99. Sehgal M, Swanson JW, DeRemee RA, Colby TV. Neurologic manifestations of Churg–Strauss syndrome. *Mayo Clin Proc* 1995; **70**:337–41.

100. Lanham JG, Elkon KB, Pusey CD, Hughes GR. Systemic vasculitis with asthma and eosinophilia: a clinical approach to the Churg–Strauss syndrome. *Medicine (Baltimore)* 1984; **63**:65–81.

101. Cravioto H, Feigin I. Noninfectious granulomatous angiitis with a predilection for the nervous system. *Neurology* 1959; **9**:599–609.

102. Calabrese LH, Mallek JA. Primary angiitis of the central nervous system. *Medicine (Baltimore)* 1988; **67**:20–39.

103. Wiggelinkhuizen J, Cremin BJ. Takayasu arteritis and renovascular hypertension in childhood. *Pediatrics* 1978; **62**:209–17.

104. Lupi-Herrera E, Sanchez-Torres G, Marcushamer J, Mispireta J, Horwitz S, Vela JE. Takayasu's arteritis: clinical study of 107 cases. *Am Heart J* 1977; **93**:94–103.

105. Kerr GS, Hallahan CW, Giordano J, Leavitt RY, Fauci AS, Rottem M, Hoffman GS. Takayasu arteritis. *Ann Intern Med* 1994; **120**:919–29.

106. Hoffman GS. Takayasu arteritis: lessons from the American National Institutes of Health experience. *Int J Cardiol* 1996; **54**(suppl):S99–102.

107. Hall S, Barr W, Lie JE et al. Takayasu arteritis: a study of 32 North American patients. *Medicine* 1985; **64**:89–99.

108. Rosser E. Takayasu's arteritis as a differential diagnosis of systemic juvenile chronic arthritis. *Arch Dis Child* 1979; **54**:798–800.

109. Hall S, Nelson AM. Takayasu's arteritis and juvenile rheumatoid arthritis. *J Rheumatol* 1986; **13**:431–3.

110. Sharma BK, Jain S, Sagar S. Systemic manifestations of Takayasu arteritis: the expanding spectrum. *Int J Cardiol* 1996; **54**(suppl):S149–54.

111. Morales E, Pineda C, Martinez-Lavin M. Takayasu's arteritis in children. *J Rheumatol* 1991; **18**:1081–4.

112. Lee KS, Sohn EY, Hong CY et al. Primary arteritis (pulseless disease) in Korean children. *Acta Paediatr Scand* 1967; **56**:526–36.

113. Takayasu M. Case with unusual changes of the central retinal vessels. *Acta Soc Ophthalmol Jpn* 1908; **12**:554.

114. Lande A, Gross A. Total aortography in the diagnosis of Takayasu's arteritis. *Am J Roentgenol Rad Ther Nucl Med* 1972; **116**:165–78.

115. Hata A, Numano F. Magnetic resonance imaging of vascular changes in Takayasu arteritis. *Int J Cardiol* 1995; **52**:45–52.

116. Yamada I, Numano F, Suzuki S. Takayasu arteritis: evaluation with MR imaging. *Radiology* 1993; **188**:89–94.

117. Fraga A, Mintz G, Valle L, Flores-Izquierdo G. Takayasu's arteritis: frequency of systemic manifestations (study of twenty-two patients) and favorable response to maintenance steroid therapy with adrenocorticosteroids (twelve patients). *Arthritis Rheum* 1972; **15**:617–24.

118. Shelhamer JH, Volkman DJ, Parrillo JE et al. Takayasu's arteritis and its therapy. *Ann Intern Med* 1985; **103**:121–6.

119. Hoffman GS, Leavitt RY, Kerr GS, Rottem M, Sneller MC, Fauci AS. Treatment of glucocorticoid-resistant or relapsing Takayasu arteritis with methotrexate. *Arthritis Rheum* 1994; **37**(4):578–82.

120. Chugh KS, Jain S, Sakhuja V et al. Renovascular hypertension due to Takayasu's arteritis among Indian patients. *Q J Med* 1992; **85**: 833–43.

121. Hunder GG, Allen GL. Giant cell arteritis: a review. *Bull Rheum Dis* 1978; **29**:980–6.

122. Amato MBP, Barbas CSV, Delmonte VC, Carvalho CRR. Concurrent Churg–Strauss syndrome and temporal arteritis in a young patient with pulmonary nodules. *Am Rev Respir Dis* 1989; **139**:1539–42.

123. Tomlinson FH, Lie JT, Nienhuis BJ, Konzen KM, Groover RV. Juvenile temporal arteritis revisited. *Mayo Clin Proc* 1994; **69**:445–7.

124. Ammann AJ, Johnson A, Fyfe G et al. Behçet's syndrome. *J Pediatr* 1985; **107**:41–3.

125. Chamberlain MA. Behçet's syndrome in 32 patients in Yorkshire. *Ann Rheum Dis* 1977; **36**:491–9.

126. Sarica R, Gülsevim A, Köse A, Disçi R, Övül C, Kural Z. Juvenile Behçet's disease among 1784 Turkish Behçet's patients. *Int J Dermatol* 1996; **35**:109–11.

127. O'Duffy JD, Goldstein NP. Neurologic involvement in seven patients with Behçet's disease. *Am J Med* 1976; **61**:170–8.

128. Dilsen AN. Sacroiliitis and ankylosing spondylitis in Behçet's disease. *Scand J Rheumatol* 1975; suppl 9:abstract 20.

129. McCalmont TH, Jorizzo JL. Behçet's disease. In: *Systemic Vasculitis* (Churg A, Churg J, eds). Igaku-Shoin: New York, 1991:219–28.

130. Yazici H. Behçet's syndrome. In: *Oxford Textbook of Rheumatology* (Maddison PJ, Isenberg DA, Woo P et al, eds). Oxford University Press: Oxford, 1993:884–9.

131. Cogan DGL. Syndrome of nonsyphilitic interstitial keratitis and vestibuloauditory symptoms. *Arch Ophthalmol* 1945; **33**:144–9.

132. Kundell SP, Ochs HD. Cogan syndrome in childhood. *J Pediatr* 1980; **97**:96–8.

133. Hammer M, Witte T, Mügge A et al. Complicated Cogan's syndrome with aortic insufficiency and coronary stenosis. *J Rheumatol* 1994; **21**(3):552–5.

11

Pain syndromes

David D Sherry

INTRODUCTION

Pain is a ubiquitous human experience. It is part of our existence throughout life and, for the most part, serves to protect us by alerting us to tissue damage. Pain is the most common reason for visiting a physician. Most painful experiences are due to direct noxious stimulation and are relatively short lived. Treatment of such pain is generally rewarding for both patient and physician, since either the cause of the pain is discovered and addressed, or the pain is readily controlled by supportive care and first-line agents. Chronic pain, however, is entirely different as it does not remit and is not biologically useful. Chronic pain is a perplexing problem with a host of physiological and psychological ramifications far beyond those of acute pain. Chronic pain arising from ongoing arthritis, destroyed joints, cancer or persistent nerve injury is generally amenable to treatment of the underlying disorder or standard pain therapies and, because it originates from known disease, is more easily understood by both patient and physician. However, many patients have chronic pain without discernible cause, or have pain out of proportion to known disease. These patients are much more disconcerting and tax the diagnostic and therapeutic skills of the physician.

Pain is purely subjective and, therefore, almost without exception, is to be accepted at face value.[1] The International Association for the Study of Pain defines pain as 'an unpleasant sensory and emotional experience associated with actual or potential tissue damage, or described in terms of such damage'.[1]

The measurement and characterization of pain is difficult at best. Because pain is subjective, the measurement of pain is also subjective. This makes the scientific study of pain extremely complex; animal models are, at best, unsatisfactory, especially regarding chronic pain. The amount of pain does not equate with the amount of noxious stimulation.[2] Confounding factors include pain thresholds, suffering, disability, fear, dependency, real and imagined losses, and a host of overt and covert psychological variables. The measurement of pain in children is not reviewed here. In addition, the lack of controlled studies and patient selection variables considerably bias the majority of studies dealing with disproportional musculoskeletal pain in adolescence.

In this chapter the spectrum of patients with chronic disproportional musculoskeletal pain presenting to a paediatric rheumatology service is characterized and a therapeutic approach outlined. It is necessary to define specific terms and conditions because there is a confusing array of classification schemes and terms (see Appendix 1 at the end of this chapter). Before doing so, it is important to realize that children with chronic, disproportional (or amplified) musculoskeletal pain are on a continuum and are not easily categorized.[3–6] The nomenclature developed over the years (Table 11.1) is wanting – it presumes pathophysiological aetiology, confuses adult disease with that which occurs in childhood and adolescence, and uses terms that

Table 11.1   Various names for the disproportional musculoskeletal pain syndromes

- Disproportional musculoskeletal pain with overt autonomic dysfunction:
  - reflex sympathetic dystrophy
  - reflex neurovascular dystrophy
  - algodystrophy
  - complex regional pain syndrome, types I and II
  - Sudeck's atrophy
  - shoulder–hand syndrome
  - traumatic angiospasm
  - algoneurodystrophy
  - causalgia, major or minor
  - localized idiopathic pain syndrome

- Disproportional musculoskeletal pain without overt autonomic dysfunction, continuous:
  - psychogenic musculoskeletal pain
  - psychosomatic musculoskeletal pain
  - pseudodystrophy
  - diffuse idiopathic pain syndrome
  - localized idiopathic pain syndrome

- Disproportional musculoskeletal pain without overt autonomic dysfunction, intermittent:
  - psychogenic musculoskeletal pain
  - psychosomatic musculoskeletal pain
  - ? growing pains

- Disproportional musculoskeletal pain with painful points:
  - fibromyalgia
  - fibrositis
  - diffuse idiopathic pain syndrome

- Disproportional musculoskeletal pain due to hypervigilance
  - psychogenic musculoskeletal pain
  - psychosomatic musculoskeletal pain
  - ? growing pains

are emotionally laden.[5–8] The presentation, manifestations and consequences of these conditions in adolescents differ significantly from those in adults with these conditions, so applying what we know about adults is not necessarily best. Rather than a pedagogic classification scheme, a descriptive approach has been adopted. Even this may be a source of confusion, since patients will overlap the arbitrary divisions between conditions or have a variety of these conditions (Figure 11.1). One reason to group these patients together is that most paediatric patients respond well to a vigorous exercise treatment programme, regardless of classification type. However, in order to be faithful to the literature, when quoting studies directly the author's term will be used.

Disproportional musculoskeletal pain syndromes can be divided into the following major categories: those with overt autonomic signs, those without overt autonomic signs (continuous pain or intermittent pain subtypes), those with widespread pain with painful points at fibromyalgia locations, and those with hypervigilance. Conditions with overt autonomic signs have commonly been called reflex sympathetic dystrophy, reflex neurovascular dystrophy, algodystrophy, idiopathic regional pain or, more recently, complex regional pain syndrome, type I. The latter is the preferred term in adults.[1,7] Causalgia, or complex regional pain syndrome, type II, is rare in childhood and is a subset of those conditions with overt autonomic signs.[1] Conditions without overt autonomic signs have been called psychogenic pain, psychosomatic pain, idiopathic regional or idiopathic diffuse pain, pseudodystrophy or growing pains.[3,6,9] Fibromyalgia, as defined by the American College of Rheumatology (ACR)[10] or by Yunus and Masi,[11] exists in adolescents and pre-adolescents, but the name is unhelpful since the treatment is similar to that for the other adolescent disproportional musculoskeletal pain syndromes and differs from that for adults with fibromyalgia. Children with overt autonomic signs (complex regional pain syndrome, type I) are also distinct from adult patients. Children much less frequently have major

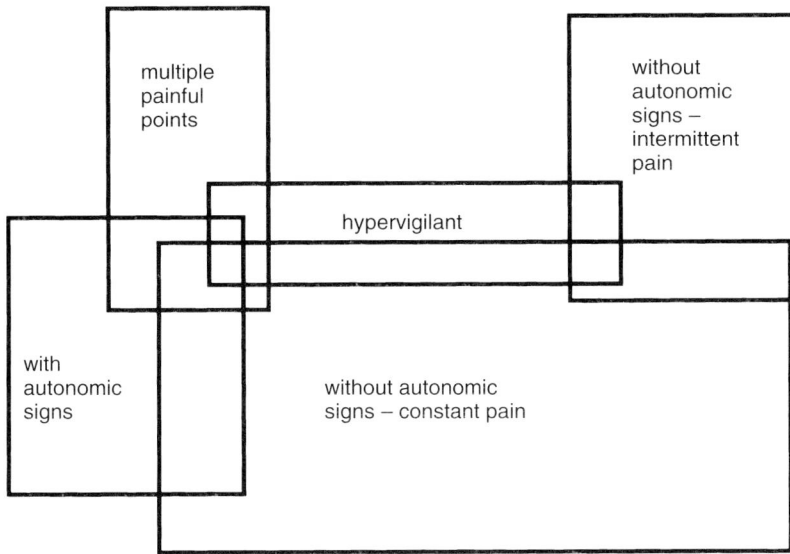

Figure 11.1 Overlapping nature of the disproportional musculoskeletal pain syndromes in children and adolescents.

trauma preceding the condition, have predominantly lower extremity (as opposed to upper extremity) disease, have a different technetium bone-scan pattern, and respond well to exercise therapy alone.[5,12–18] Thus, labelling a paediatric patient with fibromyalgia, complex regional pain syndrome, type I, reflex sympathetic dystrophy, or psychogenic pain can confuse the patient and family.

Historical notes

The first modern description of childhood limb pains not readily attributed to recognized pathology was given by Naish and Apley.[19] In this classic description, the authors recognized two large groups of patients: one with emotional disturbances and a frequent family history of rheumatic disease, and another group who were emotionally stable but had a family history of similar pains. A smaller group was identified as having psychological pain without other associations. In these children the term 'limb pain' was preferred over 'growing pain', and limb pain was defined as pain existing at least 3 months, not specifically located to the joints, and of sufficient

severity to interrupt normal activities. 'Growing pains' is a poorly defined term referring to a wide variety of vague limb pains and is not associated with growth.[19] This term was distinctly disliked by Apley, who later wrote: 'growing does not hurt but growing up can hurt like hell'.[20] Subsequent studies of limb pain in childhood looked at the frequency of complaints in schoolchildren, which was about 20%.[21] In 1991, the first large group of children with severe musculoskeletal pain who were referred to a paediatric rheumatology centre were described in detail, and exercise treatment with psychological evaluation was suggested.[5]

Overt autonomic disease, as one would expect, was recognized early in the modern era of medicine. Mitchell, Morehouse and Keen[22] are credited with the first description of causalgia in their treatise of nerve injuries sustained in gunshot victims of the American Civil War. Over the next half century a vast array of diagnoses were used for a wide variety of disproportional musculoskeletal pain syndromes. In 1947, Evans[23] coined the term 'reflex sympathetic dystrophy'. It was not until 1971 that the first description of reflex sympathetic dystrophy in a young child appeared.[24] Then, in 1978 Bernstein et al[12] described the first large group of children with reflex neurovascular dystrophy, and outlined a very successful exercise treatment.

Non-articular chronic rheumatism was a vague term used in the nineteenth century. Early in the twentieth century the term 'fibrosis' was introduced, but was not widely used until the 1960s. In the following decade, the term 'fibromyalgia' was preferred, due to the lack of demonstrable inflammation. The first large group of patients with fibromyalgia was described in 1981 by Yunus et al,[25] and in 1985 Yunus and Masi reported on 33 children.[11] In 1990, the ACR published criteria for classification of fibromyalgia.[10] However, the standardization of the determination of a painful point is quite recent.[26]

EPIDEMIOLOGY

In virtually all series, children with amplified, disproportional musculoskeletal pain are predominantly female (80%). This may be a selection bias since, at least in adults, women more frequently seek medical advice for pain than do men. Given the degree of pain and dysfunction this is probably not a major factor in paediatric patients. Although not formally studied, it is the impression of many that these conditions occur more frequently in those of higher socio-economic status and, in the USA, that proportionally more Caucasians are diagnosed.[16]

The age of onset of these conditions peaks, in paediatric clinics, in pre- and early adolescents (mean age generally around 12 or 13 years). The relatively fewer older adolescents with chronic pain syndromes may reflect referral patterns. The youngest children with pain syndromes reported are 3 years old, and they are generally considered rare under the age of 7 years.[12,13,27,28] Very careful consideration needs to be given before young children are diagnosed with disproportional musculoskeletal pain.

In schoolchildren, the prevalence of musculoskeletal pain, but not disproportional musculoskeletal pain, has been reported to be as high as 20% for back pain,[29] 16% for limb pain[21,30] and 6%

for fibromyalgia.[31] In North American rheumatology centres, about 6% of new patients have a disproportional musculoskeletal pain syndrome, excluding hypermobility and growing pains.[32,33]

Pain syndromes have been reported in siblings, as well as in parent/child pairs (usually mother/daughter)[34–37] and spouses.[38] In one study of 17 adults with fibromyalgia, all patients had other family members involved.[39] No in-depth human leucocyte antigen (HLA) or other genetic studies have been done, except one involving 15 women with reflex sympathetic dystrophy in which levels of A3, B7 and DR2 were increased over controls.[40] Interestingly, those with DR2 did not respond to routine treatment.

AETIOLOGY

The aetiology of disproportional musculoskeletal pain in children is not known. In some it seems to be causally related to injury, illness or psychological distress.

Injury

In adults with overt autonomic signs, major trauma frequently precedes the onset of the disproportional pain and autonomic signs. In two studies a quarter of adults who had a Colles' wrist fracture were found to have features of algodystrophy at 9 weeks[41] and at 10 years[42] following the injury. Reflex neurovascular dystrophy in adults has been described after surgery, usually surgery on the musculoskeletal system. It is uncommon in childhood for significant trauma to be a primary causal agent, although it does occur. Usually the trauma is not subtle and includes injury due to intramuscular injection, musculoskeletal surgery or injury to the central nervous system.[43–46] However, in many children minor trauma plays a role in localizing the area of the body affected by the disproportional pain. Minor trauma due to hypermobility has been associated with the presence of fibromyalgia in schoolchildren.[47] Determining if injury is a causal agent in any individual child with one of these syndromes is quite difficult, since disproportional musculoskeletal pain can arise in the absence of trauma, and children and adolescents experience some degree of trauma almost daily. Post-traumatic stress disorder may be a further complication in those with significant trauma or emotional upset.[48,49] The problem seems to be compounded when courts or insurance companies are involved in lawsuits or claims arising from an alleged causal injury.

Illness

In adult patients, pain syndromes, especially those with overt autonomic signs, have followed myocardial infarction or other acute illness.[50] Many relate this to the trauma associated with medical care. This kind of response to acute illness has not been reported in children, with the exception of one patient with repeated reflex sympathetic dystrophy with systemic lupus erythematosus.[51]

A whole array of prior and concurrent illnesses in adolescents with disproportional musculoskeletal pain has been observed. Illness may obfuscate the diagnosis of disproportional musculoskeletal pain, and it is difficult, at best, to determine if the illness itself was a causal agent, a coincidental finding or in some other fashion predisposed the patient to develop a disproportional musculoskeletal pain syndrome. In my experience, various juvenile chronic arthritides (both active arthritis and a history of arthritis) have been the most common. I have, in addition, seen adolescents with cerebral palsy, leukaemia and muscular dystrophy who have developed a disproportional musculoskeletal pain syndrome.

Psychological distress

The majority of children or families with pain syndromes seem to manifest various degrees of psychopathology, although no controlled studies have been done.[12,27,34,52–54] It is not clear whether the abnormal psychodynamics displayed in these families are the cause or an effect of the pain syndrome. Factors implicated include a neglect-like syndrome, helplessness, post-traumatic stress disorder, anxiety disorder, depression, affective loss, fear avoidance and role models.[34,48,49,55–61] Other studies have failed to find a psychological aetiology for the disproportional musculoskeletal pain syndromes.[52,53,62] Whether they are the cause or an effect of pain syndromes, I think it is mandatory for the physician and team to pay attention to the psychodynamics involved as well as the psychological impact of the diagnosis and treatment. Most patients should have a psychological evaluation investigating all the realms of their lives (see below).[3,5,12,27]

Other factors

There may be age, genetic, hormonal and environmental causes of pain syndromes that are not fully elucidated at present. Paediatric patients with temporomandibular joint dysfunction and facial pain were more likely to have a primary psychopathology than were adults (25% vs 7%, respectively).[63] Chronic pain occurs more frequently if there is a family history of similar pain or conditions, and tends to be more prevalent in Caucasians.[16,19,21,34,64–67] Whether the pain is due to role models for pain or specific genetic causes has not been determined. Pre-adolescents and adolescents develop pain syndromes much more frequently than do younger children.

That specific hormonal factors may be involved is, at present, speculation at best, and the reason more females have these conditions is unknown. Pain thresholds in females are lower than in males. The reasons for this are not clear. Sleep disorders have been related to the development of fatigue and painful points, as has hypermobility, which also is more frequent in females. Physiological differences, cultural expectations or coping may be part of the difference between the sexes.[68–70] As mentioned above, women are more likely to seek medical attention for pain. In addition, females have a higher incidence of conditions thought to be manifestations of psychological distress, such as anorexia nervosa, irritable bowel syndrome, depression, headache, conversion disorders and suicide attempts. If psychological distress proves to be a significant cause of these conditions, it seems reasonable that they would manifest during the pre-adolescent and adolescent years, given the psychological tasks imposed in western societies on this age group and given the psycho-developmental changes that adolescents undergo.

PATHOPHYSIOLOGY

Pain is the end result of a complex pathway starting at peripheral nociceptors, transmission through a variety of nerves and spinal-cord tracts, and final processing in the thalamus and cerebral cortex.[71] Pain is modulated by a host of factors, including chemical mediators and descending pathways under the influence of the central nervous system at multiple levels.[72]

Although we know much about the nervous pathways, transmitters and modulators, the reasons for the activation and perpetuation of the pain in disproportional musculoskeletal pain syndromes are poorly understood.[2,58,71,73–76] Some of these conditions, especially those with overt autonomic signs, are a direct consequence of either increased sympathetic nerve activity or an increased α-adrenoceptor responsiveness.[77] This has been measured by a variety of methods including thermography, thermal stress testing, resting sweat output and differential skin potential responses.[78–81] These patients are likely to have an initial response to sympathetic nerve blockade, but this is highly variable.[78] Even in this small subset of patients, different primary afferents have been implicated in the pain response.[73] Less is known about the pathways involved in those conditions without overt autonomic signs. However, some of these patients have had prior or subsequent episodes of disproportional musculoskeletal pain with overt autonomic signs, and therefore the mechanism may be similar but not to the same degree. Therefore, if present, the autonomic abnormalities are below the level of clinical detection.[5]

If, at some level, sympathetic nervous system overactivity is present in these conditions, the common final pathway may be ischaemia. A few children with overt autonomic signs have had biopsies of the affected areas and ischaemic

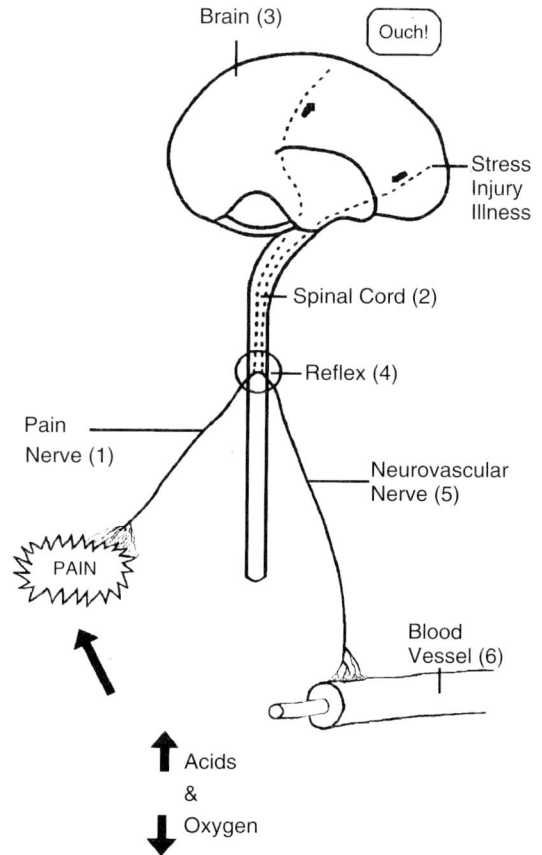

Figure 11.2 Model for the aetiology and pathogenesis of disproportional musculoskeletal pain in adolescents. A painful signal goes from the pain nerves (1) up the spinal cord (2) and to the brain (3), where the signal is interpreted as painful. In this condition, there is an abnormal short circuit in the spinal cord (4) to the nerves (5); these neurovascular nerves go to the blood vessels (6). These nerves make the blood vessels to the bones, muscle, skin and other tissues smaller, decreasing the amount of oxygen that these tissues receive. The lack of oxygen and build up of acids cause intense pain. The pain then goes back up the pain nerves, up to the spinal cord, across the abnormal reflex, and back to the neurovascular nerves. This vicious cycle goes on and on, amplifying the pain.

changes have been noted.[82] Decreased blood flow on both the blood pool and delayed images of technetium-99 radionucleotide scans lend support to ischaemia as a factor in the production or maintenance of pain. However, a number of patients have either normal or increased uptake of technetium-99 on bone scans. Nuclear magnetic resonance spectroscopy showed a significant increase in the pH of affected muscles due to either cellular hypoxia or decreased oxygen utilization.[83] Arteriograms may be normal or show decreased perfusion.[15,84] Some studies in adults with fibromyalgia have suggested ischaemic muscles, although this is not a uniform finding.[85–87]

A model for the pathophysiology of disproportional musculoskeletal pain based on sympathetically mediated pain amplification has been developed (Figure 11.2). This model gives the patient and family a tangible framework within which to understand the amplification and perpetuation of pain. It also allows the clinician to discuss the various possible aetiological factors with the patient and family and introduce the therapeutic plan.

CLINICAL MANIFESTATIONS

The clinical presentation of children with pain syndromes is remarkably consistent. As the physician obtains the medical history and examines the patient a characteristic pattern is seen, as detailed below. The history of present illness and physical examination of the skin and musculoskeletal systems varies with the subset of the condition, but the rest of the history and physical features are fairly similar between subtypes.

History of present illness

Disproportional musculoskeletal pain with overt autonomic signs
Most of these patients will remember precisely, or close to precisely, when the pain started. The pain is more common in the lower extremity and frequently minor trauma is either recalled or supposed, such as 'I must have twisted my ankle because it hurt after playing basketball'. The pain is not as intense or as disabling at first, but over a few days (or, occasionally, over a few hours) insidiously increases to such a point that medical care is sought. It is generally in these first few days that colour and temperature changes are noted; the vast majority describe the limb as looking purple, blue or grey, and being cool or cold to the touch, distinctly different from the contralateral limb. A patient will rarely complain of perspiration changes between the limbs. It is distinctly unusual for children to develop heat and redness as an initial sign of autonomic dysfunction. Oedema is not uncommon. Allodynia develops over the first few days, and most patients will be unable to wear shoes and socks, tolerate bedcovers, touch their foot to the floor (or hold a pen if the hand is involved) or adequately wash the limb. Some patients even complain that drafts from opening doors or people walking by cause extreme pain.

The intensity of the pain is marked, with most rating the pain as 9–10 out of 10 (with 10 being the most intense pain imaginable). It is not uncommon for the pain to be rated higher than 10. The location of the pain may spread over time and may occur in different sites, but this is more common in those without overt autonomic signs.

By this time most patients have become increasingly dysfunctional and are unable to attend school, do simple household chores or participate in social activities, and they may even lose the ability to perform the daily activities of living. Those with lower extremity pain will not bear weight and will get around either by using crutches or hopping. Many will report that they crawl to get around the house, which, in our experience, is almost unique to those with disproportional musculoskeletal pain.

Initial home remedies such as ice or heat and over-the-counter medications are usually not successful. Tension bandages or immobilization with a splint or cast usually leads to increased pain or, at minimum, no diminution in pain.

By this time initial medical care has been sought and first-line treatments have failed. Analgesics (including those containing opioids), non-steroidal agents, splints and casts have no lasting effect. I have seen patients who have failed prior intravenous morphine, epidural blocks, multiple sympathetic blocks and a host of chronic pain medications such as antidepressants and anticonvulsants. However, I do have a selection bias for those who have failed therapy. A few patients do not tolerate any sort of medicine due to persistent and severe subjective side-effects. The severity of pain continues to increase despite these measures.

Disproportional musculoskeletal pain without overt autonomic signs, continuous pain

The history of these patients is very similar to that of patients who do have overt autonomic signs, except that there is no history of colour, temperature or perspiration changes to the affected limb. The exact time of onset of the pain may not be recalled. More frequently there may be multiple painful sites, and some patients have total body pain (even complaining of severe pain when their hair is lightly touched). A number of these patients will have more centrally located pain, including the head, jaw, teeth, back, chest, abdomen, buttocks or genitals. Those with more widespread pain are among the most severely disabled; some cannot perform the most basic of daily activities such as feeding and toileting themselves.

Disproportional musculoskeletal pain without overt autonomic signs, intermittent pain

These patients report that, on the night after an active day, such as playing a sport, and for the next several days they experience severe, widespread musculoskeletal pain that prohibits school attendance or other activities. They usually have obvious pain behaviours, such as crying that will keep the household awake at night. The amount of disability is marked; many are unable to walk or care for themselves during these few days. The pain resolves without residua, only to recur in either a predictable manner after activity or, at times, randomly.

Disproportional musculoskeletal pain without overt autonomic signs but with multiple painful points

These patients report similar increasing pain over time as the patients with disproportional

musculoskeletal pain without overt autonomic signs. Trauma may coincide with the onset of these pains. About half of these patients report fatigue as a major factor in their disability, and poor sleep, or at least, not feeling rested after rising in the morning (even if allowed to sleep in). Feelings of melancholia and frank depression are reported more frequently in this subset of disproportional musculoskeletal pains.

Disproportional musculoskeletal pain with multiple painful points in the paediatric age group may be different from fibromyalgia in adults. Differences include outcome, treatment response, prevalence of comorbid conditions such as depression, chronic fatigue syndrome (which, some have argued, should not be diagnosed in childhood), irritable bowel syndrome and sleep disorders.[11,88,89] Therefore, applying both the label and the prognosis may be a disservice to the patient.

Disproportional musculoskeletal pain due to hypervigilance

These patients generally function well but have pain when paying attention to the body part in question.[6] They complain of pain that is generally fleeting, lasting a few seconds to less than 30 minutes. The pain may be more frequent and severe following activity. The activity associated with pain may be a normal activity; for example, 'I sprain my ankle every time I walk'. The pain usually occurs in a variety of areas over time. Patients frequently report that they do not notice the pain until they stop and think about it. Occasionally they have short-lived dysfunction, again when focused on either the pain or the activity; for example, 'I can walk unless I think about how to'. I have had two adolescents report very short-lived pain from feeling their blood flow through their veins. Patients with other forms of disproportional musculoskeletal pain may become hypervigilant to new sensations, especially as they start exercising. Inquiry about what they fear may be causing the pain may be quite revealing, since anxiety seems to be a common feature among these patients. Some of these patients have had prior major illnesses, and their disproportional musculoskeletal pain may be a manifestation of vulnerable child syndrome.[90]

Past history and review of systems

Most of these children have been well except for the usual childhood illnesses. Notable exceptions include prior evaluation, frequently without definitive diagnosis, for chronic abdominal pain and headaches. These are usually not a significant ongoing problem at the presentation of disproportional musculoskeletal pain. Breathing problems, such as reactive airway symptoms, feeling short of breath and episodes of hyperventilation, are not uncommon. A notable few will identify symptoms with every body system. Fatigue is common in those with painful points and, at times, is the major reason for disability. Not necessarily in conjunction with fatigue, patients may complain of poor sleep in that they are not rested after adequate hours of sleep. Insomnia and frequent waking are common complaints. It is not uncommon for the child to be described as a poor healer, meaning that simple lacerations and fractures take an inordinate amount of time to heal.

Conversion symptoms such as paralysis, numbness and even blindness tend to be more common in those without overt autonomic signs and those with painful points. In these subsets, there tend to be more psychiatric diagnoses, especially depression, as well as suicide attempts, and anxiety or adjustment disorders. Eating disorders have been seen in all pain syndrome subtypes.

Family history

The family history may be remarkable in two areas. First, there may be a role model for a very similar pain or chronic musculoskeletal pain in the family or a close family friend.[5,11,27,36,37,56] Again, no controlled studies are available, so it is possible that the presence of a chronic pain in the patient may indicate a higher family prevalence. The onset of the family member's pain may closely precede the child's; for example, a father suffering a fractured foot a couple of months before the onset of foot pain in the adolescent daughter. Secondly, there may be a family member with a recently diagnosed major illness. This can medically sensitize family members to be more aware of body aches and pains and also be a source of anxiety about one's health. Sibling illness has been associated with an increase in somatic complaints.[91]

Social history

It is helpful to know the major life events of the patient that have occurred within the last few years.[70,92–95] These may centre on school and peer interactions, family changes, including interpersonal interactions, or extracurricular activities. Many of these children are quite accomplished, both in school and in extracurricular areas. Of particular interest is the occurrence of these syndromes in high-level athletes, including dancers.[96,97] The patient's sport may complicate the diagnosis and treatment (stress fractures, overuse syndromes and the patient's performance expectations). Generally these patients are perfectionists who internalize their feelings and go out of their way to win approval from adults and peers.[27,56] They sacrifice meeting their own needs in order to meet the needs of others.

While obtaining a social history, it is important to discuss the role that psychological stress plays either in augmenting the pain or as a consequence of the pain. For those children for whom psychological stress does play a significant role, it is important to have all these issues discussed initially rather than later. This will avoid the appearance that psychological factors were an afterthought.

Physical examination

Most children with pain syndromes do not have underlying secondary illness, and therefore the absence of any signs of organic disease is paramount. Careful attention to the neurological examination is mandatory. In addition, a complete examination is reassuring to both patient and parent that other subtle illnesses have not been overlooked.

One of the most striking features of pain syndromes is the incongruent affect that most of these children display.[5,27,56] They will describe hyperbolic pain and rate it a 10 out of 10 with aplomb. There are a few children with marked pain behaviours, such as crying or screaming when the affected body part is touched or moved, but this is rare. Most children will allow repeated touching or use of their limb without observable pain behaviours, and appear to be quite cheerful. The typical child will have allodynia (pain generated by normally non-painful stimuli). This is ascertained by light touch or gently pinching a fold of skin between the skin between the forefinger and thumb. The border of allodynia will vary during the examination, sometimes by as much as 10 cm. Not uncommonly, if a blood sample is obtained, hyperalgesia with great dramatics ensues. The distribution of pain is non-anatomic in that it does not follow the distribution of either the nerve root or a peripheral nerve. In children with overt autonomic signs the limb will be cyanotic, dusky and cold, and, not uncommonly, will show mild diffuse oedema (Figure 11.3). Occasionally, perspiration is increased. Rarely, there are dystrophic skin changes with hyperkeratosis, increased coarse hair growth, a waxy brawny thickness to the skin and diminished peripheral pulses (Figure 11.4). Frequently the autonomic signs are best revealed after the limb is used.

When describing their symptoms, the majority of children with display *la belle indifference*. They seem unconcerned regarding the amount of pain and disability they are experiencing. They may refer to their limb as 'it' and will neglect it.[55,70]

Another striking phenomenon exhibited by the majority of patients is that of compliance. Patients who are non-ambulatory on presentation due to foot pain will repeatedly walk when requested to do so. This can surprise not only the parents, but also the patient. The degree of compliance I have seen in this condition is much greater than with other worrying illnesses such as arthritis, osteomyelitis, septic joints, leukaemia and myositis.

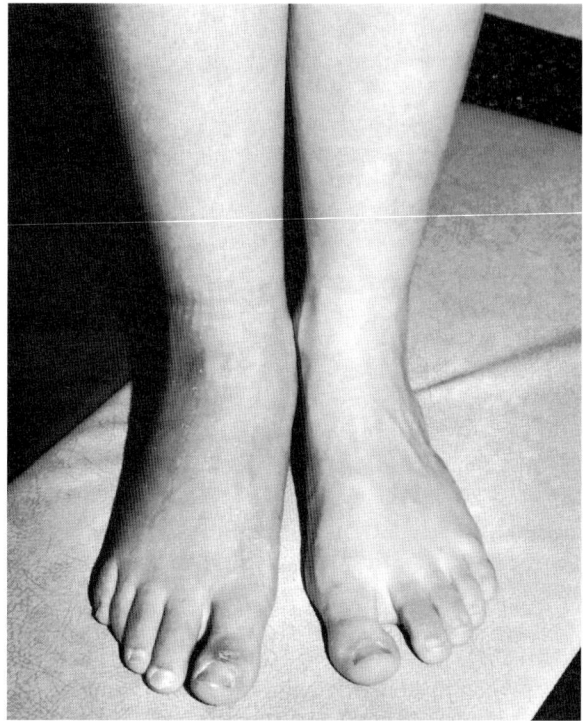

Figure 11.3 Overt autonomic dysfunction. The foot is oedematous, cold and cyanotic. This adolescent girl had marked allodynia (it took several minutes before she would touch the mat with her painful foot) and was completely asymptomatic after 2 weeks of exercise therapy.

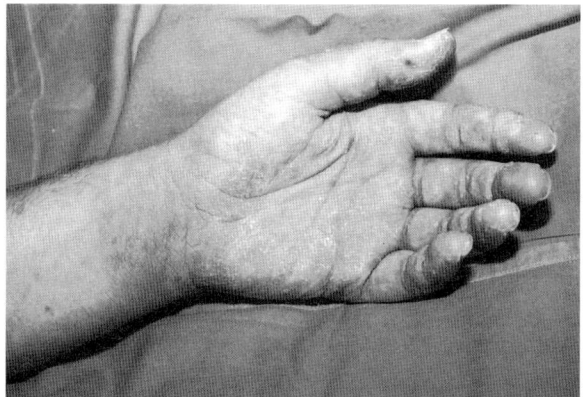

Figure 11.4 Dystrophic changes in the hand of an adolescent with disproportional musculoskeletal pain with overt autonomic dysfunction. The patient had not moved his hand for 3 months and was completely asymptomatic after 3 days of exercise therapy.

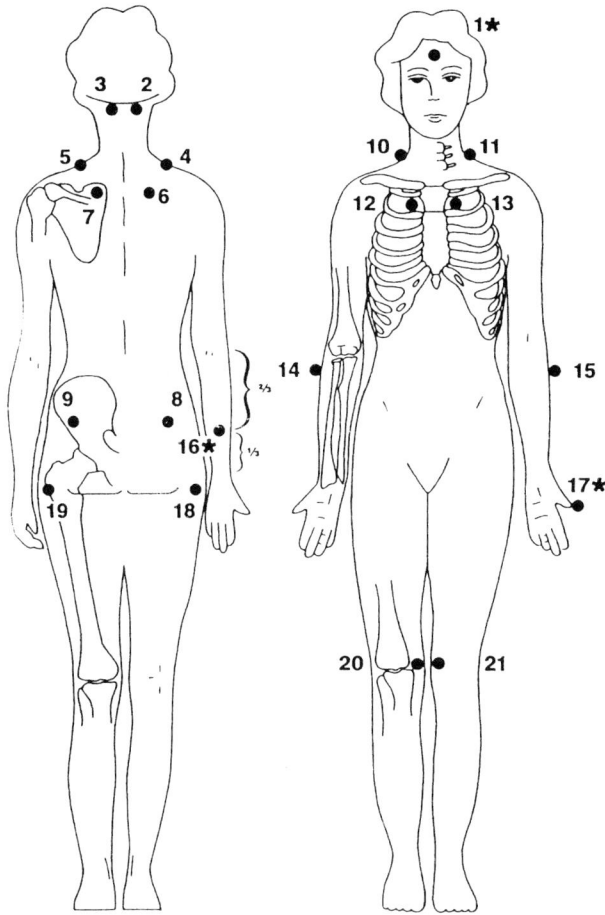

Survey and Control* Sites

SEATED	Right	Left
Mld-Forehead(*):	1.__*__	
Occiput: Suboccipital muscle insertions	2.____	3.____
Trapezius: Midpoint of upper border	4.____	5.____
Supraspinatus: Above medial border of scapular spine	6.____	7.____
Gluteal: Upper outer quadrant of buttocks	8.____	9.____
Low Cervical: Anterior aspect of intertransverse space of C5-7	10.____	11.____
2nd Rib: 2nd costochondral junction	12.____	13.____
Lateral Epicondyle: 2 cm distal to epicondyle	14.____	15.____
Dorsum R Forearm(*): Junction of proximal ⅔ & distal ½	16.__*__	
L Thumbnail (*):		17.__*__
SIDE		
Greater Trochanter: Posterior to trochanteric prominence	18.____	19.____
SUPINE		
Knee: Medial fat pad proximal to the joint line	20.____	21.____

Figure 11.5 The painful points in fibromyalgia as defined by the American College of Rheumatology.[10] (See Appendix 1.) From Okifuji et al,[26] with permission.

Painful points should be examined in all patients presenting with a disproportional pain. In adults the standard is for the examiner to use his or her thumb to apply perpendicularly 4 kg of pressure on each spot. It has been suggested by one author that 3 kg may sufficiently discriminate these spots in children.[31] Painful points have been described over multiple body areas. According to the 1990 ACR[10] criteria for fibromyalgia in adults there are 18 discriminating spots, 11 of which should be reported as painful, not just uncomfortable (Figure 11.5). Okifuji et al[26] have described a standardized examination of these spots. Yunus and Masi[11] suggested 5 of 59 spots (Figure 11.6).

In addition to the painful spot determination, control spots should also be examined such as the thumbnail, forearm, outer third of the clavicle, forehead or shin. Some patients report pain at every place where their body is touched. Whether one views these patients as having the painful spot subset of this condition is debatable. I prefer to classify them as having disproportional pain without overt autonomic signs rather than as those with specific painful points, as no one spot is any more painful than another.

Hypermobility has been related to disproportional musculoskeletal pain with painful points.[47] The classic signs of hypermobility include the ability to passively touch the forearm with the

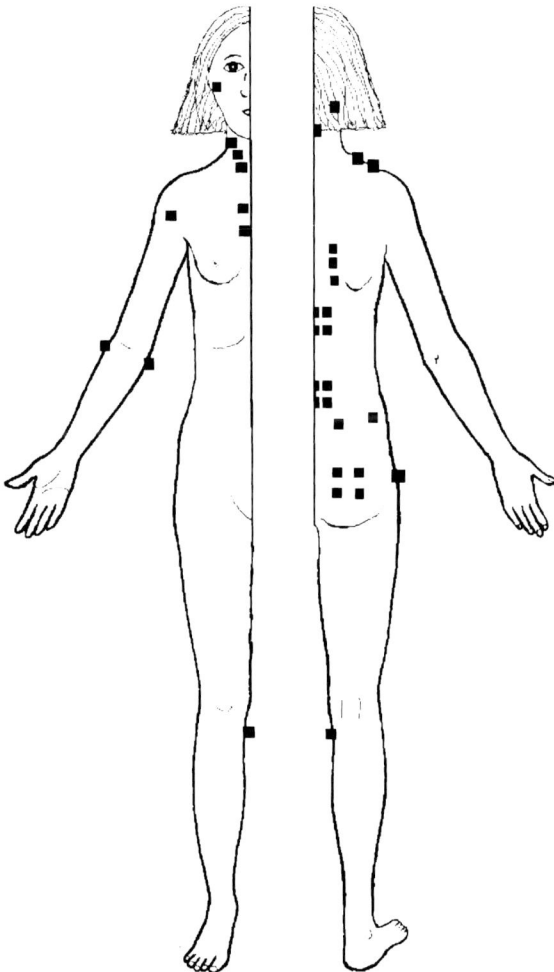

Figure 11.6 The painful points of fibromyalgia as defined by Yunus and Masi.[11]

body habitus may need ophthalmological and cardiac surveillance for dislocated lenses and aortic aneurysms.

Back pain can be quite a perplexing problem in adolescents, although it occurs in up to 21% of schoolchildren.[29,34,98,99] Back pain in adolescents and children should always be taken seriously as, more often than is the case in adults, it is due to non-trivial illness; neoplasias are not unusual. When evaluating the back, one should specifically check for non-organic back signs. These include axial loading, distracted straight-leg raising, passive rotation, allodynia and overreaction.[100] Axial loading is performed with the patient standing and the examiner applying downward pressure on the patient's head. If positive (non-organic), the patient reports back pain (some mild neck pain can be normal). A positive distracted straight-leg raising test is one in which the patient reports back pain when the hip is flexed with the knee extended when supine but not when seated and attention is diverted away from the back. Overreaction includes exaggerated wincing, loudly saying ouch, or collapsing in pain.

Patients with hypervigilance will, during the course of the interview and examination, complain of very fleeting short-lived body pains. These can arise without any stimulation or may be identified as painful when the examiner is touching or manipulating that area of the body. These pains cause no specific dysfunction and are associated with no other symptoms or signs.

During the history and examination one frequently observes inappropriate interaction between the parent (usually the mother) and child indicating emotional enmeshment (skewing of personal boundaries so the mother's and daughter's emotional lives are overly involved with one another).[5,27] Manifestations of this include secret communication between parent and child with body language, overtly close physical contact, expressions of pain and suffering of the parent because of the child's symptoms, and the parent frequently speaking for the child inappropriately. The parent's obsession with the child's illness is manifest by extensive documentation and research. Rarely do families of adolescents with

ipsilateral thumb, extend the metacarpal phalange joint to parallel the forearm, extend the elbow and knee beyond 10° of hyperextension, and place the palms on the floor while bending forward with the knees straight. Other signs include flexible flat feet, increased hip rotation, and passively touching the elbows behind the back. Small joint effusions may be present. It is important in hypermobile patients to look for signs of one of the more significant forms of Ehlers–Danlos syndrome. Those with hyperelastic skin, thin, cigarette paper scars, or abnormal inflammatory rheumatic conditions bring such dossiers to the visit. A major reason to be especially circumspect in the labels we apply to these patients is the parent's need for information. They confuse lay and professional information, and information on adult and paediatric patients, and try to apply information from patient groups (or single case reports) to their individual situation. Although this is an attempt to be helpful, it can undermine the diagnosis and treatment.

Laboratory evaluation

Patients with very typical disproportional musculoskeletal pain with or without overt autonomic signs and no other signs of underlying disease can be confidently diagnosed at the first visit. Further testing is contraindicated, as focusing on the possibility that some disease is going to be discovered undermines the diagnosis and treatment of the disproportional musculoskeletal pain. Abnormal tests, even if totally unrelated to possible causes of the pain, serve to divert attention, increase costs and can generate new worries for the family. Therefore, any testing should be done only if clear indications are present.

However, most patients have undergone prior testing. Blood counts, indexes of inflammation (erythrocyte sedimentation rate and C-reactive protein), and serological tests are normal or reflect background levels unless there is an underlying organic illness or condition. The most common finding is a low titre antinuclear antibody (ANA) test, which represents normal background and should be discounted. In some laboratories, 10% of children will have a slightly positive ANA test; repeating it only leads to doubt, anxiety and delay.

Radiographs are normal or, depending on the duration of disuse, will show generalized osteoporosis. The spotty osteoporosis seen in adults with complex regional pain syndromes has not been reported in adolescents. Serendipitously discovered bone lesions, such as a fibrous bone cyst, may focus the patient's and family's attention to that area and a new disproportional musculoskeletal pain may develop. Reassurance by an orthopaedic surgeon may be required to

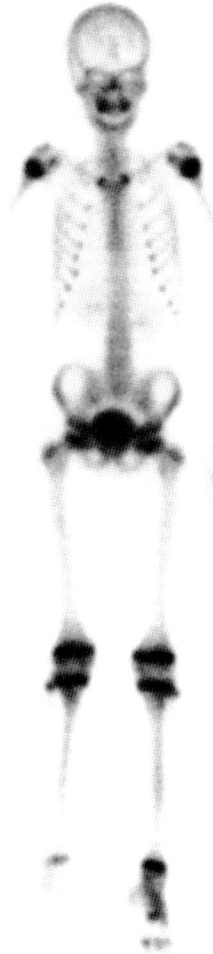

Figure 11.7 A bone scan showing decreased uptake of technetium-99 in the symptomatic foot.

allay anxiety about treatment possibly aggravating the cyst or the cyst causing the pain.

Probably the most useful study, if in doubt, is a technetium-99 radionucleotide bone scan.[16,101] A normal scan gives reassurance that there is no occult pathology such as an osteoid osteoma or stress fracture. The most common abnormality seen in adolescents is decreased uptake in the affected limb (Figure 11.7). Less common is the spotty increased uptake pattern that is characteristic of the complex regional pain syndromes in adults.[18]

Magnetic resonance images are generally normal. Nerve conduction velocities can be normal or slightly slowed in the limb affected by disproportional musculoskeletal pain with overt autonomic signs.[15,102] They have not been studied in the other forms of disproportional musculoskeletal pain in adolescents.

Psychological evaluation

The psychological aspects of pain syndromes have been commented on since the first case report in a child.[24] In most patients an individual evaluation and evaluation of family psychodynamics are warranted and, if the history is suggestive, a school evaluation should also be made.[5,12,27,28,93,95,103] The patient and family should have a psychological interview with either a skilled social worker or psychologist. In our clinic, they fill in a battery of psychological measures to evaluate individual distress, family environment and marital adjustment. Our hospital's school teacher obtains both first-hand reports from the patient's school teachers and standardized test results to determine if further testing is warranted to discover if a learning difficulty is present or if the child is in inappropriate advanced placement.[5,27,56,95] Individual judgement should be exercised in determining the extent of psychological evaluation and intervention.

DIFFERENTIAL DIAGNOSIS

In some patients the diagnosis cannot be readily made, as several conditions can imitate disproportional musculoskeletal pain. The diagnosis in those adolescents referred for disproportional musculoskeletal pain who have an inflammatory rheumatic disease is usually obvious from the history and physical examination. The exception to this are those children with spondyloarthropathy manifested mostly by enthesalgia, fatigue and pain after activity causing them to drop out of sports and physical education classes (see Chapter 6).

Patients who have severe musculoskeletal pain as a chief complaint that may be confused with a pain syndrome include the following.

Fabry's disease

Fabry's disease is an X-linked deficiency in α-galactosidase A, leading to deposition of galactosylgalactosylglucosyl ceramide in skin, nerves, kidneys and blood vessels.[104] The neuropathy causes episodic excruciating burning pain in the distal extremities in childhood that increases in frequency and intensity in adolescence. These episodes usually last a few days and are associated with fever, anhydrosis and abdominal pain. Exercise or rapid environmental temperature changes can trigger episodes. During the attacks the erythrocyte sedimentation rate is usually elevated. Angiokeratoma appear in childhood and increase with age. Examination reveals cold sensitivity and purple to blue maculopapular hyperkeratotic lesions clustered on the lower trunk and perineum. Low plasma or leucocyte levels of α-galactosidase or specific gene mutation analysis confirm the diagnosis. Prophylactic phenytoin is effective in preventing attacks of the painful acroparaesthesias.

Neoplasia

Occasionally a child will be referred for disproportional pain that actually is bone pain due to an underlying neoplasia. Symptoms and signs suggestive of leukaemia include episodic or migratory pain or arthritis, generalized malaise, anorexia and bone pain. The complete blood count can be normal initially, but usually the erythrocyte sedimentation rate is elevated. In such cases, there is usually some decrease in the white blood cell count and platelet count that would not be expected given the amount of inflammation reflected by the erythrocyte sedimentation rate. The degree of anaemia may also be surprising. Radiographs of the long bones may reveal osteoporosis or leukaemic lines and a technetium-99 bone scan can show diffuse spotty increased uptake or uptake by an unsuspected neuroblastoma. A bone marrow is indicted in patients in whom leukaemia is suspected. I have seen one patient with disproportional musculoskeletal pain involving the knee in whom a sarcoma in the popliteal space was found.

Spinal cord, sacral and bone tumours may present as back pain.[105,106] Findings include abnormal neurological examination, altered gait and spinal curvature. An adult with a cervical cord mass associated with a subacute haematoma presented with findings typical of reflex dystrophy of the hand, including technetium-99 bone scan results.[107]

Erythromelalgia

Erythromelalgia presents with episodic burning pain with accompanying erythematous, warm, swollen hands or feet (or both) that is eased by cold and elevation.[108] These patients will refuse to remove ice from their affected limbs. Exercise or heat (even wearing socks) can precipitate an attack. It may precede or coincide with a myeloproliferative disease. The erythrocyte sedimentation rate is normal. Familial, early childhood onset disease may be resistant to treatment, but later onset disease can be controlled with daily administration of acetylsalicylic acid.

Pernio (chilblains)

Pernio presents as a burning pain, with associated red to purple, swollen, papules (or even blisters) of exposed fingers or toes.[109] It is a cold injury, not quite frostbite, that is seen in cold damp climates or after exposure to cold water or snow. A history of exposure and typical skin changes establish the diagnosis. Treatment with nifedipine may be beneficial.

Raynaud's phenomenon

Raynaud's phenomenon is a tricolour change in the distal extremities, usually in response to cold, vibration or, rarely, emotional upset.[110] The initial phase is white (ischaemic), followed by blue (cyanotic due to slow blood flow and oxygen desaturation) and then red (reactive hyperaemia). It is short lived and generally benign, although it can be a sign of an underlying rheumatic condition such as scleroderma or systemic lupus erythematosus, especially if antinuclear antibodies are present. Raynaud's phenomenon can be associated with tingling, but pain is not a major complaint.

Hypermobility

Hypermobility, as defined previously in this chapter, is usually associated with intermittent nocturnal pains that may occur after certain activities. It usually occurs in children aged 3–10 years, not adolescents.[111] Only rarely is a child dysfunctional. Mild joint effusions may be observed. Children with hypermobility may be at a higher risk of developing disproportional musculoskeletal pain with painful points, so careful examination of these points, as well as control points, should be made in the older hypermobile child complaining of chronic widespread pain.[47] Hypermobility alone is generally treated with reassurance; very few children will need to change their activities because of it.

Restless leg syndrome

Restless leg syndrome is characterized by a feeling of discomfort in the legs, especially the calves, at night after resting or going to bed. It is usually relieved by activity and frequently leads to insomnia. Paraesthesias are common, as are periodic movements of the limb during sleep. These usually last less than a minute and rarely cause the patient to awaken. This is more common in older adults, but has been reported in children and adolescents.[112] Treatment includes reducing caffeine intake, along with a wide variety of medications, including quinine sulphate.

Myofascial pain

Myofascial pain syndromes are due to sustained contraction of part of a muscle and can occur in a variety of muscles, usually those about the head, jaw and upper back.[113,114] The pain is generally quite localized and is reproduced when that part of the muscle is palpated. Treatment with physical therapy modalities is generally all that is required. Some will respond to dry needling or tender point injection (with local anaesthetics or steroids).

Chronic recurrent multifocal osteomyelitis

Chronic recurrent multifocal osteomyelitis is a sterile inflammation of bone that leads to chronic musculoskeletal pain.[115,116] Children and adolescents are affected much more commonly than are adults. The tibia is most commonly involved, but virtually any bone can be involved. Usually there is specific point tenderness. If initial radiographs are normal, computed tomography or a technetium-99 bone scan will usually reveal the lesion(s). The lesions are unresponsive to antibiotic treatment, but most respond to non-steroidal or steroidal anti-inflammatory medication.

Chronic compartment syndrome

Chronic compartment syndrome is seen most commonly in the lower leg in athletes.[117] Classically, the athlete will have pain after exercising for a given amount, such as a runner consistently developing pain after the fourth kilometre. This is thought to arise from insufficiency of the compartmental space to accommodate the muscle mass, which enlarges during exercise and causes a decrease in blood flow and resulting ischaemia. Treatment is usually surgical.

Progressive diaphyseal dysplasia

Progressive diaphyseal dysplasia (or Camurati–Engelmann disease) is an autosomal dominant condition involving severe leg pain, fatigue, headaches, weight loss or decreased appetite, weakness and an abnormal, waddling gait.[118] The bone pain may be chronic or intermittent, and usually starts in early to late adolescence. Radiographs show cortical thickening and sclerosis of the diaphysis of the long bones. Many patients respond to corticosteroid treatment (analgesics usually do not help).

Peripheral mononeuropathy

Three adult patients with mononeuropathy (neuroma, irritative lesion and entrapment) after trauma presented with allodynia and autonomic signs.[119] Electrophysiological studies were normal and the diagnosis was suspected after a local nerve anaesthetic block relieved the symptoms.

Transient migratory osteoporosis

Transient migratory osteoporosis is a painful, rapidly developing, osteoporosis of unknown aetiology.[120] One adolescent has been reported to have this condition; it was thought to be a variant of reflex sympathetic dystrophy.

Vitamin D deficiency

Five debilitated patients with multiple reasons for vitamin D deficiency presented with hyperaesthetic pain that did not respond to analgesics but promptly remitted with vitamin D therapy.[121]

DISPROPORTIONAL MUSCULOSKELETAL PAIN AS A COMPLICATION OF OTHER ILLNESSES

Patients with underlying illness can develop a disproportional musculoskeletal pain syndrome. It may be extremely difficult to ascertain whether or not the pain is proportional to the amount of pain explained by the illness.[51,56] The illnesses are not necessarily limited to those affecting the musculoskeletal system but, in our experience, there seems to be an increased number of patients with an underlying musculoskeletal problem who develop a disproportional musculoskeletal pain syndrome. These underlying problems include chronic arthritis, enthesopathy syndromes, cerebral palsy, cystic fibrosis, surgery on the limbs, chronic recurrent multifocal osteomyelitis and muscular dystrophy. The underlying illness may be active or inactive at the time of the disproportional musculoskeletal pain. Recognizing that the pain is disproportional is the first step; one should then treat each condition individually.

Psychological conditions can complicate a disproportional musculoskeletal pain syndrome. Depression occurs in about 10% of patients with and without overt autonomic signs; however, it is more common in those with painful points.[27,61]

Antidepressant medication usually suffices, although an occasional patient needs more intensive therapy for depression. Suicide attempts (and, rarely, suicide) are distinct possibilities and should be discussed with the depressed adolescent with disproportional musculoskeletal pain. Eating disorders have been reported with disproportional musculoskeletal pain in children, but it is not clear that they are more common in these patients than in the population at large.[122,123] Other psychological conditions can compromise the patient's (and family's) ability to understand and comply with the treatment programme (e.g. borderline personality disorder or frank psychoses).

TREATMENT

The first step in treating children with disproportionate pain is to establish trust. A complete history and thorough physical examination is critical so that every question and symptom can be addressed. After the diagnosis is clear, it is important to be fully confident about both the diagnosis and the treatment goals. I have found that explaining the pain and treatment using the model presented is extremely helpful (see Figure 11.2). I use this same model for all subtypes. These patients have often had their symptoms questioned as real, and this model and the exercise therapy acknowledges the extreme amount of pain they are experiencing. It presents an understandable reason for the pain and, along with the exercise therapy, allow patients to become well gracefully. In addition, it emphasizes the point that using their extremity is going to be painful but not damaging. After this explanation, most patients will immediately become more functional.

Although various authors have reported a diversity of treatments over the years, there are very few data from controlled, double-blind studies of treatment.[54] The sheer number and disparate nature of treatments attests to the fact that both the aetiology and pathophysiology of disproportional pain are unknown, and that researchers tend to study it from their own perspective. The nature of these conditions, even within one subset, may be heterogeneous. For example, in adults with fibromyalgia, three different subsets have been described based on psychosocial and behavioural responses to pain, while others have divided these patients into primary and either secondary[124] or reactive[125] subtypes. In reflex neurovascular dystrophy, HLA DR2 positive women were found to be resistant to treatment.[40] These and other variables, such as referral bias, publishing bias toward positive studies, access to care, seeking of physician help, obtaining a proper control or comparison group and valid measures of improvement, all limit our ability to interpret treatment and outcome studies. It is likely that multiple other unknown factors have a direct bearing on treatment and outcome. Most treatments are first used in adults and later applied to children. As these pain syndromes are significantly different in adolescents, it stands to reason that the treatment of adolescents should not necessarily be the same as it is for adults.

Given the above, the treatments (either singly or in combination) most often reported to be of benefit in children and adolescents with disproportional musculoskeletal pain with overt autonomic signs include exercise therapy, transcutaneous electrical stimulation and sympathetic blocks.[12–15,27,28,37,44,102,103,126–130] The majority of these patients have been treated successfully with aggressive physical therapy. Other treatments used in a few children with highly variable results include steroids,[28,43] tricyclic antidepressants, opioids, anticonvulsants, sympathectomy, immobilization, biofeedback, behavioural treatment and a coping approach.[28,43,131,132] Non-steroidal agents have not been helpful.[28,103] In many of the studies, psychological support or treatment was ongoing during other therapies.[5,12,28] Wilder et al[28] treated 70 children with an advancing algorithm including multiple modalities, such as sympathetic blocks, transcutaneous nerve stimulation, and multiple medications; pain was resolved in less than half of patients.[28] I have treated 103 patients with overt autonomic signs with an intense exercise programme and psychological evaluation and support, with 92% becoming pain free.

The use of many other agents, modalities and surgery have been reported in adult patients (and tried to a much lesser degree in adolescents). Medications used include: intravenous reserpine,[133] intravenous guanethidine (although two recent studies did not show it to be effective),[134,135] nifedipine,[136,137] calcitonin,[28,102] phenoxybenzamine,[136] gabapentin,[138] bisphosphonates,[139,140] intrathecal morphine,[141,142] intramuscular steroids[143] and dimethylsulphoxide.[144] Less frequently used modalities include diapulse,[145] acupuncture,[146] ultrasound[147] and and temperature biofeedback.[148] Surgery is a rare option; reports include sympathectomy[36,149] and amputation.[36,84]

Few studies report treatment on children with disproportional musculoskeletal pain without overt autonomic signs. An intense exercise therapy programme was used along with psychological evaluations (and psychotherapy, if indicated) in 100 children with both continuous and intermittent symptoms.[5] Initially 78% were cured and 97% were restored to full function. Those with intermittent pain usually exercised for 5 days without experiencing marked pain and subsequently did well. Herregods et al[9] report a single 12-year-old girl with pseudodystrophy (defined as a reflex sympathetic dystrophy like presentation without radiographic or bone scintigraphic changes of adult disease) who resolved all pain with physical therapy, hydrotherapy, slight doses of non-steroidal anti-inflammatory medication and psychological support.

Patients with disproportional musculoskeletal pain with painful points are generally more difficult to treat due to depression, unrestorative sleep and poor cardiovascular conditioning. A plethora of diverse treatments has been reported in adults. Most recommend combined treatment with education, a mild exercise programme and a low-dose tricyclic antidepressant combined with a non-steroidal anti-inflammatory agent.[150] Small trials have advocated fluoxetine and amitriptyline in combination,[151] intravenous lignocaine[152] and cyclobenzaprine.[153,154] Several trials, however, have shown various levels of exercise therapy to be of benefit both in the short and long term.[155–158]

In the adolescents I see, the term 'fibromyalgia' is eschewed and treatment with an intense exercise programme, as described for the other forms of disproportional musculoskeletal pains, is prescribed. Initially, over 90% of patients resolve all symptoms. The duration of exercise therapy is somewhat prolonged (2–3 weeks) due to the poor cardiovascular fitness of most patients. Medication is avoided unless depression is diagnosed, in which case either a serotonin reuptake inhibitor or a tricyclic antidepressant is used. A short course of non-steroidal anti-inflammatory medication may be tried in those patients with tender entheses.

Patients with disproportional musculoskeletal pain due to hypervigilance generally need reassurance that there is no underlying serious condition and that they should not discontinue activities because of these pains.[6] A few will need a formal exercise programme to perform when they have an episode of pain.

The role of psychotherapy is generally not primary, but several reports, some in adolescents, have reported success with behaviour therapy, a coping approach and hypnosis.[48,131,132] In adults, psychotherapy as the sole therapy is rarely reported, but, as noted above, it frequently forms part of the therapeutic regimen. The type of psychotherapy reported to be successful is hypnotherapy, including classic visualization and self-hypnosis as well as ego-state integration (where different ego-states (or a 'family of self') are induced under hypnosis and personality dimensions including behaviour, affect, sensation and knowledge are integrated).[48,159] Psychological support, relaxation training and coping are frequently part of the overall therapy programmes reported, as the medical and exercise therapies intrinsically cause great stress. Many patients and families need extra psychological support during this time.

Details of the exercise therapy are outlined in Appendix 2 to this chapter. Our philosophy is to begin immediate mobilization and desensitization with aggressive, continuous aerobic exercises that are focused on function. As most patients are compliant, they are quite motivated to improve speed and quality of function. However, for the few with marked pain behaviours, this can be quite an arduous task for all involved. Pain behaviours should not dictate the intensity or duration of exercise therapy. The therapists acknowledge the pain but ignore it while strongly encouraging improved performance and quality of movement on the patient's part. In like manner, while exercising, the patient may complain of multiple other pains such as headaches, abdominal pains, chest pains and subjective, but not objective, breathing difficulties (frequently diagnosed as reactive airway disease) which, if allowed to continue, can interfere with therapy. Once again, if the patient has no underlying complicating illness, the symptoms are acknowledged and ignored. Not uncommonly the pain will migrate before it resolves, a painful foot will be just about resolved and the hand will start to hurt. When this happens, the patient is reassured that the new pain is the same as the original pain and exercises incorporating the new site are started. Treatment requires a committed team of non-judgmental, sympathetic occupational and physical therapists, along with psychologists, social workers, nurses and school personnel.

Because of the family psychodynamics involved in most cases of children with a disproportional musculoskeletal pain syndrome, parents are not allowed in the physiotherapy gym after the initial visit. This can present a problem for the especially enmeshed parent who discovers that separation is particularly difficult. Ready availability of the team social worker or psychologist is mandatory in such situations.

Highly motivated patients who are compulsive about performing a rigorous home exercise programme can resolve their symptoms without a formal outpatient or inpatient programme, but the majority of patients find the programme too painful to do so. At present, the majority of patients are treated on a daily outpatient basis unless functional impairment prohibits activities of daily living, there are marked pain behaviours (especially pain after a day of activities), or if outpatient therapy has failed. Removing the patient from the home environment can be very therapeutic, although there is a risk that they will become emotionally dependent on the hospital environment and thus have no incentive to become well.

OUTCOME

Untreated, the duration of symptoms can be years, but no natural history studies are available. Those patients who end up in tertiary referral centres have already been selected not to have self-limited disease and are treated with a variety of therapies. Many children diagnosed with a disproportional musculoskeletal pain syndrome have apparently had a similar episode in the past that has resolved spontaneously. There is one study of schoolchildren diagnosed with fibromyalgia during a prevalence study.[160] After 30 months, 11 of 15 children serendipitously found to have fibromyalgia had become well. In contrast, 12 adolescents diagnosed with fibromyalgia after referral to a paediatric rheumatologist were advised to obtain counselling, biofeedback, and a conditioning physical therapy programme in their home community, but, on follow-up 15–60 months later, 92% reported still having significant pain.[161]

Our experience with over 100 children with overt autonomic signs, several hundred without overt autonomic signs, and over 20 with painful points is very favourable. Almost all were treated with an intensive exercise programme and psychotherapy. The rapidity of functional improvement is remarkable. Patients with disproportional musculoskeletal pain with and without autonomic dysfunction did extremely well, with 90–95% regaining full function within a week or two, regardless of the duration of symptoms or degree of dysfunction. After function has been restored, most patients will experience resolution of pain within the first month.

For those with disproportional musculoskeletal pain and multiple painful points the long-term outcome is a little poorer. Over 90% became free of pain, fatigue and sleeping problems at the end of the exercise programme, but after 5 years only half were completely asymptomatic. Most of the symptomatic patients are fully functional but continue to need to exercise at home. In adults, one study showed that after 10 years more than half reported doing well, but 55% had moderate to severe pain, 79% took medication and 69% exercised regularly.[162] Psychological variables loom large in outcome studies in both adults and children with fibromyalgia. Better functional outcomes are reported with healthy coping[163] and higher levels of self-efficacy (belief that one can cope with difficult situations).[164] Few long-term studies have been done. In our experience the relapse rate is fairly low, with only about 15% of patients needing formal retreatment; relapses may take various forms.[5,165,166] Another 5% of patients develop another predominantly psychological condition such as a non-organic pain (eye pain, sinus pain or disabling headache), conversion reaction (paralysis or blindness), panic attacks, suicide attempt or an eating disorder.

Between 5% and 8% of patients do not do well during the exercise programme. In these, formal, intense psychotherapy has been efficacious for those who have persevered.

SUMMARY

Adolescence is a unique time in our lives; one is at the cusp between childhood and adulthood. It is a time fraught with physical and psychological challenges which, for the adolescent in pain, challenges the physician to determine the proper cause and most appropriate and efficacious treatment. Disproportional musculoskeletal pain is common in this age group and may assume one of several distinct patterns. Once recognized, treatment can begin; psyche and soma need to be addressed individually. Treatment is usually successful, although it is arduous for both the adolescent and the treatment team. When all is said and done, the adolescent and his or her family may have a whole new outlook on life, healthier relationships with each other, and a very real sense of accomplishment.

ACKNOWLEDGEMENT

The author gratefully acknowledges the support of Barbara and David Kipper and the Chas and Ruth Levy Foundation for his work on disproportional musculoskeletal pain in adolescents.

REFERENCES

1. Merskey DM, Bogduk N (eds). *Classification of Chronic Pain. Descriptions of Chronic Pain Syndromes and Definitions of Pain Terms*, 2nd edn. International Association for the Study of Pain: Seattle, 1994.
2. Garcia J, Altman RD. Chronic pain states: pathophysiology and medical therapy. *Semin Arthritis Rheum* 1997; **27**:1–16.
3. Malleson PN, al-Matar M, Petty RE. Idiopathic musculoskeletal pain syndromes in children. *J Rheumatol* 1992; **19**:1786–9.
4. Croft P, Burt J, Schollum J, Thomas E, Macfarlane G, Silman A. More pain, more tender points: is fibromyalgia just one end of a continuous spectrum? *Ann Rheum Dis* 1996; **55**:482–5.
5. Sherry DD, McGuire T, Mellins E, Salmonson K, Wallace CA, Nepom B. Psychosomatic musculoskeletal pain in childhood: clinical and psychological analyses of 100 children. *Pediatrics* 1991; **88**:1093–9.
6. Sherry DD. Musculoskeletal pain in children. *Curr Opin Rheumatol* 1997; **9**:465–70.
7. Stanton-Hicks M, Janig W, Hassenbusch S, Haddox JD, Boas R, Wilson P. Reflex sympathetic dystrophy: changing concepts and taxonomy. *Pain* 1995; **63**:127–33.
8. Dotson RM. Causalgia – reflex sympathetic dystrophy – sympathetically maintained pain: myth and reality. *Muscle Nerve* 1993; **16**:1049–55.
9. Herregods P, Willems J, Chappel R. Pseudodystrophy at the lower limb in children. *Clin Rheumatol* 1997; **16**:425–8.
10. Wolfe F, Smythe HA, Yunus MB et al. Criteria for the classification of fibromyalgia. Report of the Multicenter Criteria Committee. *Arthritis Rheum* 1990; **33**:160–72.
11. Yunus MB, Masi AT. Juvenile primary fibromyalgia syndrome. A clinical study of thirty-three patients and matched normal controls. *Arthritis Rheum* 1985; **28**:138–45.

12. Bernstein BH, Singsen BH, Kent JT et al. Reflex neurovascular dystrophy in childhood. *J Pediatr* 1978; **93**:211–5.

13. Silber TJ, Majd M. Reflex sympathetic dystrophy syndrome in children and adolescents. Report of 18 cases and review of the literature. *Am J Dis Child* 1988; **142**:1325–30.

14. Ruggeri SB, Athreya BH, Doughty R, Gregg JR, Das MM. Reflex sympathetic dystrophy in children. *Clin Orthop* 1982; **163**:225–30.

15. Ashwal S, Tomasi L, Neumann M, Schneider S. Reflex sympathetic dystrophy in children. *Pediatr Neurol* 1988; **4**:38–42.

16. Goldsmith DP, Vivino FB, Eichenfield AH, Athreya BH, Heyman S. Nuclear imaging and clinical features of childhood reflex neurovascular dystrophy: comparison with adults. *Arthritis Rheum* 1989; **32**:480–5.

17. Kavanagh R, Crisp AJ, Hazelman BL, Coughlan RJ. Reflex sympathetic dystrophy in children. Dystrophic changes are less likely. *Br Med J* 1995; **311**:1503.

18. Turpin S, Taillefer R, Lambert R, Leveille J. 'Cold' reflex sympathetic dystrophy in an adult. *Clin Nucl Med* 1996; **21**:94–7.

19. Naish JM, Apley J. 'Growing pains': a clinical study of non-arthritis limb pains in children. *Arch Dis Child* 1951; **26**:134–40.

20. Apley J. One child. In: *One Child* (Apley J, Ounsted C, eds). JB Lippincott: Philadelphia, 1982:23–47.

21. Oster J. Recurrent abdominal pain, headache and limb pains in children and adolescents. *Pediatrics* 1972; **50**:429–36.

22. Mitchell SW, Morehouse GR, Keen WW. *Gunshot Wounds and Other Injuries of Nerves*. JB Lippincott: New York, 1864.

23. Evans JA. Reflex sympathetic dystrophy: report on 57 cases. *Ann Intern Med* 1947; **26**:417–26.

24. Matles AI. Reflex sympathetic dystrophy in a child. A case report. *Bull Hosp Joint Dis* 1971; **32**:193–7.

25. Yunus M, Masi AT, Calabro JJ, Miller KA, Feigenbaum SL. Primary fibromyalgia (fibrositis): clinical study of 50 patients with matched normal controls. *Semin Arthritis Rheum* 1981; **11**:151–71.

26. Okifuji A, Turk DC, Sinclair JD, Starz TW, Marcus DA. A standardized manual tender point survey. I. Development and determination of a threshold point for the identification of positive tender points in fibromyalgia syndrome. *J Rheumatol* 1997; **24**:377–83.

27. Sherry DD, Weisman R. Psychologic aspects of childhood reflex neurovascular dystrophy. *Pediatrics* 1988; **81**:572–8.

28. Wilder RT, Berde CB, Wolohan M, Vieyra MA, Masek BJ, Micheli LJ. Reflex sympathetic dystrophy in children. Clinical characteristics and follow-up of seventy patients. *J Bone Joint Surg Am* 1992; **74**:910–9.

29. Payne WK III, Ogilvie JW. Back pain in children and adolescents. *Pediatr Clin North Am* 1996; **43**:899–917.

30. Abu-Arafeh I, Russell G. Recurrent limb pain in schoolchildren. *Arch Dis Child* 1996; **74**:336–9.

31. Buskila D, Press J, Gedalia A et al. Assessment of nonarticular tenderness and prevalence of fibromyalgia in children. *J Rheumatol* 1993; **20**:368–70.

32. Bowyer S, Roettcher P. Pediatric rheumatology clinic populations in the United States: results of a 3 year survey. Pediatric Rheumatology Database Research Group. *J Rheumatol* 1996; **23**:1968–74.

33. Malleson PN, Fung MY, Rosenberg AM. The incidence of pediatric rheumatic diseases: results from the Canadian Pediatric Rheumatology Association Disease Registry. *J Rheumatol* 1996; **23**:1981–7.

34. Balague F, Skovron ML, Nordin M, Dutoit G, Pol LR, Waldburger M. Low back pain in schoolchildren. A study of familial and psychological factors. *Spine* 1995; **20**:1265–70.

35. Buskila D, Neumann L, Hazanov I, Carmi R. Familial aggregation in the fibromyalgia syndrome. *Semin Arthritis Rheum* 1996; **26**:605–11.

36. Erdmann MW, Wynn-Jones CH. 'Familial' reflex sympathetic dystrophy syndrome and amputation. *Injury* 1992; **23**:136–8.

37. Rush PJ, Wilmot D, Saunders N, Gladman D, Shore A. Severe reflex neurovascular dystrophy in childhood. *Arthritis Rheum* 1985; **28**:952–6.

38. Buskila D, Neumann L. Fibromyalgia syndrome (FM) and nonarticular tenderness in relatives of patients with FM. *J Rheumatol* 1997; **24**:941–4.

39. Pellegrino MJ, Waylonis GW, Sommer A. Familial occurrence of primary fibromyalgia. *Arch Phys Med Rehabil* 1989; **70**:61–3.

40. Mailis A, Wade J. Profile of Caucasian women with possible genetic predisposition to reflex sympathetic dystrophy: a pilot study. *Clin J Pain* 1994; **10**:210–17.

41. Atkins RM, Duckworth T, Kanis JA. Algodystrophy following Colles' fracture. *J Hand Surg (Br)* 1989; **14**:161–4.

42. Field J, Warwick D, Bannister GC. Features of algodystrophy ten years after Colles' fracture. *J Hand Surg (Br)* 1992; **17**:318–20.

43. Kozin F, Haughton V, Ryan L. The reflex sympathetic dystrophy syndrome in a child. *J Pediatr* 1977; **90**:417–19.

44. Richlin DM, Carron H, Rowlingson JC, Sussman MD, Baugher WH, Goldner RD. Reflex sympathetic dystrophy: successful treatment by transcutaneous nerve stimulation. *J Pediatr* 1978; **93**:84–6.

45. Wainapel SF. Reflex sympathetic dystrophy following traumatic myelopathy. *Pain* 1984; **18**:345–9.

46. Gangi A, Dietemann JL, Gasser B et al. Interstitial laser photocoagulation of osteoid osteomas with use of CT guidance. *Radiology* 1997; **203**:843–8.

47. Gedalia A, Press J, Klein M, Buskila D. Joint hypermobility and fibromyalgia in schoolchildren. *Ann Rheum Dis* 1993; **52**:494–6.

48. Gainer MJ. Somatization of dissociated traumatic memories in a case of reflex sympathetic dystrophy. *Am J Clin Hypnosis* 1993; **36**:124–31.

49. Lebovits AH, Yarmush J, Lefkowitz M. Reflex sympathetic dystrophy and posttraumatic stress disorder. Multidisciplinary evaluation and treatment. *Clin J Pain* 1990; **6**:153–7.

50. Veldman PH, Reynen HM, Arntz IE, Goris RJ. Signs and symptoms of reflex sympathetic dystrophy: prospective study of 829 patients. *Lancet* 1993; **342**:1012–6.

51. Ostrov BE, Eichenfield AH, Goldsmith DP, Schumacher HR. Recurrent reflex sympathetic dystrophy as a manifestation of systemic lupus erythematosus. *J Rheumatol* 1993; **20**:1774–6.

52. Lynch ME. Psychological aspects of reflex sympathetic dystrophy: a review of the adult and paediatric literature. *Pain* 1992; **49**:337–47.

53. Bruehl S, Carlson CR. Predisposing psychological factors in the development of reflex sympathetic dystrophy. A review of the empirical evidence. *Clin J Pain* 1992; **8**:287–99.

54. White KP, Harth M. An analytical review of 24 controlled clinical trials for fibromyalgia syndrome (FMS). *Pain* 1996; **64**:211–9.

55. Galer BS, Butler S, Jensen MP. Case reports and hypothesis: a neglect-like syndrome may be responsible for the motor disturbance in reflex sympathetic dystrophy (complex regional pain syndrome – 1). *J Pain Symptom Management* 1995; **10**:385–91.

56. Vandvik IH, Forseth KO. A bio-psychosocial evaluation of ten adolescents with fibromyalgia. *Acta Paediatr* 1994; **83**:766–71.

57. Van Houdenhove B, Vasquez G. Is there a relationship between reflex sympathetic dystrophy and helplessness? Case reports and a hypothesis. *Gen Hosp Psychiatry* 1993; **15**:325–9.

58. Van Houdenhove B, Vasquez G, Onghena P et al. Etiopathogenesis of reflex sympathetic dystrophy: a review and biopsychosocial hypothesis. *Clin J Pain* 1992; **8**:300–6.

59. Van Houdenhove B. Neuro-algodystrophy: a psychiatrist's view. *Clin Rheumatol* 1986; **5**:399–406.

60. Rose MJ, Klenerman L, Atchison L, Slade PD. An application of the fear avoidance model to three chronic pain problems. *Behav Res Ther* 1992; **30**:359–65.

61. Mikkelsson M, Sourander A, Piha J, Salminen JJ. Psychiatric symptoms in preadolescents with musculoskeletal pain and fibromyalgia. *Pediatrics* 1997; **100**:220–7.

62. Reid GJ, Lang BA, McGrath PJ. Primary juvenile fibromyalgia: psychological adjustment, family functioning, coping, and functional disability. *Arthritis Rheum* 1997; **40**:752–60.

63. Pillemer FG, Masek BJ, Kaban LB. Temporomandibular joint dysfunction and facial pain in children: an approach to diagnosis and treatment. *Pediatrics* 1987; **80**:565–70.

64. Selbst SM, Ruddy RM, Clark BJ, Henretig FM, Santulli T Jr. Pediatric chest pain: a prospective study. *Pediatrics* 1988; **82**:319–23.

65. Livingston R, Witt A, Smith GR. Families who somatize. *J Dev Behav Pediatr* 1995; **16**:42–6.

66. Garralda ME. Somatisation in children. *J Child Psychol Psychiatry* 1996; **37**:13–33.

67. Walker LS, Garber J, Greene JW. Somatic complaints in pediatric patients: a prospective study of the role of negative life events, child social and academic competence, and parental somatic symptoms. *J Consult Clin Psychol* 1994; **62**:1213–21.

68. Brazier DK, Venning HE. Conversion disorders in adolescents: a practical approach to rehabilitation. *Br J Rheumatol* 1997; **36**:594–8.

69. Cicuttini F, Littlejohn GO. Female adolescent rheumatological presentations: the importance of chronic pain syndromes. *Aust Paediatr J* 1989; **25**:21–4.

70. Prazar G. Conversion reactions in adolescents. *Pediatr Rev* 1987; **8**:279–86.

71. Willis WD, Westlund KN. Neuroanatomy of the pain system and of the pathways that modulate pain. *J Clin Neurophysiol* 1997; **14**:2–31.

72. Markenson JA. Mechanisms of chronic pain. *Am J Med* 1996; **101**:6S–18S.

73. Price DD, Long S, Huitt C. Sensory testing of pathophysiological mechanisms of pain in patients with reflex sympathetic dystrophy. *Pain* 1992; **49**:163–73.

74. Drummond PD, Finch PM, Smythe GA. Reflex sympathetic dystrophy: the significance of differing plasma catecholamine concentrations in affected and unaffected limbs. *Brain* 1991; **114**:2025–36.

75. Ecker A. Norepinephrine in reflex sympathetic dystrophy: an hypothesis. *Clin J Pain* 1989; **5**:313–5.

76. Gracely RH, Lynch SA, Bennett GJ. Painful neuropathy: altered central processing maintained dynamically by peripheral input. *Pain* 1992; **51**:175–94. Erratum. *Pain* 1993; **52**:251–3.

77. Arnold JM, Teasell RW, MacLeod AP, Brown JE, Carruthers SG. Increased venous α-adrenoceptor responsiveness in patients with reflex sympathetic dystrophy. *Ann Intern Med* 1993; **118**:619–21.

78. Chelimsky TC, Low PA, Naessens JM, Wilson PR, Amadio PC, O'Brien PC. Value of autonomic testing in reflex sympathetic dystrophy. *Mayo Clin Proc* 1995; **70**:1029–40.

79. Cronin KD, Kirsner RL, Fitzroy VP. Diagnosis of reflex sympathetic dysfunction. Use of the skin potential response. *Anaesthesia* 1982; **37**:848–52.

80. Herrick A, el-Hadidy K, Marsh D, Jayson M. Abnormal thermoregulatory responses in patients with reflex sympathetic dystrophy syndrome. *J Rheumatol* 1994; **21**:1319–24.

81. Procacci P, Francini F, Maresca M, Zoppi M. Skin potential and EMG changes induced by cutaneous electrical stimulation. II. Subjects with reflex sympathetic dystrophies. *Appl Neurophysiol* 1979; **42**:125–34.

82. Nickeson R, Brewer E, Person D. Early histologic and radionuclide scan changes in children with reflex sympathetic dystrophy syndrome (RSDS). *Arthritis Rheum* 1985; **28**(suppl):S72.

83. Heerschap A, den Hollander JA, Reynen H, Goris RJ. Metabolic changes in reflex sympathetic dystrophy: a ³¹P NMR spectroscopy study. *Muscle Nerve* 1993; **16**:367–73.

84. Eyres KS, Talbot IC, Harding ML. Amputation for reflex sympathetic dystrophy. *Br J Clin Pract* 1990; **44**:654–6.

85. Bengtsson A, Henriksson KG, Larsson J. Reduced high-energy phosphate levels in the painful muscles of patients with primary fibromyalgia. *Arthritis Rheum* 1986; **29**:817–21.

86. Bennett RM, Clark SR, Goldberg L et al. Aerobic fitness in patients with fibrositis. A controlled study of respiratory gas exchange and xenon-133 clearance from exercising muscle. *Arthritis Rheum* 1989; **32**:454–60.

87. Lund N, Bengtsson A, Thorborg P. Muscle tissue oxygen pressure in primary fibromyalgia. *Scand J Rheumatol* 1986; **15**:165–73.

88. Simms RW. Fibromyalgia syndrome: current concepts in pathophysiology, clinical features, and management. *Arthritis Care Res* 1996; **9**:315–28.

89. Smith MS, Mitchell J, Corey L et al. Chronic fatigue in adolescents. *Pediatrics* 1991; **88**:195–202.

90. Thomasgard M, Metz WP. The vulnerable child syndrome revisited. *J Dev Behav Pediatr* 1995; **16**:47–53.

91. Daniels D, Miller JJ, Billings AG, Moos RH. Psychosocial functioning of siblings of children with rheumatic disease. *J Pediatr* 1986; **109**:379–83.

92. Poikolainen K, Kanerva R, Lonnqvist J. Life events and other risk factors for somatic symptoms in adolescence. *Pediatrics* 1995; **96**:59–63.

93. Dunger DB, Pritchard J, Hensman S, Leonard JV, Lask B, Wolff OH. The investigation of atypical psychosomatic illness. A team approach to diagnosis. *Clin Pediatr (Philadelphia)* 1986; **25**:341–4.

94. Greene JW, Walker LS, Hickson G, Thompson J. Stressful life events and somatic complaints in adolescents. *Pediatrics* 1985; **75**:19–22.

95. Schmitt BD. School phobia – the great imitator: a pediatrician's viewpoint. *Pediatrics* 1971; **48**:433–41.

96. Pillemer FG, Micheli LJ. Psychological considerations in youth sports. *Clin Sports Med* 1988; **7**:679–89.

97. Dvonch VM, Bunch WH, Siegler AH. Conversion reactions in pediatric athletes. *J Pediatr Orthop* 1991; **11**:770–2.

98. Hollingworth P. Back pain in children. *Br J Rheumatol* 1996; **35**:1022–8.

99. Kristjansdottir G. Prevalence of self-reported back pain in school children: a study of sociodemographic differences. *Eur J Pediatr* 1996; **155**:984–6.

100. Waddell G, McCulloch JA, Kummel E, Venner RM. Nonorganic physical signs in low-back pain. *Spine* 1980; **5**:117–25.

101. Laxer RM, Allen RC, Malleson PN, Morrison RT, Petty RE. Technetium-99m–methylene diphosphonate bone scans in children with reflex neurovascular dystrophy. *J Pediatr* 1985; **106**:437–40.

102. Lemahieu RA, Van Laere C, Verbruggen LA. Reflex sympathetic dystrophy: an underreported syndrome in children? *Eur J Pediatr* 1988; **147**:47–50.

103. Stanton RP, Malcolm JR, Wesdock KA, Singsen BH. Reflex sympathetic dystrophy in children: an orthopedic perspective. *Orthopedics* 1993; **16**:773–80.

104. Desnick RJ, Eng CM. Fabry disease: α-galactosidase A deficiency. In: *The Molecular and Genetic Basis of Neurological Disease.* 2nd edn. (Rosenberg RN, Prusiner SB, DiMauro S, Barchi RI, eds). Butterworth-Heinemann: Boston, 1997:443–69.

105. Parker AP, Robinson RO, Bullock P. Difficulties in diagnosing intrinsic spinal cord tumours. *Arch Dis Child* 1996; **75**:204–7.

106. Burger EL, Lindeque BG. Sacral and non-spinal tumors presenting as backache. A retrospective study of 17 patients. *Acta Orthop Scand* 1994; **65**:344–6.

107. Bhatnagar A, Chakraborty K, Mehndiratta MM, Jena A, Soni NL, Mondal A. Cervical mass lesion presenting as reflex sympathetic dystrophy of the hand. *Clin Exp Rheumatol* 1997; **15**:101–4.

108. Kurzrock R, Cohen PR. Erythromelalgia: review of clinical characteristics and pathophysiology. *Am J Med* 1991; **91**:416–22.

109. Goette DK, Chilblains (perniosis). *J Am Acad Dermatol* 1990; **23**:257–62.

110. Blunt RJ, Porter JM. Raynaud syndrome. *Semin Arthritis Rheum* 1981; **10**:282–308.

111. Gedalia A, Press J. Articular symptoms in hypermobile schoolchildren: a prospective study. *J Pediatr* 1991; **119**:944–6.

112. Walters AS, Picchietti DL, Ehrenberg BL, Wagner ML. Restless legs syndrome in childhood and adolescence. *Pediatr Neurol* 1994; **11**:241–5.

113. Fine PG. Myofascial trigger point pain in children. *J Pediatr* 1987; **111**:547–8.

114. Escobar PL, Ballesteros J. Myofascial pain syndrome. *Orthop Rev* 1987; **16**:708–13.

115. Martin JC, Desoysa R, O'Sullivan MM, Silverstone E, Williams H. Chronic recurrent multifocal osteomyelitis: spinal involvement and radiological appearances. *Br J Rheumatol* 1996; **35**:1019–21.

116. Laxer RM, Shore AD, Manson D, King S, Silverman ED, Wilmot DM. Chronic recurrent multifocal osteomyelitis and psoriasis – a report of a new association and review of related disorders. *Semin Arthritis Rheum* 1988; **17**:260–70.

117. Mannarino F, Sexson S. The significance of intra-compartmental pressures in the diagnosis of chronic exertional compartment syndrome. *Orthopedics* 1989; **12**:1415–18.

118. Naveh Y, Alon U, Kaftori JK, Berant M. Progressive diaphyseal dysplasia: evaluation of corticosteroid therapy. *Pediatrics* 1985; **75**:321–3.

119. Thimineur MA, Saberski L. Complex regional pain syndrome type I (RSD) or peripheral mononeuropathy? A discussion of three cases. *Clin J Pain* 1996; **12**:145–50.

120. Mailis A, Inman R, Pham D. Transient migratory osteoporosis: a variant of reflex sympathetic dystrophy? Report of 3 cases and literature review. *J Rheumatol* 1992; **19**:758–64.

121. Gloth FMD, Lindsay JM, Zelesnick LB, Greenough WBD. Can vitamin D deficiency produce an unusual pain syndrome? *Arch Intern Med* 1991; **151**:1662–4.

122. Silber TJ. Anorexia nervosa and reflex sympathetic dystrophy syndrome. *Psychosomatics* 1989; **30**:108–11.

123. Silber TJ. Eating disorders and reflex sympathetic dystrophy syndrome: is there a common pathway? *Med Hypoth* 1997; **48**:197–200.

124. Turk DC, Okifuji A, Sinclair JD, Starz TW. Pain, disability, and physical functioning in subgroups of patients with fibromyalgia. *J Rheumatol* 1996; **23**:1255–62.

125. Greenfield S, Fitzcharles MA, Esdaile JM. Reactive fibromyalgia syndrome. *Arthritis Rheum* 1992; **35**:678–81.

126. Stilz RJ, Carron H, Sanders DB. Reflex sympathetic dystrophy in a 6-year-old: successful treatment by transcutaneous nerve stimulation. *Anesth Analg* 1977; **56**:438–43.

127. Kesler RW, Saulsbury FT, Miller LT, Rowlingson JC. Reflex sympathetic dystrophy in children: treatment with transcutaneous electric nerve stimulation. *Pediatrics* 1988; **82**:728–32.

128. Doolan LA, Brown TC. Reflex sympathetic dystrophy in a child. *Anaesth Intensive Care* 1984; **12**:70–2.

129. Lightman HI, Pochaczevsky R, Aprin H, Ilowite NT. Thermography in childhood reflex sympathetic dystrophy. *J Pediatr* 1987; **111**:551–5.

130. Hood-White R, Gainor J. Reflex sympathetic dystrophy in an 8-year-old: successful treatment by physical therapy. *Orthopedics* 1997; **20**:73–4.

131. Alioto JT. Behavioral treatment of reflex sympathetic dystrophy. *Psychosomatics* 1981; **22**:539–40.

132. Schulman JL. Use of a coping approach in the management of children with conversion reactions. *J Am Acad Child Adolesc Psychiatry* 1988; **27**:785–8.

133. Chuinard RG, Dabezies EJ, Gould JS, Murphy GA, Matthews RE. Intravenous reserpine for treatment of reflex sympathetic dystrophy. *South Med J* 1981; **74**:1481–4.

134. Jadad AR, Carroll D, Glynn CJ, McQuay HJ. Intravenous regional sympathetic blockade for pain relief in reflex sympathetic dystrophy: a systematic review and a randomized, double-blind crossover study. *J Pain Symptom Management* 1995; **10**:13–20.

135. Yasuda JM, Schroeder DJ. Guanethidine for reflex sympathetic dystrophy. *Ann Pharmacother* 1994; **28**:338–41.

136. Muizelaar JP, Kleyer M, Hertogs IA, DeLange DC. Complex regional pain syndrome (reflex sympathetic dystrophy and causalgia): management with the calcium channel blocker nifedipine and/or the α-sympathetic blocker phenoxybenzamine in 59 patients. *Clin Neurol Neurosurg* 1997; **99**:26–30.

137. Prough DS, McLeskey CH, Poehling GG et al. Efficacy of oral nifedipine in the treatment of reflex sympathetic dystrophy. *Anesthesiology* 1985; **62**:796–9.

138. Mellick GA, Mellick LB. Reflex sympathetic dystrophy treated with gabapentin. *Arch Phys Med Rehabil* 1997; **78**:98–105.

139. Schott GD. Bisphosphonates for pain relief in reflex sympathetic dystrophy? *Lancet* 1997; **350**:1117.

140. Cortet B, Flipo RM, Coquerelle P, Duquesnoy B, Delcambre B. Treatment of severe, recalcitrant reflex sympathetic dystrophy: assessment of efficacy and safety of the second generation bisphosphonate pamidronate. *Clin Rheumatol* 1997; **16**:51–6.

141. Berry H. Re: Long-term treatment of intractable reflex sympathetic dystrophy with intrathecal morphine. *Can J Neurol Sci* 1996; **23**:156–7.

142. Becker WJ, Ablett DP, Harris CJ, Dold ON. Long term treatment of intractable reflex sympathetic dystrophy with intrathecal morphine. *Can J Neurol Sci* 1995; **22**:153–9.

143. Grundberg AB. Reflex sympathetic dystrophy: treatment with long-acting intramuscular corticosteroids. *J Hand Surg (Am)* 1996; **21**:667–70.

144. Geertzen JH, de Bruijn H, de Bruijn-Kofman AT, Arendzen JH. Reflex sympathetic dystrophy: early treatment and psychological aspects. *Arch Phys Med Rehabil* 1994; **75**:442–6.

145. Comorosan S, Pana I, Pop L, Craciun C, Cirlea AM, Paslaru L. The influence of pulsed high peak power electromagnetic energy (Diapulse) treatment on posttraumatic algoneurodystrophies. *Rev Roum Physiol* 1991; **28**:77–81.

146. Fialka V, Resch KL, Ritter-Dietrich D et al. Acupuncture for reflex sympathetic dystrophy. *Arch Intern Med* 1993; **153**:661, 665.

147. Portwood MM, Lieberman JS, Taylor RG. Ultrasound treatment of reflex sympathetic dystrophy. *Arch Phys Med Rehabil* 1987; **68**:116–18.

148. Blanchard EB. The use of temperature biofeedback in the treatment of chronic pain due to causalgia. *Biofeedback Self Regulation* 1979; **4**:183–8.

149. Olcott CT, Eltherington LG, Wilcosky BR, Shoor PM, Zimmerman JJ, Fogarty TJ. Reflex sympathetic dystrophy – the surgeon's role in management. *J Vasc Surg* 1991; **14**:488–95.

150. Russell IJ. Fibromyalgia syndrome: approaches to management. *Bull Rheum Dis* 1996; **45**:1–4.

151. Goldenberg D, Mayskiy M, Mossey C, Ruthazer R, Schmid C. A randomized, double-blind crossover trial of fluoxetine and amitriptyline in the treatment of fibromyalgia. *Arthritis Rheum* 1996; **39**:1852–9.

152. Bennett MI, Tai YM. Intravenous lignocaine in the management of primary fibromyalgia syndrome. *Int J Clin Pharmacol Res* 1995; **15**:115–9.

153. Carette S, Bell MJ, Reynolds WJ et al. Comparison of amitriptyline, cyclobenzaprine, and placebo in the treatment of fibromyalgia. A randomized, double-blind clinical trial. *Arthritis Rheum* 1994; **37**:32–40.

154. Norregaard J, Volkmann H, Danneskiold-Samsoe B. A randomized controlled trial of citalopram in the treatment of fibromyalgia. *Pain* 1995; **61**:445–9.

155. Martin L, Nutting A, MacIntosh BR, Edworthy SM, Butterwick D, Cook J. An exercise program in the treatment of fibromyalgia. *J Rheumatol* 1996; **23**:1050–3.

156. Wigers SH, Stiles TC, Vogel PA. Effects of aerobic exercise versus stress management treatment in fibromyalgia. A 4.5 year prospective study. *Scand J Rheumatol* 1996; **25**:77–86.

157. Burckhardt CS, Mannerkorpi K, Hedenberg L, Bjelle A. A randomized, controlled clinical trial of education and physical training for women with fibromyalgia. *J Rheumatol* 1994; **21**:714–20.

158. McCain GA, Bell DA, Mai FM, Halliday PD. A controlled study of the effects of a supervised cardiovascular fitness training program on the manifestations of primary fibromyalgia. *Arthritis Rheum* 1988; **31**:1135–41.

159. Gainer MJ. Hypnotherapy for reflex sympathetic dystrophy. *Am J Clin Hypnosis* 1992; **34**:227–32.

160. Buskila D, Neumann L, Hershman E, Gedalia A, Press J, Sukenik S. Fibromyalgia syndrome in children – an outcome study. *J Rheumatol* 1995; **22**:525–8.
161. Rabinovich CE, Schanberg LE, Stein LD, Kredich DW. A follow up study of pediatric fibromyalgia patients. *Arthritis Rheum* 1990; **33**(suppl):S146.
162. Kennedy M, Felson DT. A prospective long-term study of fibromyalgia syndrome. *Arthritis Rheum* 1996; **39**:682–5.
163. Schanberg LE, Keefe FJ, Lefebvre JC, Kredich DW, Gil KM. Pain coping strategies in children with juvenile primary fibromyalgia syndrome: correlation with pain, physical function, and psychological distress. *Arthritis Care Res* 1996; **9**:89–96.
164. Buckelew SP, Huyser B, Hewett JE et al. Self-efficacy predicting outcome among fibromyalgia subjects. *Arthritis Care Res* 1996; **9**:97–104.
165. Veldman PH, Goris RJ. Multiple reflex sympathetic dystrophy. Which patients are at risk for developing a recurrence of reflex sympathetic dystrophy in the same or another limb? *Pain* 1996; **64**:463–6.
166. Barrera P, van Riel PL, de Jong AJ, Boerbooms AM, Van de Putte LB. Recurrent and migratory reflex sympathetic dystrophy syndrome. *Clin Rheumatol* 1992; **11**:416–21.
167. American Psychiatric Association. *Diagnostic and Statistical Manual of Mental Disorders*, 4th edn. APA: Washington, DC, 1994.

APPENDIX 1

The language we use to describe pain is fundamental in order to communicate. The International Association for the Study of Pain has published definitions of pain terms and descriptions of chronic pain syndromes as has the American Psychiatric Association.[1,167] However, in dealing with adolescents, the conditions described therein are inadequate, since our patients with chronic pain cover the full spectrum of these syndromes. Any artificial division of this spectrum inevitably fails. Useful, standard terms and conditions include the following:

allodynia Pain due to a stimulus that does not normally provoke pain.

anaesthesia dolorosa Pain in an area or region that is anaesthetic.

causalgia A syndrome of sustained burning pain, allodynia and hyperpathia after traumatic nerve lesion, often combined with fascial motor and sudomotor dysfunction and, later, trophic changes.

central pain Pain initiated or caused by primary lesion or dysfunction in the central nervous system.

dysaesthesia An unpleasant abnormal sensation, either spontaneous or provoked.

hyperaesthesia An increased sensitivity to stimulation, excluding the special senses (includes both *allodynia* and *hyperalgesia*).

hyperalgesia An increased response to a stimulus that is normally painful.

hyperpathia A painful syndrome characterized by an abnormally painful reaction to a stimulus, especially a repetitive stimulus, as well as an increased threshold.

hypoaesthesia Decreased sensitivity to stimulation, excluding the special senses.

hypoalgesia Diminished pain in response to an abnormally painful stimulus.

neuralgia Pain in the distribution of a nerve or nerves.

neuritis Inflammation of a nerve or nerves.

neurogenic pain Pain initiated or caused by a primary lesion, dysfunction, or transitory perturbation in the peripheral or central nervous system.

neuropathic pain Pain initiated or caused by primary lesion or dysfunction in the nervous system.

neuropathy A disturbance of function or a pathological change in a nerve: in one nerve, *mononeuropathy*; in several nerves, *mononeuropathy multiplex*; if diffuse and bilateral, *polyneuropathy*.

nociceptor A receptor preferentially sensitive to a noxious stimulus or to a stimulus that would become noxious if prolonged.

noxious stimulus   A noxious stimulus is one that is damaging to normal tissues.

pain   An unpleasant sensory and emotional experience associated with actual or potential tissue damage or described in terms of such damage.

pain threshold   The least experience of pain that a subject can recognize.

pain tolerance level   The greatest level of pain that a subject is prepared to tolerate.

paraesthesia   An abnormal sensation, either spontaneous or provoked.

peripheral neurogenic pain   Pain initiated or caused by a primary lesion or dysfunction of or transitory perpetuation in the peripheral nervous system.

peripheral neuropathic pain   Pain initiated or caused by a primary lesion in or dysfunction of the peripheral nervous system.

Complex regional pain syndrome, type I

1. The presence of an initiating noxious event, or a cause of immobilization.
2. Continuing pain, allodynia or hyperalgesia, with which the pain is disproportionate to any inciting event.
3. Evidence at some time of oedema, changes in skin blood flow, or abnormal sudomotor activity in the region of the pain.
4. This diagnosis is excluded by the existence of conditions that would otherwise account for the degree of pain and dysfunction.

Note: Criteria 2–4 must be satisfied.

Complex regional pain syndrome, type II

1. The presence of continuing pain, allodynia or hyperalgesia after a nerve injury, not necessarily limited to the distribution of the injured nerve.
2. Evidence at some time of oedema, changes in skin blood flow or abnormal sudomotor activity in the region of the pain.
3. This diagnosis is excluded by the existence of conditions that would otherwise account for the degree of pain and dysfunction.

Note: All three criteria must be satisfied.

Classification criteria for primary and concomitant fibromyalgia

For classification purposes, patients will be said to have fibromyalgia if both of the criteria described below are satisfied. Widespread pain must have been present for at least 3 months. The presence of a second clinical disorder does not exclude the diagnosis of fibromyalgia.

1. History of widespread pain. *Definition:* Pain is considered widespread when all of the following are present: pain in the left side of the body, pain in the right side of the body, pain above the waist and below the waist. In addition, axial skeletal pain (cervical spine or anterior chest or thoracic spine or low back) must be present. In this definition, shoulder and buttock pain is considered as pain for each involved side. 'Low back' pain is considered lower segment pain.

2. Pain in 11 of 18 tender point sites on digital palpation. *Definition:* Pain, on digital palpation, must be present in at least 11 of the following 18 tender point sites:
   - Occiput: bilateral, at the suboccipital muscle insertions.
   - Low cervical: bilateral, at the anterior aspects of the intertransverse spaces at C5–C7.
   - Trapezius: bilateral, at the midpoint of the upper border.
   - Supraspinatus: bilateral, at origins above the scapula spine near the medial border.
   - Second rib: bilateral, at the second costochondral junctions, just lateral to the junctions on upper surfaces.
   - Lateral epicondyle: bilateral, 2 cm distal to the epicondyles.
   - Gluteal: bilateral, in upper outer quadrants of buttocks in anterior fold of muscle.
   - Greater trochanter: bilateral, posterior to the trochanteric prominence.
   - Knees: bilateral, at the medial fat pad proximal to the joint line.

Digital palpation should be performed with an approximate force of 4 kg. For a tender point to be considered 'positive', the subject must state that the palpation was painful. 'Tender' is not to be considered painful.

Diagnostic criteria for somatization disorder

1. A history of many physical complaints beginning before age 30 years that occur over a period of several years and result in treatment being sought or significant impairment in social, occupational or other important areas of functioning.
2. Each of the following criteria must have been met, with individual symptoms occurring at any time during the course of the disturbance:
   (a) Four pain symptoms: a history of pain related to at least four different sites of functions (e.g. head, abdomen, back, joints, extremities, chest, rectum, during menstruation, during sexual intercourse or during urination).
   (b) Two gastrointestinal symptoms: a history of at least two gastrointestinal symptoms other than pain (e.g. nausea, bloating, vomiting other than during pregnancy, diarrhoea or intolerance of several different foods).
   (c) One sexual symptom: a history of at least one sexual or reproductive symptom other than pain (e.g. sexual indifference, erectile or ejaculatory dysfunction, irregular menses, excessive menstrual bleeding or vomiting throughout pregnancy).
   (d) One pseudo-neurological symptom: a history of at least one symptom or deficit suggesting a neurological condition not limited to pain (conversion symptoms such as impaired coordination or balance, paralysis or localized weakness, difficulty swallowing or lump in throat, aphonia, urinary retention, hallucinations, loss of touch or pain sensation, double vision, blindness, deafness, seizures; dissociative symptoms such as amnesia; or loss of consciousness other than fainting).
3. Either
   (a) After appropriate investigation, each of the symptoms in criterion 2 cannot be fully explained by a known general medical condition or the direct effects of a substance (e.g. a drug of abuse or a medication).
   Or
   (b) When there is a related general medical condition, the physical complaints or resulting social or occupational impairment are in excess of what would be expected from the history, physical examination or laboratory findings.
4. The symptoms are not intentionally produced or feigned (as in factitious disorder or malingering).

Diagnostic criteria for undifferentiated somatoform disorder

1. One or more physical complaints (e.g. fatigue, loss of appetite, or gastrointestinal or urinary complaints).
2. Either
   (a) After appropriate investigation, the symptoms cannot be fully explained by a known general medical condition or the direct effects of a substance (e.g. a drug of abuse or a medication).
   Or
   (b) When there is a related general medical condition, the physical complaints or resulting social or occupational impairment is in excess of what would be expected from the history, physical examination or laboratory findings.
3. The symptoms cause clinically significant distress or impairment in social, occupational or other important areas of functioning.
4. The duration of the disturbance is at least 6 months.
5. The disturbance is not better accounted for by another mental disorder (e.g. another somatoform disorder, sexual dysfunction, mood disorder, anxiety disorder, sleep disorder, or psychotic disorder).

6. The symptom is not intentionally produced or feigned (as in factitious disorder or malingering).

Diagnostic criteria for conversion disorder

1. One or more symptoms or deficits affecting voluntary motor or sensory function that suggest a neurological or other general medical condition.
2. Psychological factors are judged to be associated with the symptom or deficit because the initiation or exacerbation of the symptom or deficit is preceded by conflicts or other stressors.
3. The symptom or deficit is not intentionally produced or feigned (as in factitious disorder or malingering).
4. The symptom or deficit cannot, after appropriate investigation, be fully explained by a general medical condition, or by the direct effects of a substance, or as a culturally sanctioned behaviour or experience.
5. The symptom or deficit causes clinically significant distress or impairment in social, occupational or other important areas of functioning, or warrants medical evaluation.
6. The symptom or deficit is not limited to pain or sexual dysfunction, does not occur exclusively during the course of somatization disorder, and is not better accounted for by another mental disorder.

Diagnostic criteria for pain disorder

1. Pain in one or more anatomical sites is the predominant focus of the clinical presentation and is of sufficient severity to warrant clinical attention.
2. The pain causes clinically significant distress or impairment in social, occupational or other important areas of functioning.
3. Psychological factors are judged to have an important role in the onset, severity, exacerbation or maintenance of the pain.
4. The symptom or deficit is not intentionally produced or feigned (as in factitious disorder or malingering).

5. The pain is not better accounted for by a mood, anxiety or psychotic disorder, and does not meet criteria for dyspareunia.
   Acute pain disorder: duration of less than 6 months.
   Chronic pain disorder: duration of 6 months or longer.

Diagnostic criteria for hypochondriasis

1. Preoccupation with fears of having, or the idea that one has, a serious disease based on the person's misinterpretation of bodily symptoms.
2. The preoccupation persists despite appropriate medical evaluation and reassurance.
3. The belief in criterion 1 is not of delusional intensity and is not restricted to a circumscribed concern about appearance (as in body dysmorphic disorder).
4. The preoccupation causes clinically significant distress or impairment in social, occupational, or other important areas of functioning.
5. The duration of the disturbance is at least 6 months.
6. The preoccupation is not better accounted for by generalized anxiety disorder, obsessive–compulsive disorder, panic disorder, a major depressive episode, separation anxiety or another somatoform disorder.

APPENDIX 2

A typical day of exercise therapy is as follows:

08.00–09.00   *Routine morning chores.* Dressing, grooming one's self and eating breakfast before therapy begins.

09.00–09.50   *Therapy pool.* Most patients are seen in small groups, although younger patients require one-to-one supervision for safety and compliance. Patients who compete with each other for greater degrees of pain and dysfunction are supervised on a one-to-one basis. Pool activities include: weight-bearing laps in shallow water such as hopping, running or jumping, 20 minutes of water aerobics, jogging while wearing a waist float or treading water for 5 minutes, flutter kicking laps with a kick board, upper extremity resistive exercises wearing hand paddles, swimming laps and water polo. Motivators such as choosing to eliminate one or two activities later in the day are used to increase effort and speeds during pool activities.

10.00–11.00 *Occupational therapy*. Patients are seen on a one-to-one basis. Timed activities are used to measure functional progress. For example: a 100-foot walk, a 900-foot walk, stepping in and out of bathtub 10 times, loading and unloading a dishwasher, and removing and replacing all the dishes from a cupboard. Non-timed activities include: washing the wall with dry towels 10 times in each direction (up and down, side to side, clockwise, counterclockwise and in a 10-foot arc – to require shifting of weight from foot to foot), ball aerobics for 10 minutes, writing or kitchen activities (such as folding 25 towels). These activities are frequently done while standing only on the involved foot with the other foot elevated. The quality of movement is monitored continuously by the therapist, who frequently gives verbal cues to correct abnormal gait or arm movements. Regions of allodynia are treated with contrast baths, towel rubs (from 30 seconds to 2 minutes), and ice or lotion massage. Patients are encouraged to do the desensitization, but early on most are unable to do so. Patients time themselves and are

otherwise encouraged to take an active role in the therapy programme.

11.00–12.00 *Physical therapy*. Patients are seen on a one-to-one basis. Endurance exercises are selected with the patient's interest, independence and symptoms in mind. Sessions begin with the relevant sport stretches and maximum active range of motion of the involved joints. Endurance exercises include: stationary bicycling with varying resistances, treadmill jogging and running at various speeds and inclines, mini-trampoline jumping using aerobic dance and skiing jumps to give maximum weight-shifting and balance reactions, skipping with a rope, and calisthenics such as jumping jacks, squat thrusts, mountain climber steps, push-ups and sit-ups. Every effort is made to simulate physical education or sport-specific activities, especially those that result in pain. The exercises are frequently done using a mirror or videotaping for visual feedback and to assist with compliance.

12.00–13.00 *Lunch*.

13.00–14.00 *Occupational therapy*. Desensitization exercises are repeated, increasing the pressure and the amount of texture and time up to 10 minutes as the programme progresses. The timed activities of the morning are repeated, and if goals to decrease times are not met, the activities are repeated until they are. Additional activities include: timed scooter board races with a therapist (prone for upper extremity involvement, sitting for lower extremity involvement), timed animal walks for 100 feet (bear walk on all fours, frog hop by squatting with one hand touching the floor on each hop, one-legged bunny hop using two hands and the involved foot, crab walk in supine with both hands and feet weight-bearing), sitting activities for those with pain on sitting (writing and computer games for up to 20 minutes).

14.00–15.00   *Psychological evaluation time.*

15.00–16.00   *Physical therapy.* The patient's functional mobility is re-evaluated. All timed activities are repeated with goals to improve times. Activities are repeated if the time goals are not met. Endurance training, as in the morning, is resumed with the final 20 minutes being soccer drills or other sport-specific activities of the patient's choice.

16.00–17.00   *Free patient and family swim.* During this time the patient independently performs an exercise programme based on the morning pool session. Time is allowed for play and relaxation in the therapy pool.

Evening   *Home programme.* This consists of 30–40 minutes worth of activities from both physical therapy and occupational therapy and is done independently by the patient. A checklist is provided to indicate compliance. If the patient experiences increased pain during the evening or night, they repeat the programme. Patients are strongly encouraged to pick active recreational activities such as walks, shopping and sightseeing, and to do routine household chores (if an outpatient), rather than watching television or videotapes.

Schoolwork is generally put on hold and catch-up work done once the adolescent returns to the classroom. Some schoolwork can be done during break times and in the evenings, but most patients are too exhausted to do much. Rarely, a patient will have missed so much school before being diagnosed and treated that a school year is lost.

12

Rehabilitation and recreation

Carol B Lindsley

INTRODUCTION

According to one USA paediatric rheumatology database, adolescents comprise approximately 36% of children with rheumatic disease (S Bowyer, personal communication). A majority of these patients will require or will benefit from some aspect of rehabilitation during the course of their disease. Adolescents may even have an higher prevalence of rheumatic disease than the overall paediatric population. In a study done in Belgium, the overall prevalence was 167 per 100 000 with definite arthritis and up to 301 per 100 000 with possible arthritis.[1] Milder and remitting cases may contribute to the higher than average prevalence figures.

'Rehabilitation' is an umbrella term encompassing activities ranging from therapeutic exercise and heat to the use of minimal-to-extensive joint support or corrective devices. Many of the commonly used methods of treatment lack proof of efficacy. This chapter presents generally accepted approaches currently used by paediatric rheumatologists.

The spectrum of disability affecting the adolescent depends on the specific disease, its severity and previous therapy. Successful rehabilitation includes four key factors:

- careful assessment of musculoskeletal status
- access to a team of professionals with the necessary expertise to provide treatment
- good communication (or even a contract) with the patient and family about the goals of the therapy
- a programme with specific definitions of realistic expectations, time lines for improvement, etc.

The team of professionals ideally includes a paediatric rheumatologist, physical therapist, occupational therapist, nurse and social worker, with consultation available as needed from a psychologist, psychiatrist, dietician, orthopaedist, ophthalmologist and orthodontist.

REHABILITATION

Generic issues

Both the level of pain as well as pain tolerance varies with the individual. Optimal therapy cannot be accomplished when the teenager has substantial pain. With new-onset disease in particular, a minimal programme of joint protection and isometric exercises may be all that is tolerable until the disease is better controlled with medication and a more comprehensive and progressive programme can be instituted. Conversely, most patients with any degree of joint inflammation have stiffness, which is usually worse in the early morning. Stiffness is relieved by proper medication and, often, heat application. Timing of the therapy sessions is important, and they should not occur in the early morning, when patients are stiff, or late in the day, when they are fatigued. Even in patients with mild or inactive disease, early morning stretching is helpful. Fatigue occurs as a result of numerous factors, including poorly controlled disease, intercurrent infections, poor nutrition, inadequate rest and, especially in teenagers, overscheduled and stressed life-styles. Optimal therapy does not occur with fatigued patients, so attempts to identify the relevant factors in individual patients should be made by the appropriate team members.

General principles

Assessment

Careful comprehensive musculoskeletal assessment includes assessment of all joints, including measured range of motion in all involved joints. This should be done using a goniometer, both at baseline and at periodic re-evaluations thereafter. Care should be taken to do measurements on a typical day if possible. In addition, evaluation should include:

- assessment of gait with attention to stride, limping, asymmetry
- assessment of muscle strength, both distal and proximal, using a standard scale[2]
- assessment of posture and the axial skeleton, including scoliosis, lordosis, leg length and pelvic obliquity (pelvic tilt)
- assessment of activities of daily living as appropriate.

Realistic treatment programme

It is increasingly uncommon for children with arthritis to be hospitalized for rehabilitation, but this varies from country to country. Therefore, almost all therapeutic regimens may be on an outpatient or home basis. Therapy is likely needed at some point for almost every patient with active arthritis. Most patients will not tolerate therapy sessions of longer than 30 minutes on a long-term basis. Therefore, recommended items of the programme need to be prioritized. An exercise programme should be demonstrated, and written or video instruction provided. Early in the course of treatment, periodic occupational therapy or physical therapy supervision is often needed to complement the home programme. In situations where the parents and child do not tolerate the stress of home therapy regimens, the school therapist, if available, can play an important role. As an alternative, the patient can be managed by regular outpatient clinic visits. Even if therapy is carried out solely in the outpatient clinic or school setting, patients will still need to be educated on a home joint protection programme.

Emphasis on extension

Since inflammation results in tenderness and swelling of joints, the tendency is for the patient to place their joints in a 'position of comfort', which is almost always flexion. This preference for a position of flexion leads to complications, including flexion contractures, extensor tendon atrophy, muscle shortening and spasm, abnormal posture and fatigue from inefficient muscle mechanics.

Prevention of contractures and deformities

Prevention of contractures and deformity are important components of rehabilitation. Key factors include:

- adequate medical therapy for good disease control
- a regular exercise programme to maintain muscle strength and mobility
- adequate time for injury healing
- protection of involved or vulnerable joints (especially wrists, knees or ankles) during sports or recreational activities
- a daily stretching programme prior to any sports participation.

Therapeutic exercises

A regular exercise programme in the patient with arthritis is required to maintain range of motion and minimize deformity. The ongoing inflammation is a constant force toward joint flexion and loss of range, associated atrophy and ultimate deformity. General activities, such as bicycling or swimming, although desirable, are not a substitute for a therapeutic exercise programme.

The goal of the exercise programme is to maintain or regain lost range of motion, and to prevent or reverse muscle atrophy. Maintaining function or regaining lost functional skills is always a priority, and is frequently motivation for the teenager to adhere to the exercise programme. The categories of exercise are listed in Table 12.1. Generally, in a patient with actively inflamed joints, the regimen begins slowly, with few repetitions and passive–assistive exercises or isometrics. As the arthritis becomes better controlled, the regimen gradually progresses to active exercises with or without resistance. Resistive exercises with free weights should be used cautiously, if at all, during active disease, as loading of an inflamed joint can increase the inflammatory

Table 12.1 Categories of exercise

- Passive: therapist provides all movement
- Passive–assistive: therapist provides some of movement, assisted, as tolerated, by patient
- Isometrics: no movement of joint, but muscle contraction
- Active: patient provides all movement
- Resistive: movements are resisted by therapist or weights

response. Exercise programmes carried out in water will often decrease the discomfort and are an ideal way to initiate an exercise programme in a patient with very active disease.

Heat and other modalities

Heat is the most commonly used therapeutic modality and will almost always relieve pain and joint stiffness to some degree.[3] Heat can be applied to local areas by means of hot packs, hot towels, microwave packs or heating pads (less desirable). These are particularly helpful prior to beginning an exercise programme or to relieve morning stiffness, especially of the cervical spine. More generalized heat is also beneficial, and can be accomplished with the use of an electric blanket, outdoor-rated sleeping bag, heated waterbed and morning showers or a warm bath. Waterbeds are particularly helpful in improving the quality of sleep in patients who awaken multiple times during the night due to stiffness or joint pain.

Paraffin baths have long been used for hand and wrist arthritis. Hands are dipped in warm wax several times until a layered effect is achieved and then wrapped in a towel for 15–20 minutes. This procedure is particularly helpful prior to a hand exercise programme, but the effect is not long lasting. The time required may be problematic for adolescents.

Deep heat, such as ultrasound or diathermy, is frequently used in adults with acute arthritis, but has not been effective in chronic arthritis. It has not been shown to be effective in younger patients, and should be used with caution even in adolescents. In ultrasound treatment, high-frequency sound waves increase the temperature primarily at the muscle–bone interface, with little effect on superficial tissues. This modality is potentially useful in therapy for hip involvement and for stretching bands of fibrous tissue.[4]

Cold application (cold packs, ice packs or frozen vegetable packages) is of benefit primarily in acute injury or postoperatively as a means of minimizing swelling and providing mild analgesia. Cold occasionally is also beneficial for the treatment of muscle spasms or severe episodic pain. Caution must be used in the application of heat or cold in patients with impaired sensation or with impaired vascular perfusion. The optimal temperature for heat therapy is 40–45°C.[3]

Other modalities include transcutaneous electrical stimulation (TENS), which is the application of an electric current through the skin to the muscle. This technique can be helpful for limited periods of time to increase muscle strength, after injury or during the later phases of rehabilitation of reflex sympathetic dystrophy.[5]

Splinting

Splints can be very useful adjuncts to therapy in order to rest a joint experiencing a disease flare and to maintain or occasionally regain motion in an involved joint. The most commonly used splints in adolescents are the individually fabricated wrist cock-up splints, soft 'gauntlet'-type wrist splint and cervical collars. Lower extremity posterior knee extension shells and ankle splints have very limited use in this age group. Splints can be divided into three categories according to their function: resting splints, corrective splints and functional splints.[6]

Resting splints. These are used in the active stage of disease and can initially be worn for long hours; however, as disease control improves, they are generally worn as night resting splints only. The most common position is 20° of wrist extension in the cock-up splint, usually without finger extension in the adolescent (Figure 12.1).

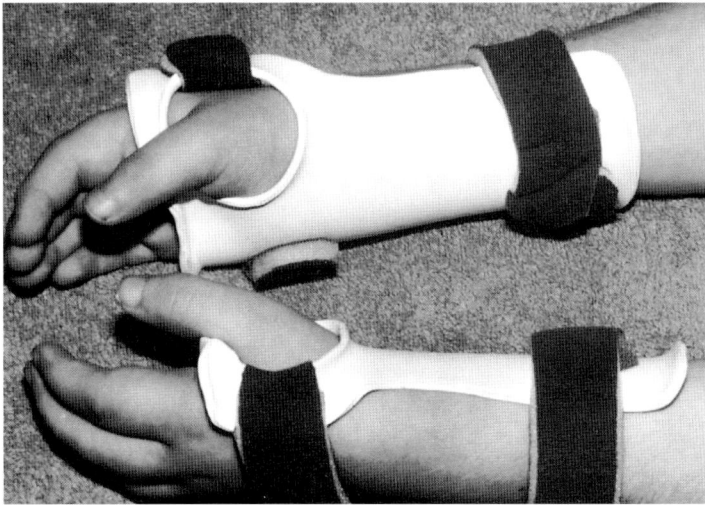

Figure 12.1 Wrist 20° cock-up splints without finger extension.

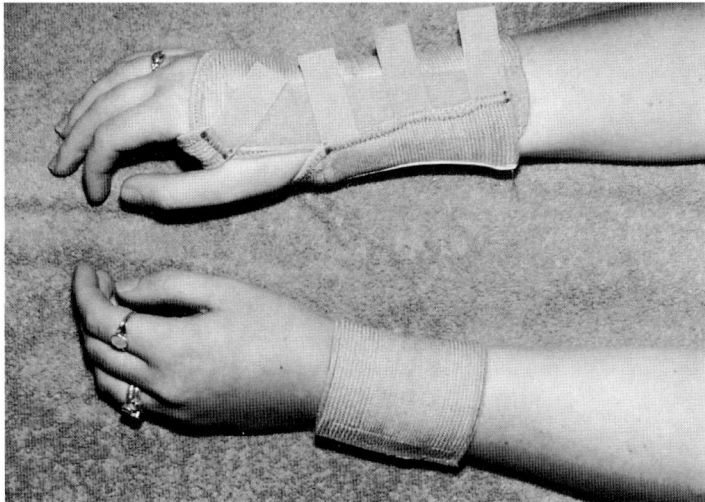

(a)

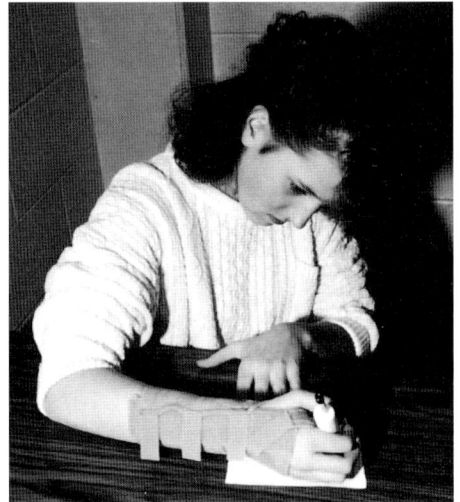

(b)

Figure 12.2 (a) Gauntlet-style functional splint (top) and wrist wrap (bottom). (b) These can be worn during writing or other functional activities.

Functional splints. In active adolescents who require wrist splinting during the day or for joint protection, the gauntlet splint (functional splint) is a good option (Figure 12.2). It can be worn at school during periods of writing or exercise on an as-needed basis, and is generally well accepted. Simple wrist wraps can also provide support. Other functional splints include ankle–foot orthoses. These can be a custom-made ankle–foot orthosis or a simple laced ankle support. These are usually helpful in teenage boys with persistent ankle pain and ankle valgus. For feet needing just some additional medial support, a soft moulded shoe insert can be helpful. For patients with fasciitis and heel tenderness, heel cushions or cups offer relief (Figure 12.3). Silver Ring Splints™ are also in the functional category (Figure 12.4).

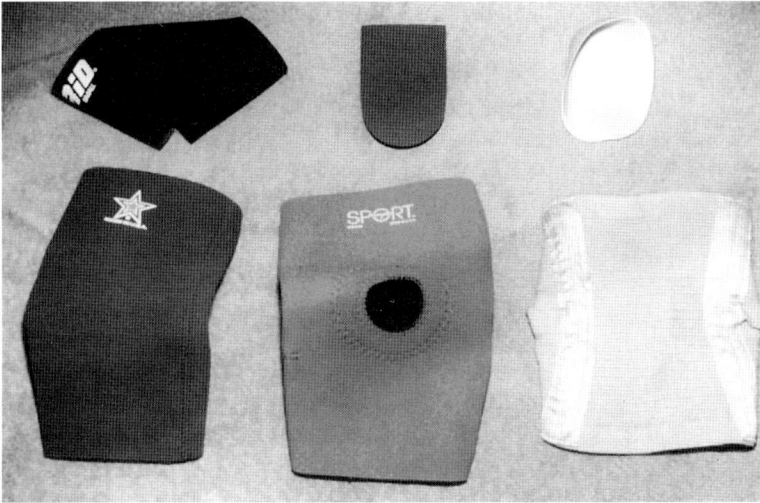

Figure 12.3 Soft supports/cushions (clockwise from upper left): neoprene ankle; heel cushion; heel cup; neoprene knee; neoprene knee with patellar cut-out; rayon x-action knee sleeve. All can be used for light joint support or joint protection.

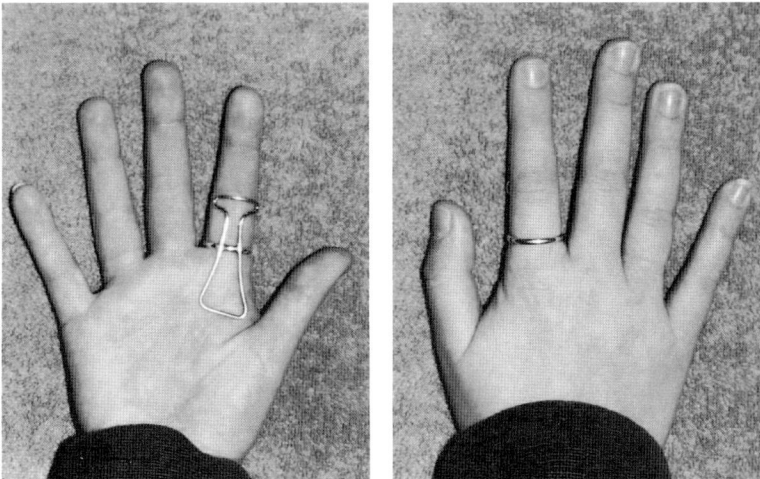

Figure 12.4 Silver Ring Splints™ for (a) 'trigger finger' and (b) 'boutonniere' deformity (middle finger) and 'swan-neck' deformity (ring finger) worn with true ring.

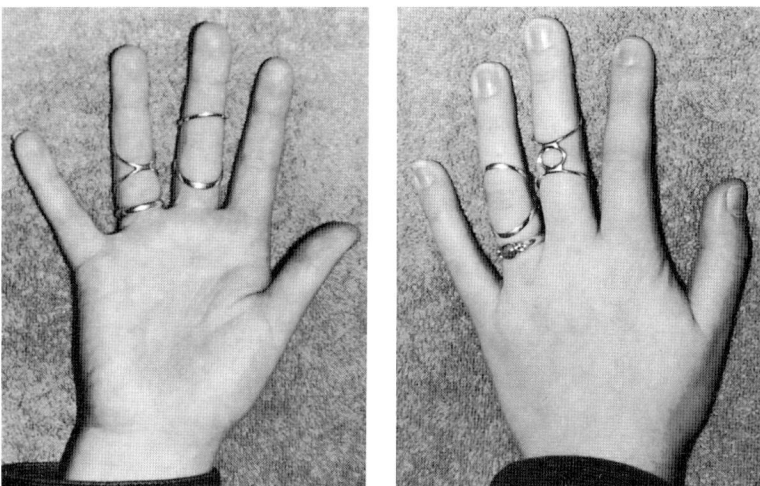

(a)

(b)

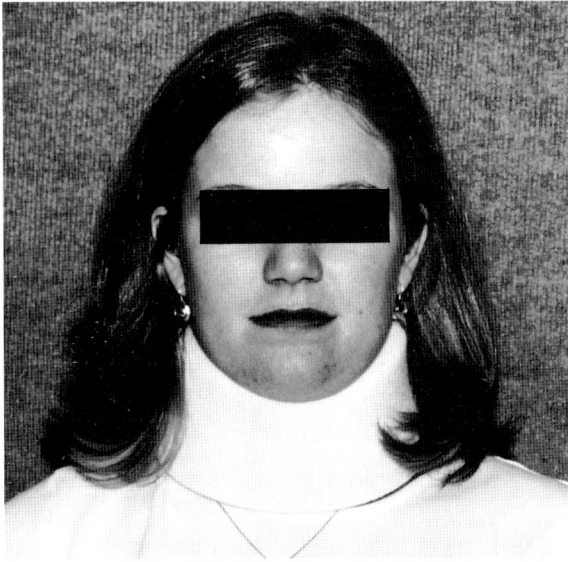

Figure 12.5 A soft cervical collar (neck held at neutral position) used to reduce pain and maintain position.

Corrective splints (including both serial casting and dynamic splints). Serial casting is rarely used in adolescents, but is helpful in younger patients in reducing long-standing contractures. The more commonly used corrective splint for adolescents is the dynamic wrist extension splint used to increase range of motion, especially postoperatively. Dynamic splints contain rubber bands or springs that provide a constant extension force on the wrist.

Cervical collar. Many teenagers with arthritis have limited cervical spine motion and neck pain. A fitted soft cervical collar tailored so that the chin just rests on the top of the collar can provide excellent pain relief and help maintain a good head position, avoiding the tendency toward increasing flexion and contracture (Figure 12.5). These collars can be purchased in sporting goods stores or medical supply stores and modified to fit the individual. They can be especially helpful during long study periods, while watching TV in the evenings or when travelling in a car.

There are few scientific data addressing the efficacy of splinting. Unfortunately, no controlled studies in comparable populations of adolescents with arthritis have been made. However, wrist splints have been shown to improve writing performance in 60% of children with arthritis.[7] A recent study in children over 10 years of age compared the orthoplast cock-up splint with the ready-made work splint, a gauntlet-type splint.[8] Both splints were worn during the day and performed well at reassessment at 3 and 6 months. The ready-made splint was preferred for comfort but the orthoplast splint demonstrated better joint position at the end of the study. Both splint types improved wrist extension, and correction of ulnar deviation was also accomplished.

Mobility aids and adaptive equipment

Independence is of prime importance to the adolescent. The largest threat to these patients' independence is hip disease. For limited periods, full or partial weight-bearing crutches (axillary or platform) can provide pain relief and potentially prevent further hip deterioration. Crutches are particularly helpful if wrist and elbow involvement is minimal. Care must be taken to fit the crutches correctly and to instruct in proper usage. The older adolescent or young adult with severe irreversible disability may need a powered mobility scooter or wheelchair in order to navigate the workplace or college campus. For long-term pain and disability, total hip replacement is the best option.

Adaptive equipment most useful to teenagers includes loose clothing, warm-up style outfits, early use of a keyboard or computer for writing and pencil adapters (larger circumference). However, most adolescents resist any adaptive equipment that sets them apart from their peers.

Specific joints

Upper extremities
The wrist and fingers are the most frequently affected joints in polyarticular disease. With active arthritis, the tendency is toward volar

(palmar) wrist flexion, flexion of proximal inter-phalangeal joints and metacarpal phalangeal joints and ulnar deviation. In joints without flexion deformity, a regular exercise programme involving range of motion (including pronation and supination) and resistive exercises for intrinsics is helpful in preventing contractures and atrophy. Exercises should be done on a daily basis. Gripping devices or hand-strengthening devices can further strengthen the hand musculature. These may be simple foam rubber or devices like 'Silly Putty', and the exercises can be done at times convenient to the patient on an ad hoc basis. The patient who presents with contractures or limitation of extension requires splinting of the wrist with or without the fingers included. Night resting splints in a position of function are best. With severe contractures, work splints or dynamic splints for daytime use may be added. The lightweight 'gauntlet-style' work splints may be used for light support and protection during vigorous activity. For the wrist with severe flexion deformity, serial casting may be used. Local steroid injection for severe tenosynovitis may also be useful.

Finger deformities often occur, especially the loss of extension, boutonniere (metacarpal phalangeal joint hyperextension, proximal inter-phalangeal joint flexion and distal interphalangeal joint hyperextension) and 'swan-neck' deformities (proximal interphalangeal joint hyperextension with distal interphalangeal joint flexion). Finger splints of orthoplast may be helpful for flexion deformities; however, the splints most readily accepted by adolescents are the Silver Ring Splints™, which can look like jewellery (see Figure 12.4). These can be worn for up to 24 hours per day, and must be customized. Overall hand weakness and, especially, thumb abduction can lead to problems with activities of daily living.[9] A paraffin bath prior to exercise can be especially effective in reducing hand stiffness.

The elbow is also frequently involved, and limitation of extension can occur early. It is best prevented with regular range-of-motion exercises. Once contracture occurs, active progressive strengthening, often with light weights (less than 2 lb or 0.9 kg) can be helpful. A posterior elbow splint or serial casting can also be used in severe disease. With more chronic changes, limitation of flexion also occurs. This often limits important activities such as hair washing and combing.

The shoulder is involved in juvenile arthritis and spondyloarthropathy. Severe limitation of abduction of the glenohumeral joint can occur. Large effusions and even dissecting cysts of that joint may present with anterior bulging. Range-of-motion exercises, often aided by the use of a pulley, are crucial to maintaining function. Shoulder exercises should be done supine in order to stabilize the scapula and encourage the shoulder motion. Use of aids, such as Theraband or even light weights can make exercises more enjoyable and efficient. Disintegration of the rotator cuff can occur and severely impair shoulder function. Magnetic resonance imaging can identify this complication, which may be amenable to surgical repair.

The temporomandibular joint (TMJ) is involved in over 50% of patients with juvenile arthritis and less commonly in those with spondyloarthropathy.[10] This leads to 'popping', pain with chewing, a decreased oral aperture and, often, problems with dental occlusion. In addition, micrognathia, secondary to growth disturbances involving the mandible, may be present. Gum chewing may increase TMJ problems and should be discouraged.

The TMJ can be exercised by regular stretching. Monitoring by a dentist or orthodontist is important. Night-time splints or mouth guards can be most helpful in relieving jaw pain and helping maintain good dental occlusion.

Spine – cervical region

Most patients with childhood-onset arthritis and many with spondyloarthropathy have cervical spine involvement. Pain leads to flexion deformities, as well as limitation of lateral rotation and lateral flexion. Poor posture often results, and important teenage activities such as driving a car and washing hair are adversely affected.

Hot packs and range-of-motion exercises can help prevent deformity. If severe pain is present, a soft, fitted cervical collar will provide relief. Attention to posture, adjusting chair or table height when studying, use of wide mirrors when driving and avoidance of carrying heavy loads are important.

Ankylosis of one or more cervical vertebrae occurs in up to one-third of patients with juvenile arthritis[11] and the goal is for the joints to fuse in as functional a position as possible. Atlantoaxial joint subluxation accompanied by neurological symptoms is uncommon in juvenile arthritis. If neurological symptoms do occur, surgical fusion is indicated.

Lumbar spine and sacroiliac joints
Both the lumbar spine and sacroiliac joints are frequently involved in spondyloarthropathies and, to a milder degree, the sacroiliac joints in juvenile arthritis. Loss of normal lordosis, with a straightening of the lumbar spine, decreased flexion (as measured by the Schober's test), loss of lateral flexion and loss of extension all occur.

Regular exercise programmes focusing on flexion and extension will help relieve symptoms and prevent loss of motion, as well as abdominal flexor and back extensor muscle weakness. A therapeutic regimen should include abdominal muscle strengthening and chest-expansion exercises, swimming (if possible) and education regarding back protection. The key component of back protection includes good body mechanics, with proper lifting (bending the knees), sitting positions with a maximum of hip flexion (e.g. with the car driver's seat forward) and, often, use of a light back support. Most teenagers prefer support in the form of compression shorts or Spandex biking shorts. These are often worn by their peers for sports-related reasons and do not make the adolescents with arthritis feel conspicuous. They should be worn under regular clothing.

Scoliosis may complicate the inflammatory joint changes if leg-length discrepancy or other causes of pelvic tilt occur. Correction with a shoe lift is usually made to 50–75% of normal. Back evaluation and scoliosis screening should be a regular part of the evaluation of a teenager with arthritis.

Lower extremities
Severe hip involvement is painful and usually the most limiting of all joint involvement in both juvenile arthritis and spondyloarthropathy. Early signs of involvement are increasingly limited motion, especially internal rotation and extension. Mild flexion contractures can occur insidiously, and contribute further to abnormal body mechanics.

Range-of-motion exercises, especially flexion, extension and abduction exercises, are helpful. The pelvis must be stable during the exercises. Prone lying for 20–30 minutes per day with full hip and knee extension will help prevent contractures. With severe involvement, adaptive equipment, including a cane, crutches or walker, can be helpful in relieving acute symptoms.

In spite of overall good disease control, disease progression often occurs in the hip joint. Maintaining as good a joint position and muscle strength as possible is important even if tissue-release procedures or total hip arthroplasty is later required.[12] Acetabuloprotrusio is seen in some patients with significant hip involvement.

Hydrotherapy and swimming are excellent activities for reversing mild flexion deformities and should be strongly encouraged. The natural buoyancy of the water lessens the resistance and hence the strength and energy required to perform joint movement.

The knee is the most frequently involved joint in adolescents with arthritis and is often the initial site of symptoms. Effusions can occur abruptly and markedly limit ambulation. Baker's cysts can also occur, causing pain and occasionally rupturing. Chronic inflammation tends to:

- weaken supporting ligaments and soft-tissue structures, increasing the tendency toward knee valgus
- weaken knee extensors, leading to flexion contractures (further enhanced if hip flexion contractures are present)
- lead to leg-length discrepancy and muscle asymmetry if one knee is more severely involved than the other.

Regular assessment of the knee range of motion, muscle strength, joint stability and leg

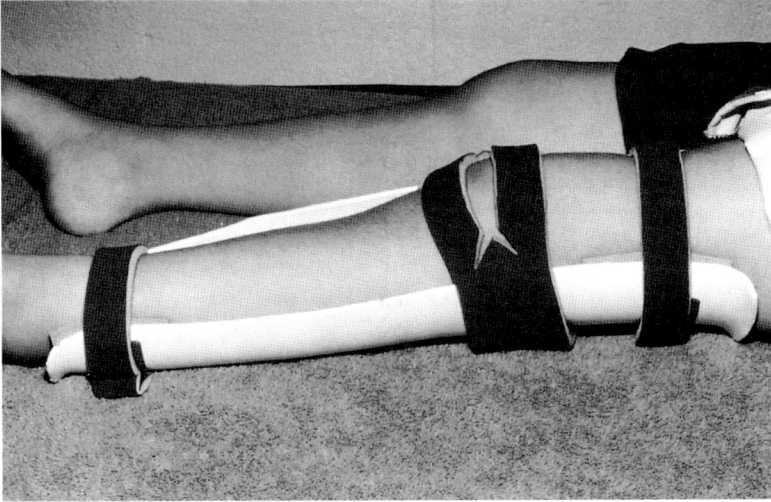

Figure 12.6 Posterior knee splint (shell) of orthoplast, with padding to decrease knee valgus.

length are important. Knee effusions are usually resolved with appropriate antirheumatic medication, which may include local corticosteroid injections.

Regular quadriceps strengthening exercises, initially isometrics and then progressing to light weights, should be used to maintain muscle strength. Iliotibial band and hamstring stretching are important. Posterior knee splints (shells) (Figure 12.6) or serial casting are occasionally used to reduce more severe flexion contractures. Joint protection from injury is extremely important. Soft neoprene or elastic knee sleeves worn during exercise periods or sports are very helpful. If chondromalacia patella is a component of the adolescent's disease, knee sleeves with patellar cut-outs should be used. Occasionally, bracing with an adjustable metal hinge is required to maximize stability after injury or surgery.

Ankle involvement is often heralded by pain, effusion or limitation of dorsiflexion associated with a weak heel strike. Progressive valgus deformity may be seen. Involvement of the talus is particularly painful. Depending upon the severity of involvement, varying degrees of support are indicated. For mild disease, range-of-motion and inversion exercises coupled with good medial shoe support (high-top tennis shoes) will relieve pain and maintain position. For more severely involved joints, customized ankle–foot orthoses will provide more stability. Heel pain is common and is usually relieved by using heel cups or cushions. Arch pain may be secondary to uneven wear on the internal shoe cushion.

Foot involvement, especially of the metatarsophalangeal (MTP) joints, often leads to a painful gait and a weak push-off. It can be exacerbated by wearing high-heeled shoes or western 'cowboy' boots. Careful attention should be paid to the toe box when the teenager purchases shoes, and the wider or more square the toes the better. Hammer and 'claw toe' deformities can be discouraged by wide-toed shoes of adequate length. In severely painful MTP joints, metatarsal bars applied to the sole of the shoe can relieve symptoms. Exact placement is important. Internal bars or pads are usually not helpful because they decrease the internal shoe volume. Occasionally, surgical fusion of the first MTP to realign the joint in severe hallux valgus is helpful and will allow use of more comfortable footwear.

School function

Adolescents spend the majority of their waking hours in school. It is an environment where

Table 12.2 Common school problems
• Gross motor (gelling, standing)
• Fine motor (writing, hand strength)
• Self-care (morning slowness, afternoon fatigue)
• Physical education (running, team sports)
• Social (reluctance to ask for help)

success or failure can have a major impact on the rest of their life. Our studies have shown that approximately 30% of children with juvenile arthritis need some type of modification or assistance with regard to their school routine.[13]

The major problems are listed in Table 12.2. Many of these problems can be solved with simple modifications. The routine history should include questions regarding school problems or adjustments. Often, rearranging class schedules to avoid physical education in the early morning, for example, can make a major difference. Arranging classes on one level to minimize stair-climbing, use of two sets of books (one at school, one at home) to avoid transporting heavy books between home and school, and avoidance of heavy food trays or long periods of standing in line are all other specific helpful modifications. Handwriting is a common problem due to pain, decreased motion and weakness. Decreasing the number and extent of writing assignments or use of a computer or tape recorder are appropriate alternatives. Physical education remains the most problematic of all school activities, and heavy contact sports need to be avoided for most teenagers with active disease. Clear communication between the physician or team member and school personnel can clear the way for 'participation to tolerance' in many activities and avoid total non-participation. For example, walking instead of running laps and stretching instead of strengthening exercises, can make the physical education experience more tolerable. Also high-impact aerobic exercises such as jumping jacks or push-ups need to be monitored and, if problematic, restricted.

Patients with arthritis frequently have reduced aerobic capacity[14] and will benefit from even moderate exercise. Care must be taken to avoid overuse and injury. Nonetheless, risks of total inactivity are far worse, and include muscle weakness, joint contractures, poor endurance and easy fatiguability, and osteoporosis. Heavy weights, overhead lifts, some gymnastics manoeuvres, distance running and heavy contact sports should be avoided. Wrist protection is often needed, particularly in volleyball. Adolescents with moderate or severe disability should have an individual education plan (IEP) or 504 plan (Section 504 of the US Rehabilitation Act[15]) and all patients and family members should be cognizant of the legal rights of children and adolescents.[16] Fatigue and concentration problems secondary to active disease are common complicating factors. Disease symptoms may fluctuate throughout the day or from week to week and school performance may vary accordingly. This fluctuation can be confusing to school personnel if good communication has not occurred.

Adherence and behaviour

Adolescents often have difficulty adhering to long-term medical regimens. There is a tendency to want to discontinue medication when they feel well, and to even overdose on bad days.[17] As most medications used for arthritis take weeks to show maximal effect and when discontinued are not immediately excreted from the body, the long-term benefits of medications are not immediately apparent to most teenagers. Ongoing education and support by the rheumatology team is important. Rehabilitation regimens including daily exercise programmes, splint wearing or joint protection procedures often have similar adherence problems. Some of the simple approaches that the rheumatologist or other team member can take are listed in Table 12.3. Appropriate education of the patient and family is the important initial step. This is particularly essential when the rehabilitation regimen increases family stresses and

Table 12.3   Approaches to improving adherence to treatment

- Simplify medication regimen
- Simplify rehabilitation regimen:
  - prioritize exercises
  - total duration of 10–30 minutes or less
  - provide written, graphical or video instruction
  - maximize comfort of splints
  - help family provide positive reinforcement (e.g. family contract)
  - provide regular follow-up visits for re-evaluation and reinforcement
  - combine rehabilitation activities with fun activities (e.g. prone-lying with TV watching, exercise programmes joined by other family members)
  - choose a convenient time for both the patient and the family for the exercises

impairs parent–child communication. Ultimately, professional consultation with a behavioural psychologist may be needed.

Joint protection

Joint protection is a concept that is important to all adolescents with arthritis. No matter how good their disease control, the involved joints are vulnerable to overuse or injury. Wrists, knees and ankles are particularly at risk and, to a lesser degree, the low back, especially in polyarticular arthritis and the spondylo-arthropathies. Simple elastic joint sleeves can provide adequate joint support and warmth, and add stability during sports and other activities. Compression shorts can provide increased low-back support, and are usually cosmetically acceptable to teenagers. Patients with Raynaud's phenomenon should wear gloves in cold

weather and avoid handling cold objects in order to decrease the risk of cold injury.

Desensitization

Reflex sympathetic dystrophy can accompany arthritis, injury or be idiopathic. The involved extremity(s) is exquisitely sensitive to touch or manipulation. As an initial step in rehabilitation the use of different textures by the occupational therapist in a structured desensitization process can be important. Jelly, jam, rice and beans are examples that can be used in a stepwise process with, or prior to, initiation of a graduated exercise regimen.

RECREATION

Summer camp

Summer camps offer adolescents with arthritis an opportunity to be outdoors, participate either as campers or counsellors and improve their self-image. In one study, campers improved during a 7-day camping experience in both self-image and locus of control.[18] Repeat campers did even better. In addition to physical and psychosocial benefits, the campers gain independence from parents and can meet new friends that may share their health-related problems. Increasing independence will in turn foster disease-management capabilities.[18]

Weekend retreats and family meetings

Two- or three-day retreats for the whole family have been increasingly popular. Data from American Juvenile Arthritis Organization regional conferences have shown significant educational and psychological benefits for participants.[19] These families are often unable, due to financial limitations, to travel to the larger national conferences and other meetings. Other retreats focus on improving coping skills. Three-day sessions in the form of a weekend family retreat have been found to be an effective multidisciplinary method of improving the child's and family's coping skills.[20]

Aquatic sports/water exercise

Water exercise has many general health benefits as well as psychosocial and physical benefits.[21] For patients with arthritis, it is both a safe and an effective means of exercise.[22] In a study of adults with rheumatoid arthritis, participants in a water exercise programme had less disability, pain, anxiety, depression, disease severity and higher grip strengths than did clinic controls.[23] Adolescents should be encouraged to swim regularly and improve swimming techniques so that this beneficial exercise is a fun, life-long habit, not just a prescribed exercise. The various swimming strokes focus on extension, the motion most often compromised in active arthritis. Those patients with back and neck involvement will particularly benefit. Swimming for 30 minutes 2–3 times a week is recommended. Swimming can often be substituted for required gym or physical education class or more formal therapy programmes. Most water facilities have specific times when the water is warmer, at least to 84–86°F or even higher in therapeutic pools (92–98°F). This lessens the effect of cold intolerance that patients may have.[24] An arthritis water exercise class offers specific stretching and strengthening exercises for every joint, and frequently has an aerobic component included. Group exercise classes also function as a support group, which encourages regular and consistent participation.

Other sports

Other sports that can be fun and beneficial are golf, cycling, walking and non-contact forms of karate (e.g. tai chi). Active golfers may benefit from a special handle design.[25] Cycling is an excellent indoor or outdoor aerobic sport that utilizes the large lower extremity muscle groups. It can be both an individual or a group sport. Participants should use proper equipment and avoid overuse, particularly if knee pain is experienced. Specific guidelines should be reviewed.[26]

Competitive or distance running should be done with caution. However, short-distance running and, particularly, walking are excellent aerobic exercises. Proper footwear is important, and intensity and distances should be increased gradually (by approximately 5% per week).[27]

Patient partner programme and other educational programmes

Adolescents may also find recreation and fun through participation in educational projects related to arthritis. In a university-based patient partner programme, two of the nine patient partners were adolescents with arthritis. The adolescents were found to be as effective educators as adults in teaching the musculoskeletal joint examination to medical students and gained in terms of both knowledge and satisfaction from participation.[28]

SUMMARY

Adolescents comprise a significant portion of the paediatric population with arthritis and often have different rehabilitation needs than young children or adults. Communication with both adolescents and their family members is important in order to ensure adherence to the prescribed programme. A multidisciplinary approach is necessary to meet the variety of rehabilitation needs, as is integration of the therapeutic programme into the patient's daily routine if an optimal outcome is to be achieved.

REFERENCES

1. Mielants H, Veys EM, Maertems M et al. Prevalence of inflammatory rheumatic diseases in an adolescent urban student population, age 12 to 18, in Belgium. *Clin Exp Rheumatol* 1993; **2**:563–7.
2. Lovell D. *Childhood Muscle Assessment Scale*. 1998; in press.
3. Lehman JD (ed). *Therapeutic Heat and Cold*. Williams & Wilkins: Baltimore, 1982:82–100.
4. Emery HM, Bowyer SL. Physical modalities of therapy in pediatric rheumatic diseases. *Rheum Dis Clin North Am* 1991; **17**:1001–13.
5. Michlovitz SL. The use of heat and cold in the management of rheumatic diseases. In: *Thermal*

Agents in Rehabilitation (Micholovitz SL, ed), 2nd edn. FA Davis: Philadelphia, 1990:258–74.

6. Donovan WH. Physical measures in the treatment of juvenile rheumatoid arthritis. *Arthritis Rheum* 1977; **20**:553–7.

7. Silver R, Lawton S, Ansell BM. A comparison of Vitrathene moulded with Tweeklon ready-made wrist work splints in juvenile chronic arthritis. *Intl Rehabil Med* 1982; **4**:97–100.

8. Eberhard BA, Sylvester KL, Ansell BM. A comparative study of orthoplast cock-up splints versus ready-made Droitwich work splints in juvenile chronic arthritis. *Disabil Rehabil* 1993; **15**:41–3.

9. Athreya BH. The hand in juvenile rheumatoid arthritis. *Arthritis Rheum* 1977; **20**(suppl):573–4.

10. Olson L, Eckerdal O, Hallonsten AL. Craniomandibular function in juvenile chronic arthritis. A clinical and radiographic study. *Swed Dental J* 1991; **15**:71–2.

11. Fried JA, Athreya BH, Gregg JR et al. The cervical spine in juvenile rheumatoid arthritis. *Clin Orthop Rel Res* 1982; **179**:102–7.

12. Swann M. Management of lower limb deformities. In: *Surgical Management of Juvenile Chronic Polyarthritis* (Arden GP, Ansell BM, eds). Academic Press: London, 1978:97–116.

13. Wright SJ, Lindsley CB, Olson NY. Elementary school function screening tool in JRA. *Arthritis Care Res* 1992; **5**:52.

14. Giannini MJ, Protas EJ. Aerobic capacity in juvenile rheumatoid arthritis patients and healthy children. *Arthritis Care Res* 1991; **4**:131–5.

15. Spencer CH, Zubay Fife R, Rabinovich CE. The school experience of children with arthritis. Coping in the 1990s and transition into adulthood. *Pediatr Clin North Am* 1995; **42**:1285–98.

16. Cassidy JT, Lindsley CB. Legal rights of children with musculoskeletal disabilities. *Bull Rheum Dis* 1997; **45**:1–5.

17. Rapoff MA, Lindsley CB, Olson NY et al. Prevention of medication non-adherence in children with juvenile rheumatoid arthritis. *Arthritis Rheum* 1996; **39**:S314.

18. Stefl ME, Shear ES, Levinson JE. Summer camps for juveniles with rheumatic disease: do they make a difference? *Arthritis Care Res* 1989; **1**:10–15.

19. Kunkel LA, Lindsley CB, Olson NY et al. Regional juvenile arthritis family conferences promote development of advocacy skills to empower families for positive outcomes. *Arthritis Rheum* 1994; **37**:S363.

20. Hagglund KJ, Doyle NM, Clay DL et al. A family retreat as a comprehensive intervention for children with arthritis and their families. *Arthritis Care Res* 1996; **9**:35–41.

21. Tork SC, Douglas V. Arthritis water exercise program evaluation. A self-assessment survey. *Arthritis Care Res* 1989; **2**:28–30.

22. Kirchheimer JC, Wanivenhaus A, Engel A. Does sport negatively influence joint scores in patients with juvenile rheumatoid arthritis. An 8-year prospective study. *Rheumatol Int* 1992; **12**:239–42.

23. Meyer CL, Hawley DJ. Characteristics of participants in water exercise programs compared to patients seen in a rheumatic disease clinic. *Arthritis Care Res* 1994; **7**:85–9.

24. McNeal RL. Aquatic therapy for patients with rheumatic disease. *Rheum Dis Clin N Am* 1990; **16**:915–29.

25. Cahalan TD, Cooney WP, Tamai K et al. Biomechanics of the golf swing in players with pathologic conditions of the forearm, wrist and hand. *Am J Sports Med* 1991; **19**:288–93.

26. Namey TC. Adaptive bicycling. *Rheum Dis Clin North Am* 1990; **16**:871–86.

27. Allen ME. Arthritis and adaptive walking and running. *Rheum Dis Clin North Am* 1990; **16**:887–914.

28. Wright SW, Kunkel A, Lindsley HB, Lindsley CB. Demonstration of the total body musculoskeletal exam to students and physicians is a positive experience for patients with rheumatic disease. *Arthritis Rheum* 1996; **39**:S167.

13

Surgical management of adolescents with rheumatic disease

Stephen J Drew, Brian Cohen and Johan D Witt

INTRODUCTION

This chapter principally deals with the surgical management of adolescents with chronic arthritis although other common problems encountered in the adolescent such as soft tissue and sports injuries will also be covered. The majority of patients with chronic arthritis will be primarily under the care of rheumatologists. They generally present with joint pain and stiffness. Instability is a late feature. Chronic arthritis is rare, affecting approximately 1 in a 1000 children. However, if untreated, especially in the lower limb, it can lead to severe crippling in adolescence and adulthood. The role of orthopaedic surgery in the management of the adolescent with chronic arthritis is limited. Two major factors support a conservative attitude towards surgery: age and growth potential. However, in selected circumstances, especially those associated with pain and mechanical instability, early surgical intervention is indicated. Close consultation between the rheumatologist, therapist and surgeon is essential to identify the indications for and aims of surgical intervention.

There is no universal agreement about the role of surgery in the treatment of patients with chronic arthritis. However, in the case of the growing child, surgical intervention is usually limited to prophylactic procedures. Reconstructive procedures often used in adults are not appropriate, as epiphyseal arrest may ensue. Prophylactic procedures such as splinting, tenosynovectomy and joint synovectomy (usually carried out arthroscopically) still need to be considered, despite the active use of local steroid injections. Reconstructive procedures such as joint resections, osteotomies and arthroplasties are very rarely performed on patients under the age of 16 years. The generalized aims of surgery are to maintain normal function as well as normal physical growth of the affected joint.

The pattern of presentation of adolescents with soft-tissue or sports-related injuries is more variable. They may present acutely or with more chronic conditions and may appear in a variety of clinics, including fracture clinics, sports injuries clinics, orthopaedic clinics and rheumatology clinics. The indications for surgical intervention in individual conditions are discussed.

THE SHOULDER

Chronic arthritis

The shoulder is the least frequently involved large joint and, consequently, until relatively recently has more or less been ignored. In recent years a more active approach has been followed. The incidence of shoulder involvement varies according to the type of chronic arthritis. In pauciarticular-onset chronic arthritis shoulder involvement is virtually absent, while in the polyarticular-onset form the incidence is approximately 50% and in the systemic-onset form the incidence rises to about 80%.[1] In 95% of cases in which there is shoulder involvement the disease is bilateral.

The musculoskeletal pathology is similar to that seen in adult rheumatoid arthritis, with synovial hyperplasia and, in severe cases, pannus formation and erosion of articular cartilage and adjacent bone. Chronic arthritis not only involves the synovium of the glenohumeral joint but can also involve the distal third of the clavicle and acromioclavicular joint, the subacromial bursa, the rotator cuff tendons and the surrounding muscles.[2]

Unless specifically sought for, shoulder involvement may go unrecognized, since the onset is often insidious, the shoulder joint is deeply seated and synovial swelling can, therefore, escape notice. The hallmarks of shoulder involvement are pain and limitation of movement, with internal rotation the most commonly and severely limited motion, followed by abduction.[1] Patients with involvement of the subacromial bursa and rotator cuff tendons will often demonstrate a painful arc, as well as having positive impingement signs.

In examining the shoulder joint radiographically, circumscribed erosive lesions on the superolateral aspect of the humeral head are more commonly seen in adolescent-onset arthritis (44%) than other forms of inflammatory arthropathy.[3] Posterior erosions are better visualized on an axillary view. However, recently magnetic resonance imaging (MRI) appears to be the most sensitive method for evaluating shoulder involvement, since, not only are osseous abnormalities of the glenoid and humeral head readily detected, but soft-tissue abnormalities such as involvement of the rotator cuff tendons and subacromial bursae, joint effusion, and muscular atrophy are easily depicted.[4]

Conservative management of the shoulder involves:

- physiotherapy with daily range-of-motion exercises to preserve good function and muscle strength while, in particular, preventing loss of internal rotation and abduction
- local corticosteroid injections either into the glenohumeral joint or the subacromial bursa.

Surgical intervention may involve either prophylactic or reconstructive procedures.

Prophylactic surgery

SYNOVECTOMY ± BURSECTOMY
The rationale for joint synovectomy is to:

- remove destructive inflamed synovium and pannus tissue
- reduce inflammation by removing fibrin and other debris
- relieve pain by denervation.

There are, however, arguments against synovectomy in children and adolescents. These include problems with patient cooperation after surgery and fears that synovectomy may harm the cartilage, disturb epiphyseal blood circulation and growth, or even cause the disease to progress. An experienced physiotherapist who can win the child's trust and improve cooperation is essential. In addition, it is known that if an appropriate atraumatic technique is used, no cartilage or circulatory disturbance should result.[5]

The indications for synovectomy are:

- little or no erosive changes as seen on radiographs
- no instability or contracture
- failed conservative treatment (i.e. resistant synovitis).

Since arthroscopic synovectomy of the shoulder is a recent addition to the armament in the treatment of synovitis, little is known about its long-term prophylactic effect. However, this is likely to be similar to synovectomy of other large joints, in which good short-term relief of pain is obtained with little influence on disease progression. In the short term, good pain relief and improved mobility have been obtained.[6] However, Ovregard et al[7] have shown that the initial good results following synovectomy in chronic arthritis in children, for a variety of joints, deteriorate significantly after 3 years. It should be noted that most published series of the results of synovectomy involve open synovectomy. The long-term results of arthroscopic synovectomy, which is the usual method of synovectomy now employed, are not known. Synovectomy is contraindicated in patients with indolent dry disease in whom it would be tantamount to performing an arthrodesis.

Arthroscopic shoulder surgery is usually performed through two portals; a posterior portal for the camera and an anterior or working portal for the instruments used for debridement and synovectomy. This allows access to the synovium of the glenohumeral joint, the articular surfaces of the humeral head and glenoid, the long head of the biceps tendon and the undersurface of the rotator cuff tendons. An additional lateral working portal allows debridement of the subacromial bursa, the undersurface of the acromium and the bursal surface of the rotator cuff.

Reconstructive surgery

These operations are rarely indicated before skeletal maturity.

OSTEOTOMY

Where there is moderate to severe bony destruction an osteotomy of the humeral neck combined with a similar osteotomy of the glenoid neck, as originally described by Benjamin,[8] has been shown to give excellent relief of pain, although range of movement is often unaffected. It is becoming less popular with the advent of successful shoulder arthroplasty.

ARTHRODESIS

This is rarely indicated in a disease where stiffness itself is a problem, and even less so now because of the advances made with shoulder arthroplasty. It is largely reserved for use as a salvage operation after the failed arthroplasty.

ARTHROPLASTY

This is rarely necessary in patients less than 16 years old in whom the epiphyses have not closed. It is indicated in patients after skeletal maturity with resistant pain, marked limitation in function and radiological evidence of joint destruction (Figure 13.1). As with other joint replacements in the patient with chronic arthritis, the bone architecture is often small, so that custom-made components may be required. There are no published series of results in patients with chronic arthritis alone; however, in adult patients with rheumatoid arthritis (including a number of patients with chronic arthritis) the results are good, with good or excellent pain relief in 80–90%, improvement in the range of abduction by at least 20° (despite a significant number having rotator cuff tears) and over 90% survival at 11 years.[9–11] The results differ from those for osteoarthritis in only one major respect. The gain in range of motion postoperatively in patients with rheumatoid arthritis is significantly less due to the associated rotator cuff disease.

Other causes of shoulder pain in the adolescent

Shoulder pain is commonly seen in adolescent athletes, particularly those involved in sports requiring overhead actions such as swimming and tennis. The pain is usually secondary to rotator cuff tendinitis, especially the distal aspect of the supraspinatus tendon underlying the coracoacromial arch, although the rest of the rotator cuff and the long head of the biceps tendon may be involved. There is a close relationship between rotator cuff tendinitis, impingement and glenohumeral instability. Both impingement of the rotator cuff on the undersurface of the coracoacromial arch and glenohumeral instability can lead to secondary rotator cuff tendinitis and the differentiation between the two causes can be very difficult.

In patients with shoulder laxity or instability the static stabilizers (glenohumeral ligaments and capsule) are relatively incompetent, and therefore the rotator cuff and shoulder girdle muscles must work harder to limit glenohumeral translation. This may lead to overuse tendinosis. This has been documented in competitive swimmers.[12] In athletes in sports requiring overhead actions, neuromuscular imbalance may also cause rotator cuff tendinitis.[13] Neuromuscular imbalance between either

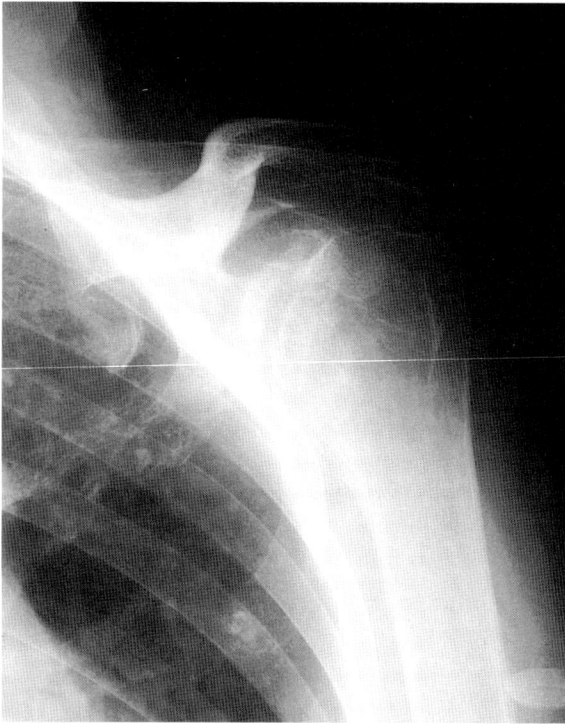
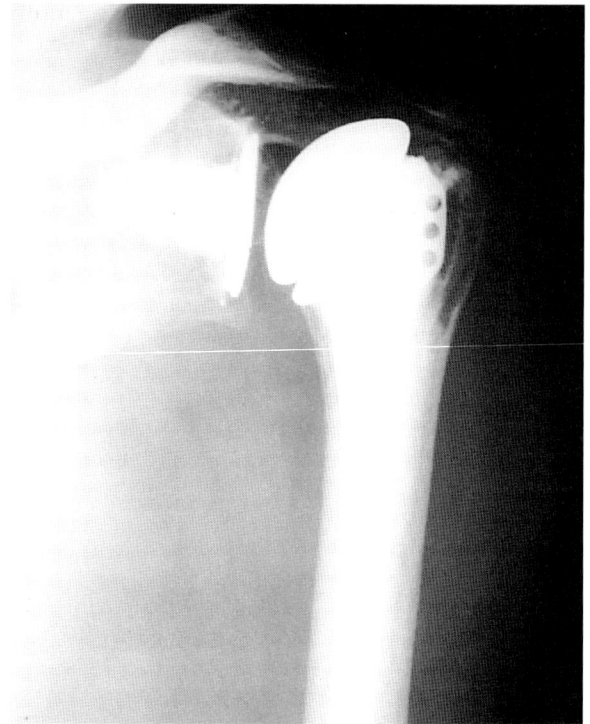

(a)   (b)

Figure 13.1   (a) Radiograph of the left shoulder in a 25-year-old female with chronic arthritis. (b) Radiograph of the same patient treated with a total shoulder replacement.

the internal and external rotators, or between the upper and lower fibres of the trapezius can alter glenohumeral and scapulothoracic dynamics, leading to secondary impingement of the humeral head on the undersurface of the coracoacromial arch and, consequently, rotator cuff tendinitis. Other causes of secondary impingement include poor postural habits and a stiff thoracic spine.

Assessment
The commonest presenting symptom of rotator cuff tendinitis is pain, although other symptoms such as catching, clicking, weakness or feelings of instability may be present. It should be noted that cervical spine and shoulder disorders often have overlapping symptoms and may exist concomitantly.

A thorough shoulder and cervical spine examination is imperative, starting with inspection and leading on to palpation, assessment of range of movement, strength testing, neurological assessment and, finally, performance of special provocative tests. Loss of the normal scapulothoracic and glenohumeral rhythm or scapular winging suggests underlying scapulothoracic dysfunction secondary to shoulder instability, muscle imbalance or fatigue. The range of movement and the arc at which pain occurs should be noted. Loss of internal rotation may indicate posterior capsule contraction, which is often associated with glenohumeral instability. The impingement sign and the impingement test[14] are often positive regardless of the cause of the rotator cuff tendinitis. The tests of Yergason and Speed[14] may indicate long head of biceps pathology. Instability can be very difficult to verify, but several provocative tests are available, including the anterior apprehension sign and relocation test[14] and the posterior stress test.[14] The presence of a sulcus sign[14] may indicate multidirectional instability. If a diagnosis of instability is being considered, generalized ligamentous laxity should be excluded. A formal examination under anaesthesia may be needed to assess the amount of glenohumeral translation in the anterior, posterior and inferior directions.

Treatment
Regardless of the aetiology of the rotator cuff tendinitis most patients can be managed with an appropriate rehabilitation programme. This consists of:

- Pain control by rest, activity modification and the use of non-steroidal anti-inflammatory drugs (NSAIDs).
- Formal assessment by a physiotherapist. A biofeedback machine may be helpful in confirming muscle imbalance. Instigation of a rehabilitation programme aimed at correcting muscle imbalance by re-education, restoration of range of movement and a muscle strengthening programme.
- Subacromial injections of steroids should be reserved for those not responding to NSAIDs and physiotherapy.

If the patient fails to respond to an appropriate rehabilitation programme then consideration should be given to surgical intervention.

The use of shoulder arthroscopy has enhanced the ability to diagnose and evaluate shoulder pathology more accurately. Patients demonstrating primary mechanical impingement may benefit from an arthroscopic (or open if arthroscopy is not available) subacromial decompression, consisting of resection of the coracoacromial ligament and an anterior acromioplasty. It should be noted that postoperative recovery is slow, with only 28% of patients having relief of symptoms at 3 months, although 85% have relief of symptoms at 12 months.[15]

For instability, various procedures are available. The procedure chosen is determined by the underlying pathology. Those patients who have had formal anterior shoulder dislocation commonly have a tear of the anterior glenoid labrum, and in those patients with recurrent symptoms of dislocation or instability a Bankart repair,[16] which is now often combined with a capsulorrhaphy, gives excellent results. In those patients in whom the instability is largely due to capsular laxity, a capsular shift procedure to reduce the redundant capsule also gives excellent results.[17]

Acromioclavicular joint dislocation
The acromioclavicular joint is classically injured by a fall onto the point of the shoulder. The peak incidence is in the adolescent and young adult, and it is far more common in males, especially those involved in contact sports. Although complex classifications are available, it can be simply classified into complete and incomplete dislocation, depending on the integrity of the acromioclavicular and coracoclavicular ligaments. The patient usually presents acutely with localized pain and tenderness over the acromioclavicular joint and, if the injury involves complete disruption of the acromioclavicular and coracoclavicular ligaments, the distal clavicle appears to be displaced superiorly as the scapula and shoulder complex droop inferomedially.

The treatment of an incomplete dislocation is rest, NSAIDs, and a sling for support for approximately 2 weeks until symptoms start to subside, followed by a gradual rehabilitation programme.

The treatment of complete dislocations is more controversial, with both surgical and non-surgical methods having enjoyed cyclical popularity. Non-surgical methods are again based on the use of a sling and a rehabilitation programme. Some surgeons have recommended the use of a harness/strapping, although this is not currently favoured by most surgeons. Surgical treatment is currently only recommended for patients who perform heavy manual tasks or overhead sporting activities. Numerous procedures have been described, the majority of which involve repair of the coracoclavicular

(a)

(b)

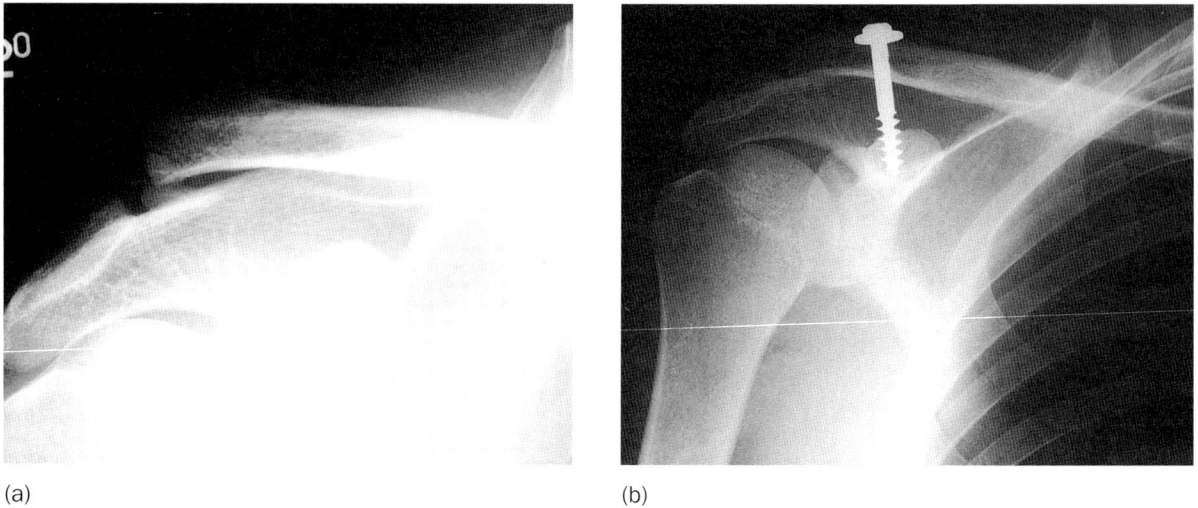

Figure 13.2 (*a*) An 18 year old male with complete (grade 3) dislocation of acromioclavicular joint. (*b*) Radiograph following repair of the coracoclavicular ligament and insertion of coracoclavicular screw.

ligaments combined with temporary internal fixation with either a coracoclavicular screw or sling to protect the repair (Figure 13.2). Later reconstructive procedures are available for those treated conservatively and who have ongoing pain from the acromioclavicular joint.

THE ELBOW JOINT

Chronic arthritis

Approximately 25% of patients with chronic arthritis exhibit early symptoms in the elbow joint and 45% have some residual joint symptoms. One of the earliest signs seen with elbow involvement is loss of full extension, which often occurs before the patient complains of pain or there is palpable synovitis. The number of procedures performed on the elbow is very low. There are several possible explanations for this:

- although the overall incidence of early symptoms in the elbow is high the prognosis for the elbow joint is often good
- local medical treatment may have a more

beneficial effect on the elbow than on other joints
- there is a limited number of surgical procedures available and few patients fulfil the criteria for these procedures.

While total elbow replacement has been successful in providing pain relief and functional improvement in advanced disease, synovectomy has been the traditional treatment for early stages of involvement after conservative measures have failed.

Synovectomy ± radial head excision
The indication for and rationale of elbow synovectomy are as listed for the shoulder joint. Ovregard et al[7] reported on a series of 394 joint synovectomies in children with chronic arthritis over a 12-year period, and in their series only 15 were carried out on the elbow. Arden[18] has stated that elbow synovectomy is a valuable procedure for suitably selected patients. The radial head is usually preserved in the skeletally immature patient so as to prevent postoperative deformity as growth continues. There are no

large series of cases published for patients with chronic arthritis; however, synovectomy in rheumatoid arthritis is usually done in combination with radial head excision (due to erosive damage to the radiocapitellar joint). Most authors regard the operation as reliable in terms of pain relief in the short term.[19,20] The results with regard to movement are more variable, with some authors reporting significant gains in flexion and extension and others reporting minimal improvement or even loss of movement.[21] The longer term results are mixed. Gendi et al[22] reported that only approximately 50% of patients had little or no pain at 6 years. Tulp and Winia[23] reported that 67% had a satisfactory result at 6 years. Others report a significant incidence of instability following radial head excision and synovectomy.[21,24] Again it should be noted that most of the published series are on the results of open synovectomy. Arthroscopic synovectomy is being increasingly used. Lee and Morrey[25] have reported on a series of 14 arthroscopic synovectomies, with 93% achieving a good or excellent rating in the short term. After an average of 42 months, however, only 57% maintained this rating, with four patients having gone on to require a total elbow replacement.

Reconstructive surgery

This is indicated in the skeletally mature patient with debilitating pain, loss of function or radiological evidence of joint destruction.

INTERPOSITION ARTHROPLASTY

This is an infrequently used procedure in which the joint is resurfaced by clothing the joint surface either with strips of fascia lata or epidermal skin. It is indicated in patients with debilitating pain and stiffness, and may be more applicable in the younger patient, in whom there is more concern about early loosening of a prosthetic replacement. There are no reports of its use in patients with chronic arthritis alone, but it has been shown to give good relief of pain and improved range of movement in both rheumatoid arthritis and post-traumatic arthritis.[26,27]

DISTRACTION ARTHROPLASTY

This technique was developed for younger patients with post-traumatic arthritis in whom there was significant stiffness and intra-articular damage. Again it may have a place in the treatment of younger patients with chronic arthritis. The device used allows the elbow joint to be distracted, but maintains a constant distance between the surfaces of the trochlear and the ulna notch, allowing the ulna to rotate around a single axis. Following capsular release and fascial grafting, a combination of the distraction device and continuous passive motion gave significant relief of pain and improved range of movement.[28]

PROSTHETIC REPLACEMENT

A total elbow replacement is reserved for end-stage disease (Figure 13.3). There are no reported series of patients with chronic arthritis, but in patients with rheumatoid arthritis there are good early reports, with both the unconstrained surface replacements, such as the capitellocondylar prosthesis,[29,30] and the semi-constrained/'sloppy hinge' type, such as the Coonrad–Morrey prosthesis.[31] Both types of replacement have been shown to consistently provide relief of pain as well as improved function and range of movement. The survival of the prosthesis to date is in excess of 80% at 5.5 years.

Soft-tissue injuries involving the elbow joint

Throwing injuries of the elbow are well documented. They are most commonly seen in baseball pitchers, hence the title 'little leaguer's elbow', but other throwing activities can lead to similar lesions. The mechanism of injury is excessive valgus force applied to the elbow as it is rapidly extending. This causes tension on the medial side and compression on the lateral side. Similar lesions on the medial side are also produced in patients who play racquet sports, in which the forehand stroke creates excessive stress on the medial elbow structures.

Both soft tissue and bony components are seen, depending on the age of the patient. In younger children fatigue fractures of the medial

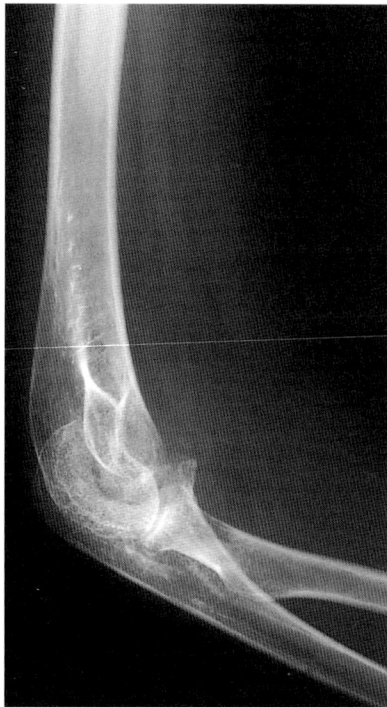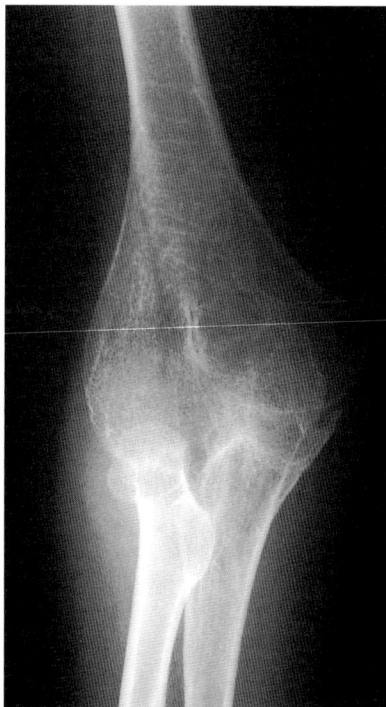

(a)

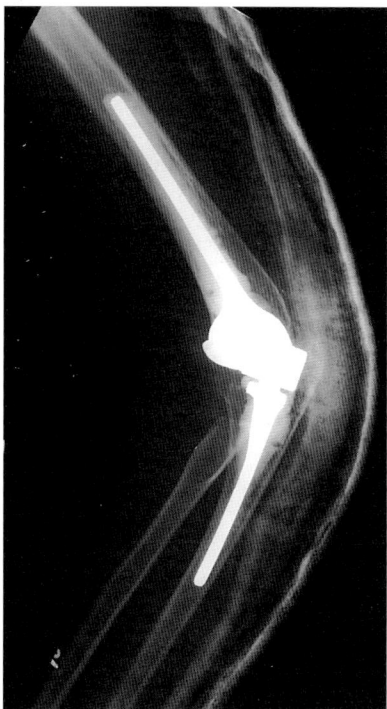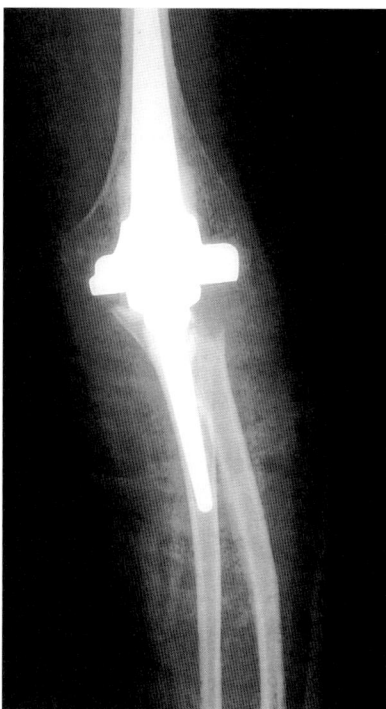

(b)

Figure 13.3 (*a*) Radiograph of patient with polyarticular chronic arthritis demonstrating severe disease affecting the elbow joint. (*b*) Postoperative radiography following total elbow replacement.

epicondyle cause localized pain and swelling. In adolescents and young adults the medial injury is usually a medial epicondylitis and medial tendinitis in the tendons of pronator teres and flexor carpi radialis. Repeated stress on the medial structures may stretch or tear the medial collateral ligament, leading to long-term instability. On the lateral side osteonecrosis of the capitellum may occur, leading to loose body formation and, later, secondary osteoarthritis with osteophyte formation. The extension overload causes either a triceps strain or an avulsion fracture of the olecranon.

The most important component of management is prevention and teaching of correct technique. In addition, throwing activities should be stopped if pain is present. Once pain and inflammation are present, treatment is started to reduce inflammation and swelling with rest, ice, NSAIDs and physiotherapy.

Osteonecrosis is treated purely symptomatically, although if loose fragments are present they may cause locking and impingement, in which case they must be excised either arthroscopically or by an open procedure.

Long-term medial collateral instability that fails to respond to conservative treatment may require a reconstructive procedure.

THE WRIST JOINT

Chronic arthritis

The wrist is one of the most commonly affected joints in patients with chronic arthritis. An early sign of wrist involvement is loss of extension. In cases of persistent, progressive synovitis a fixed flexion contracture often results, associated with ulnar deviation at the carpus (Figure 13.4a). This is in contrast to the typical radial carpal translation seen in the adult with rheumatoid arthritis.

The key to successful management of the wrist is to maintain the joint in a functional position with splinting. This usually involves the use of a night splint, but in difficult cases a daytime splint may also be needed. Occasionally, serial casting is required.

In children, dorsal tenosynovitis is less frequent and less troublesome than in the adult.

It is usually easier to remove, and recurrent synovitis is less common. However, in about 20% of cases wrist-joint disease is a major problem.

As previously stated, synovitis initially causes loss of extension followed by loss of other wrist movements. In progressive synovitis the articular surface of the radius develops a volar tilt and the carpus subluxes towards the ulna (Figure 13.4a). The growth plate of the radius may fragment and early closure of the ulna growth plate occurs, leading to relative shortness of the ulna, which increases the ulna malposition.

Prophylactic surgery

The vast majority of operations on the wrist are prophylactic.

SYNOVECTOMY

The indications for this procedure are:

- persistent synovitis despite aggressive medical management and physiotherapy
- no instability or contracture
- minimal or no erosive changes as seen on radiographs.

This may involve tenosynovectomy as well as wrist synovectomy. In Ovregard et al's series,[7] the wrist was the second commonest joint in which synovectomy was undertaken, with 75 out of a total of 394 over a 12-year period. Kvien et al[5] compared synovectomy with no synovectomy in patients with juvenile rheumatoid arthritis over a 2-year period. The synovectomy group showed decreased swelling, decreased disease activity and decreased pain compared to the non-synovectomy group, although joint motion was slightly reduced for the synovectomy group for the first 6 months. The improvement seen in the synovectomy group continued for at least 2 years.

Hanff et al[32] studied synovectomy in 20 wrist joints of patients with juvenile chronic arthritis. At 3 years, 60% were improved in terms of pain and grip strength, although range of movement had decreased. In total, 20% of the patients went on to require an arthrodesis.

CARPAL TUNNEL DECOMPRESSION

Symptoms of carpal tunnel syndrome are easily missed in patients with chronic arthritis, as younger patients may not complain of pain or sensory disturbance. Therefore, the symptoms must be actively sought for. It is often associated with flexor tenosynovitis, and a volar synovectomy may be needed in combination with the carpal tunnel decompression. A carpal tunnel decompression should be considered in any patient when there is bulging volar synovitis or thenar muscle atrophy. It should be noted that the latter is a late sign of median nerve compression and signifies prolonged compression. The thenar muscle atrophy is unlikely to recover even after decompression. Over the last 10 years local injections of steroid have decreased the frequency of carpal tunnel decompression.[6]

Reconstructive surgery

OSTEOTOMY

Length discrepancies of the forearm bones at the wrist may require a shortening osteotomy of the radius or lengthening of the ulna.

EXCISION OF THE DISTAL ULNA (DARRACH PROCEDURE)

This is indicated in patients with significant disease of the distal ulna and distal radioulnar joint when associated with significant pain and limitation of rotatory movements of the forearm. The ulna should not be excised unless the growth plate is closed. The results in patients with rheumatoid arthritis are very good. Complications following the procedure include instability of the distal ulna, with pain.

TENDON RECONSTRUCTION

Tendon rupture is much less common in the adolescent with chronic arthritis than in the adult with rheumatoid arthritis. Tendon rupture, if it does occur, should be treated by side to side suturing if possible. If this is not possible, tendon transfer or tendon grafting may be necessary, depending on the tendon involved and the residual function.

WRIST ARTHROPLASTY

Indications for this procedure are severe wrist joint disease with intact flexor and extensor tendons. Some surgeons feel that it is only indicated in bilateral wrist disease, where an arthroplasty is performed on one side and an arthrodesis on the other side. The most frequently used implant has been the Swanson implant, a stemmed silicone elastomer spacer. A limited range of motion, perhaps 40–60°, is sought around the neutral replacement. The results with this implant in adults are generally good. Fatti et al[33] showed that 75% of 58 wrists showed good pain relief at 2.5 years. However, while successful in adults, the implant is not currently recommended for use in children or young adults because of concerns over implant loosening, migration and fracture, as well as microparticulate silicone synovitis.

ARTHRODESIS

This has been the reconstructive procedure of choice for many surgeons in patients with disabling wrist pain and severe destructive changes seen radiographically (Figure 13.4). Although fusion is necessary in some patients, spontaneous fusion occurs in a significant proportion of patients with chronic arthritis. The arthrodesis can be secured by a variety of means, the commonest methods being with an intramedullary pin passing from the third metacarpal shaft into the radius or a plate and screws applied dorsally. The results are very good. Kobus and Turner[34] reported on 87 wrist fusions after an average follow-up period of 6 years and showed that 97% had good or excellent relief of pain following the procedure.

Other causes of wrist pain in adolescents

The ligamentous anatomy of the wrist consists of both extrinsic (radiocarpal) and intrinsic (intercarpal) ligaments. The intrinsic ligaments are much thicker and maintain stability between individual carpal bones within the wrist. Those of the proximal row are the strongest and the most elastic, allowing for most motion. Rupture of these intrinsic ligaments will lead to dissociation of individual carpal bones and, if combined with injury to the extrinsic ligaments, can result in various carpal dislocations. Dislocation of the

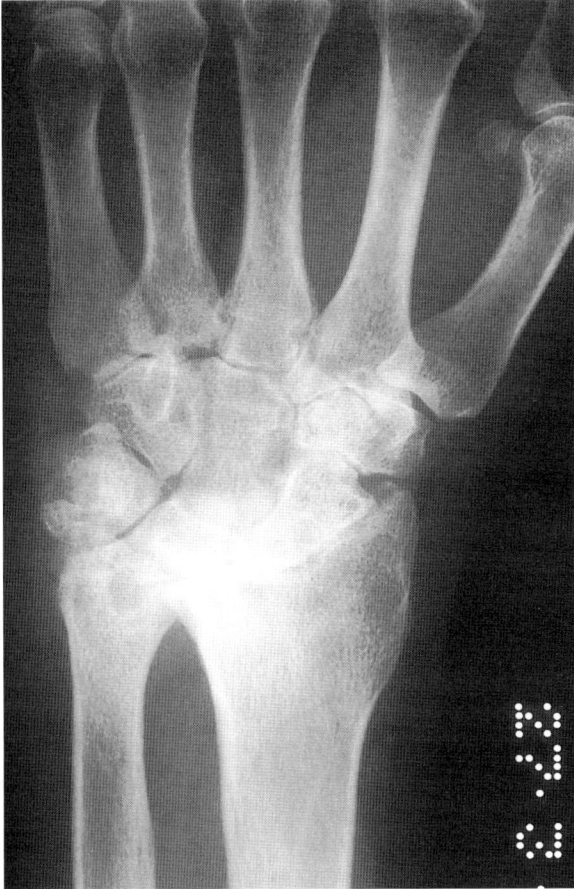

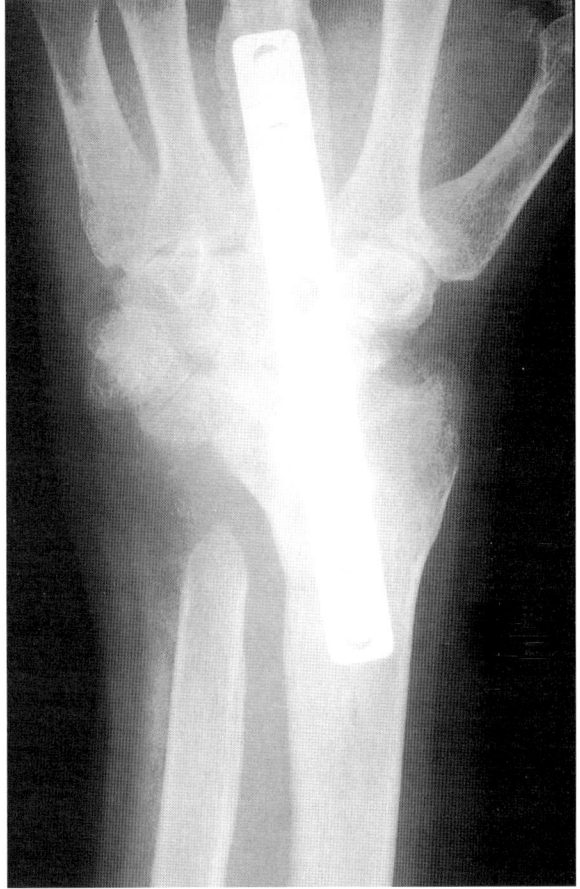

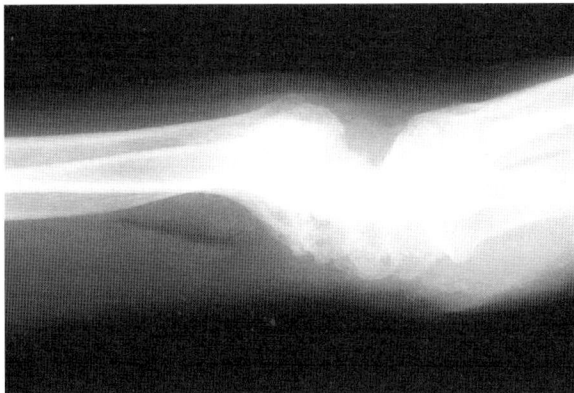

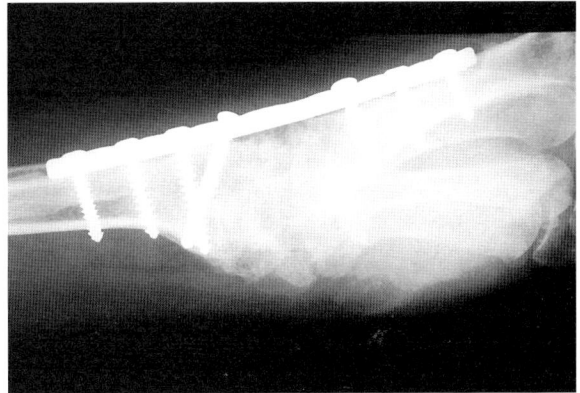

(a)   (b)

Figure 13.4   (a) Radiographs showing severe chronic arthritis involving the wrist joint. (b) Postoperative radiographs demonstrating shown arthrodesis.

carpus usually arises as a result of a high-velocity fall onto the hyperextended wrist, such as may occur in sport. These injuries are usually diagnosed immediately and treated with closed or open reduction, often combined with pinning. However, more commonly, carpal instability is the result of unrecognized isolated ligamentous injury to the wrist, which often presents as a chronic cause of wrist pain.

Patients with carpal instability will often complain of pain, weakness, clicking, snapping or a clunk. Pain is hard to localize, but certain provocative tests such as a scaphoid shift test or ballotment test[35] can aid diagnosis.

Another cause of wrist pain in adolescents is that associated with injury to the triangular fibrocartilage complex (TFCC), which is associated with distal radioulnar joint instability. Pain is usually located around the distal ulna, with point tenderness at this site. Rotatory movements of the forearm are often painful, and a click or snap may be heard.

A series of radiographs of the wrist consisting of posteroanterior images in neutral, radial and ulnar deviation, a clenched fist anteroposterior view and a lateral view, is usually taken if carpal instability is suspected, although a posteroanterior and lateral view will suffice for distal radial ulnar joint instability. Carpal instability may be apparent on the radiographs, with the lunate and scaphoid axis being tilted relative to the distal radius on the lateral. Further investigation may include MRI, which may show a tear in the TFCC, although at the present point in time MRI does not demonstrate the intrinsic ligaments well enough to be of major help in investigating carpal instability. Wrist arthrograms used to be used in assessing the integrity of the intrinsic and extrinsic ligaments of the wrist, but arthroscopy of the wrist has recently become far more widely used.

Treatment of acute carpal ligament injuries consists of open repair of the torn ligament through a dorsal approach. Far more commonly, however, these patients present with chronic wrist pain, and the treatment then may consist of a capsulodesis or ligament reconstruction or even a limited wrist arthrodesis, depending on the ligaments damaged and the patient's symptoms. Treatment of chronic TFCC lesions consists of either debridement (arthroscopically) or repair (open or arthroscopically).

THE HAND

Chronic arthritis

Hand involvement in patients with chronic arthritis is characterized by progressive stiffness and loss of flexion at both the metacarpophalangeal (MCP) and proximal interphalangeal (PIP) joints. In addition, the child with chronic arthritis may develop deformity with ulnar deviation of the metacarpals and radial deviation of the fingers, in marked contrast to the typical deformity in the adult with rheumatoid arthritis who develops radial deviation of the metacarpals and ulnar deviation of the fingers.

At the MCP joints, in addition to radial deviation, loss of flexion without loss of extension is often seen. This contrasts with the case of adults with rheumatoid arthritis in whom extension deficits and ulnar and volar drift are common. Boutonniere deformities are common, as are fixed flexion deformities of the interphalangeal (IP) joints. Swan-neck deformities are seen far less often than in adult rheumatoid arthritis, probably because most swan-neck deformities occur secondary to MCP volar subluxation (which is infrequent in patients with chronic arthritis) rather than PIP joint synovitis. Intrinsic tightness, so common in the adult with rheumatoid arthritis, is rarely seen in chronic arthritis.

Treatment of MCP and IP joint involvement is focused on prevention of functional deficits, and includes physiotherapy, hydrotherapy, dynamic and static splinting and occasional steroid injections. Surgery is indicated for established deformity. If the deformity is flexible (i.e. passively correctable), then a soft-tissue procedure is indicated. For fixed deformities, arthroplasty or arthrodesis may be needed.

TENOSYNOVECTOMY
Indications include: bulging synovium over the tendons/joints, presence of a palpable bony

spur or prominence, or presence/risk of tendon rupture. Again, prevention of ruptures by the judicious use of synovectomy and removal of the spur is far better than repair of ruptures or frayed tendons.[36]

Flexor tenosynovitis is far more likely to require surgery than extensor tenosynovitis, although the need for surgery is declining due to better prevention with conservative management.[6]

For trigger fingers, an injection into the tendon sheath is effective in about 60% of cases.[37] If this fails, synovectomy with/without removal of a slip of the flexor digitorum superficialis tendon is preferred where there is established radial deviation of the fingers, since release/removal of a segment of the A1 pulley increases the radial pull and may increase the deviation of the fingers.

SYNOVECTOMY

The indications are: resistant synovitis in a joint with well-preserved movement and minimal erosive changes on radiography. Ovregard et al[7] performed synovectomies on 107 MCP and PIP joints out of their series of 394 synovectomies in children with chronic arthritis. Results were good for 3 years and then steadily declined. Other authors have not found synovectomy of the MCP and PIP joints to be particularly successful, due to the propensity for loss of movement.[38]

ARTHROPLASTY

This is indicated in the MCP joint with severe pain and/or deformity in which the radiograph shows severe destruction. It is not indicated before skeletal maturity. The most frequently used implant is the flexible Swanson interpositional silastic implant (Figure 13.5). The results are good,[39,40] as defined by relief of pain, increased grip strength and function with active flexion to about 60°. Early postoperative physiotherapy is essential. Active flexion is gradually lost at the rate of approximately 5° every 2–3 years.

Arthroplasty is not currently recommended for severe PIP joint disease, especially in the younger patient.[38]

ARTHRODESIS

This is the current treatment of choice for the severely destroyed PIP joint with significant pain and/or deformity not tolerated by the patient. Arthrodesis is performed in a functional position of about 40° of flexion, and is regarded as a reliable procedure with good relief of pain and acceptable function.[36]

Boutonniere deformity

These should initially be managed with splinting to achieve maximal range of motion at both the PIP and DIP joints. If deformity persists with a preserved passive range of movement then a soft tissue procedure is indicated. This involves:

- reconstruction of the thinned central slip of the extensor tendon
- reconstruction of the lateral bands of the extensor tendon which have migrated towards the volar plate
- lengthening/division of the extensor tendon distally to prevent a mallet finger.

Numerous procedures have been employed.[41]

For the rigid fixed deformity which is not tolerated by the patient, PIP joint arthrodesis may be indicated in the skeletally mature.

Thumb deformities

Thumb deformities are usually better tolerated than those in the other fingers. The most common thumb deformity encountered is a pseudo-boutonniere deformity with hyperflexion at the MCP joint and hyperextension at the IP joint. This should initially be managed with appropriate medical treatment of the synovitis and extension splinting of the MCP joint. If deformity persists but the MCP joint movement is well preserved, then an extensor pollicis longus tendon rerouting may be useful.[42] For severe MCP joint destruction arthrodesis is recommended.

Soft-tissue injuries

The commonest soft-tissue injury involving the hand that is likely to present with a chronic

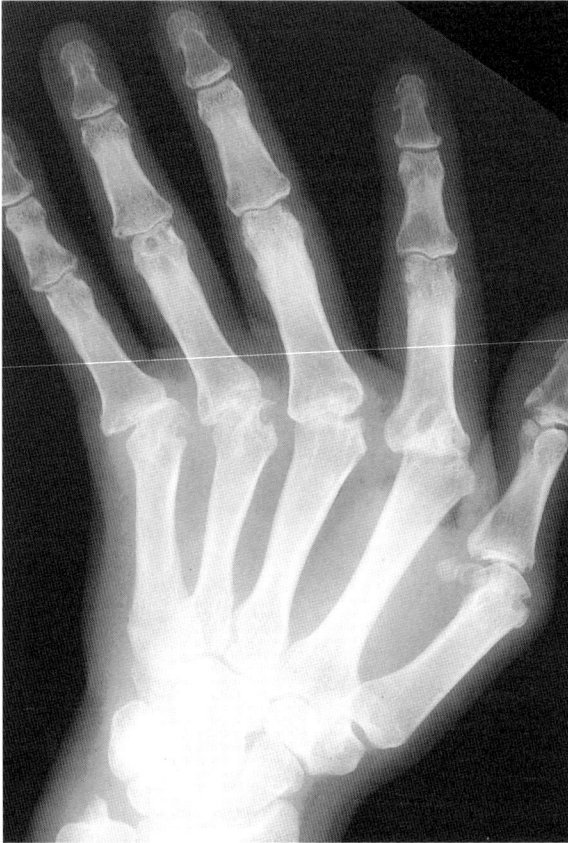

(a)

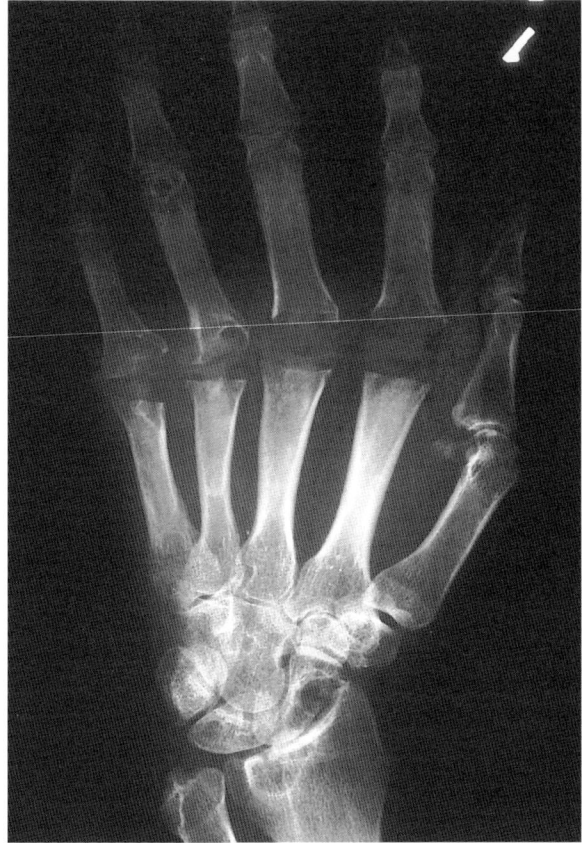

(b)

Figure 13.5 (*a*) Radiograph of a 25-year-old female with chronic arthritis involving the MCP joints of the fingers. (*b*) Radiographs of the same patient following MCP joint replacements with Swanson implants.

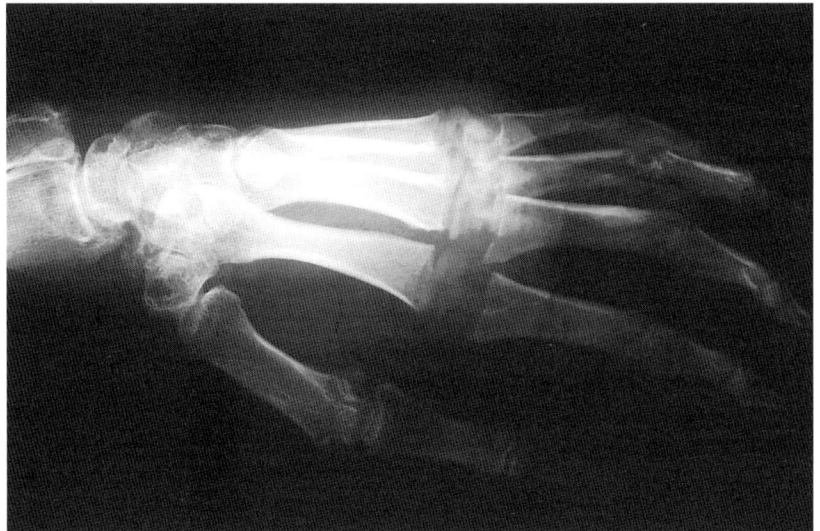

(b)

problem is that of damage to the ulnar collateral ligament of the thumb. It is commonly known as skier's thumb acutely and gamekeeper's thumb when it presents chronically. The patient presents with pain around the MCP joint of the thumb, weakness of pinch and, possibly, a feeling of instability. Examination may reveal tenderness over the ulnar collateral ligament of the MCP joint, excessive opening up of the joint compared to the uninvolved side when stressed, and weakness of pinch. The major indications for chronic repair of the ligament are pain, functional instability and weakness of pinch. If the ulnar collateral ligament is missing or atrophic at attempted repair, then a free tendon graft may be needed for reconstruction.

Other soft-tissue injuries that may present chronically are those involving the PIP joints. There is usually a history of trauma to the hyper-extended finger which, if the force was sufficient, will have resulted in dislocation. If the force applied was less, then injury may still have been caused to the collateral ligaments and/or volar plate. Injuries to the collateral ligaments may present with chronic pain and swelling of the PIP joint, instability and stiffness. If symptoms are sufficient and instability is present a ligament reconstruction may be needed.

In volar plate injuries a pseudo-boutonniere deformity may result. This resembles a true boutonniere deformity, but disruption of the central slip is not present. Examination reveals a flexion contracture of the PIP joint, which is more resistant to correction by passive extension than the true boutonniere, slight hyperextension of the DIP joint and flecks of calcification at the distal end of the volar plate seen on radiography. Treatment should consist of serial splinting to correct the flexion contracture but, if this is greater than 45°, surgical intervention is often required. Surgery involves release of the scarred proximal volar plate and distal advancement.

Infections

Bone and joint infections of the upper limb are very rare in adolescents. Osteomyelitis will present with localized pain, a febrile illness, loss of function of the involved limb, and, most importantly, localized bone tenderness. Investigation includes a full blood count, erythrocyte sedimentation rate, C-reactive protein, blood cultures, and radiography (although radiographically detectable demineralization does not occur for at least 10 days). A bone scan used to be the confirmatory investigation of choice, but now MRI is increasingly being used since it has the added advantage of demonstrating any intraosseous or subperiosteal collections of pus. Once the diagnosis of osteomyelitis has been made, aspiration of the bone should be performed to identify the pathogen. *Staphylococcus aureus* is the most common cause and an anti-staphylococcal antibiotic should be started while awaiting blood culture results. Any collection of pus identified requires surgical drainage. Antibiotics should be continued for a minimum of 6 weeks.

Septic arthritis presents in a similar fashion, except that the pain and tenderness are centred over the involved joint, there is an effusion (of pus) in the joint and the joint is often held rigidly with only a few degrees of movement possible. *Staph. aureus* is again the most common organism. Treatment consists of urgent washout of the joint, preferably arthroscopically, and commencement of antibiotics once a specimen for culture has been sent. In the sexually active adolescent gonococcal arthritis may occur. Arthritis develops 2–4 weeks following the initial infection. The patient should always be asked about urethral discharge. One or several joints may be involved, including the knees, ankles, wrists and sternoclavicular joints. Destruction of articular cartilage occurs rapidly, and immediate treatment with penicillin is very effective.

Other infections seen are those involving the hand. A pulp space infection or felon is an abscess of the terminal phalanx pulp. It presents with a painful, red, swollen and tense pulp that is exquisitely tender. It is usually secondary to a penetrating injury, although an untreated paronychia or subungal abscess may result in a felon. If seen early, antibiotics and elevation may be sufficient, but most cases require surgical drainage, with the incision not being placed too volar in order to avoid the neurovascular structures.

Tendon sheath infections may also present in this age group and often follow puncture wounds or lacerations. This closed-space infection can lead to chronic finger stiffness as a result of destruction of the pulley system, adhesions, and liquefaction of the tendon itself. Therefore, prompt recognition with immediate surgical drainage is essential. Diagnosis is based on Kanavel's four classic signs:[43] tenderness over the involved tendon sheath, pain on passive finger extension, the finger is held in flexion and a fusiform swelling of the finger. *Staph. aureus* is again the commonest organism, although about 20% of these infections are due to Gram-negative bacteria. Antibiotics may be curative if employed early, but, if there is no improvement in 24 hours, incision, drainage and irrigation of the tendon sheath should be performed.

Other infections seen in the hand include web-space infections at the base of the fingers, and deep-space infections, such as thenar and midpalmar space infections. Again both are usually caused by direct puncture of the overlying skin, and present with marked swelling, pain and overlying tenderness. The treatment is urgent incision and drainage, ensuring there is no extension to other closed spaces.

THE NECK

Chronic arthritis

When the cervical spine is involved, the neck is usually painful, neck mobility is limited, torticollis may develop and, in advanced cases, neurological deficit may be encountered.

The diagnosis of an inflammatory torticollis (where the head is tilted to one side and the chin rotated to the opposite side) such as may occur in chronic arthritis is usually readily made as most patients have involvement of multiple joints. If an acute torticollis develops one should rule out fracture of the odontoid process secondary to erosion by the hypertrophic synovium of the adjacent joints.[44] If a torticollis is neglected, the patient will be left with a permanent disability. Often a general anaesthetic is needed to overcome the muscle spasm, together with the application of a firm cervical orthosis to hold the spine in a better alignment.

Early ankylosis of the cervical spine is a relatively common outcome for the child and adolescent with chronic arthritis. Fusion of the whole cervical spine may occur, although it is more common from the C2/C3 level downwards. A soft collar helps to relieve pain and muscle spasm and may need to be worn for most of the day in the adolescent with severe neck problems.

Atlantoaxial instability, which is a common lesion in adult patients with involvement of the cervical spine, is also seen in the adolescent. Atlantoaxial instability may be totally asymptomatic and be accidentally discovered in routine cervical spine radiography. Symptoms vary from mild to severe neck pain and limitation of movement of the cervical spine to neurological deficit resulting from impingement on the spinal cord by the anterior body of the axis and the base of the odontoid process. Physical signs include those of an upper motor neuron lesion with motor weakness, sensory dysfunction, hyper-reflexia, ankle clonus, an extensor plantar response, and bladder and bowel dysfunction. In atlantoaxial instability cervical spine radiographs reveal an atlantodens interval (ADI) of greater than 4–5 mm in flexion and a reduced space available for the spinal cord (SAC; which should normally be twice the diameter of the odontoid). Treatment involves the medical management of the chronic arthritis, as well as local treatment. A simple cervical orthosis may stabilize the neck and prevent progressive subluxation. However, atlantoaxial subluxation in association with neurological deficit is an absolute indication for cervical fusion. This is especially true when the childhood-onset arthritis develops in a patient with pre-existing ligamentous laxity, as seen in conditions such as Down's syndrome or Ehlers–Danlos syndrome.

Involvement of the cervical spine is of particular concern to the anaesthetist with regard to management of the airway. The combination of a rigid neck and a small airway may make intubation impossible except by means of the fibre-optic laryngoscope. Atlantoaxial instability may be equally hazardous, as injudicious intubation could cause spinal cord damage.

THE TEMPOROMANDIBULAR JOINTS

Involvement of the temporomandibular joints is very common, especially in adolescents with polyarthritis. If these joints are affected early in life then the growth of the mandible can be severely impaired, leading to micrognathia. This causes distortion of the physical appearance of the face, as well as malocclusion. Arthritis affecting the temporomandibular joints causes pain on both opening and closing of the mouth, together with reduced opening of the mouth. This can again be of particular concern to the anaesthetist with regard to intubation.

Treatment of temporomandibular joint arthritis may involve passive mobilizing techniques if the range of movement of the joint is limited, although this is relatively contraindicated if the joint is actively inflamed. The help of a dentist and/or orthodontist may be needed to improve occlusion and function by means of jaw or dental regulation. In severe cases of bony ankylosis, surgical intervention may be needed to create a gap between the mandible and the skull to allow free movement. The gap may be left open or filled with a foreign material such as sialastic.

THE HIP

Causes of deformity

Involvement of the hip occurs in 30–63.5% of patients with juvenile chronic arthritis,[45–48] and this is the most common cause of limited mobility.[47] Inflammatory synovitis leads to pain and muscle spasm, with the inevitable development of joint contractures if this cycle is not broken. The tendency to contracture is greater in seronegative patients, often with minimal effusion, whereas seropositive patients tend to experience a proliferative synovitis more like that seen in adults.

An effusion in the joint will cause pain, and the tendency will be for the joint to be held in the position in which the capsule has the maximum capacity, thereby reducing the pressure within the joint. In the hip this position is in neutral rotation with about 45° of flexion.[49] In time, with the persistence of an inflammatory synovitis and pannus formation, the articular cartilage degenerates. This is exacerbated by the stiff, contracted nature of the joint, which impairs the normal mechanisms of cartilage nutrition.[50,51] In addition, periarticular inflammation induces regional osteopaenia, which is compounded by the muscle weakness and relative immobility of these patients.

A combination of regional hyperaemia and abnormal mechanical forces on the hip induces growth abnormalities and a failure of the normal remodelling process of the proximal femur. The exact pattern of the deformity is related to the age of onset and the duration of the disease.[46] Children below 9 years of age tend to develop coxa magna, where the femoral head is enlarged and there is an elongated valgus femoral neck with marked anteversion, and an acetabulum that appears dysplastic. In children over the age of 9 years, coxa magna often occurs, but frequently with premature fusion of the growth plate of the femoral head, producing a short and varus femoral neck. Continued growth of the trochanteric epiphysis contributes to the varus deformity. A protrusio pattern of deformity is another feature that may develop in the older child.

In time, narrowing and irregularity of the joint space occurs, with bone erosions, destruction and sometimes subluxation of the femoral head. In a proportion of cases there is evidence of avascular necrosis of the head. This was seen in 10 of 72 hips in 36 children with hip disease, and a further 20 showed suspected late sequelae of the ischaemic process.[52] This is thought to occur secondary to a tamponade of the joint resulting from the synovitis and effusion, as the nutrient vessels to the capital epiphysis are largely intracapsular.

The typical deformity of the affected hip that ultimately develops is one of fixed flexion, adduction and internal rotation.[53] Both hips are not necessarily involved to the same extent, but a fixed flexion deformity in one hip will tend to induce the same in the other. As a consequence of the hip deformity, patients develop an excessive lumbar lordosis and also a tendency towards fixed flexion deformities of the knees. The fixed adduction at the hip leads to the development of a genu valgum deformity, and this combined with internal rotation may lead to external tibial torsion.

Surgical management

Intra-articular steroids
In the early stages of hip involvement, patients may present with acute irritability of the hip but with no changes seen radiographically. Examination will reveal a flexion deformity and adductor spasm. Some cases may respond to appropriate analgesics and anti-inflammatory medication combined with a physical therapy programme, including traction, aimed at preventing fixed deformities.

In those that do not respond, it is worth performing a gentle examination under anaesthetic. In these circumstances it is possible to determine if a fixed deformity has developed, but often the deformity disappears and there is no limitation of movement. A steroid injection can then be performed. In our practice, confirmation of localization of the hip joint is made by performing an arthrogram at the time. Postoperatively, traction should be continued while the irritability persists, interspersed with physiotherapy. Prone lying is encouraged for part of each day to help overcome the fixed flexion deformity. In the meantime the other involved joints should continue to be treated.

Synovectomy and soft-tissue release
The role of synovectomy of the hip by itself is not clear, as usually it is combined with some sort of soft-tissue release procedure. There is evidence that it is effective in reducing pain, but possibly at the expense of losing some range of motion.[54] A soft-tissue release procedure is indicated when there is an established flexion contracture with limitation of range of motion, and where a joint space can still be demonstrated.

The majority of cases can be managed with a release of the tight adductors and the psoas through a small incision in the groin. Swann and Ansell[55] reported an improvement in the flexion contracture from an average of 26° before surgery to 9° at 1 year, and this was maintained in 46 of 89 hips at 3 years. In addition, this was associated with marked pain relief, which is probably due to decompression of the joint.[56] However, the longer term improvement is likely to reflect changes in disease activity. For patients with more severe fixed flexion deformities a more extensive release procedure has been described[57] where the muscles are stripped from their attachments to the ilium, and which is also combined with a partial synovectomy. Using this procedure the average preoperative flexion contracture in 31 hips was reduced from 35° to 9.5° at 1 year and at 3 years it was 18°. In some cases it was noted that there was an improvement in the appearance of the hip on radiography, with a reduction in the degree of porosis, a clearer definition of the joint line and a widening of the joint space.

The postoperative management is extremely important in order to maintain the improved range of motion. Traction with the hips in abduction is commenced together with range-of-motion exercises immediately postoperatively, and hydrotherapy once the wounds have healed. As the hips become more comfortable, patients are mobilized, with traction continued at night.

Osteotomy
Theoretically, osteotomy would be indicated in cases where there is marked femoral neck valgus associated with a dysplastic acetabulum and subluxation of the hip. However, owing to the porotic bone and restricted range of motion usually present it is rarely appropriate. It may occasionally be used in a patient whose disease is no longer active and who still has a good range of motion with a preserved joint space.

Total hip replacement
Pain in patients with severely destroyed joints is the main indication for total hip replacement.

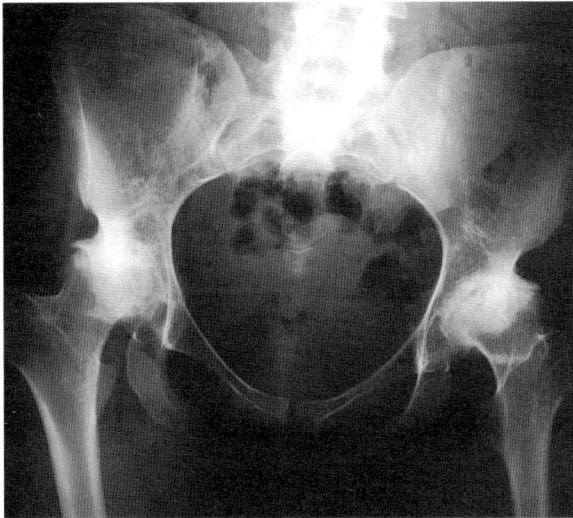
(a)

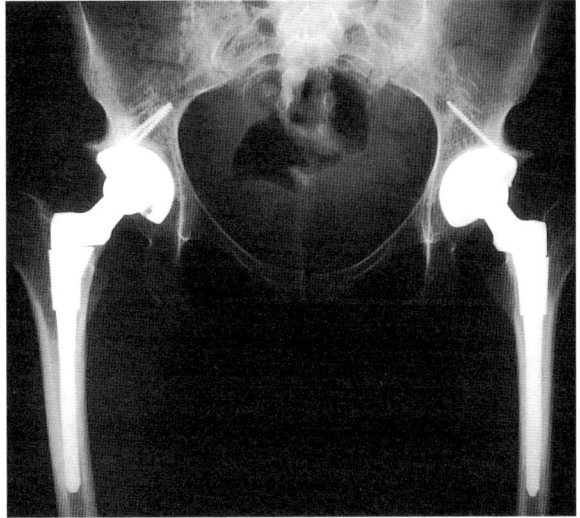
(b)

Figure 13.6 Radiograph of a 24-year-old female with polyarticular juvenile chronic arthritis wheelchair bound because of severe hip disease and very restricted hip abduction allowing only 9 cm separation at the ankles (b) Radiographs of hips treated with bilateral uncemented modular hip replacements.

Less commonly, the indication may be for anky-losis in a poor position leading to functional impairment and secondary deformity of other joints. The results in a number of series have demonstrated a marked reduction in pain and a major improvement in functional ability. However, the rate of loosening and the subse-quent problems associated with revision hip surgery are of concern. Witt et al,[58] in a study on 92 hip replacements in patients with juvenile chronic arthritis, found that 25% of hips had been revised after an average follow-up of 11.5 years. Chmell et al[59] reviewed 66 hips and found that 15% of femoral components and 35% of acetabu-lar components required revision for aseptic loosening after an average follow-up of 12 years.

There are significant technical problems asso-ciated with total hip replacement in this group of patients. The bones may be extremely porotic and, with considerable proximal femoral defor-mity, insertion of standard components may not be possible. The disappointing medium-term results in terms of loosening rates in cemented hip replacements has led to the use of unce-mented implants. These may need to be custom made for the individual; specialized modular implants are also available. The implants have a porous coating applied to them to allow bone ingrowth to occur, or have an hydroxyapatite coating that bonds directly to bone. Although there is limited follow-up on this type of implant, the early clinical and radiographic results are encouraging (Figure 13.6).

THE KNEE

The knee is commonly involved in all forms of juvenile chronic arthritis. Inflammation results in the joint being held in a position of flexion, and hamstring spasm will prevent straighten-ing. In time, resistant flexion contractures may develop as the periarticular structures undergo fibrosis, and extra-articular and intra-articular adhesions progressively limit joint movement. It is important to identify factors that may exacer-bate the deformity, such as ipsilateral hip involvement and contralateral knee involvement. Because the knee's two epiphyseal growth plates account for 70% of lower extremity growth, it is not surprising that involvement leads to growth abnormalities. Simon et al[60] published a detailed study of leg-length discrepancies in 100 cases of monoarticular disease in juvenile chronic arthritis. It was noted that if the disease began before the age of 9 years the involved side was always the longer one and the final discrepancy was rarely more than 3 cm. None of the patients with disease beginning before the age of 9 years had premature epiphyseal closure. If the disease had its onset after that age, rapid premature growth-plate closure was evident and leg-length differences of up to 5.9 cm were observed. The medial side of the growth plate seems to have the propensity to be stimulated to a greater extent, and this is one of the causes of a valgus deformity.

Surgical treatment

Steroid injection and synovectomy

Physiotherapy and rest splints are indicated in the early stages of the disease. If the flexed position is resistant to treatment with a vigorous conservative programme including reversed dynamic traction, then an examination under anaesthetic and intra-articular steroid injection is valuable. If a fixed flexion deformity persists, then a programme of serial plastering is started to gradually correct this.

The role of synovectomy in the management of symptoms, the most appropriate timing for the procedure and the influence on disease progression have not been determined. Because of the thick articular cartilage in children, subchondral cysts and erosions are late to appear on radiographs, and cartilage destruction seen at operation often far exceeds that seen on radiographs. In general, better results are likely in patients with oligoarticular or monoarticular disease.[61,62]

Soft-tissue release

In instances where a fixed flexion deformity persists and has been resistant to serial casts, it may be necessary to release the contracted tissues surgically. This may allow complete correction of the deformity, but may also require serial casts or reversed dynamic traction in order to gain and maintain full correction. To perform a release, posteromedial and posterolateral incisions are needed. The hamstring tendons are lengthened and the posterior capsule of the knee joint is exposed by blunt dissection. Taking care to protect the neurovascular bundle, the posterior capsule is incised transversely so that the joint is entered. Postoperatively, patients are maintained in a cast for 2–3 days. This is then bivalved and range-of-motion exercises are commenced.

In one series of 31 knees (19 patients), a mean fixed flexion deformity of 38° was reduced to 12° at the 6-month follow-up. This correction was maintained until the 3-year follow-up, and then tended to deteriorate.[63] Rydholm et al[64] reported on 29 releases in 23 children, with 21 knees having a flexion contracture greater than 15°. At a mean follow-up of 3.9 years only eight knees had a flexion deformity exceeding 15°.

Osteotomy

In those cases in which the deformity is fixed and associated with more advanced joint destruction it may be appropriate to perform a supracondylar femoral extension osteotomy, and any valgus deformity can be corrected at the same time. This creates a second deformity which masks the first. Because of the porosity of the bone, stable internal fixation is not usually possible; therefore, these patients require a cast postoperatively. This is removed as early as possible, usually at about 4 weeks, to try to avoid too much stiffness, and range-of-motion exercises are commenced.

Forty knee osteotomies in 24 patients aged 16 years or less resulted in the satisfactory correction of the deformity and bone union in all cases.[65] Relapse of the deformity occurred in five patients and osteotomies had to be repeated in three. Four knees lost movement following surgery.

Although there clearly is a place for osteotomy, this should be reserved for the younger child and in the older child should perhaps only be performed when a reasonable joint surface remains and where the disease is less active. The reason for this is that performing an osteotomy makes the subsequent operation of a knee replacement much more difficult because of the distorted anatomy. The results of current-design total knee replacements are extremely good, and, therefore, if it can be predicted that a patient will end up requiring a knee replacement, an osteotomy should probably be avoided if at all possible.

Epiphyseodesis
Epiphyseodesis has been used to correct valgus deformity and leg-length discrepancy.[66] Its use is probably best confined to monoarticular disease in juvenile chronic arthritis. Simon et al[60] reported on the results in 15 patients out of 35 followed to skeletal maturity, and showed satisfactory results.

Total knee replacement
The indication for total knee replacement is primarily pain, but this is often associated with significant deformity resulting in major functional incapacity. Skeletal immaturity is not necessarily a contraindication to surgery. Considerable preoperative planning is required because of the small sizes of the knees in many cases and because of the distorted local anatomy. A further concern is the degree of osteoporosis that is present, and great care has to be taken when operating to release the fibrous intra- and extra-articular adhesions in order to expose the joint without fracturing the bone.

The results of current designs of condylar resurfacing total knee replacements in adults with rheumatoid arthritis are extremely good, with a predicted survival rate of 91% at 15 years.[67] Early results of total knee arthroplasty in juvenile chronic arthritis are also very encouraging (Figure 13.7). Sarokhan et al[68] reported results in 29 knees in 17 patients with an average age of 23 years and a follow-up of 2–11 years (average 5 years). Pain relief was present in all cases; there was one late deep infection, but no patients required revision for aseptic loosening. Carmichael and Chaplin[69] reported on 21 total knee replacements in 11

patients with an average age of 20.1 years. At a mean follow-up of 61 months no revisions were required, and no infections or loosenings occurred. Others have reported similar results,[70] and uncemented implants have also been used in very selected cases.[71]

THE FOOT AND ANKLE

Virtually any conceivable combination of deformities can occur in juvenile chronic arthritis.[72] Pronation of the foot with valgus of the heel is a frequent finding. Clawing of the toes is common, with or without a cavus deformity of the forefoot. A varus hindfoot, hallux valgus and hammer toe deformities also occur. Tarsal joint involvement is common, with a tendency to early ankylosis. The key to the management of these problems is to try to prevent fixed deformities from developing and to preserve as great a range of motion as possible. It is most important to try to preserve neutral alignment of the foot and ankle. In children with more proximal joints involved and who may be partly wheelchair bound there is a tendency for the ankle and foot to drift into equinus due to gravity.

Non-surgical treatment

The arthritic foot should be well supported most of the time. Careful attention to footwear, with prescription of appropriate heels, sole wedges, lasts, arch supports and metatarsal weight-relieving inserts, is important. Deformity of the foot and ankle should be corrected by serial plastering and maintained subsequently with the use of orthotic devices at night. Intra-articular injections of steroids may also help control active synovitis.

Surgical treatment

Soft-tissue release
Resistant equinus of the ankle may be corrected by lengthening the achilles tendon and capsulotomy of the ankle and subtalar joints. Varus deformities of the hindfoot can be corrected by performing a posteromedial release similar to

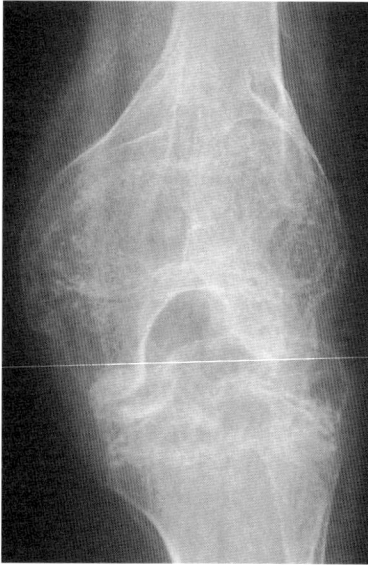
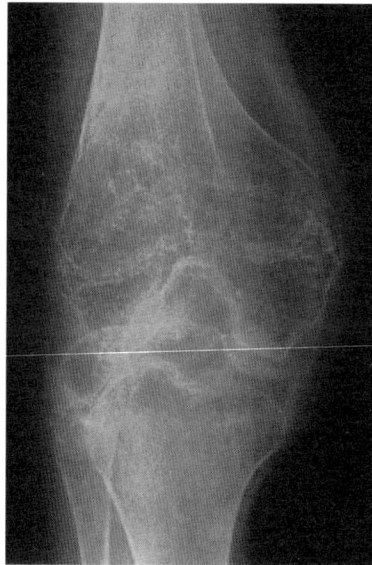

(a)

Figure 13.7 (a) A 15-year-old male with juvenile spondyloarthropathy and severe knee involvement. Knee radiographs show extreme osteoporosis and evidence of previous bilateral supracondylar femoral osteotomies.
(b) Postoperative radiographs showing bilateral cemented knee replacements. The previous osteotomies make the surgery technically much more difficult.

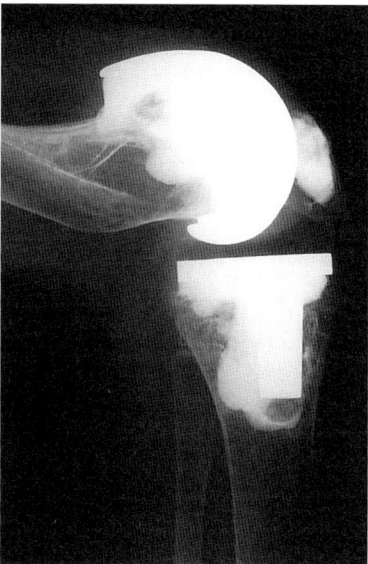
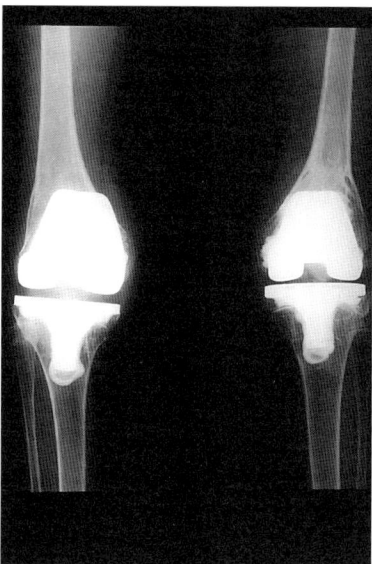
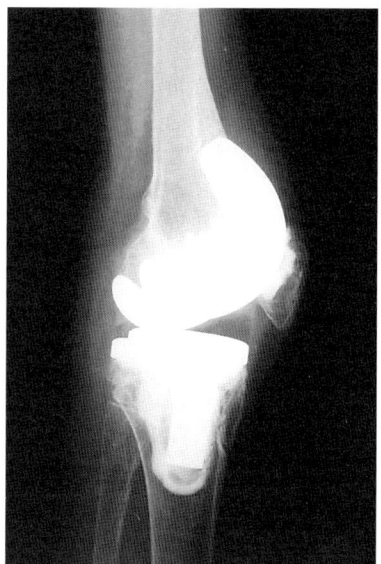

(b)

the procedures developed for clubfoot. Similarly a variety of release procedures may allow correction of a cavus foot or claw toes.

Osteotomies
Occasionally, a calcaneal osteotomy may allow correction of fixed hindfoot varus while retaining movement in the adjacent joints. Midtarsal osteotomies usually combined with a dorsal wedge resection allow correction of equinus at the midtarsal joints where these have ankylosed (Figure 13.8). First metatarsal osteotomies for hallux valgus are sometimes appropriate, although if there are severe lesser toe deformities

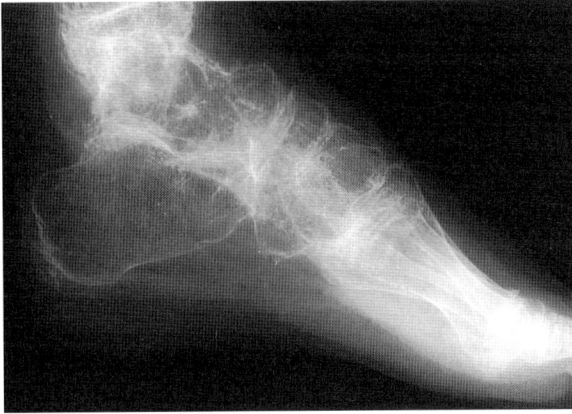

(a)

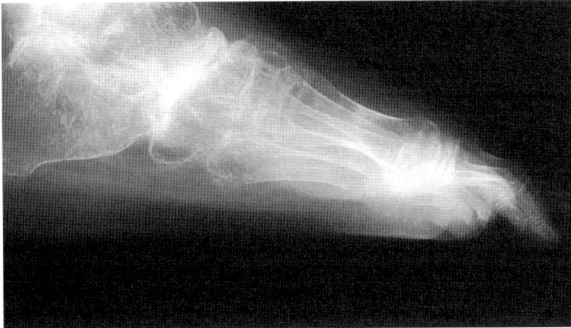

(b)

Figure 13.8 (a) Radiograph showing fixed equinus deformity at the mid-tarsal joints in a 15-year-old male with juvenile chronic arthritis. (b) Radiograph following dorsal wedge excision osteotomy with correction of deformity.

with dorsal and lateral subluxation then arthrodesis is often a better alternative.

Arthrodesis
Once children reach the age of 12–14 years, fixed deformities of the hindfoot may be best corrected by performing a triple arthrodesis, although if the subtalar joint alone is involved then a subtalar fusion may be sufficient. Occasionally, an isolated talonavicular joint

fusion may be appropriate where this joint is painful, and conversion to a triple arthrodesis is possible should this be required. If the ankle joint is painful and clinically and radiographically deformed then an ankle fusion is the recommended procedure (Figure 13.9).

Resection arthroplasty
In the majority of cases, subluxation and dislocation of the metatarsophalangeal joints can be managed with suitable footwear. Once all the epiphyses around the metatarsals and phalanges have fused, excision arthroplasty can be considered. The long-term results of these procedures are disappointing,[73] with recurrence of deformity in 8–10 years, and so are best put off for as long as possible.

GENERAL CONSIDERATIONS

Surgery in patients with juvenile idiopathic arthritis may provide the anaesthetist with some very difficult problems to overcome. A number of factors conspire to make intubation in these patients a formidable task. There may be cervical spine involvement, the mandible is frequently micrognathic and the temporomandibular joints may also be involved and have a very poor range of motion. Fibre-optic intubation may be necessary and the use of a laryngeal mask has proved invaluable. Peripheral venous access is also often difficult and may require the insertion of a central venous line. An anaesthetist experienced in dealing with the problems peculiar to these patients is very important.

Postoperative therapy needs to take into account overall disease activity and adjacent joint deformity. Patients in the perioperative period are vulnerable to stress ulceration, particularly when they are on steroid medication, and careful observation for the development of this complication is required, as early symptoms may be minimal and rather non-specific.

The functional results in this group of patients following appropriate surgery is most gratifying and allows them to maintain some degree of independence and quality of life.

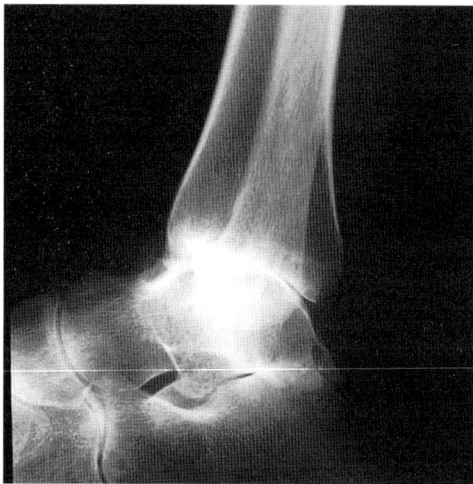

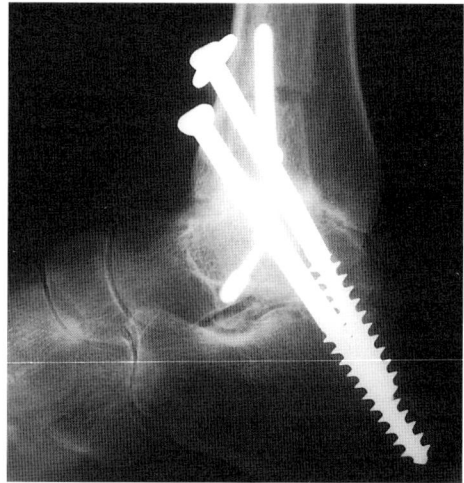

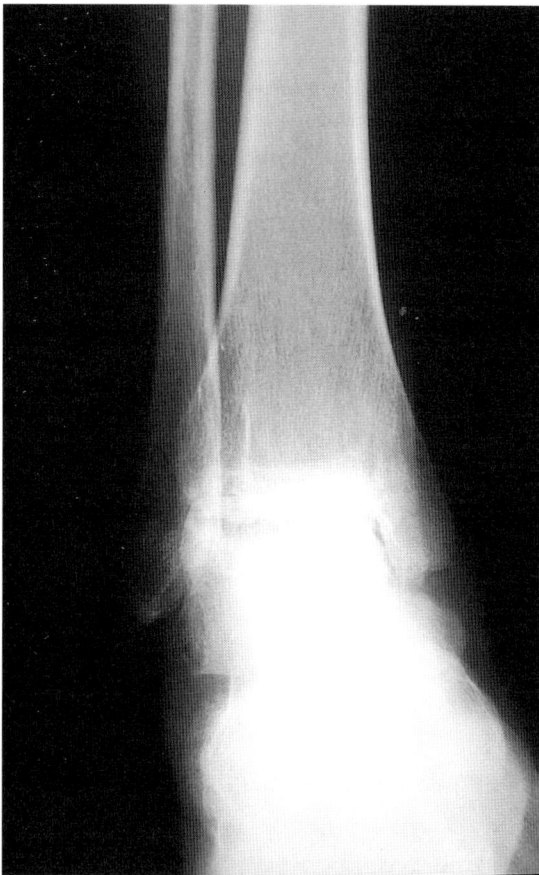

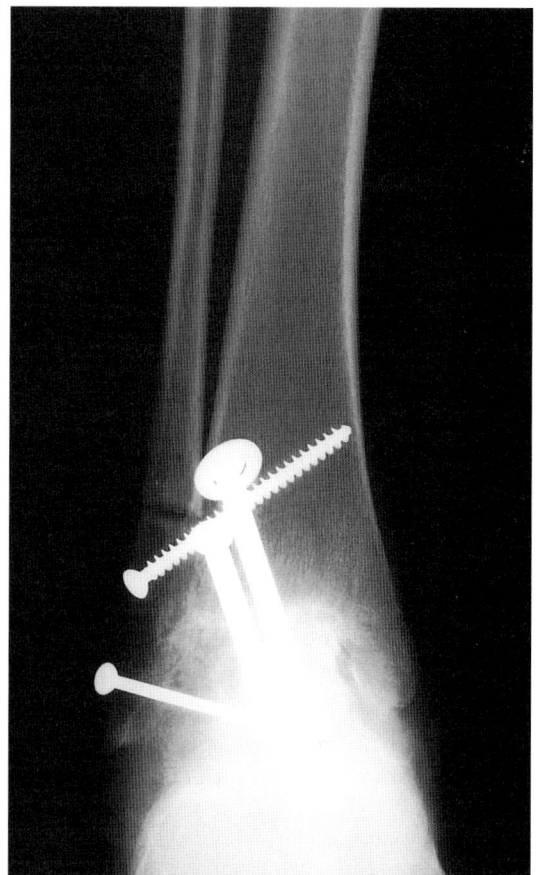

(a)

(b)

Figure 13.9 (a) A 19-year-old female with polyarticular juvenile chronic arthritis. Radiographs show disease affecting the ankle and subtalar joint. (b) Postoperative radiographs showing ankle and subtalar arthrodesis.

OTHER CAUSES OF PAIN AND SYMPTOMS IN THE LOWER LIMB

It should of course be recognized that a variety of conditions may present with lower limb symptoms in adolescents, not least because this age group has a high involvement in sporting activities. It is particularly important to remember that hip pathology may present as pain in the knee and patients frequently present with knee pain and a limp. Failure to routinely examine the hip in these instances will inevitably result in missed diagnoses and inappropriate treatment.

Septic arthritis

Infection of a joint is a surgical emergency. Once bacteria have gained access, the processes of bacterial phagocytosis, synovial proliferation, granulation tissue formation, and bone and cartilage destruction begin. This destruction is mediated by the direct toxic effects of the bacteria and by the pressure that develops within the joint cavity.

The diagnosis is based on the history and any predisposing factors, such as rheumatoid disease, diabetes mellitus, sickle cell anaemia and haemophilia. Any joint infected will be extremely painful to move and associated with severe muscle spasm. The patient is usually febrile with a raised white cell count and raised erythrocyte sedimentation rate. Aspiration of the joint should be performed in a sterile manner and the synovial fluid examined for bacteria and crystals. A white cell count in the synovial fluid above 50 000 cells/mm^3 in an immune competent host strongly suggests the presence of infection.

Parenteral antibiotics should be initiated as soon as material for culture has been obtained. The aim of treatment is to decompress the joint and to remove the inflammatory debris. In the hip this is accomplished by open drainage, and in the knee the joint can be decompressed and irrigated arthroscopically.

Transient synovitis of the hip

This is a benign, self-limited condition of the hip of unknown aetiology which presents as hip or knee pain, restriction of movement and a limp. It usually presents in young children (average 6–7 years), but occasionally may present in adolescents. The most important aspect in diagnosis is to differentiate it from septic arthritis and Perthes' disease. The presence of a temperature, and a raised erythrocyte sedimentation rate and white cell count would tend to indicate an infection. However, if there is any doubt aspiration of the hip is indicated.

In transient synovitis radiographs are normal. An effusion may be demonstrated on ultrasound but this is somewhat operator dependent. Bone scan and MRI have not proven particularly useful for diagnosis.[74] Treatment is symptomatic, and there is no evidence that transient synovitis leads to Perthes' disease.

Perthes' disease

This disorder remains poorly understood and most commonly presents in males aged 4–8 years. However, presentation may occur later owing to the aftermath of the effect of the disease on the hip. The pathology of the condition involves fragmentation of the capital femoral epiphysis, possibly related to multiple episodes of infarction. The end result may produce significant residual deformity of the femoral head, predisposing the hip to the early development of osteoarthritis. The principle of treatment in the early stages of the disease is 'containment', whether by splintage or surgery, to maximize the congruity of the femoral head as this undergoes reossification and remodelling. In the later stages certain types of femoral osteotomy may be appropriate to improve symptoms and delay the onset of osteoarthritis.

Slipped capital femoral epiphysis

The aetiology of this condition is generally considered to be idiopathic, but may be due to a subtle endocrinopathy. It is more common in males than females and most commonly affects the 10- to 16-year age group. Presentation usually occurs as pain in the groin or knee. The condition is bilateral in 20% of patients. The diagnosis is made by radiography, where it is essential to have anteroposterior and lateral views. Slips may be classified as acute, chronic, or acute on chronic. Treatment is aimed at minimizing the progression of the slip by pinning the capital epiphysis in situ. A realignment osteotomy may be necessary in those cases which have progressed significantly. However, this surgery is technically demanding and carries with it a significant risk of the development of osteonecrosis of the femoral head.

Developmental dysplasia of the hip

Acetabular dysplasia may become symptomatic during adolescence. The typical symptoms would be of pain felt in the groin or the knee, particularly after exercise. The condition is much more common in females than males. Sometimes there may be episodes of locking of the hip associated with a sharp pain in the groin; the so-called acetabular rim syndrome.[75] These symptoms come about because of the abnormal stresses on the shallow margins of the acetabulum, and in time will result in the development of osteoarthritis.[76]

Treatment is aimed at reorientating the acetabulum to improve the coverage of the femoral head and reduce the shear stresses on the superolateral margins of the acetabulum, thereby delaying the onset of osteoarthritis.

Knee ligament injuries

Ligamentous injuries of the knee in children and adolescents are being recognized with increasing frequency, and tears of both cruciate and collateral ligaments have been reported. A haemarthrosis without fracture implies a significant soft-tissue injury. A study reporting the arthroscopic evaluation of haemarthrosis in children reported that 47% had anterior cruciate ligament (ACL) tears and 47% had meniscal tears, with 6% having both ACL and meniscal tears.[77] Data from a number of studies have shown a high failure rate of rehabilitation and bracing if the repair of ACL tears has not been

satisfactory. Reconstruction may have to be considered in this group of patients, especially as they may suffer recurrent meniscal injuries as a result of continued instability.[78]

Meniscal injuries

Diagnosis of meniscal lesions may be difficult in adolescents because they may not be good historians. A history of a twisting injury followed by the development of an effusion with episodes of locking point to the diagnosis. A haemarthrosis may develop in cases of a peripheral tear through the vascular zone of the meniscus. MRI may be helpful in making the diagnosis in equivocal cases. Treatment should be aimed at preserving as much meniscus as possible, and in cases of peripheral tears the meniscus can be reattached using arthroscopic techniques. Patient compliance is extremely important following meniscal repair and a supervised rehabilitation programme should be followed.

Discoid meniscus

This is an infrequent congenital anomaly of the knee where the lateral meniscus is discoid in shape rather than having the normal crescentic configuration. Presentation usually occurs in children younger than 6–8 years, but may occur in adolescents. The symptoms include a history of snapping, clicking, catching or giving way at the knee. MRI usually gives information about the size and shape of the meniscus.

The preferred treatment is partial menisectomy or sculpting of the meniscus to a more normal shape if there are symptoms of internal derangement of the knee.

Osteochondritis dissecans

This is a condition in which a portion of the articular cartilage together with the subchondral bone becomes separated from the remaining articular cartilage. The aetiology is uncertain, but may include both ischaemia and trauma to that area of the femoral condyle. The most common site is the intercondylar region of the medial femoral condyle; the weight-bearing areas of the medial and lateral femoral condyles are less commonly affected.

Clinical symptoms usually include pain, knee effusion and, occasionally, symptoms of locking or catching of the knee when the fragment has separated and become a loose body. The diagnosis can be made on radiographs and more clearly delineated on MRI. In adolescents, when the lesion has not separated, treatment is directed at healing of the lesion, with cast immobilization in the first instance. If the fragment has separated or has failed to heal, surgical intervention is indicated. Arthroscopic drilling to stimulate union may be required, or refixation of loose fragments with pins. Excision of irregular defects with currettage of the underlying bone may be of value, and a number of techniques for regenerating articular cartilage are currently under evaluation.[79]

Anterior knee pain

A variety of disorders involving the patellofemoral joint can give rise to pain. These most commonly include patellofemoral instability, malalignment, quadriceps tendinitis, distal patellar tendinitis and patellofemoral arthrosis. The standard treatment is conservative care. Careful evaluation for evidence of patella maltracking is very important. This may be associated with relative external tibial torsion, and increased Q angle, genu valgum and overall joint laxity. The clinical lateral patella tilt, ability to evert the lateral edge of the patella, the dynamic Q angle, seated 90° Q angle, apprehension signs and the flexibility of the quadriceps and hamstrings are all important components of the clinical examination.

In general, patients should exhaust conservative measures before surgical treatment is considered. Arthroscopic lateral release may be considered for patients with lateral patellar tilt and pain and who have minimal articular surface damage. Lateral release is generally ineffective in patients with more severe patellofemoral chondromalacia. Realignment procedures may be suitable for patients with increased Q angles and subluxation or recurrent dislocation.

Tarsal coalition

This condition arises through a failure of differentiation and segmentation of primitive mesenchyme in the foot. Presentation is usually with pain and stiffness or a flat-foot deformity, where subtalar joint motion is resisted by peroneal muscle spasm. Calcaneonavicular bars are the most common variety (53%), followed by talocalcaneal (37%). Talonavicular bars are always associated with other congenital foot anomalies. The age at presentation varies closely with the age at which each type ossifies. Ossification of the calcaneonavicular bar occurs at 8–12 years, and symptoms tend to develop at around 16 years of age. Talocalcaneal bar ossification occurs at 12–16 years, with symptoms developing around 18 years of age.

Treatment is initially aimed at reducing physical activity, and immobilization in a cast for 6 weeks may be necessary. If symptoms continue, surgical treatment consists of resecting the abnormal segment of bone with measures to prevent it from reforming. Results tend to be better before secondary adaptive changes have occurred in the foot.

Sever's disease

This condition is a traction apophysitis at the insertion of the tendo achilles. The patient complains of pain localized to the heel that is exacerbated by running and jumping. Symptoms are eased by rest. Examination reveals tenderness at the insertion of the tendon on the calcaneus, usually without swelling. Radiographs are usually normal, but occasionally may show increased fragmentation of the calcaneal apophysis, but this may also be a normal variant.

Treatment begins with activity modification, a heel cushion, icing and a stretching programme. This can be combined with administration of anti-inflammatory medication. In severe cases it may be necessary to immobilize the foot in a below-knee cast for a period of time. The condition is self-limiting and the patient can return to normal activities when symptoms allow.

Freiberg's infraction

This condition is believed to be due to aseptic necrosis of the second metatarsal head. It is usually seen in adolescents, and 75% of cases occur in girls. Symptoms usually consist of anterior metatarsalgia and may be bilateral. Although the second metatarsal head is most commonly involved, other metatarsals may also be affected. On examination the affected joint is slightly swollen, with restriction of movement. Radiographs reveal irregularity and flattening of the metatarsal head.

Non-surgical treatment may require the application of a below-knee cast to relieve symptoms and the use of a metatarsal pad. If symptoms persist, surgery in the form of a dorsal closing wedge osteotomy to remove the abnormal section of the metatarsal head and to rotate up more normal articular surface provides good results.

REFERENCES

1. Libby AK, Sherry DD, Dudgeon BJ. Shoulder limitation in juvenile rheumatoid arthritis. *Arch Phys Med Rehabil* 1991; **72**:382–4.
2. Harris ED. Rheumatoid arthritis: the clinical spectrum. In: *Textbook of Rheumatology* (Kelley WN, Harris ED, Ruddy S, Sledge CB, eds). WB Saunders: Philadelphia, 1981:928–63.
3. Babini JC, Gusis SE, Babini SM, Cocco JA. Superolateral erosions of the humeral head in chronic inflammatory arthropathies. *Skeletal Radiol* 1992; **21**:515–7.
4. Kieft GJ, Dijkmans BAC, Bloem JL, Kroon HM. Magnetic resonance imaging of the shoulder in patients with rheumatoid arthritis. *Ann Rheum Dis* 1990; **49**:7–11.
5. Kvien TK, Pahle JA, Hoyeraal HM, Sandstad B. Comparison of synovectomy and no synovectomy in patients with juvenile rheumatoid arthritis. *Scand J Rheumatol* 1987; **16**:81–91.
6. Hamalainen M. Surgical treatment of juvenile rheumatoid arthritis. *Clin Exp Rheumatol* 1994; **12**(suppl 10):S107–12.
7. Ovregard T, Hoyeraal HM, Pahle JA, Larsen S. A 3 year retrospective study of synovectomies in children. *Clin Orthop* 1990; **259**:76–82.
8. Benjamin A. Double osteotomy of the shoulder. *Scand J Rheumatol* 1987; **3**:65–70.
9. Brenner BC, Ferlic DC, Clayton ML, Dennis DA. Survivorship of unconstrained shoulder arthroplasty. *J Bone Joint Surg (Am)* 1989; **71**:1289–96.
10. Stewart MPM, Kelly IG. Total shoulder replacement in rheumatoid disease. *J Bone Joint Surg (Br)* 1997; **79**:68–76.
11. Thomas BJ, Amstutz HC, Cracchiolo A. Shoulder arthroplasty for rheumatoid arthritis. *Clin Orthop* 1990; **265**:125–8.
12. Fowler PJ, Webster MS. Shoulder pain in highly competitive swimmers. *Orthop Trans* 1983; **7**:170.
13. Glouseman R, Jobe F, Tibone J, Moynes D, Antonelli D, Perry J. Dynamic electromyographic analysis of the throwing shoulder with glenohumeral instability. *J Bone Joint Surg (Am)* 1988; **70**:220–6.
14. Rodosky MW, Bigliani LU. The shoulder joint and girdle. In: *Principles of Orthopaedic Practice* (Dee R, Hurst LC, Gruber MA, Kottmeier SA, eds). McGraw-Hill: New York, 1997:1041–104.
15. Nutton RW, McBirnie JM, Phillips C. Treatment of chronic rotator cuff impingement by arthroscopic subacromial decompression. *J Bone Joint Surg (Br)* 1997; **79**:73–6.
16. Rowe CR, Zarins B. Recurrent transient subluxation of the shoulder. *J Bone Joint Surg (Am)* 1981; **63**:863–72.
17. Neer CS II, Foster CR. Inferior capsular shift for involuntary inferior and multidirectional instability of the shoulder: a preliminary report. *J Bone Joint Surg (Am)* 1980; **62**:897–908.
18. Arden GP. Surgical treatment of juvenile rheumatoid arthritis. *Ann Chir Gynaecol* 1985; **198**(suppl):103–9.
19. Inglis AE, Ranawat CS, Staub LR. Synovectomy and debridement of the elbow joint in rheumatoid arthritis. *J Bone Joint Surg (Am)* 1971; **53**:622–52.
20. Copeland SA, Taylor JG. Synovectomy of the elbow in rheumatoid arthritis. *J Bone Joint Surg (Br)* 1979; **61**:69–73.
21. Brumfield RH, Resnick CT. Synovectomy of the elbow in rheumatoid arthritis. *J Bone Joint Surgery (Am)* 1985; **67**:16–20.
22. Gendi NST, Axon JMC, Carr AJ, Pile KD, Burge PD, Mowat AG. Synovectomy of the elbow and

radial head excision in rheumatoid arthritis. *J Bone Joint Surg (Br)* 1997; **79**:918–23.

23. Tulp NJ, Winia WP. Synovectomy of the elbow in rheumatoid arthritis: long term results. *J Bone Joint Surg (Br)* 1989; **71**:664–6.

24. Vahvanen V, Eskola A, Peltonen J. Results of elbow synovectomy in rheumatoid arthritis. *Arch Orthop Trauma Surg* 1991; **110**:151–4.

25. Lee BPH, Morrey BF. Arthroscopic synovectomy of the elbow for rheumatoid arthritis. *J Bone Joint Surg (Br)* 1997; **79**:770–2.

26. Vainio K. Arthroplasty of the elbow and hand in rheumatoid arthritis. In: *Synovectomy and Arthroplasty in Rheumatoid Arthritis* (Chapchal G, ed). Thieme Verlag: Stuttgart, 1976:66–70.

27. Froimsen A, Silva JE, Richley WG. Cutis arthroplasty of the elbow joint. *J Bone Joint Surg (Am)* 1976; **58**:863–5.

28. Morrey BF. Post-traumatic stiffness: distraction arthroplasty. *Orthopaedics* 1992; **15**:863–9.

29. Ewald FC, Simmons ED, Sullivan JA. Capitellocondylar total elbow replacement in rheumatoid arthritis. *J Bone Joint Surg (Am)* 1993; **75**:498–507.

30. Weiland AJ, Weiss APC, Willis RP, Moore JR. Capitellocondylar total elbow replacement: a long term follow-up study. *J Bone Joint Surg (Am)* 1989; **71A**:217–22.

31. Morrey BF, Adams RA. Semi-constrained arthroplasty for the treatment of rheumatoid arthritis of the elbow. *J Bone Joint Surg (Am)* 1992; **74**:479–90.

32. Hanff G, Sollerman C, Elborogh R, Pettersson H. Wrist synovectomy in juvenile chronic arthritis. *Scand J Rheumatol* 1990; **19**:280–4.

33. Fatti JF, Palmer AK, Greenky S et al. Long-term results of Swanson interpositional wrist arthroplasty II. *J Hand Surg* 1991; **16**:432–7.

34. Kobus RJ, Turner RH. Wrist arthrodesis for treatment of rheumatoid arthritis. *J Hand Surg* 1990; **15**:541–6.

35. Schefer AJ, Garrowaay RY, McCue FC III. Ligamentous injuries of the wrist and hand. In: *Principles of Orthopaedic Practice* (Dee R, Hurst LC, Gruber MA, Kottmeier SA, eds). McGraw-Hill: New York, 1997:1201–6.

36. Feldon P, Millender LH, Nalebuff. Rheumatoid arthritis in the hand and wrist. In: *Operative Hand Surgery* (Green DP, ed), 3rd edn. Churchill Livingstone: New York, 1993:1587–690.

37. Anderson B, Kaye S. Treatment of flexor tenosynovitis of the hand ('trigger finger') with corticosteroids: a prospective study of the response to local injection. *Arch Intl Med* 1991; **151**:153–6.

38. Dennis DA, Clayton ML. Management of juvenile rheumatoid arthritis. In: *Surgery for Rheumatoid Arthritis* (Smith CJ, Clayton MJ, eds). Churchill Livingstone: New York, 1992:373–88.

39. Nalebuff EA. Rheumatoid hand surgery – update. *J Hand Surg* 1983; **8**:678–82.

40. Beckenbaugh RD. Implant arthroplasty in the rheumatoid hand and wrist. *J Hand Surg* 1983; **8**:675–8.

41. Nalebuff EA, Millender LH. Surgical treatment of the boutonniere deformity in rheumatoid arthritis. *Orthop Clin North Am* 1975; **6**:753–64.

42. Nalebuff EA. Restoration of balance in the rheumatoid thumb. In: *La Main Rheumatoide* (Tubiana R, ed). Expansion Scientifique Francaise: Paris, 1969:197.

43. Kanavel AB. *Infections of the Hand*, 7th edn. Lea & Febiger: Philadelphia, 1943:chap 1.

44. Fried JA, Athreya B, Gregg JR, Das M, Doughty R. The C-spine in juvenile rheumatoid arthritis. *Clin Orthop* 1983; **179**:102–6.

45. Isdale IC. Hip disease in juvenile rheumatoid arthritis. *Ann Rheum Dis* 1970; **29**:603–8.

46. Rombouts JJ, Rombouts-Lindemans C. Involvement of the hip in juvenile rheumatoid arthritis. *Acta Rheumatol Scand* 1971; **17**:248–67.

47. Ansell BM. Heberden oration 1977. Chronic arthritis in childhood. *Ann Rheum Dis* 1978; **37**:107–20.

48. Jacqueline F, Boujot A, Canet L. Involvement of the hips in juvenile rheumatoid arthritis. *Arthritis Rheum* 1961; **4**:500–13.

49. Rydholm U, Wingstrand H, Egund N et al. Sonography, arthroscopy, and intracapsular pressure in juvenile chronic arthritis of the hip. *Acta Orthop Scand* 1986; **57**:295–8.

50. Ekholm R, Norback B. On the relationship between articular changes and function. *Acta Orthop Scand* 1951; **21**:81–98.

51. Salter RB, Field P. The effects of continuous compression on living articular cartilage: an experimental investigation. *J Bone Joint Surg (Am)* 1960; **42**:31–49.

52. Kabayakawa M, Rydholm G, Wingstrand H, Pettersson H, Lindgren L. Femoral head necrosis in juvenile chronic arthritis. *Acta Orthop Scand* 1989; **60**:164–9.

53. McCullough CJ. Surgical management of the hip in juvenile chronic arthritis. *Br J Rheumatol* 1994; **33**:178–83.

54. Mogensen B, Brattstrom H, Ekelund L, Svantesson H, Lidgren L. Synovectomy of the hip

in juvenile chronic arthritis. *J Bone Joint Surg (Br)* 1982; **64**:295–9.

55. Swann M, Ansell BM. Soft-tissue release of the hips in children with juvenile chronic arthritis. *J Bone Joint Surg (Br)* 1986; **68**:404–8.

56. Soto-Hall R, Johnson LH, Johnson RA. Variations in the intra-articular pressure of the hip joint in injury and disease: a probable factor in avascular necrosis. *J Bone Joint Surg (Am)* 1964; **46**:509–16.

57. Witt JD, McCullough CJ. Anterior soft tissue release of the hip in juvenile chronic arthritis. *J Bone Joint Surg* 1994; **76**:267–70.

58. Witt JD, Swann M, Answell BM. Total hip replacement for juvenile chronic arthritis. *J Bone Joint Surg (Br)* 1991; **73**:770–3.

59. Chmell MJ, Scott RD, Thomas WH, Sledge CB. Total hip arthroplasty with cement for juvenile rheumatoid arthritis. Results at a minimum of ten years in patients less than thirty years old. *J Bone Joint Surg* 1997; **79**:44–52.

60. Simon S, Whiffen J, Shapiro F. Leg-length discrepancies in monoarticular and pauciarticular juvenile rheumatoid arthritis. *J Bone Joint Surg* 1981; **63**:209–15.

61. Kampner S, Ferguson AB. Efficacy of synovectomy in juvenile rheumatoid arthritis. *Clin Orthop* 1972; **88**:94–109.

62. Rydholm U, Elborgh R, Ranstam J, Schroder A, Svantesson H, Lidgren L. Synovectomy of the knee in juvenile chronic arthritis. A retrospective, consecutive follow-up study. *J Bone Joint Surg (Br)* 1986; **68**:223–8.

63. Moreno Alvarez MJ, Espada G, Maldonado-Cocco JA, Gagliardi SA. Longterm follow-up of hip and knee soft tissue release in juvenile chronic arthritis. *J Rheumatol* 1992; **19**:1608–10.

64. Rydholm U, Brattstrom H, Lidgren L. Soft tissue release for knee flexion contracture in juvenile chronic arthritis. *J Pediatr Orthop* 1986; **6**:448–51.

65. Swann M. Juvenile chronic arthritis. *Clin Orthop* 1987; **219**:38–49.

66. Rydholm U, Brattstrom H, Bylander B, Lidgren L. Stapling of the knee in juvenile chronic arthritis. *J Pediatr Orthop* 1987; **7**:63–8.

67. Rodriguez JA, Saddler S, Edelman S, Ranawat CS. Long-term results of total knee arthroplasty in class 3 and 4 rheumatoid arthritis. *J Arthroplasty* 1996; **11**:141–5.

68. Sarokhan AJ, Scott RD, Thomas WH, Sledge CB, Ewald FC, Cloos DW. Total knee arthroplasty in juvenile rheumatoid arthritis. *J Bone Joint Surg (Am)* 1983; **65**:1071–80.

69. Carmichael E, Chaplin DM. Total knee arthroplasty in juvenile rheumatoid arthritis. A seven-year follow-up study. *Clin Orthop* 1986; **210**:192–200.

70. Stuart MJ, Rand JA. Total knee arthroplasty in young adults who have rheumatoid arthritis. *J Bone Joint Surg* 1988; **70**:84–7.

71. Boublik M, Tsahakis PJ, Scott RD. Cementless total knee arthroplasty in juvenile onset rheumatoid arthritis. *Clin Orthop* 1993; **286**:88–93.

72. Rana NA. Juvenile rheumatoid arthritis of the foot. *Foot Ankle* 1982; **3**:2–11.

73. Tillman K. Surgery of the rheumatoid forefoot with special reference to the plantar approach. *Clin Orthop* 1997; **340**:39–47.

74. Royle SG. Investigation of the irritable hip. *J Pediatr Orthop* 1992; **12**:396–7.

75. Klaue K, Durnin CW, Ganz R. The acetabular rim syndrome. A clinical presentation of dysplasia of the hip. *J Bone Joint Surg (Br)* 1991; **73**:423–9.

76. Ganz R, Klaue K, Vinh TS, Mast JW. A new periacetabular osteotomy for the treatment of hip dysplasias. Technique and preliminary results. *Clin Orthop* 1988; **232**:26–36.

77. Stanitski CL, Harvell JC, Fu F. Observations on acute knee haemarthrosis in children and adolescents. *J Pediatr Orthop* 1993; **13**:506–10.

78. Graf BK, Lange RH, Fugisaki CK et al. Anterior cruciate ligament tears in skeletally immature patients: meniscal pathology at presentation and after attempted conservative treatment. *Arthroscopy* 1992; **8**:229–33.

79. Brittberg M, Lindahl A, Nilsson A et al. Treatment of deep cartilage defects in the knee with autologous chondrocyte transplantation. *N Engl J Med* 1994; **331**:889–95.

14

Educational and vocational planning – the key to success in adulthood

Patience H White

INTRODUCTION

Working is an activity of primary importance to the lives of millions of people around the world. Holding a job helps provide the financial support needed for themselves and their families, engages them in a regular routine, and allows for an experience of job satisfaction and feelings of self-esteem. Most of us live in a work-orientated society, yet many members of our societies with a variety of disabling conditions remain either unemployed or are in jobs that do not make full use of their skills and abilities.

This chapter discusses the importance of work as it relates to adolescents with disabilities, workforce participation by adolescents with disabilities, and what an adolescent with a disability will need to be competitive in the future work environment. A review of the research on adolescent developmental tasks as they relate to career development and how disabilities affect that development will follow. The final section outlines the necessary components of a pre-vocational readiness programme and suggests what the health professional can do to maximize vocational readiness in the adolescent with chronic illness and disabilities.

THE IMPORTANCE OF WORK

Work, a career, a job, employment. Short clear words in the vocabulary. They mean so much. Most of our lives are spent working. School years and retirement flank work like book ends. Work is an important dimension to life both to the individual and to society as a whole. Yet, ask a disabled youth how often he or she has been asked by relatives or professionals, 'what are you going to be when you grow up?' Chances are, they will respond, 'Never.' People seem afraid to ask such a question for fear of focusing attention on the child's disability and limitations. The conditioning that results for all concerned is a negative feeling about eventual employment.[1]

When adolescents with disabilities are asked what they want for their future, they are clear that they want jobs. This was demonstrated by one of the largest American surveys of young people with disabilities, conducted in 1995 by the PACER Center in Minneapolis, Minnesota. Over 11 000 households where young adults with disabilities lived were mailed a survey that asked questions about what these young people wanted in transition services. A total of 1314 teenagers aged 14–18 years (range 14–25 years) with a variety of disabilities (learning disabilities, chronic illness, mental health problems, physical disabilities, arthritis and sensory impairments) responded (Table 14.1). All groups identified job training as the most important, with independent living skills and college or vocational guidance close behind.[2] Few felt medical issues were the priority, yet most transition programmes focus on medical transition services to adult health care not vocational preparation skills. This concept was reinforced by another American survey in 1997, conducted by the Schriners Hospital for Children, of 297

Table 14.1   Teenagers with disabilities rank areas of importance for transition to adulthood[2]

- Job training
- Independent living
- College or vocational counselling
- Social issues
- Medical issues

families and 315 teenagers with disabilities. Eighty-eight per cent of the teenagers wanted a job in 5 years (unpublished results). A third study of 106 graduates of a school for adolescents with physical disabilities found that they most desired more guidance counselling, especially in areas of job placement, and additional training for upgrading job skills.[3]

WORK PARTICIPATION AND LONG-TERM OUTCOME

Even with this interest in work, the long-term outcome of the workforce participation by young adults with disabilities is poor. In the USA, a 1998 Harris Poll again found that two-thirds of Americans with disabilities and aged 16–64 years were unemployed, and of these 72% wanted to work.[4] In long-term outcome studies of children with juvenile inflammatory arthritis, both English[5] and American[6] studies have found that adults with a history of childhood-onset arthritis are less likely to be employed, and have more disability, pain, and fatigue, as well as a poorer perception of their health and physical functioning than do age- and sex-matched controls, and this was found despite equal or higher levels of education. A Canadian study found that young adults with inflammatory arthritis had higher levels of education and equal employment compared to national norms, and had good job satisfaction; but higher numbers of criminal convictions and poorer health.[7] In studies of

psychosocial outcome it can be difficult to compare employment rates to controls or national statistics, as was done in the Canadian study. For example, in the USA, employment is highly related to the highest education level attained.[8] In studies, cases must match with controls for highest level of education attained to ascertain if employment rates are appropriate or low with respect to educational level attained. Some studies choose not to look at employment as an outcome variable for performance as an adult. Such a study was done in Norway. It looked at psychosocial outcome, but did not mention employment rates.[9] Unemployment also is found when outcome studies are done on those individuals with a variety of physically disabling conditions. Several authors have pointed out that specific issues, such as career development for young adults with disabilities, are generic and not disease specific. The authors concluded it is valid to include diverse groups of disabilities when discussing specific outcome parameters such as employment rates, career maturity[10–12] or emotional well-being. The follow-up study of 106 graduates of a school for adolescents with physical disabilities (orthopaedic and neurological problems and cerebral palsy) previously mentioned, found a 25% unemployment rate.[3] Again this study did not look at education level and compared the study subjects with national norms. In general, studies of people with disabilities show a similar relationship of educational level to workforce participation, but their level of employment at each level of education attained is lower by 50%.

Assessing long-term outcomes of children with disabilities is becoming a priority in many countries. Increased survival rates over the past 20 years for children with diseases such as systemic lupus erythematosus[13] and the resultant financial toll on society for non-participation of those with disabilities in the workforce is now being realized. These members of society are minimally contributing to the economy because they are often in welfare programmes and living in poverty. Statistics find that the prevalence of chronic illness and disability among children and youth is estimated to be as high as 30%,[14] with 4% of the paediatric population sustaining significant limitation in functioning.[15] Today, in the industrialized countries, 90% of those born with a disability will reach their twentieth birthday.[14] In rheumatic diseases the development of disability has been documented by 12 functional outcome studies in patients with juvenile inflammatory arthritis.[16] The studies documented that an average of 20% (range 3–48%) of children with this diagnosis who had been followed for an average of 16 years (range 3–38 years) had limited functional capability to the point of inability to perform self-care. It has also been shown that the longer the follow-up the worse the functional state as measured by Steinbrocker functional class.[17]

DEVELOPMENTAL TASKS OF ADOLESCENCE

The problem of unemployment begins in adolescence. Data in the USA on participation in the workforce of adolescents with disabilities show that they are twice as likely as their non-disabled counterparts to be unemployed. This lack of work experience delays one of the most important developmental tasks of adolescence, finding a vocation.

Adolescence is a time marked by changes occurring biologically, emotionally and socially. In moving toward adulthood, adolescents face four major tasks, and the attainment of these tasks can be adversely affected by having a chronic illness or disability.[18] These major tasks are:

- to consolidate his or her identity
- to establish relationships outside the family
- to achieve independence from parents
- to find a vocation.

Each of the first three tasks is essential to achieving the fourth goal of independence in the work force.

To become comfortable with one's identity, one should be confident in one's body image and have the ability to dream about different roles and identities. Exposure to the world is key

in broadening the choices that children try on in their dreaming about their career identity.[19] Experimenting with independence can be hampered by growth retardation and pubertal delay, both of which can be seen in juvenile arthritis and other chronic illnesses. Dreaming about future roles is essential in shaping the directions one takes in adulthood. Expanding the horizons of a child with a disability is often hampered by physical and social isolation. This social isolation has been documented in many studies of children with rheumatic diseases, and most recently in a study done in England. This study found that children with inflammatory arthritis were treated differently by their peers, had little autonomy due to health regimens, had less peer involvement due to limited mobility and that social adjustment was more difficult for adolescents than for younger age groups.[20]

The majority of jobs today are still obtained via the family/friend network,[4] and employers feel the ability to fit in with coworkers is essential to being a valued employee. The capacity to be an accepted member of a peer group becomes a crucial milestone in attaining employment. The later a young person joins a peer group, the later the attainment of independent milestones toward adulthood.[21] Similarly, like all children and adolescents, young people with disabilities need to be exposed to multiple role models in order to expand their horizons and explore how they eventually will find a satisfying career.[19]

Overprotectiveness by parents, teachers and health professionals often results in a delay in the adolescent separating from their family and challenging authority. Both are necessary to achieve independence from parents. To succeed in the competitive workplace environment, personal responsibility, a sense of self-reliance and commitment is essential. Personal autonomy must be encouraged within the home and in educational and medical environments.[22] The need for all involved to treat the young person with dignity like their non-disabled peers is emphasized throughout this book. Often it is the health professional who can lead the way by anticipatory guidance around these developmental tasks for parents and other adults in the child's life. Close attention to their career-development milestones is needed because the timely and sequential attainment of these tasks makes future employment more likely. Attempting to address a later task before attaining an earlier one increases risk of dysfunction and failure in the competitive marketplace. For example, data show that it is difficult to become employed without prior work experience during the secondary school years.[23]

THE FUTURE WORKPLACE AND HOW TO PREPARE

The social context coupled with the functional capabilities of the individual can determine the extent of the disability.[18] The previous sections in this chapter have discussed some important tasks that need to be accomplished by the young person with a disability in order for them to be ready for employment. Another key part of the equation to becoming employed is understanding the future workplace. What does an employee need to know to survive in the workplace of the future? The world of work today is undergoing a monumental change that, social scientists say, is equivalent to the disrupting changes that came with the industrial revolution.

> Mobility, Empowerment, Teams, Cross training, Virtual Offices, Telecommuting, Re-engineering, Outsourcing. If these buzzwords don't sound familiar, they should. They are changing your life. The last decade, perhaps more than any other time since the advent of mass production, has witnessed a profound redefinition of the way we work.[24]

By the year 2006 the Bureau of Labor Statistics in the USA forecasts that there will be an increase in professional (12.4%), managerial (30%) and technical (8.3%) jobs.[8] Nearly one in every two jobs added to the economy will be in the service industry (health, business and social). Most jobs requiring high skill levels will increase, whereas the low-skill jobs will decline. There will be labour efficiency, with better technology, better processes and fewer, better educated workers. The employee of the future with continual retraining can expect life-long employability, not employment. The essential components of jobs are shared responsibility and constant training. The employee, like business, must be reinvented to keep up with new technology. The technology explosion makes the workplace more friendly to people with disabilities, allowing flexible hours and locations for work. In this fast-changing, global economy, the US Department of Labor suggests that workers will need to:

- get as much education as possible
- keep upgrading their skills (retrain)
- sharpen career exploration/development skills to remain employed in this changing global economy
- change careers – not just jobs – three to four times during their working years.[24]

Education is essential in today's knowledge-based economy. Studies today still show that the level of education attained is directly related to life-time earnings and who becomes employed.[8] The relationships hold up for those with disabilities as well. This means that in the USA, for example, in order for an individual with disability to have access to health insurance through employers, they must be employed in a high-skill job requiring as much education as possible beyond high school. Thus, counselling to make post-secondary education a reality for young people with disabilities is central to their success. This is exemplified by the fact that 32% of individuals with disabilities say it is their lack of skills, education and training that accounts for their lack of employment.[4]

Early work experience is equally important. A 1996 survey from the *New York Times* of 300 employers revealed the top three qualities that counted with employers were attitude, communication skills and previous work experience. In the USA, a study was conducted that showed over 53% of 13 year olds without disabilities were involved in a work experience outside their homes once a week. The average age at which parents felt children without disabilities should start work was 13 years (SD 1.9 years).[25] A recent study of 14–17 year olds in North Carolina revealed that over 95% of the sample had worked for pay for someone outside their family, with 32% of the sample getting paid for work before the age of 14 years. The majority of the youth reported having worked in the retail trade and the service sector, especially in the food industry. A consequence of work is on-the-job injury. Over half of the respondents in that study had been injured at work at least once. These injuries resulted from being cut (29%), burned (25%), or hit by an object or person (10%).[26]

Part-time work in middle adolescence has become the norm, but a debate is growing that work may be detrimental.[27] Researchers in the field have reasoned that secondary school work experience should be one of the most important elements of the transition to adulthood[28] and facilitate exploratory activity that helps in the development of self-concepts and career choice.[29] Yet this has not been supported in studies of how adolescent work affects vocational development. In fact, vocational development may be unaffected by part-time work experience because most of these jobs are low-level, unchallenging, entry-level sales, service or manual positions that pay 40% of an adult wage.[30] A large study of 483 high-school students in the USA showed a lack of connection between assuming a part-time work role and making future occupational plans and decisions.[31] The national longitudinal study on adolescent health of 12 118 adolescents in grades 7 to 12 in the USA showed that working more than 20 hours per week was associated with more emotional distress and more health-risk behaviours such as drinking and drug use.[12] Thus the debate has centred on hours worked rather than work experience. These studies have important implications for vocational guidance and career counselling. Part-time work experience should be done in association with careful counselling that asks what the adolescent is learning about his or her likes and dislikes and abilities as they think of future work choices.

In light of the above data for adolescents without disabilities, data on adolescents with disabilities show that they have fewer employment/career experiences and are less career mature than their non-disabled counterparts. This immaturity was statistically related to their parents' expectations that a first work experience should occur at least 1–2 years later (i.e. at 14–16 years of age) than adolescents of the same age without disabilities.[32] Thus teenagers with disabilities had less experience and knowledge of the workplace and exposure to vocational choices than their non-disabled peers. Given that prior work experience is essential to employers, their lack of prior work experience makes it difficult to secure that first job. Given the debate around part-time work for teenagers without disabilities discussed above, those with disabilities need even more attention to the planning of early work experience that is framed by knowledgeable career counsellors and parents.

Work environments for youth with disabilities should be tailored to their cognitive and developmental capacity. Health professionals should be familiar with the options available within their own countries. For example, options available in the USA include: (a) day care or independent living programmes for severely disabled young adults who would not succeed in any paid employment setting; (b) sheltered workshops for those with mental impairments but normal physical capabilities, where the environment is sheltered and controlled; (c) supported employment, where a vocational rehabilitation counsellor works with a person with a disability, tailoring job activities to the individual's capabilities and the support continues with job support personnel indefinitely; and (d) competitive employment, which is possible for those with disabilities who can gain the education and independence required.[33]

CAREER DEVELOPMENT RESEARCH

Given the predictions of the future work-environment requirements and the current problems with employment of people with disabilities, what is known about career development that can be used to improve the employment outcome of adolescents with disabilities? Many of the theoretical writings on vocational development of disabled persons focus on: (a) models of work adjustment in a particular job, and do not address

---

Table 14.2 Factors important for career development

- Intrinsic:
  - Define self-concept
  - Develop autonomy
- Extrinsic:
  - Develop career maturity at same rate as non-disabled peer
  - Exposure to vocation/career challenges
  - Exposure to work and work experiences
  - Acquire skills to manage vocational/career choices/planning
  - Expectation for employment by health professional, parents, educators and society

---

Table 14.3 Hurdles to workforce participation for adolescents with chronic illness and disability

- Social isolation of adolescent and family
- Late incorporation into peer groups
- Undeveloped self-concept
- Lower expectations by those around them
- Little planning for transition
- Less exposure to vocation/career tasks and information
- Less exposure to the world of work and role models
- Less higher educational attainment
- Less and later workforce participation
- Career immaturity
- Limited knowledge by parent, educational and health professionals on how to assist with the process of employment readiness

---

patterns of vocational development throughout their lifetime; and (b) theories that have been developed for traumatically disabled rather than congenitally or acquired during childhood

disabled persons. Super[34] is one of the few authors whose writing discusses the implications of disability on vocational development. Super was the first to point out that there may be social forces (i.e. attitudes, values and stereotypes) that play a predominant role in shaping vocational development of disabled persons because they are not exposed to vocational choices, and that most vocational theorists did not distinguish between pre-career and midcareer issues. Thus, many other vocational theorists assumed that self-concept is well established by early adulthood, whereas this may not be true for disabled persons (Table 14.2). Super concluded that for the great majority of occupations, handicaps result in erecting hurdles (Table 14.3), not imposing barriers, and since vocational development requires the attainment of a self-concept, the counselling of a person with a disability must begin with the task of defining self-concept.[30]

Conte summarizes the pre-career development research that has been published in studies of deaf children:

- people with disabilities must have exposure to vocational challenges and tasks early in life if they are to develop adequate vocational maturity to become successful employed adults
- young people lag significantly behind their non-disabled peers in acquiring vocational experiences, thus vocational services are provided too late in life and should be provided in early adolescence.[35]

Lichert studied 106 graduates of a special school for those with severe physical disabilities. He found that involvement with a vocational rehabilitation counsellor before secondary school graduation was related to attainment of employment, while post-secondary contact was not.[3] This study also reflects the importance of early intervention.

In 1967, Allen[36] also studied physically disabled youth. His results showed that there was no significant difference in the vocational aspirations/expectations of physically disabled and non-disabled youth when they were

Table 14.4 Two models of disability[38]	
Medical model	**Interactional model**
• Disability is a deficiency or abnormality	• Disability is a difference
• Being disabled is a negative	• Being disabled is, in itself, neutral
• Disability resides in the individual	• Disability derives from the interaction between the individual and society
• The remedy for disability-related problems is cure or normalization of the individual	• The remedy for disability-related problems is a change in the interaction between the individual and society
• The agent of remedy is the professional	• The agent of remedy could be the individual, an advocate or anyone who effects the arrangements between the individual and society

matched for cumulative grade-point average and level of father's occupation, but as a whole disabled seniors had lower grades and socio-economic status than did non-disabled high-school seniors. Thus the author concluded that extrinsic factors more than intrinsic factors resulted in lower vocational development. These conclusions were supported by Brolin,[37] who concluded that extrinsic environmental factors were much more important than internal traits and must receive attention if normal vocational development is to occur.

Health professionals tend to focus on finding a way to 'fix' the individual with a disability, and this approach often is not shared by the child with a disability. A study showed that the longer the child had had their disability, the less likely they were to opt for a surgical 'cure'.[33] Recently, the community of people with disabilities has articulated several observations about the medical model, in which most health professionals are trained and work. They feel it should be changed to a more interactive model, as outlined in Table 14.4.[38] The need to change from a medical model to an interactive model for health professionals and society is demonstrated by the following quote from a psychiatrist with a disability who is chair of a large rehabilitation

department: 'Most of the negative consequences of having a disability are not the result of the illness or disabling condition but rather by the way those without disabilities related to their disabled peers'.[19]

Osipow[39] has also commented that professionals working with people with disabilities have a number of erroneous practices and assumptions about people with disabilities. Examples of some of these assumptions are: (a) career development is not important for the disabled; (b) the disability overrides the person's other characteristics in determining career behaviour; (c) career options are very limited for those with disabilities; (d) career development is arrested; and (e) career development of the disabled is influenced by chance and is unsystematic. Osipow viewed health and rehabilitation professionals as hindering the development of persons with disabilities by their low expectations for and by stereotyping and segregating people with disabilities. This view that the professionals may inhibit the vocational development of individuals with disabilities implies that the health professional should recognize they have a significant, and possibly determining, impact on the individual's success or failure in the world of work. This is substantiated by the 1997 Schriners

Hospital for Children CHOICES project survey of 297 parents of young adults with disabilities. Seventy per cent of parents felt that the medical professional should take a leading role in the vocational planning and development of their disabled teenager (unpublished data). These data and the other studies discussed here have major implications on what should be included in the medical transition services offered to teenagers with a disability, and what role the health professional should play in the vocational/career development of the adolescent with a disability.

Many researchers have suggested that vocational decision-making may be more complicated than for the general non-disabled population, that the process of career counselling with various populations with disabilities is more generic than specialized, and that vocational challenges are important in the development of vocational maturity and future employment.[40] From a developmental perspective, it is generally accepted that vocational choice and career awareness are shaped by childhood experiences.[41] Early career experiences are the framework for vocational development of individuals with disabilities. Inability to participate in decision-making and to test self-competencies can be the outcome of limited early experiences and can impede career development. This was demonstrated in the results of the Career Maturity Inventory when given to 100 disabled youths aged 12–24 years. These young people scored statistically below their age-matched non-disabled peers in all areas, and the greatest difference was found in orientation ('I know very little about the requirements of jobs'), decisiveness ('I have so many interests its hard to choose any one occupation') and independence ('You should decide for yourself what kind of work to do'). Interestingly, they scored closest to the norm on involvement ('There is no point in deciding on a job when the future is so uncertain'), demonstrating that teenagers with disabilities are not fatalistic and want to take risks to be in the workforce.[32] Thus, as Super implied,[34] teenagers with disabilities need to explore, learn about and try out work in preparation for their future career choices and complete these experiences with guided, systematic career-development sessions.

Another area of active research in determining the long-term psychosocial and employment outcome is in defining the characteristics of resilient individuals with disabilities. Those with resilience have the capacity to spring back from a difficult situation. For many years studies focused on the negative differences between those with disabilities and those without disabilities, until recently when the researchers began to focus on resilient traits of individuals. These are the individuals whom many would say are functioning well in adulthood despite their disability. These recent studies have outlined factors for children with disabilities that foster resilience, not vulnerability. For those involved with adolescents with disabilities, a goal of interventions would be to shift the balance toward resilience and away from vulnerability. At any stage the balance can shift, often turning a well-compensated child into an adolescent with an emotional or behavioural problem. This possibility for psychosocial change in the adolescent years was observed in a psychosocial outcome study in children with arthritis.[9] The characteristics that have been associated with resilience in studies of non-disabled children are outlined in Table 14.5.[42,43] In persons with a disability factors associated with resilience also include: self-perception as not handicapped; involvement with household chores; having a network of friends who are disabled and non-disabled; family and peer support; and parental support without overprotectiveness.[44] Professionals caring for a child with a disability often do not realize that it is the lack of the resilience factors and the characteristics of the chronic condition rather than the diagnosis that makes coping with a disability difficult. Thus those with invisible illnesses, unstable courses, unpredictable symptoms and an uncertain prognosis often find it more difficult to cope. Many of the paediatric rheumatic diseases are examples of unpredictable illnesses. It is often this group of teenagers with non-disfiguring and unpredictable diseases that need counselling, even

Table 14.5   Factors that foster resilience in children[42,43]

• Dispositional attributes of the individual:
   – active engagement with environment (extracurricular activities)
   – responsiveness to others (peer relationships)
   – cognitive skills
   – communication skills
   – internal locus of control
 • Familial factors:
   – warmth
   – cohesion
   – family role model present if parent not available
   – concern for well-being of the child
   – expectation of success at taking personal responsibility (household chores)
 • External support systems:
   – other role models outside family
   – caring community/agency
   – reward individual competencies

though they resist identifying themselves for services such as special education or career counselling. Assisting the adolescent to maintain competent attributes under stress is important. Social and work competence, despite ongoing emotional distress, remain indicators of resilience.[43]

CAREER AND VOCATIONAL ASSESSMENTS

Adolescents with disabilities are rarely assessed for career and vocational information that could be used for transition planning and counselling. Levinson[45] reported that students with disabilities in special education are provided with an annual evaluation that incorporates medical, psychological, social, cultural, educational and economic assessments. Few data specifically related to career and vocational aptitudes, interests and work-related adaptive habits and behaviours are obtained. The latter type of assessment should be made available, not only for those in special education, but for all adolescents with disabilities.[46]

Assessments of career and vocational aptitude and experience should be a part of any information obtained in planning the future of an adolescent with a disability. Several tools are available. Examples are: APTICOM, Goldberg Scale of Vocational Development (adolescent form), OFFER Self-image Questionnaire Revised, Myers–Briggs, and the Career Maturity Inventory. Much of the outcome assessment of children with chronic illnesses, such as idiopathic arthritis, focus on functional status (juvenile artyhritis functional assessment report (JAFAR), childhood arthritis impact measurement scales (CHAIMS), childhood health assessment questionnaire (CHAQ), juvenile arthritis self-report index (JASI)) or overall health-related quality of life (functional independence measure for children (WeeFIM), juvenile arthritis quality of life questionnaire (JAQQ), childhood arthritis health profile (CAHP), paediatric evaluation of disability inventory (PEDI)).[47] Like the status of many functional assessment tools, the tools for assessing vocational maturity and work readiness vary in what they measure, and therefore each tool has its own advantages and disadvantages (Table 14.6). In long-term studies of chronic arthritis, there appears to be no correlation between the measurement of functional status and employment.[9,48] For example, in a study of disabled adolescents there appeared to be no relationship of functional status as measured by using Scales of Independent Living and career maturity.[32] Because the functional measures do not assess vocational maturity or attitude toward or experience in work, this type of assessment is needed to help the adolescents plan for their future workforce participation.

EDUCATIONAL AND VOCATIONAL PLANNING

Vocational planning for children and adolescents with disabilities is rarely incorporated into

Table 14.6   Examples of career/vocational assessment tools

Tool	Age	Measures	Advantages	Disadvantages
APTICOM	Adolescents to adulthood	Vocational interests, general aptitude	Provides immediate feedback; portable-computer based	Not appropriate for all disabilities (e.g. visual)
Goldberg Scales, adolescent form	Adolescents	Career plans, work values, origins of work, interests, rehabilitation outlook following disability	First test developed	Scoring relies on judgment of rater
OFFER Self-image	Adolescents, 13–18 years	Personality inventory: vocational altitudes, self-confidence, body image, social and family functions	Good validity/reliability compared with measures in adolescents of same age	Useful for limited age range; if chronologically older, need to judge if is appropriate
Myers–Brigges	Adolescents to adulthood	Identifies differing styles of perception, judgment, lifestyles	Leads to greater self-understanding; useful in evaluating team dynamics	Subjective, relies on rater's accurate self-report
Career Maturity Inventory	Adolescents to young adults	Attitude to vocation and career	Validated to age-matched norms	Not normalized to contemporary youth experiences

the treatment plan available in medical clinics, hospitals and schools. Likewise, parents and society often offer little planning guidance.[49] Brunner[50] has stressed the need for planning:

The decision to delay vocational or job decisions until comparatively late in the life cycle inevitably makes fuzzy one's definition of ones self as an adult. The neuroses of the young are far more likely to revolve around work than around sex. Therefore the first order of business in the transformation of our mode of educating is to revolutionize and revivify the idea of vocation or occupation.[50]

In the USA there are rehabilitation centres for the vocational planning and rehabilitation of the severely disabled adult. These centres rely on the concepts that adults have a prior work experience and knowledge that needs to be rehabilitated. A child has little or no experience with the world of work and needs a habilitative process geared to their lack of self-awareness. Most of the adult centres for rehabilitation are unprepared to offer vocational planning and assistance to the disabled child. Current disability laws in the USA focus on the need for a vocational development service.[33] An example is the requirement, at as early an age as 14 years, for a transition plan as part of the Individual Education Program (IEP) for students in special education. Yet many students with disabilities do not have a plan that was created by those with appropriate expertise in the current world of work; therefore, it is difficult for such teams to create a realistic, comprehensive plan with appropriate early intervention. An even larger number of students with chronic illnesses and disabilities are not in special education, and therefore have no protective laws to mandate access to vocational planning services.

Usbane[49] proposed five processes for the child with a disability that he felt were essential to promote entry and participation in the workforce. First is the socialization process, which includes attainment of social skills. The presence or lack of social skills is one of the better predictors of future vocational success either in training classes or in the actual job itself.[51] As discussed previously, loneliness and the lack of experience in group relationships for children with disabilities is the norm. Practice in job-interview skills for adolescents with disabilities has been inadequate and is needed.

The second process is the evaluation process, which includes early introduction of occupational information and awareness of possible requirements for accommodation that is needed in various job settings. As early as grade 4, children without disabilities express a concern about their vocational future.[52] During the elementary grades career planning should emphasize the world of work and to widen the child's exposure to future possibilities. Involvement of business in this process and availability of information on current occupational needs and requirements is essential.[53,54] Interests in occupations often stems from the games children play that deal with occupations, elementary school hobbies and actual work experiences.[55]

The third process is the exploration process which includes an up-to-date resource room that can be identified as a meeting ground for social, vocational and educational needs. Actual developmental tasks geared to occupational skills based on real work examples should be available. This allows the child with a disability the opportunity to attain a level of accomplishment with non-disabled peers.

The fourth process, is the ambulatory process, where the young person with a disability learns independence in travelling to a real work experience. This could begin with taking a tour through the local environment, such as the school or hospital, to identify different occupations and then reporting back to parents, school personnel or health professionals. Educational requirements for the occupations viewed could be discussed to reinforce the need for continued education. These trips could be expanded into visiting work sites and businesses.

The fifth process is the guidance and counselling process. This should include group experiences. This would allow socialization, which equalizes the many medical one-to-one relationships for treatment of medical problems. Counselling often deals with the here and now questions about the work environment and outlines long-term plans for education and training tailored to disease characteristics, disease stage and the developmental stage of the adolescent. Knowledge about adolescent development is a prerequisite for counsellors, and counsellors with this expertise can be hard to find in adult-oriented vocational systems.

The health professional should collaborate with the counsellor, giving him or her information on developmental issues and suggesting the above discussed steps of the planning process. An example of a life-centred career educational curriculum is outlined in a paper by Brolin.[56] A comprehensive paper by Roessler[54] outlines the need for a national agenda in the USA to address the barriers to those with disabilities in the federal systems (e.g. social security disability income and tax disincentives).

An important component of career planning is obtaining post-secondary education. The future

Table 14.7   Post-secondary education for persons with chronic illness/disability elements of effective transition planning[57]

Assess the impact of illness on the student:

- Educationally:
  - Has the illness necessitated any special accommodations at school?
  - Was the class missed at certain times of day to perform a health-care routine?
  - Did the illness affect attendance?
  - Did medication affect ability to concentrate or participate in school? (Was the student more alert at certain times of the day? Were frequent breaks from class required to take medications or rest?)
  - Was extra time necessary to complete class work, tests or homework?
  - Was technology, such as computers, used in the classroom or at home to fulfil academic requirements?
  - Was in-class assistance required, such as a person to take notes?
- Medically:
  - Are any activities restricted?
  - Does the student require specialized medical care (e.g. dialysis)?
  - Does the student require the coordinated care of many health-care providers?
  - Does the student have a care routine that must be performed at a specific time of day?
  - Does the student have a care routine that can only be done by a specially trained individual, such as a physical therapist, respiratory therapist or nurse?
  - Is there a medication schedule that must be strictly adhered to?
  - Are required drugs difficult to find?
  - Is the care of a medical specialist required? How frequently?
- Environmentally:
  - Do certain environmental factors such as heat, cold, moulds, dust, odours and humidity affect the student's health and well-being?
  - Does the student need to limit exposure to noise and distractions?
  - Does the student require a special living environment?
  - Are certain activities such as walking long distances or climbing stairs difficult?
- On activities of daily living:
  - Is assistance with getting out of bed required?
  - Is assistance with food preparation/eating needed?
  - Does the student require a special diet?
  - Does the student need assistance with bathing or using the bathroom?
  - Is assistance with dressing necessary?
  - Is assistance with mobility required?

workplace will be a knowledge-based economy requiring skilled labour. Thus careful planning must be done so that the move from a secondary school to post-secondary school environments occurs and the student succeeds in completing the educational path desired. Careful consideration should be given to when to disclose illness-related issues to college/university staff and

Table 14.8   Transition to post-secondary education/employment timeline checklist[58]

- Four years prior to leaving secondary education:
  - identify career interests and skills, explore them
  - seek a counsellor to discuss appropriate post-secondary education/employment options
  - learn to communicate your interests, preferences and needs effectively
  - learn when, where and how to disclose information about your illness/disability
- Three years prior to leaving secondary education:
  - match career skills and interests with vocational course work
  - obtain work experience or continue work experiences
  - determine eligibility for financial support, if appropriate
  - practice personal communication skills (e.g. interview skills for job/school)
  - meet counsellor to discuss entrance exams and plan visits to post-secondary institutions to assess the need for and availability of medical- and disability-related support (e.g. visit infirmary and disability student services)
  - learn advocacy skills and take responsibility for yourself
  - practice assuming management of health concerns
  - learn to complete curriculum vitae, if necessary
- Two years prior to leaving secondary education:
  - start application process for post-secondary education job/school
  - consider when to disclose illness in application process
  - think about accommodations needed for post-secondary school/job
  - visit schools/jobs
  - identify community supports
  - plan transition of medical care to new providers, if necessary
  - explore legal status with regard to decision-making prior to age of majority
  - go to medical appointments and/or meet with your physician on your own
- One year prior to leaving secondary school:
  - identify post-secondary education institutions or job, and complete any final applications
  - assume full responsibility for management of medical condition
  - complete any necessary medical transition tasks, if necessary
  - practice effective communication skills (e.g. interviewing skills)
  - become knowledgeable about relevant laws that protect individuals with disability

what accommodations might be needed. Questions to assist in assessing the impact of chronic illness on the student are given in Table 14.7. Issues and resources for the transition to post-secondary education can be found in *Maximizing Success for Young Adults with Chronic Health Related Illness*, published by the American Council on Education.[57]

To ensure appropriate planning, several organizations have outlined what steps should be taken during high school to improve employment outcome. An example of an outline is given in Table 14.8.[58] One can never start too early in planning the transition process. In a survey of state programme directors, directors of programmes for children with special health care needs, vocational rehabilitation counsellors and adolescent health coordinators in the USA, all cited insufficient transition planning as the most important factor limiting successful transition.[59]

PARENTS' ROLE

The parents' role in the vocational planning process is essential. Often career development in secondary school is seen as inferior to developing proficiency in an academic area. Similarly, in many school systems, any systematic career development programmes are left unattended or, as often the case in the USA, are directed by guidance counsellors who are overwhelmed by large student caseloads and many other pressing issues such as teenage pregnancy or school violence. It is a poor assumption for parents to assume that the laws enacted at a national level mean that schools know best how to provide for the career development needs of their disabled children. Parents should be actively involved to:

- set the expectation that their child can and will work
- learn the basic factors of vocational development
- ensure the attainment of basic career exploration goals and objectives in conjunction with an IEP process or on their own
- keep the attainment of functional living skills and the development of autonomy and self-advocacy skills as close as possible to the timetable of developmental milestones attained by their non-disabled peers
- enable their child to obtain career exploration and early work experiences in elementary and secondary school

- be aware of the resources and technology available and understand the disability rights laws of their country.

Professionals should provide access to resources and information at appropriate times in the course of the child's development to assist parents in fulfilling their important role. This proactive action by the health professional will assist the family to be less overprotective and more willing to be flexible as the child matures. Transition programmes should integrate parents into the transition process of their child,[60] and the adolescent with the disability.

CAREER READINESS AS AN ESSENTIAL COMPONENT OF TRANSITION PROGRAMMES

In a national survey of over 300 transition programmes in the USA, four different transition models were identified.[61] Surprisingly, less than 9% of these programmes offered vocational planning, despite vocational/job training issues being the major concern of young people with disabilities.[62] Recent vocational literature also strongly supports the need for the development of comprehensive programmes that include the following components: early intervention (before age 14 years), transition planning services, career development and exploration services, early work exposure with quality not quantity experiences, post-secondary education counselling, and service components for parents.[63,64] These services must be age and disease-stage appropriate for the adolescent. Today, secondary-school systems in the USA may provide individual service components, but they do not provide: (a) continuity across activities throughout the 4-year curriculum; (b) services that specifically focus on the impact of disability and its relationship to career education planning, while promoting choice for students with disabilities; or (c) a component that provides parents with the information they need to foster career development, effective transition planning and ultimate choice for their child. With over 10 years' experience from a pre-vocational programme for adolescents with chronic illnesses and disabilities in Washington, DC, the staff of the Adolescent Employment Readiness Program have found several additional services to be worthwhile. These services include: (a) availability of up-to-date information on the future workforce requirements; (b) involvement of employers who can give advice on services offered such as job seeking skills, participate in career exploration and offer job experience; and (c) having services in convenient locations. In the USA, school personnel have a difficult time identifying students with disabilities who do not look disabled or self identity through an IEP. Therefore, the pre-vocational service may need to be located near the medical service providers that teenagers with chronic illnesses frequently visit.[65]

WHAT A HEALTH PROFESSIONAL CAN DO

If the health professional is going to care for youth with chronic illness and disability, he or she has an obligation to identify these young people and play an important role in placing emphasis on the need for pre-vocational guidance, while also caring for their medical illness needs. As the child with a disability grows up, the issues discussed in this chapter come to play a major role in the outcome obtained. Health providers can foster resilience in the adolescent and family by assisting the teenager and parents to improve their understanding of the chronic illness, the teenager's capacity and the future prognosis of the illness. With this knowledge, all involved can set achievable employment goals. This can be accomplished in part by giving anticipatory guidance to the adolescent and family in areas identified as important for future employability. Some examples are:

- Assist the family to allow the adolescent to develop autonomy (e.g. during medical visits talk directly to the adolescent, and/or see the adolescent without the parents present).

- Foster career exploration (e.g. discuss occupations observed by adolescent throughout their day or while watching their favourite TV programmes).
- Foster expectation of future employment (e.g. ask 'What will you be when you grow up?').
- Foster personal responsibility and reward individual competencies (e.g. similar participation in household chores as non-disabled siblings).
- Foster the adolescent's involvement with a peer group that has disabled and non-disabled participants.
- Reinforce the need to attain the highest level of education possible so that the adolescent will be able to compete in the future workforce.
- Know and assist the family and teenager in attaining, at the appropriate time, the developmental milestones important for career development.
- Alert the family to the need for early planning, and plan with the adolescent, family and counsellors for transitions from school to work or post-secondary education well in advance.
- Know the laws and resources available to assist the adolescent and family in the transition process from school to work (e.g. lists of resources available in the USA can be found in Conte,[34] Edelman et al,[57] White,[66] Council of Chief State School Officers,[67] National Information Center for Children and Youth with Disabilities,[68] and Arthritis Foundation[69]).

CONCLUSION

Outcome data for children with chronic illnesses such as rheumatic disease demonstrate the need for assistance in career and vocational planning. Work plays a central role in all our lives. Attaining that important goal is dependent upon knowing the developmental needs of adolescents with disabilities that affect future employment and understanding the future workplace. Vocational/career planning plays a key role in the transition process. A knowledgeable health professional can foster this planning process by being a catalytic consultant that urges the adolescent and family forward. The result of this help can be an adolescent that successfully navigates the transition process and has a meaningful life as an adult, despite their disability or chronic illness.

REFERENCES

1. Hippolitus P. Employment opportunities and services for youth with chronic illnesses. In: *Issues in Care of Children with Chronic Illness* (Hobbs, Novel, Perrin, eds). Jossey-Bass: San Francisco, 1985.
2. Wright B. Teens say job training their top need. In: *Point of Departure*. Act Project, PACER Center, Minneapolis, 1996:2:8.
3. Liehart D, Lutsky L, Gottlieb A. Post secondary experiences of young adults with severe physical disabilities. *Exceptional Children* 1990; Sep:56–63.
4. *NOD/Harris Survey of People with Disabilities Study*, No. 942003, Louis Harris Association, Inc: Washington DC, 1998.
5. Martin K, Woo P. Outcome in juvenile chronic arthritis. *Rev Rhum (Engl Edn)* 1997; **10**:S242.
6. Petersen LS, Mason T, Nelson AM, Fallon W, Gabriel SE. Psychosocial outcomes and health studies in adults who have had juvenile arthritis: a controlled population based study. *Arthritis Rheum* 1997; **40**:2235–40.
7. Wirrell E, Lang B, Canfield C. Social outcomes in young adults with juvenile arthritis: implications for the development of transition clinics. *Arthritis Rheum* 1995; **38**:S184.
8. Oslkaloosa IA. *Post Secondary Education Opportunity Newsl* 1997; **66**:14.
9. Aasland A, Flato B, Vondivik LH. Psychosocial outcome in juvenile chronic arthritis: a nine year follow-up. *Clin Exp Rheumatol* 1997; **15**:561–8.
10. Stein RE, Jessup DJ. A non categorical approach to chronic childhood illness. *Public Health Rep* 1982; **97**:354–62.
11. Wolman C, Resnick MD, Harris LJ, Blum RW. Emotional well-being among adolescents with and without chronic caditias. *J Adolesc Health* 1994; **15**:199–204.
12. Resnick MD, Bearman PS, Blum RW et al. Protecting adolescents from harm. Findings from the National Longitudinal Study on Adolescent Health. *JAMA* 1997; **278**:823–32.
13. Lehman TJA. Long-term outcome in SLE in childhood. What is the prognosis? *Rheum Dis Clin North Am* 1991; **17**:921–30.
14. Newacheck PH. Adolescents with special health needs: prevalence, severity and access to health services. *Pediatrics* 1989; **84**:872–81.
15. Newacheck PH, Budetti PP, Halfin N. Trends in activity-limiting chronic conditions among children. *Am J Public Health* 1986; **76**:178–84.
16. Anderson-Gare BA, Fasth A. The natural history of juvenile chronic arthritis: a population based cohort study. II: Outcome. *J Rheumatol* 1995; **22**:308–19.
17. Laaksonen AL. A prognostic study of juvenile arthritis. *Acta Pediatr Scand* 1966; **166**(suppl):9–91.
18. Blum RW, Gehn O. Chronically ill youth. In: *Textbook of Adolescent Medicine* (McAnarney ER, Kreipe RE, Orr DP, Comerci GO, eds). WB Saunders: London, 1992:222–8.
19. Strax TE. Psychosocial issues faced by adolescents and young adults with disabilities. *Pediatr Ann* 1991; **20**:501–6.
20. Barlow JH, Shaw KL, Harrison K. Psycho-social impact of juvenile chronic arthritis. *Br J Rheum* 1997; **36**(suppl 1):139.
21. Hassan G. Transition to independent living: a family life cycle approach to the separation of physically disabled adolescents and their families. Dissertation, California School of Professional Psychology at Berkeley, CA, 191, DA 9209149.
22. Wall WD. *Adolescents in School and Society*. National Foundation for Educational Research: Windsor, 1968.
23. Hasazi SB, Gordon LR, Roe CA. Factors associated with the employment status of handicapped youth exiting high school from 1979 to 1983. *Exceptional Children* 1985; **51**:455–69.
24. Hammonds KH, Kell K, Thurston K. Rethinking work. *Business Week* 1994:Oct:76–87.
25. Philips S, Sandston KL. Parental attitudes toward work. *Youth Society* 1990; **22**:160.
26. Dunn KA, Runyan CW, Cohen LR, Schulman D. Teens at work: a statewide study of jobs, hazards and injuries. *J Adolesc Health* 1998; **22**:19–25.
27. Gallo N. How the work ethic works against teens. *Family Circle* 1997; Feb:72–95.
28. Skorikov VB, Vondracek PW. Career development in the commonwealth of independent states. *Career Dev Q* 1993; **41**:314–29.
29. Vondracek FW, Lerner RM, Scholenberg SE. *Career Development: A Life Span Approach*. Erlbaum: Hillsdale, NJ, 1986.

30. Stern D, Nakata Y. Characteristics of high school students paid jobs and employment experience after graduation. In: *Adolescents and Work, Influences of Social Structure, Labor Markets and Culture* (Stern D, Eichorn P, eds). Erlbaum: Hillsdale, NJ, 189–233.

31. Skorikov VB, Vondracek FW. Longitudinal relationships between part-time work and career development in adolescents. *Career Dev Q* 1997; **45**:221–35.

32. White PH, Gussek DG, Fisher B. Career maturity in adolescents with chronic illnesses. *J Adolesc Health Care* 1990; **11**:372.

33. Hallum A. Disability and the transition to adulthood: issues for the disabled child, the family and the pediatrician. *Curr Probl Pediatr* 1995; **25**:12–50.

34. Super DE. Assessment in career guidance: toward truly developmental counseling. *Personnel Guidance J* 1983; **61**:555–62.

35. Conte LE. Vocational development theories and the disabled person: oversight or deliberate omission? *Rehab Counselor Bull* 1983; **26**:316–28.

36. Allen GH. Aspirational expectations of physically impaired high school seniors. *Personnel Guidance J* 1967; **46**:59–62.

37. Brolin DE. *Vocation Preparation of Retarded Citizens.* Charles E. Merril: Columbus, OH, 1976.

38. Gill C. *Vocational Development.* Institute of Disability Research, Rehabilitation and Training Research Center: Chicago, IL, 1996.

39. Osipow SH. Vocational development problems of the handicapped. In: *Contemporary Vocational Rehabilitation* (Rusalen H, Malikin O, eds). New York University Press: New York, 49–61.

40. Curnow TC. Vocational development of persons with a disability. *Career Dev Q* 1989; **37**:269–78.

41. Neff WF. *Work and Human Behavior.* Alcline: Chicago, 1968.

42. Werner EE. High risk children in young adulthood: a longitudinal study from birth to 32 years. *Am J Orthopsychiatry* 1989; **59**:72–81.

43. Garmezy N. Research in children's adaptation to negative life events and stressed environments. *Pediatr Ann* 1991; **20**:459–66.

44. Patterson J, Blum RJ. Risk and resilience among children and youth with disabilities. *Arch Pediatr Adolesc Med* 1996; **150**:692–8.

45. Levinson EM. Vocational assessment and programming of students with handicaps: a need for school counselor involvement. *School Counselor* 1987; **35**:6–8.

46. Omizo SA, Omizo MM. Career and vocational assessment, information for proper planning and counseling for students with disabilities. *School Counselor* 1992; **40**:32–9.

47. Duff CM, Watanabe KN. Health assessment in rheumatic diseases of childhood. *Curr Opinion Rheumatol* 1997; **9**:440–7.

48. Baildam EM, Holt PJL, Conway SC, Morton MJS. The association between physical function and psychological problems in children with juvenile chronic arthritis. *Br Med J* 1995; **34**:470–7.

49. Usdane WM. Vocational planning for the handicapped child. In: *The Child with Disability Illness: Principles of Rehab* (Usdane WM, ed). 569–78.

50. Brunner J. Continuity of learning. *Saturday Review* 1973; **Mar**:21–23.

51. *Training Guide for Vocational Rehabilitation, SRS Demonstration Project, RD-1525.* Jewish Employment and Vocational Service, St Louis, MO, 1966.

52. Bennett ME. *Guidance in Groups.* McGraw Hill: New York, 1955.

53. Lifton WM. *Working in Groups.* Wiley: New York, 1961.

54. Roessler RT. Work, disability and the future: promoting employment for people with disabilities. *J Counseling Dev* 1987; **66**:188–9.

55. Edgerton AH. *Report: National Guidance Evaluation Studies.* University of Wisconsin: Madison, WI, 1959.

56. Brolin DE, Gysbers NC. Career education for students with disabilities. *J Counseling Dev* 1989; **68**:155–60.

57. Edelman A, Schyler V, White P. *Maximizing Success for Young Adults with Chronic Health-Related Illnesses: Transition Planning for Education after High School.* HEATH Resource Center, American Council on Education: Washington, DC, 1998.

58. *Transition Time Line Strategies in Career Focus.* Adolescent Employment Readiness Center: Washington, DC, 1995; vol 6, no. 2:1–2.

59. Blum RW, Okinow NA. *Teenagers at Risk: A National Perspective of State Level Services for Adolescents with Chronic Illnesses or Disabilities.* National Center for Youth with Disabilities, University of Minnesota: Minneapolis, MN, 1993.

60. Izzo MV. Career development of disabled youth: the parent's role. *J Career Dev* 1987; **13**:47–55.

61. White PH. Future expectations: adolescents with rheumatic disease and their transition into adulthood. *Br J Rheumatol* 1996; **35**:80–3.

62. *Transition Planning for the Twenty-first Century: A*

Call to Action. National Center for Youth with Disabilities: Minneapolis, MN, 1995:14.

63. Benz M, Yovanoff, Dorea B. School to work components that predict post school success for students with and without disabilities. *Exceptional Children* 1997; **63**:151–67.

64. Enright M, Conyers L, Szymanski E. Career and career-related educational concerns of college students with disabilities. *J Counseling Dev* 1996; **75**:103–14.

65. White PH. Success on the road to adulthood: issues and hurdles for adolescents with disabili-

ties. *Rheum Clin North Am* 1997; **23**:697–707.

66. White PH, Spurrier K. You are not alone: advocacy for children and young adults with rheumatic diseases. *Pediatr Clin North Am* 1995; **42**:1299–309.

67. *Including Students with Disabilities in School to Work Opportunities.* Council of the Chief State School Officers: Washington, DC, 1995.

68. *Transition Summary.* National Information Center for Children and Youth with Disabilities. Washington DC, vol 3, No. 1, March 1993.

69. *Decision Making for Teenagers with Arthritis.* Arthritis Foundation: Atlanta, GA, 1996.

15

Adolescent rheumatic disease and sexuality

David M Siegel and John Baum

INTRODUCTION

While human sexual development is a life-long process commencing in utero and encompassing the physical and psychological, many aspects of the development of adult sexuality become accentuated during adolescence. Representing a central component of normal growth, sexuality should be addressed in the overall health care of adolescents, including those with rheumatological and other chronic diseases. This chapter begins with a description of the psychosocial transitions that take place during adolescence leading toward the establishment of mature sexuality, followed by a discussion of how chronic illness can affect the normal evolution of adolescent sexuality. The specific impact of rheumatological illness on sexuality and sexual function is then presented, including practical considerations for working with these teenagers and their families. The interactions between rheumatological disease and the biological events of puberty are discussed in Chapter 16.

ADOLESCENT SEXUALITY

During childhood, young boys and girls undergo similar sexual exploration through fantasy, play and masturbation as they become aware of their bodies and gender differences.[1,2] However, in most societies it is during adolescence that the sexual behaviours of males and females begin to differentiate. This is influenced by both the neuroendocrine changes of puberty and the socio-cultural context in which the individual resides. In order to understand the impact of adolescent rheumatic disease (and other chronic illness) on sexuality it is first necessary to recognize what is considered normal development for teenagers.[1,3,4]

Adolescence is divided into three stages – early, middle and late – with the approximate chronological boundaries being 11–15 years, 15–17 years, and 17 years to early 20s, respectively. Significant developmental tasks challenge young people at each of these stages leading toward adulthood.[5] Pre-eminent in this process is a consolidation of identity, including a capacity for intimacy that is made up, in part, by sexuality. For early adolescents, puberty arises with concomitant body changes representing concrete manifestations of the physical dimension of sexuality. These young people are powerfully preoccupied with both the adequacy and attractiveness of these changes. Those who mature early and late may experience additional distress as their bodies seem to differ from their contemporaries. At the same time, the social skills necessary for successful peer interaction begin to develop, and undergo repeated practice and rehearsal with family and friends, in school and in other group settings. Toward the conclusion of middle adolescence most young people experience a slowing and completion of the bodily transformations, whereas a more sophisticated repertoire of social and cognitive abilities continue to be established. It is during this period that overt sexual activity becomes increasingly incorporated into the individual's behaviour such that, in the USA, by age 19 years,

Table 15.1   Nine processes of sexual unfolding*
1. Evolving sense of the body that is gender specific and free of body-image distortion
2. Overcome guilt, shame, fear and childhood inhibitions associated with sexual thoughts and behaviour
3. Loosening of emotional ties to parent and family
4. Learning to recognize what is erotically pleasing and displeasing and being able to communicate this to a partner
5. Resolution of sexual orientation
6. Absence of sexual dysfunction or compulsion
7. Awareness of being a sexual person and the place and value of sex in one's life, including the option of celibacy
8. Becoming responsible regarding sexuality (e.g. contraception, barriers, not using sex as a means of exploitation)
9. Increasing ability to experience eroticism as one aspect of intimacy with another person

*Adapted from Sarrel and Sarrel.[8]

over half will have experienced sexual intercourse. There is, in fact, a significant range of sexual experience as a function of age, gender, personality and socio-cultural background.[6,7]

A number of frameworks have been proposed as templates for the goals of adolescent psychosocial development that facilitate healthy adult sexuality. Sarrel and Sarrel[8] label this process 'sexual unfolding', and they have identified nine characteristics and tasks that culminate in a fully evolved, personally incorporated and gratifying adult sexuality (Table 15.1). Their observations derive from clinical work involving thousands of middle and upper middle class, American college students and must therefore be interpreted in that context. However, we feel that the general principles they have articulated provide a useful paradigm with which to view the psychology of sexuality, albeit from a Western, industrialized socio-cultural perspective. It is also important to note that mastery of each of these points is not expected or necessarily predominant, but rather a gradual (and lifelong) striving for incorporation of these attributes into one's behaviour and relationships. Obviously, the full accomplishment of these goals does not occur during adolescence, but personal development and experiences during the second decade of life lay the groundwork for one's eventual sexual adaptation and adjustment, be it heterosexual, homosexual or bisexual.

ADOLESCENT CHRONIC ILLNESS AND SEXUALITY

The presence of chronic illness during adolescence can adversely affect evolving sexuality through a variety of mechanisms.[1,3,4,9–11] Confirmation of one's maleness or femaleness is centrally invested in the expected physical attributes that identify gender. The development of these characteristics during puberty is carefully monitored by the body-preoccupied early and middle adolescent as he or she searches for signs of those changes observed or reported by peers. The chronically ill adolescent is often faced with a significant delay in growth and appearance of secondary sex characteristics, creating fear, uncertainty and decreased self-esteem. Growth delay and suppression is a striking manifestation of juvenile arthritis. In the precorticosteroid therapy era, one-third of those with systemic-onset disease experienced significant restriction of growth. Polyarticular disease also resulted in growth limitation, although not to the same extent.[12] Not only is there concern about whether adult features will ever become manifest, but attractiveness and appeal are also questioned. These young people can be resentful and distressed about their slowed (or absent) development, but they may also be convinced that peers will judge them negatively as a consequence. The overwhelming importance placed by children in early and middle adolescence on peer perception and acceptance explains the immediacy of this fear. As teenagers aspire to accept themselves, they typically display intolerance for those who appear and/or act differently. Thus, peer groups or cliques emerge, organized around patterns of speech, dress, attitude, etc. Adolescents with chronic illness find themselves readily excluded from this social organization, at least in part because of their visible differences, if not also due to their actual physical limitations.

Impairments and abnormalities suffered as a result of chronic illness affect the individual, not only among their peers, but at home as well. While adolescence is a time during which increased autonomy and independence are appropriate goals, chronic illness can present serious obstacles to their attainment. Initial diagnosis and management of diseases in adolescents is usually undertaken by parent(s). It is the adults (or adult) in the home who are expected to understand and take primary responsibility for the medical, psychosocial and therapeutic dimensions of the illness while including the adolescent patient in the informational and decision-making processes. Soon, however, the teenager is faced with the developmental and logistic need to take on increasing self-care, a transition that can conflict with parental resistance to disrupting the status quo. Furthermore, depending on the magnitude of care-taking requirements, it may not be entirely possible for the patient to adequately address the bulk of the adolescent's needs.

These impediments to individual development, independence and separation from family bear directly on sexuality. As cited by Sarrel and Sarrel,[8] part of the maturation process necessary for the establishment of adult intimacy and sexuality includes a loosening of the primary bonds to family in order to make way for the next phase of relationships. While not an easy transition for any individual, the forced dependency imposed by chronic disease renders this step a particular challenge for the handicapped or disabled teenager. The obvious difficulty in accomplishing this shift from family bonding

further exacerbates the potential problem regarding peer acceptance. That is, as the adolescent patient needs to explore ways of expressing and learning about his or her sexuality through interactions with others, these potential partners may be reluctant to pair with one who is unable to distance from parent(s). Furthermore, just being exposed to a peer who cannot begin to separate from his or her family can be threatening and create anxiety in the healthy adolescent. In addition to holding on to primary care-taking for their ageing son or daughter, for fear that he or she will otherwise lack for proper attention, parents confronted with their child's persistent physical immaturity (and dependence) are left without the usual visual and behavioural cues prodding them to recognize the coming of late adolescence and adulthood. This is particularly salient for sexuality when one considers the reluctance with which parents address the topic of sexuality even with their healthy children.[2] Thus, the chronically ill adolescent is dually burdened by problems in moving away from his or her concerned and tenacious family of origin, as well as impaired in making steps toward the progressively more autonomous, but reluctantly accepting or inviting, peer group.

Despite the intimidating potential for dysfunction among chronically ill teenagers, there are some reassuring data. In a comparison of patients with oncological, cardiac, diabetic or rheumatological disease, as well as cystic fibrosis to healthy controls, overall measures of self-esteem and trait anxiety were similar.[13,14] Conversely, in a report of 270 chronically ill children (of whom 24 (9%) had juvenile arthritis) maternal responses to a behaviour checklist indicated higher than normed references for behavioural and social competence problems. In the specific scale of 'externalizing behaviour problems', however, children with arthritis scored lower than the other disease groups (diabetes, spina bifida, haemophilia, chronic obesity and cerebral palsy).[15]

In a study of 363 children and young adults, all with juvenile arthritis, average scores on measures of self-concept revealed no differences with a normative sample of Australian children.

When analysed separately, high-school students who scored lower on the self-concept scale were, in fact, more socially isolated, including fewer close friends and less dating. There was also a direct relationship between increased disease severity and decreased psycho-social functioning and adjustment.[16] For all these young people, during periods of illness exacerbation and increased disability one can anticipate greater than normal levels of anxiety, depression and dysfunction. Interestingly, in one study children with juvenile arthritis whose disability was less visually apparent reported greater psycho-social disruption than those with more noticeable impairment.[17] Nevertheless, chronically ill adolescents do become sexually active, some (with milder impairments) at rates comparable to healthy teenagers.[18]

Rheumatic disease and sexuality

Amidst these generic issues of adolescent chronic disease and sexuality there are specific considerations for those with rheumatic disease. The literature on sexuality in adults with rheumatic disease is not voluminous, and what has been reported about adolescents (in both books and journals) is sparse and primarily inclusive only of patients with juvenile arthritis. Below, we describe what we recovered from the literature, both studies that deal with adolescents as well as those that address sexuality in adult rheumatic disease populations. Findings from the latter, we believe, have applicability to adolescents. Wilkinson[19] reported on a population of 27 adolescents with severe juvenile arthritis who were inpatients. He found 70% to be significantly socially isolated, and anxieties about lack of sexual contact, as a consequence of the isolation, were raised.

In a study of 58 individuals with juvenile arthritis, participants were asked at a mean of 14.5 years after disease onset about marital status, dating, masturbation, orgasm, coitus and limitation of coitus by pain, position or fatigue.[20,21] The study sample included 21 men and 37 women with an age range at follow-up of 19–37 years. However, age distribution was skewed toward late adolescents and young adults; 50 out of 58 patients were less than 28 years old, and 17 subjects were aged 19 or 20 years. Thus, the observations appear to be characteristic of the adolescent experience. Fifty-two of the subjects were interviewed by a gynaecologist experienced in sexual counselling, lending credence to the information gathered. When asked about frequency of coitus, marital status was a powerful determinant with all of those who were married reporting regular coitus, but only 17 out of 31 of those unmarried giving the same response. The authors stratified the group by functional class (I to IV) and found that those with greater disability (III and IV) had a lower prevalence of 'regular coitus' than did those with milder impairment (I and II). Interestingly, achievement of orgasm among the women did not differ by disease severity (9/23 with mild, 4/10 with severe disease). Limitation of coital activity due to pain, position or fatigue was a factor for all patients with functional class III or IV, and 16 out of 28 of those who were in class I or II. Thirty-eight per cent of the group desired sexual counselling. The authors, as would be expected, concluded that juvenile arthritis has an impact on sexual activity, although some of the most severely affected (two individuals confined to wheelchairs) nevertheless reported regular coitus. Intercourse does not make up the totality of sexuality, but these data certainly provide some insight into the coital dimension of sexuality for patients with juvenile arthritis.

Consistently high prevalences of loss of sexual interest and decrease in sexual desire have been reported.[22,23] Elst et al[24] utilized a standardized questionnaire to compare sexual motivation and coital position preference among adults with rheumatoid arthritis ($n = 122$) to those with ankylosing spondylitis ($n = 66$). The mean ages of the two groups were early to mid-40s. Those with ankylosing spondylitis displayed a normal tendency to want to engage in sexual interaction, whereas those with rheumatoid arthritis were abnormally averse to sexual interaction. High joint-activity indices correlated with low sexual motivation, and rheumatoid arthritis patients scored lower on length of foreplay and sexual enjoyment and were more likely to express need for help and advice regarding coital positioning. Although it is a generalization to apply these observations to teenagers, they are at risk for the same array of sexual dysfunction.

Blake et al[25] assembled an appropriate, concurrent control group (*n* = 130) to compare to 169 patients (mean age 57 years) diagnosed with rheumatoid arthritis, osteoarthritis or ankylosing spondylitis. More similarities than differences were observed. Subjects were asked about the quality of their current sexual adjustment: 36% of patients and 39% of controls indicated that they were not satisfied, whereas 35% and 33%, respectively, were satisfied. When asked to compare past (pre-arthritis for patients) and present status, 42% of controls but 58% of those with arthritis described a decrease in sexual satisfaction over time, and loss of sexual pleasure was reported by 21% of controls and 38% of patients. These findings did not differ based on marital status either within or between groups. Thus, although age was clearly a factor, living with arthritis makes an additional negative contribution.

Symptoms and concerns that can negatively impact on sexual function for patients with arthritis were also recorded. Joint pain, joint stiffness and fatigue were ranked highest by patients, although controls also reported fatigue as a problem. Loss of libido and loss of lubrication were issues identified by both groups, and it is notable that feeling unattractive was of no greater concern for patients than for controls. Finally, being receptive to sexual counselling regarding guidance on changes in coital position, mutual masturbation, masturbation and (of least interest) oral sex was comparable in both groups (independent of level of sexual satisfaction) and ranged from one-fifth to one-third of the population.

The relationship between sexual satisfaction and functional disability was examined in a mailed questionnaire comparison of 113 married couples of whom one spouse had a rheumatic disease and 37 healthy couples.[26] Patients and controls reported similar overall levels of dissatisfaction, women were more sexually dissatisfied than men, and a positive correlation between higher level of disability and increased sexual dissatisfaction was found.

These, and other, studies provide evidence that sexual function and sexuality are important in the lives of patients with rheumatic disease. Certainly more has been described about adult populations, but adolescents soon become adults (a transition with significant health-care implications[27]) and will have similar outcomes, complicated by the additional complexity of chronic illness during early development (as discussed previously). It is reasonable to conclude from available research that the presence of arthritis, particularly when severe, can interfere significantly with sexual satisfaction, although some individuals cope quite well with their disability.

This area is sufficiently important that assessment of sexual function in patients with rheumatic disease deserves a prominent place on the list of other physical and psychological parameters. A systematic review of the literature to identify valid, reliable and generalizable instruments that assess sexual function of patients with specific rheumatic diseases was recently undertaken.[28] Utilizing a comprehensive yet rigorous selection procedure, only 10 suitable articles were identified for critical appraisal. They addressed sexual function among those with systemic lupus erythematosus (three studies), rheumatoid arthritis (two studies), osteoarthritis (one study), chronic arthritis (three studies), and one paper compared those with systemic sclerosis, systemic lupus erythematosus and rheumatoid arthritis. None of these studies addressed the adolescent population and no article satisfied the quality criteria, either because the study did not describe important issues of the instrument construction or because the properties (i.e. reliability, validity, responsiveness) of the instrument used were not tested'.[28] The authors of this meta-analysis concluded that adequate questionnaire and scale development is urgently needed to evaluate sexual function in these patients.

Practical points regarding care

Given the developmental issues and literature that have been presented, the clinician participating in the care of adolescents with rheumatic disease can incorporate numerous strategies to forge a healthy compromise between the normal needs of the patient and the demands of the chronic illness.[9–11] To begin, one cannot address sexuality without introducing the subject during the patient encounter. Asking questions and soliciting information about sexuality should ideally begin just prior to early adolescence, in anticipation of puberty onset. For those with rheumatic illness, puberty onset can be delayed due to disease activity and/or medication (e.g. corticosteroids), but as 11 and 12 year olds begin to see their peers enter puberty, they will start to consider the changes in store for themselves and need the opportunity to talk about their own maturation. This is an opportunity for the paediatric rheumatologist to provide accurate information to the patient and family regarding the normal physical and psychological progression the early teenager is about to go through. In addition, deviations from the usual (as consequences of the disease) can be explained. This is also an important time for the clinician to start offering the adolescent private, one-to-one time during the visit. While general discussions about puberty can certainly take place with the patient and parent(s) together, the more specific conversation about sexuality should include time apart from other family members. This allows the teenager to speak confidentially and is also more likely to result in accurate and complete information for the provider.

Interviewing the adolescent is different from interacting with younger children or adults. Assurances of confidentiality and a non-judgmental approach are essential in soliciting sexuality related information.[29] Some patients are reluctant to bring up the topic, but almost certainly have questions and concerns to express. Reflecting on the larger peer group as an opening question is often effective with these teenagers. For example: 'Many people your age are starting to go through puberty with pubic hair around the penis or vagina, or having their period, or changes in their voice or breasts, or acne, or other new body differences. Have any of your friends been talking about that? Have you noticed changes in yourself? Are you wondering when these changes might start for you?' By bringing up this discussion in early adolescence, not only is the teenager benefited, but the family (and provider) is reminded that, even in the absence of growth and the appearance of secondary sexual characteristics, the patient is nevertheless entering a period of developmental transition and should be dealt with accordingly.

As middle adolescence is reached, further discussion should take place around an evolving capacity for intimacy and specifically regarding sexuality. It is important at this point to remain non-judgmental, especially concerning sexual orientation. It is common for physicians unwittingly to discourage rapport with gay adolescents by stereotyping their patient's partner curiosity as heterosexual. That is, asking boys only about girlfriends and girls only about boyfriends. While early dating experiences for gay adults are reported as having been heterosexual,[29] some middle and late adolescents are aware of their sexual orientation and are put off and/or alienated by heterosexual assumptions.

Problems in achieving autonomy can become more acute for the 15–17 year old with a rheumatic (or other chronic) disease, particularly if overt milestones such as obtaining a driver's license[30] or securing a part-time job are prevented or delayed by the illness. Similarly, the limitations imposed on sexual experimentation by the chronic disease deserve attention. An inability to orchestrate one's own dating activities because of disability presents an opportunity for the patient, physician and family to work out ways to allow this important psychosocial step to take place. In addition to encouraging young people to assume increasing responsibility for the management of their rheumatic disease, older adolescents should be pushed to consider their sexuality in a responsible way. Specifically, they need to think about the implications of becoming sexually active and whether the timing is appropriate for either them or their partner. If they have decided to engage in sexual intercourse then considerations of contraception (discussed in detail in Chapter 16), sexually transmitted diseases, and mechanical adjustments to allow for sexual activity must be taken into account. Some of these issues vary depending on the disease, as described below.

For adolescents and young adults with arthritis, the quantity and quality of joint involvement requires some attention regarding sexuality. Coital positioning can be very important in determining whether intercourse is painful for one or both partners, let alone pleasurable. For example, in a young woman with hip disease and limitations of abduction and rotation, the traditional heterosexual, frontal ('missionary') position may be quite uncomfortable, if not impossible.[31] Involvement of the hands and wrist can interfere with stroking, caressing and masturbation (mutual or self), which is an issue for both those who are abstinent and those who have decided to become sexually active.[32] The approach to these limitations involves both awareness and communication of preferences and capabilities, as well as education about adaptive techniques. Adolescents (and many adults) find it very difficult to express needs and choices about sexuality to their partner, and thus it is helpful for the physician or nurse to bring up the subject and support open communication, as well as the methodology to achieve sexual satisfaction.[33]

In addition to talking with one's partner about what works best for sexual gratification, manipulation of medication and timing of intercourse can also facilitate more pleasurable physical intimacy. Knowing that fatigue is a significant factor in decreased sexual satisfaction and enjoyment, the patient with a rheumatic disease may need to plan for sex and carefully pace the balance of the day's activities. Furthermore, the pain and stiffness associated with arthritis can be temporarily addressed through 'pretreatment' with heat, range of motion and anti-inflammatory and analgesic medication prior to physical closeness, stimulation and intercourse. The application of heat and gentle range-of-motion exercises can even become part of initial foreplay for the more mature, and less self-conscious older adolescent or young adult. Obviously, what is recommended

above precludes spontaneous, unplanned sexual activity, which is the typical approach of teenagers. The clinician must be aware of this and acknowledge to the patient that this may feel like yet another way in which the disease has complicated the emergence of their sexuality. On the other hand, without such strategies, sexual activity, including masturbation, may remain unpleasant, painful and frustrating.

Other rheumatic disease manifestations can also adversely affect sexuality (Table 15.2). Oral mucous membrane lesions in patients with systemic lupus erythematosus can make kissing and/or oral–genital contact painful. Patient's

Table 15.2 Rheumatic diseases and interference with sexual function

Disease	Sexuality related impairment
Juvenile arthritis	Joint limitation of motion: – hips (genital intercourse) – hands and wrists (stroking, caressing, masturbation, hygiene)
Systemic lupus erythematosus	Mucous membrane lesions
Reiter's syndrome	Urethritis, cervicitis, balanitis
Behçet's syndrome	Genital ulcers, balanitis
Sjögren's syndrome	Xerostomia, atrophic vaginitis
All diseases	Pain Stiffness Fatigue Depression Feeling unattractive Medication side-effects

with Reiter's syndrome who have urethritis, cervicitis or balanitis can find genital contact uncomfortable as can those with the ulcerative genital lesions and balanitis of Behçet's disease. Sjögren's syndrome (rare in adolescents) complicated by xerostomia and atrophic vaginitis can result in pain with either oral or genital contact. The use of condoms and lubricants can help to alleviate some of the above problems.[34]

As described, the judicious use of pain-reducing medication can be useful in facilitating pleasurable sexual activity, but drugs can also interfere. Corticosteroids may cause difficulty in attaining penile erection, but when discontinued this problem should resolve. Numerous antihypertensive agents, often necessary in treating patients with renal disease, can also cause impotence, ejaculatory abnormalities and loss of libido. Although uncommonly necessary in the management of rheumatic-disease-related pain, narcotic analgesics might contribute to fatigue, impotence and loss of libido. Non-steroidal anti-inflammatory drugs are not known to interfere with sexual desire or function. Hair loss secondary to immunosuppressive drugs (e.g. cyclophosphamide) might result in feelings of unattractiveness, but sexual function is not directly affected. These cytotoxic therapies can also cause mouth and genital ulcers, as can gold compounds. Medication considerations are also relevant in choosing a method of contraception (see Chapter 16). Adolescents with antiphospholipid antibodies (such as systemic lupus erythematosus or in the antiphospholipid antibody syndrome) are at increased risk for thromboembolic events and should therefore not be given oral contraceptive preparations. General principles of 'safer sex' apply to everyone, including those with rheumatic disease, especially in the setting of oral and/or genital ulcers that can increase the efficiency of infection transmission (i.e. gonorrhoea, chlamydia, syphilis, human papillomavirus, and human immunodeficiency virus (HIV)).

Thus there are developmental, psychological and physical aspects to sexuality in adolescents with rheumatic disease. Unlike adults who develop a rheumatic illness after having already established their sexual attitudes, expectations and behaviours, adolescents do not have a premorbid sexual status with which to compare. As an integral part of comprehensive care of the teenage patient sexuality must be included. Individuals may respond differently to various members of the health-care team, and while the paediatric rheumatologist must address these issues, some adolescents might be more comfortable with other professionals. This can be related to a desire to discuss sexuality with a professional of the same gender, or other aspects of what allows the patient to feel most comfortable and relaxed. Nurses, occupational and physical therapists, social workers, psychologists and physicians are all potential resources for the adolescent.[35] It is incumbent on those caring for these patients and their families to assess sexuality in the appropriate developmental context and provide guidance and intervention as young people move through adolescence and into adulthood. Furthermore, it is clear from our search of the literature, that adequate investigation into the area of sexuality in adolescents with rheumatic disease is sorely lacking (despite the presence of articles discussing many other psychosocial issues in these patients). Research on this topic should therefore be made a priority by those studying and participating in the care of these young people.

REFERENCES

1. Perrin EC, Gerrity PS. Development of children with a chronic illness. *Pediatr Clin North Am* 1984; **31**:19–31.
2. Zuengler KL, Neubeck G. Sexuality: developing togetherness. In: *Stress and the Family* (McCubben H, ed). Bruner/Mazel: New York, 1983:41–53.
3. McAnarney ER. Social maturation. A challenge for handicapped and chronically ill adolescents. *J Adolesc Health Care* 1985; **6**:90–101.
4. Strax TE. Psychological problems of disabled adolescents and young adults. *Pediatr Ann* 1988; **17**:756–61.

5. Hamberg BA. Psychosocial development. In: *Comprehensive Adolescent Health Care* (Friedman SB, Fisher MM, Schonberg SK, Alderman EM, eds). Mosby: St Louis, MI, 1998:38–49.

6. Rodgers JL. Development of sexual behavior. In: *Comprehensive Adolescent Health Care* (Friedman SB, Fisher MM, Schonberg SK, Alderman EM, eds). Mosby: St Louis, MI, 1998:49–54.

7. Netting NS. Sexuality in youth culture: identity and change. *Adolescence* 1992; **27**:961–76.

8. Sarrel LJ, Sarrel PM. Sexual unfolding. *J Adolesc Health Care* 1981; **2**:93–9.

9. Selekman J, McIlvain-Simpson G. Sex and sexuality for the adolescent with a chronic condition. *Pediatr Nursing* 1991; **17**:535–8.

10. Woodhead JC, Murph JR. Influence of chronic illness and disability on adolescent sexual development. *Semin Adolesc Med* 1985; **1**:171–6.

11. Frauman AC, Sypert NS. Sexuality in adolescents with chronic illness. *Mat Child Nursing* 1979; **4**:371–5.

12. Stoeber E. Corticosteroid treatment of juvenile chronic polyarthritis over 22 years. *Eur J Pediatr* 1976; **121**:141–7.

13. Kellerman J, Zeltzer L, Ellenberg L et al. Psychological effects of illness in adolescence. I. Anxiety, self-esteem, and perception of control. *J Pediatr* 1980; **97**:126–31.

14. Zeltzer L, Kellerman J, Ellenberg L, Dash J, Rigler D. Psychological effects of illness in adolescence. II. Impact of illness in adolescents – crucial issues and coping styles. *J Pediatr* 1980; **97**:132–8.

15. Wallander JL, Varni JW, Babani L et al. Children with chronic physical disorders: maternal reports of their psychological adjustment. *J Pediatr Psychol* 1988; **13**:197–212.

16. Ungerer JA, Horgan B, Chaitow J et al. Psychosocial functioning in children and young adults with juvenile arthritis. *Pediatrics* 1988; **81**:195–202.

17. McAnarney ER, Pless IB, Satterwhite B et al. Psychological problems of children with chronic juvenile arthritis. *Pediatrics* 1974; **53**:523–8.

18. Choquet M, Fediaevsky LDP, Manfredi R. Sexual behavior among adolescents reporting chronic conditions: a French national survey. *J Adolesc Health* 1997; **20**:62–7.

19. Wilkinson VA. Juvenile chronic arthritis in adolescence: facing the reality. *Intl Rehab Med* 1981; **3**:11–17.

20. Hill RH, Herstein A, Walters K. Juvenile rheumatoid arthritis: follow-up into adulthood – medical, sexual and social status. *Can Med Assoc J* 1976; **114**:790–6.

21. Herstein A, Hill RH, Walters K. Adult sexuality and juvenile rheumatoid arthritis. *J Rheumatol* 1977; **4**:35–9.

22. Ferguson K, Figley B. Sexuality and rheumatic disease: a prospective study. *Sexuality Disability* 1979; **2**:130–8.

23. Yoshino S, Uchida S. Sexual problems of women with rheumatoid arthritis. *Arch Phys Med Rehabil* 1981; **62**:122–3.

24. Elst P, Sybesma T, van der Stadt RJ, Prins APA, Muller WH, den Butter A. Sexual problems in rheumatoid arthritis and ankylosing spondylitis. *Arthritis Rheum* 1984; **27**:217–20.

25. Blake DJ, Maisiak R, Alarcon GS, Holley HL, Brown S. Sexual quality-of-life of patients with arthritis compared to arthritis-free controls. *J Rheumatol* 1987; **14**:570–6.

26. Majerovitz SD, Revenson TA. Sexuality and rheumatoid disease: the significance of gender. *Arthritis Care Res* 1994; **7**:29–34.

27. Rettig P, Athreya BH. Adolescents with chronic disease: transition to adult care. *Arthritis Care Res* 1991; **4**:174–80.

28. Quaresma MR, Goldsmith CH, Lamont J, Ferraz MB. Assessment of sexual function in patients with rheumatic disorders: a critical appraisal. *J Rheumatol* 1997; **24**:1673–6.

29. Deisher R, Remafedi G. Adolescent sexuality. In: *Adolescent Medicine* (Hofmann A, Greydanus D, eds). Prentice Hall: Englewood Cliffs, NJ, 1989:337–46.

30. Orr DP, Weller SC, Satterwhite B et al. Psychosocial implications of chronic illness in adolescence. *J Pediatr* 1984; **104**:152–7.

31. Buckwalter KC, Wernimont T, Buckwalter JA. Musculoskeletal conditions and sexuality (part II). *Sexuality Disability* 1982; **5**:195–207.

32. Malek CJ, Brower SA. Rheumatoid arthritis: how does it influence sexuality? *Rehab Nursing* 1984; **Nov–Dec**:26–8.

33. Hamilton A, Hawkins C. Sex and arthritis. In: *Reports on Rheumatic Diseases* (Hawkins C, Currey HLF, eds). The Arthritis and Rheumatism Council for Research: London, 1977:144–7.

34. Lim PAC. Sexuality in patients with musculoskeletal diseases. *Phys Med Rehab* 1995; **9**:401–15.

35. Conine TA, Quastel LN. Occupational therapists' roles and attitudes toward sexual habilitation of chronically ill and disabled children. *Can J Occup Ther* 1983; **50**:81–6.

16

Interactions of puberty with rheumatic diseases, contraception and gynaecological issues

Barbara E Ostrov and Richard L Levine

INTRODUCTION

Puberty is a time of profound change for any adolescent, especially for the teenager with a chronic disease. The usual adolescent issues, which include physical development, psychosocial changes and planning for the future, are no different for teenagers with chronic illness. However, physical changes of puberty may be delayed or altered by the disease or its treatment, and emotional development may also be hindered by the illness. Gynaecological evaluation may be indicated due to delayed puberty and potential effects of disease or medication. Future planning may be ill considered by the family and patient because of perceptions about the long-term effects of the child's illness.

In this chapter we review aspects of normal pubertal development and the interaction of rheumatic and autoimmune diseases with these processes. These rheumatic diseases are described in detail in Chapters 5–10. Unique gynaecological issues in this population are also addressed. In many instances, reference is made to other chronic illnesses that affect adults and adolescents, as few data exist that specifically address the effects of rheumatic diseases alone.

THE BIOLOGY OF PUBERTY

Endocrinological and physical aspects of puberty

Puberty is not a separate biological event, but represents a transitional period between the juvenile state and the adult state. As reviewed by Neinstein,[1] the hypothalamic–pituitary–gonadal (HPG) system starts functioning during fetal life. Gonadotropin-releasing hormone (GnRH), luteinizing hormone (LH), follicle-stimulating hormone (FSH) and the appropriate sex steroids are detectable by 10 weeks of gestation and rise between 10 and 20 weeks. During fetal life the hypothalamus is imprinted to that of a male or female centre. The male centre secretes hormones in a tonic pattern, and the female centre demonstrates a tonic and cyclic pattern of hormone secretion. Gonadotropins decrease after week 20 due to the maturation of the central nervous system and an increase in hypothalamic sensitivity. After the fall in placental sex steroids levels that occurs after birth, the concentrations of serum gonadotropins rise to midpubertal levels. Testosterone in males and oestradiol in females also rise. This may result in precocious breast development (thelarche) or premature development of pubic and axillary hair (adrenarche). However, by 9–12 months of age in males and 2 years in females, the gonadotropins and gonadal steroids fall to prepubertal levels. This involves a strong negative feedback control of FSH and LH secretion, which is highly sensitive to low levels of sex steroids (a low set point).[2]

The exact trigger for the onset of puberty is unknown, although a number of theories have been investigated.[1,3] At puberty, there is a decrease in the sensitivity of the hypothalamus and pituitary to sex steroids so that GnRH and the gonadotropins begin to rise.[1–3] In other words, the set point for negative feedback control increases. This regulatory change leads to an increase in the sex steroids, an increase in growth and the development of secondary sexual characteristics. In females a positive feedback system develops later in puberty, in which critical levels of oestrogen trigger a large release of GnRH stimulating the LH surge and leading to ovulation.[1,2] Other hormones play a role in pubertal development, including growth hormone, mediated by insulin-like growth factor 1 (IGF-1), thyroid hormone and adrenal steroids.[3]

The extent and rapidity of pubertal development can vary markedly from person to person, in both males and females.[4] However, the sequence of pubertal development follows a well-established sequence and major variations are uncommon.[4] The somatic pubertal stages have been well described by Tanner.[5] For males puberty begins with testicular development, followed within 6 months by the development of pubic hair. Phallic enlargement occurs 12–18 months after testicular development, and the peak height velocity typically occurs 2–2.5 years after testicular development. It is important to note that the peak height velocity is a later development in males. The sequence for females usually begins with the appearance of the breast bud and then linear growth acceleration. Sixteen per cent of girls develop some pubic hair prior to breast enlargement. The peak height velocity is an earlier development in females, usually in Tanner stage 3. Menarche is a later event, about 2 years after the breast bud, usually in Tanner breast and pubic hair stage 4, when linear growth is declining. Marked discordance between the stages of breast and pubic hair development is unusual and may indicate organic pathology.[4] The mean age of menarche in the USA (currently 12.7 years), has declined progressively during the twentieth century.[3,4] The exact mechanism for this is unknown, but improved nutrition has certainly been an important factor.[3] It is common for females to have irregular periods for approximately 2 years after menarche due to an immaturity of the hypothalamic–pituitary–ovarian axis and anovulatory cycles. This can result in dysfunctional uterine bleeding.

Both hormonal and non-hormonal factors can influence the progression through puberty. The non-hormonal influences include nutrition, stress, chronic systemic diseases and medications.[3,6] Few studies have specifically addressed the effect of chronic rheumatic diseases on puberty and pubertal development. One would expect that the influence of these chronic illnesses themselves as well as nutritional aberrations might result in a delay in the onset of puberty, but this has not been confirmed.[6] There has been work, however, on the effect of chronic arthritis in childhood on growth, particularly skeletal growth and bone mineral metabolism (see Chapter 17 for details).

Effect of rheumatic diseases on puberty and growth

Growth retardation is a well-described complication of children with arthritis.[7–9] Up to 30% of children with arthritis will experience generalized and/or localized growth abnormalities.[10–12] In children with systemic-onset arthritis or polyarticular arthritis, generalized growth delays are present by puberty,[8,13] and premature fusion of multiple epiphyses may develop, leading to short stature.[13] In one study, 30% of children had poor linear growth at the time when arthritis was diagnosed.[8] Short stature, generalized muscle atrophy and/or asymmetric growth abnormalities have also been reported in systemic lupus erythematosus (SLE), juvenile dermatomyositis (JDMS) and scleroderma.[14–17] Suggested causes have included disease activity and duration with direct damage to multiple joints and/or muscles, immobilization, poor nutrition and the effects of glucocorticoids.[7] Decreased nutritional intake, increased metabolic requirements, abnormal micronutrient utilization (discussed in Chapter 17) and the effects of inflammatory mediators may all play a role in the growth delays.[10,11,18] The additional metabolic and nutritional needs of puberty may further exacerbate the growth deficits.[19]

Corticosteroid use inhibits growth in height but does not affect skeletal maturation, further contributing to adult short stature.[13] Although glucocorticoids have been implicated, some researchers have demonstrated that the growth of patients with arthritis is more severely affected than those with SLE, despite comparable medication regimens.[8] This suggests an inherent problem with growth in arthritis. In addition, in arthritis, a defect in the peripheral effect of growth hormone has been hypothesized, including the demonstration of low levels of IGF-1 and other growth factors.[7,20,21] A recent study confirmed the association of growth retardation in arthritis patients who had never received corticosteroids.[7] This association was demonstrated in patients with systemic and polyarticular disease, but not those with pauciarticular arthritis. A significant negative correlation was demonstrated in affected patients between the duration of disease as well as the degree of functional joint involvement. The growth rate during the normal pubertal growth spurt was significantly affected, with a reduction in the peak growth velocity and duration of the growth spurt. This resulted in a final height below that expected. This study did not observe catch-up growth as has been reported previously by others.[13,22] Notably the pubertal development in these patients was reported to be normal.

A number of promising studies have been published that evaluated the effect of human growth hormone administration in children with chronic arthritis.[23-25] Recently, Davies et al[23] studied the growth of patients with arthritis treated with human growth hormone. They documented an increase in serial height velocity over a 1-year period. Growth improved in patients with mild to moderate disease severity and when using higher doses of human growth hormone. No significant side-effects were noted. Further long-term study is required to demonstrate a significant impact on long-term growth and final adult height. In addition, one study has suggested that the human growth hormone seems to have a beneficial impact on the activity of the disease, but the number of patients studied was small.[25]

Localized growth abnormalities are also found in children with arthritis and linear scleroderma and sometimes in JDMS (partial lipodystrophy). In pauciarticular arthritis, asymmetric growth may be most pronounced and has the greatest functional impact when involving the lower extremities. The epiphyseal plates of the knee, the most commonly involved joint in children, account for 70% of lower extremity growth.[26] Accelerated, asymmetrical growth of one knee is commonly described in patients diagnosed before 5 years of age. However, premature fusion of the epiphyseal plate may develop at puberty in children with ongoing disease activity, leading to a leg-length shortening of up to several centimetres.[26]

Temporomandibular joint (TMJ) involvement by the arthritis may lead to growth aberrations of the mandible.[27,28] In many children, bilateral TMJ involvement is noted. Hence the jaw grows poorly, ultimately leading to micrognathia, which has dental, nutritional as well as cosmetic consequences. The TMJs are involved unequally in some patients and the mandible grows suboptimally on only one side. TMJ arthritis may be associated with cervical spine involvement in these patients (Figure 16.1). In the cervical spine, fusion of the apophyseal bones can be seen on radiographs in 20–35% of such patients.[29] Decreased range of motion, especially with lateral rotation and extension, is frequent in these children. Cosmetic appearance, sports activities and car-driving, a key aspect of developing independence in adolescence, may be hindered if significant cervical spine arthritis is present.

Linear scleroderma may produce poor limb growth in 25–30% of patients.[16,17,30] Contractures are found in over half these patients,[31] and produce the most functionally significant limb shortening when involving the leg. Leg-length discrepancies of more than 1 cm are found during late adolescence or young adulthood. Orthotics or surgery, even possibly amputation, may be required in these patients.[16,17] Prostheses may then be used to improve function and ambulation.

In JDMS, late complications that may hinder normal growth include ongoing muscle inflammation or weakness, severe calcinosis and lipodystrophy. This latter process causes an abnormally reduced deposition of fat in the subcutaneous tissues, which produces an

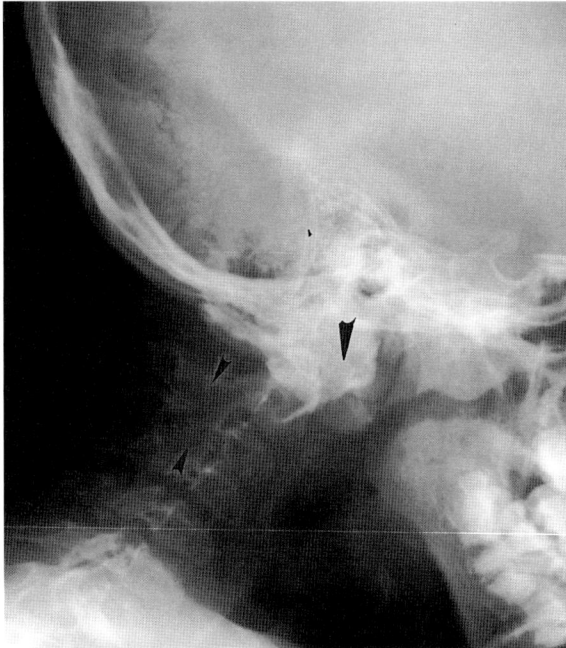

(a)

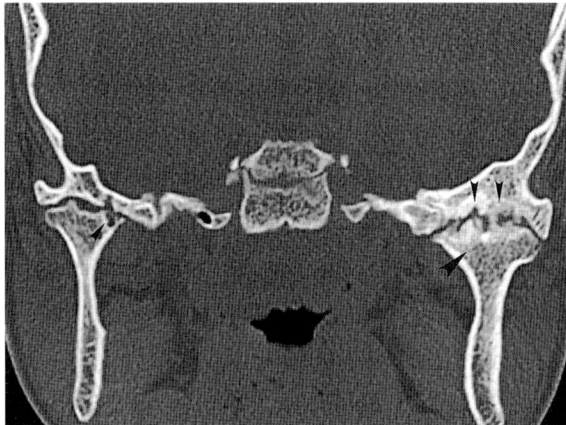

(b)

Figure 16.1 Radiographic changes of the spine and temporomandibular joint in juvenile idiopathic arthritis. (a) Cervical spine films from a 10-year-old boy with systemic onset juvenile idiopathic arthritis since 2 years of age. One centimetre C1–C2 subluxation (large arrow) and fusion of apophyseal joints (small arrows) are apparent on the films. (b) Temporomandibular joint computed tomography scan from the same patient at 14 years of age. Severe erosive arthritis (small arrows) with flattening of the mandibular head and remodelling of the ramus (large arrow) are noted.

asthenic, wasted appearance, typically in the face and arms. In some individuals, partial lipodystrophy develops and, although some areas are thin, asymmetrical fat deposition can be present. Insulin resistance and hypertriglyceridaemia are also associated with lipodystrophy.[32]

Calcinosis (subcutaneous and intrafascial deposits of calcium hydroxyapatite) develops in up to 50% of individuals 1–7 years after the onset of JDMS.[33] Small lumps are of little consequence; however, large masses or plates of dystrophic calcification may restrict joint motion, growth and ambulation. No treatment is uniformly beneficial for such patients. Colchicine may decrease the pain and inflammation that is associated with liquefication of calcinosis which sometimes occurs.[34] Recent reports suggest a role for the calcium channel blocker diltiazem in aiding the resorption of these lesions.[35]

Immunity and autoimmunity in puberty

Autoimmunity and puberty

Autoimmunity is due to a loss of normal tolerance, with formation of autologous antibodies and inability to discriminate self- from non-self-antigens. The precise combination of events that lead to the clinical expression of autoimmunity are uncertain. Several factors are thought to play a role in the development of these diseases:

- genetic predisposition
- immune function or deficiency
- environmental agents or triggers
- gender and/or neuroendocrine system
- age and developmental period.[36,37]

Many autoimmune diseases first present around the time of puberty, including SLE, seropositive rheumatoid arthritis, multiple sclerosis,[38] thyroiditis and others.[39] These diseases are manifested by the production of autoantibodies, which cause cellular dysfunction, immune-complex formation and/or further immune activation (i.e. complement activation).

In the following sections we review the literature on the development and age-related changes in the immune system. We also review the processes that may be related to neuro-endocrine changes which occur during puberty. Possible associations between these processes and the increase in autoimmunity near the time of puberty are suggested.

Immune system development during puberty
Developmental immunology is the study of the changes in the immune system during fetal and neonatal maturation through normal ageing, including senescence. Ageing does not affect all parts of the immune system similarly. B-cell function and antibody production mature primarily during the first decade of life. T-cell function and T-cell subset development evolve throughout life, with predominant changes occurring during the neonatal period, puberty and senescence. Natural killer (NK) cells, complement and cytokine production alter little during life. The developmental changes seen during puberty are summarized in Table 16.1.

Bone marrow production of B cells is relatively unaltered after childhood.[40] T-cell function, which does change significantly during adolescence (see below), regulates B-cell immunoglobulin production and secretion. Mature immunoglobulin function, isotype switching and B-cell reactivity are not achieved until at least 2–4 years of age. In many individuals serum concentrations of immunoglobulins do not reach adult levels until puberty. Total immunoglobulin G (IgG) production matures by 10 years of age.[41] IgG1 and IgG4 subclass levels are at adult values by early childhood, but IgG2 and IgG3 concentrations do not mature until the teenage years.[42] Total IgM and IgA concentrations reach maturity by 15–16 years, with IgA levels usually reaching adult levels last.[41,43,44]

Maturation patterns of immunoglobulin production are genetically based and vary with different ethnic backgrounds. Healthy Asian children have a biphasic rise in immunoglobulin levels, reaching adult concentrations of IgG and IgA in puberty.[45] Adult levels of total IgG are reached earlier in African-American children and are higher than in Caucasians.[42] However, IgG2 and IgG4 subclasses are reportedly lower

in healthy African-American children at comparable ages.[46] Diminished response to polysaccharide antigens in this population may be due to these variances in IgG2 production. In addition, the differing B-cell reactivity in these populations may partly explain the increase in some autoimmune diseases (e.g. SLE) in non-Caucasian teenagers.[47]

In contrast to humoral immunity, immuno-cellular function does decline with age, beginning at puberty. Splenic size is maximum around the time of puberty,[42] and then the thymus and lymphoid tissues begin to involute. As this happens, a decreased number of mature T cells differentiate and ten-fold fewer migrate from the thymus to the periphery.[40] Peripheral blood T lymphocyte numbers, which peak at 1–2 years of age, decrease after puberty.[48] Cytokine and macrophage influences as well as interactions with B cells and endocrine hormones also influence the T-cell functional decline seen with age.[49,50] Macrophage-derived interleukins promote proliferation and maturation of thymocytes.[49] Other cytokines as well as prostaglandins also regulate these processes. These factors rise and fall during childhood, also controlling T-cell production and maturation. These factors may also play a role in programmed cell death, or apoptosis, which is important in the ageing process and the development of autoimmunity.[49,51] In the periphery, T-cell subsets also react to these cytokines, altering effector and immunoregulatory responses.[52,53] Developmental changes in T-cell subsets may be important to the increased autoimmune phenomena seen at puberty. The response of T-lymphocyte subsets to various antigenic stimuli may also play a role in the development and perpetuation of autoimmunity.

The complement attack system and phagocytic cells function at adult capacity by approximately 6 months of age,[54] enabling the young child to handle environmental antigens. C1q and C3 both reach adult levels within the first month of life. C3 declines at puberty, rising again through adulthood.[55] Complement components are also important in immune-complex formation, which is pathogenic in many autoimmune diseases.

Table 16.1	Changes in the immune system during puberty
B cells	Total IgG levels mature by 10 years of age
	IgG2 and IgG3 levels mature during puberty
	IgM levels reach maturity by puberty
	IgA levels are the last to mature during puberty
	Common variable immunodeficiency often diagnosed during puberty
	Racial differences in timing of maturation
T cells	Decreased size of thymus, spleen and lymphoid tissues at puberty
	Thymic involution at puberty
	Fewer T cells differentiate and migrate to periphery
	Peripheral T lymphocyte numbers decrease
	Decreased prostaglandin and increased cytokine levels regulate functions as well as maturation and migration
	Target of neuroendocrine influences, especially oestrogens, prolactin and other HPG axis hormones
Complement	Deficiency syndromes often diagnosed during puberty
	C3 levels decline, rising again in adulthood
Cytokines	IL-1 and IL-6 influenced by feedback loops and pubertal changes in neuroendocrine function

HPG, hypothalamic–pituitary–gonad.

Immunodeficiency

Immunodeficiency, either acquired or inherited, and immune dysfunction related to senescence are associated with increased autoimmune phenomena. Such diseases occur with increased frequency in individuals with immunoglobulin and/or IgG subclass deficiency or dysfunction.[56] The increased incidence of some autoimmune diseases, including arthritis, vasculitis and other autoimmune rheumatic diseases, may be related to immunoglobulin defects.[15] Common variable immunodeficiency is manifested by gradually decreasing production of immunoglobulins and the occasional development of overt T-cell dysfunction. Common variable immunodeficiency is usually diagnosed in the second and third decades of life.[57,58] Infectious complications are frequently seen in these patients, but autoimmune

phenomena (colitis, cytopenias and vasculitis) may be the primary problems in such individuals.

Complement deficiencies are associated with infections as well as autoimmune diseases, particularly SLE and the vasculitic syndromes.[15,59] Autoimmunity is most often seen with heterozygous or homozygous deficiencies of C2, C3, C4 or C5.[15] These complement components are essential in promoting the solubility and clearance of immune complexes.[60] Inadequate immune-complex processing seems to be important in the development of autoimmune phenomena. Early onset or familial SLE, or atypical vasculitic syndromes should suggest the possibility of a complement deficiency.

T-cell deficiencies are strongly associated with the risk of infection (viral, human immunodeficiency virus (HIV), fungal). The normal decline in

T-cell function over a lifetime is associated with an increased risk of malignancy and infections in older adults.[61] The alterations in cellular immune function after childhood and the influence of the neuroendocrine system may, in part, explain the increase in autoimmune phenomena at puberty.[50]

Neuroendocrine and immune system interactions

Fundamental interrelationships exist between the immune and neuroendocrine systems in health and disease (Figure 16.2).[39,62–65] Both activating and suppressing pathways exist between these systems.[66] Sex-hormone receptors are present in the thymus and on activated immune system cells.[64] These relationships have important implications for the development of autoimmune disease at the time of puberty, when many endocrine changes occur, especially involving the sex hormones. The preponderance of autoimmune illness in females, especially with onset near puberty (SLE, arthritis and multiple sclerosis), strongly suggests that their development must depend to some extent on these neuroendocrine–immune system interactions.[67]

Adrenal, hypothalamic and pituitary hormones, including luteinizing hormone releasing hormone (LHRH), prolactin, growth hormone and adrenocorticotrophic hormone (ACTH) are immunomodulatory.[62,66,68] Prolactin receptors are found on both T and B cells[69] and may play a role in the gender differences in autoimmune diseases. Bromocryptine, a specific prolactin antagonist, has been used with limited success in the treatment of a few SLE patients,[70] supporting a role for prolactin in some SLE disease manifestations.

Melatonin is produced by the pineal gland and decreases at the onset of puberty.[65] Serotonin, the precursor of this hormone, has immunomodulatory effects and both chemicals influence circadian rhythm. Melatonin has been purported to play a role in the development of multiple sclerosis,[38] which often presents around the time of puberty.

Sex hormones regulate cellular and humoral immunity. Thymic hyperplasia develops in gonadectomized patients due to secondary alter-ations in pituitary hormones.[71] Sex hormone receptors are present in the thymus[64] and on immunoactive cells.[63] Oestrogens and androgens alter T-cell-mediated immunity, having different effects on various T-cell subsets.[63] The proportions of oestrogens to androgens, as well as the presence and function of sex-hormone receptors on immune cells, may be important in the gender disproportions of many of the rheumatic diseases.[67] Oestrogens seem to have a dualistic effect and may enhance B-cell activity in some disorders, such as SLE, and cause a reduction in T-cell activity in others, such as rheumatoid arthritis.[39,62]

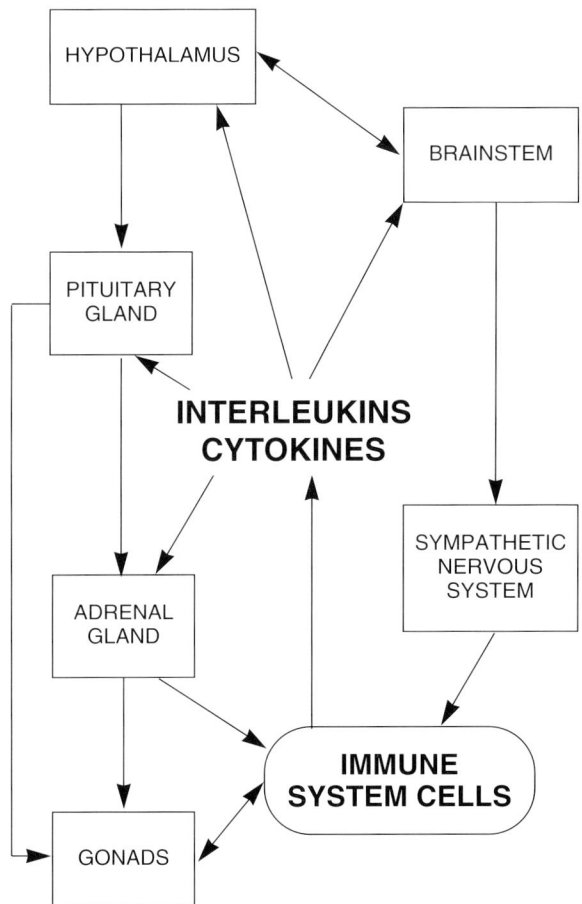

Figure 16.2 Interactions between the neuroendocrine and immune systems. Adapted from Wilder.[66]

Cytokines also play a role in the neuroendocrine–immune system interrelationship. Interleukin-1 (IL-1) and IL-6 function as bidirectional regulators of communication between these systems. IL-6, which is thought to be a key cytokine in systemic-onset JCA, also inhibits IGF-1 activity. This specific neuroendocrine–immune system interaction may partly explain the poor weight gain seen in some children with systemic-onset arthritis.[72]

PSYCHOSOCIAL ASPECTS OF ADOLESCENT DEVELOPMENT

Pubertal development is a biopsychosocial process.[73] The psychosocial aspects of puberty involve a developmental continuum in the model developed by Erikson. It is not a continuous, uniform process, but involves periods of growth and regression. Adolescents are not a homogeneous group and individual and cultural differences are significant. However, certain general observations can be made. Adolescence is often separated into three stages: early adolescence, age 11–14 years; middle adolescence, age 15–17 years (the secondary or high school years); and late adolescence, age 18–21 years (the transition from high school to college or university and work).[73,74] In the following sections we review normal adolescent development and the interaction with chronic rheumatic diseases.

Normal adolescent development

The tasks of adolescence have been characterized as achieving independence from one's parents, adopting appropriate peer codes and lifestyles, the achievement of a normal body image, and the development of a sexual ego with appropriate vocational goals and a moral identity.[73,74] Authors and clinicians have noted that the years of adolescence have been broadened in recent times, with younger pre-teenagers dealing with issues that are normally associated with older adolescents, as well as young adults in their twenties still working on the issues of independence from one's parents, especially financial independence. This transition may be especially difficult for teenagers with chronic medical conditions. In addition to the above outlined tasks of adolescence, significant cognitive development occurs in the teenage years. In Piaget's schema, cognitive development involves the progression from concrete operational thinking to more abstract formal operational thinking.

In the early adolescent years much of physical pubertal development is occurring, especially in females. Thus there is a great deal of preoccupation involving normal sexual development, anatomy and physiology. Teenagers are often anxious and uncertain about their bodies, making frequent comparison with others. In addition there is a significant shift to less dependence on one's parents and less interest in parental activities. Wide mood and behavioural swings may occur due to the emotional void created by this separation. Early adolescents become much more interested in their peers, often developing intense friendships. Cognitive maturation begins to occur. Often, however, the adolescent's attention is turned inward, with frequent daydreaming and fantasizing, and with idealistic and unrealistic vocational goals. A pattern of testing authority accompanied by a lack of impulse control may become apparent.

Middle adolescence is dominated by intense involvement by the teenager with their peer group. They are under significant pressure to conform to their peer group and their friends. They are still struggling with independence and dependence issues in the family, this often involving frequent conflicts about rules, regulations and responsibilities. Their body-image concerns often improve, with a greater acceptance of their bodies and development. Most adolescents continue to demonstrate a preoccupation with the correct clothes, make-up, etc. In relation to their identity development, middle adolescents often have feelings of invulnerability which can lead to experimentation and risk-taking behaviour. In fact, the most frequent causes of morbidity and mortality in the teenage years are accident, suicide and homicide as a result of this risk-taking behaviour. Adolescent sexual activity, with subsequent unintended pregnancies and sexually transmitted diseases, as well as alcohol and drug use, are other manifestations of such risk-taking attitudes.[75]

In the later adolescent years the situation has often improved. These years are often marked by reduced restlessness and increased integration back into the family. Body image is usually also more integrated and accepted. Peer acceptance is less important, with more emphasis on individual relationships. Usually realistic vocational goals have been developed, with the ability to compromise and delay gratification.

> By the end of adolescence, most adolescents have been emancipated from [their] parents and other adults and have attained a psychosexual identity and sufficient resources from education, family and community to begin to support themselves in a emotionally, socially, and financially satisfying way.[73]

Pubertal psychosocial development and chronic rheumatic diseases

As outlined above, the tasks of adolescent psychosocial development are challenging, especially in our current culture. The accomplishment of these tasks is even more challenging for an adolescent with a chronic disease such as chronic arthritis, SLE or fibromyalgia. A number of studies have looked at the reciprocal influences of chronic diseases such as these rheumatological conditions on adolescent development. It is very important for the physician caring for these patients to consider both the effect of the patient's illness on their adolescent psychosocial development, and the effect of adolescent development on the course and treatment of their rheumatological condition. One must take a holistic approach in the care of these challenging patients.

One may consider these reciprocal influences in a number of ways.[76] The first would be cognitive development. As previously mentioned, adolescents progress from concrete operational thinking to formal, more abstract thinking during the teenage years. Chronic illness can influence this complex process. In SLE, for example, central nervous system involvement may lead to cognitive dysfunction, and hence alter this normal developmental process in the adolescent patient.[77] Medications, including corticosteroids, can also affect the learning process. In addition, patients may miss a large amount of school secondary to their illness, which may prove a problem to academic achievement. Finally, chronic pain and fatigue may prove a hindrance to learning. The patient's cognitive development is an important consideration for the physician in determining care as well as the proper level of communication with the patient.[76] As adolescents mature they should take on more and more responsibility for the management of their illness, and this process should be facilitated by the health-care team.[76]

Second, adolescent patients with chronic illnesses face challenges in their identity development.[74,76,78–80] The traditional concept of 'normality' must undergo some modification as the teenager compares themself with their peers. This could foster emotional and behavioural problems. Disability from chronic joint disease, problems with growth and pubertal development, and constant requirements for medication, health-care visits and hospitalizations can all have a significant impact on the adolescent's body image, self-esteem and sense of identity. Health-care professionals caring for these patients need to strive to foster a positive sense of self-identity, emphasizing their individuality and self-worth. Third, family relations and achieving independence from one's parents can also be a significant challenge for adolescents with a chronic illness.[74,76,79] Both from the patient's and the parents' perspective, a number of forces work to maintain the teenager in a dependent role. This can be compounded by medical personnel and a health-care system that can also be overly controlling. It is critical that strong support for the entire family be maintained in order to maximize the outcome of these young people.[81] It is also important that adolescents with chronic medical conditions be allowed to accept increasing levels of responsibility for the care of their own illness, fostering a sense of independence and control. This offers the best chance for improved compliance with treatment and medication regimens.

The development of a healthy sexual identity can also be a difficult task for adolescents with chronic medical conditions.[74,76,79] Both from a psychosocial point of view as well as physically this can be a challenge for these teenagers. Many are sexually active, however, and it is very important for the health-care personnel to be sensitive to these issues and provide counselling and family-planning materials when appropriate. In addition, other risk-taking issues in these adolescents need to be addressed, including substance use and abuse.[76] In our society alcohol and drugs are easily available and teenagers with rheumatological conditions are as susceptible to experimentation and regular use of illicit substances as are other youth. Recent data have revealed that about 31% of teenagers with JCA have used alcohol, even when contraindicated because of medications prescribed.[82] These issues also need to be addressed in the medical evaluation and care.

A number of studies have looked at the level of psychological and social functioning in patients with rheumatological conditions.[83–91] In one study, psychological functioning of chronically ill teenagers, including 30 with rheumatological disorders such as SLE and arthritis, was assessed.[83] Interestingly, this study demonstrated no significant differences from controls in patients' levels of anxiety and self-esteem. They did, however, have significantly decreased feelings of self-determination with psychological testing, signifying that they perceived themselves to have little control over their own life (referred to as 'external locus of control'). This observation was most notable in relation to their health. Surprisingly, adolescents with chronic rheumatic diseases were more affected than the other chronically ill teenagers studied, including those with cancer and cardiac and renal diseases. Adolescents with rheumatological conditions in this study also reported more illness and treatment-related disruption of normal body image and problems with parents than did other ill teenagers and controls.[84] Patients with fibromyalgia have also been reported to have more anxiety and depressive related symptoms than healthy peers.[85]

Other work has examined the psychological problems of 42 children and adolescents with arthritis.[86] This study demonstrated that these patients had more psychological problems than controls, including problems of self-esteem and behavioural adjustment. The patients with more obvious physical disability had fewer emotional problems, while patients with disease but lesser disability did poorer on the psychological measures. The concept of marginality (those who have disease but are not visibly impaired) has been put forward to explain these results.[86] Such individuals are in a difficult, ambiguous position and do not readily identify with healthy or ill peers. Therefore, these individuals do not develop the emotional and social support of more severely affected patients.

Another group studied the use of a developmental model as a means of understanding the psychosocial functioning of young people with arthritis.[87] They demonstrated differences in psychological function depending on the age and developmental stage of the patient. Social functioning was associated with overall adjustment and level of disability in the primary and high-school students but not in the older young adults. This young adult group (18 years and older) who had been diagnosed with arthritis in childhood, were studied further by Miller et al.[88] In general, these patients were functioning well socially and in the work environment. Recent studies suggest that health status may be negatively influenced by having had arthritis,[91] but psychosocial functioning and social status are not necessarily affected by arthritis in these individuals.[90] Of concern, however, are data suggesting that fewer than one-third of young adults with a variety of physical disabilities, including JCA, receive adequate ongoing medical care.[91,92] The issues related to the transition of older adolescents to adult medical care are covered in detail in Chapter 18.

MEDICATION USE AND EFFECTS ON THE ADOLESCENT PATIENT

The management of rheumatic diseases usually requires intervention with medications, as well as the psychosocial support and education of the patient and their family. Medication non-compliance is a common risk-taking behaviour in teenagers. This issue has been most often discussed in relation to insulin use in the teenage diabetic. Adolescents with SLE or JCA may also admit to medication avoidance,[93,94] especially with those drugs which may cause outward side-effects (corticosteroids) or interfere with other potential teenage concerns (non-steroidal anti-inflammatory drugs (NSAIDs) and alcohol consumption, for example). Disease exacerbations and physiological problems due to abrupt medication withdrawal (especially chronic corticosteroids) are concerns which the adolescent patient may fail to appreciate. Medication use in the treatment of these diseases has been described in detail in Chapters 5–10, but specific issues related to puberty and medication effects will be discussed here. In the following sections we review common medications used in the management of rheumatic diseases and focus on the potential unique toxicities and issues for the adolescent patient.

Non-steroidal anti-inflammatory drugs

NSAIDs have a role in the management of the arthritides, regardless of the aetiology. These drugs function primarily via prostaglandin inhibition and anti-inflammatory effects. Many of the potential toxicities of NSAIDs are related to the disruption of normal prostaglandin functions throughout the body. This includes renal, cardiac and gastrointestinal side-effects. Experimentation with nicotine, caffeine and alcohol during the teenage years significantly increases the risk of these side-effects, especially on the stomach and liver.[82,95]

Anti-inflammatory doses of NSAIDs are generally not recommended during pregnancy due to rare reports of fetal toxicity[96] and haemorrhagic complications at delivery. Low-dose aspirin, however, appears to be safe and indicated in pregnant women with antiphospholipid syndrome[97] as well as for pre-eclampsia.[98]

Corticosteroids

Corticosteroids are essential treatment in several diseases, such as SLE and myositis. Low dosages

are preferred in such patients when possible, but occasionally, especially with more severe systemic illness, high dosages are indicated. During the management of SLE with severe glomerulonephritis, JDMS and the vasculitic syndromes, high-dose glucocorticoids are the rule during the early stages of treatment; low doses may be prescribed over years in many individuals. Side-effects of corticosteroids have been well described;[99] they are more problematic with moderate to high dosages used over months to years. The risk of chronic therapy (> 6 months) with low-dose steroids (approximately 0.25 mg/kg/day or up to 10 mg/day) is due to the bone effects, primarily osteoporosis. This has been well described in adults, but has only more recently been recognized as a complication of chronic therapy in children with rheumatic diseases.[100] Chronic inflammation, steroid use, inactivity and inadequate intake of calcium are also contributing factors in the development of osteoporosis in teenage patients. Deflazacort, a derivative of prednisolone, has anti-inflammatory effects but decreased bone and endocrine toxicities in patients with arthritis.[101,102] Although this agent seems attractive to patients, it is not available in many countries.

Gastrointestinal side-effects of steroids include heartburn, reflux and abdominal pain. Concomitant use of NSAIDs adds to these symptoms, and the risk of ulcer development increases in patients prescribed both classes of medication.[95] Alcohol use also increases these complications, and presents a major concern in adolescent patients.[82] Careful questioning of teenagers regarding the use of alcohol is imperative when prescribing these medications.

The development of Cushing's syndrome is one of the more unwelcome complications of corticosteroid use in the adolescent patient. The hypertension, hyperglycaemia, hirsutism, weight gain, acne and moodiness all disappear as the steroid dosage is lowered (typically below 0.5 mg/kg/day or 15 mg/day), but striae persist. The duration of these complications is variable, but in the teenage patient even 6 months is too long to cope with these physical changes. One can limit these steroid side-effects by: alternate-day dosing, minimizing dose recommendations, use of steroid sparing drugs, dietary salt restriction or the use of deflazacort, if available.

Growth retardation and pubertal delay are also complications of long-term, moderate to high dose (> 0.5 mg/kg/day) corticosteroid use. Growth velocity may not return to normal for age if the dose of prednisone is maintained above 4–6 mg/m^2/day (roughly the same as 0.15 mg/kg/day).[103] Menstrual irregularities and primary or secondary amenorrhoea may also develop in young women on high-dose steroids.

Slow-acting antirheumatic drugs

Steroid-sparing drugs are indicated in: teenagers with seropositive rheumatoid arthritis or progressive chronic arthritis, many vasculitic syndromes, severe SLE, and patients whose illness has responded to corticosteroids but who are experiencing unacceptable side-effects. These slow-acting antirheumatic drugs (SAARDs) are prescribed with or without concomitant glucocorticoids. These include: antimalarials (hydroxychloroquine), sulphasalazine, gold salts (myochrisine, solganol, auranofin), penicillamine and immunosuppressive agents (methotrexate, azathioprine, cyclophosphamide, cyclosporine). Each of these drugs has potential toxicities, some of which may be additive with corticosteroids or NSAIDs. Only those issues unique to the adolescent patient are reviewed here.

Antimalarial drugs are commonly used in the management of patients with childhood-onset arthritis or SLE and for some features of JDMS. These medications are usually well tolerated with few side-effects. In SLE patients, arthritis, rash, alopecia and fatigue are most benefited by the use of antimalarial therapy. SLE exacerbations can be minimized by long-term maintenance use of these drugs.[104] Definite ophthalmic toxicity is not reported when the dosages are maintained below 6.5 mg/kg/day.[105] In the teenager with significant weight fluctuations, correct calculation of antimalarial dosage must be made and adjusted based on weight gain or loss. Ophthalmological evaluations are routinely recommended on a 6–12 monthly basis.

Sulphasalazine is a SAARD which is used primarily for chronic arthritis and the seronegative spondyloarthropathies. This drug consists of sulphapyridine and salicylate moieties, the former causing most of the toxicities. Other than allergic reactions, leucopenia, headache, nausea and diarrhoea are occasional side-effects. Azospermia develops infrequently in men prescribed this drug, but may be a concern in the adolescent or adult male population. Normalization of the sperm count is the rule when therapy is stopped, and no fetal abnormalities have been reported.[106]

Immunosuppressive agents are indicated in the treatment of children with more severe rheumatic diseases such as SLE with neurological or renal involvement, JDMS, vasculitis and severe arthritis. Methotrexate is the most frequently used of these drugs.[107] Methotrexate is a folate antagonist which has mucosal, bone marrow and hepatic toxicities.[108] This drug is an abortofacient and is teratogenic.[109] It should be stopped at least 3 months before a planned pregnancy and should not be prescribed to a pregnant or nursing woman. NSAIDs increase the half-life of methotrexate, increasing the risk of side-effects. Therefore, careful monitoring is required of all patients using these medications in combination. All such patients should be warned against the use of over-the-counter NSAIDs.

Alcohol significantly increases the risk of liver toxicity in patients given methotrexate. As many as 24% of methotrexate-treated patients with chronic arthritis admitted to the use of alcohol,[87] even after repeated warnings. Unsafe sexual activities and drug use that exposes patients to hepatitis must be avoided. Careful review of current birth control, habits and potential risk-taking behaviours should be made before instituting therapy and at each visit.

Cyclophosphamide is an alkylating agent usually reserved for patients with SLE and diffuse proliferative glomerulonephritis or vasculitic syndromes (polyarteritis and Wegener's granulomatosis). Rarely, severe, treatment resistant systemic-onset arthritis has been treated with cyclophosphamide.[110] Toxicities from this drug include: alopecia, bone-marrow suppression, gastrointestinal upset, haemorrhagic cystitis and infertility. Late malignancies, primarily lymphoma and bladder carcinoma, are reported in up to 20% of long-term patients.[111] Many of these side-effects are minimized by use of intravenous monthly pulse cyclophosphamide therapy, which is quite effective in SLE.[112] However, this method of administration does not seem to be as beneficial in the long-term management of the vasculitic syndromes.[113]

Sustained amenorrhoea, and hence potential sterility, is a complication of long-term high-dose cyclophosphamide use. Sterility appears to be most problematic when cyclophosphamide is given to women over the age of 31 years, 62% of whom may become infertile. Twenty-seven per cent of women aged 26–30 years may develop infertility after using cyclophosphamide.[114] Follow-up studies of young men who had taken alkylating agents, including cyclophosphamide, for treatment of cancer between the ages of 15 and 20 years showed a 60% rate of infertility.[115] Some workers propose that progesterone-induced temporary amenorrhoea may protect the ovaries from these effects of cyclophosphamide and similar drugs, and prevent long-term sterility or infertility.[116]

The sexually active adolescent patient prescribed cyclophosphamide must use birth control, since this drug is a potent teratogen. Careful questioning about sexual activity and birth control practices must be reviewed at each office visit when prescribing this drug. Since menstrual irregularities are common in young women given cyclophosphamide, if sexually active, pregnancy tests should be part of the routine laboratory evaluation of such patients. Depomedroxyprogesterone acetate (DMPA) (see below) is safe and effective in such patients.

GYNAECOLOGICAL ISSUES IN ADOLESCENTS WITH RHEUMATIC DISEASES
Gynaecological evaluation and health maintenance issues

The indications for a routine pelvic examination in adolescent females include the initiation of sexual activity, the presence of a significant menstrual or gynaecological complaint or an age of approximately 18–21 years. These indications would also apply to adolescents with rheumatological conditions. However, some special considerations apply to these affected teenagers. Mechanically, the performance of the pelvic examination might be difficult in the presence of severe hip arthritis. Examination performed in the prone, knee–chest position may minimize this difficulty.

A recent association has been demonstrated between SLE and cervical dysplasia.[117–120] Therefore, regular PAP smears are indicated in sexually active adolescents to look for evidence of human papilloma virus (HPV) infection and subsequent cervical dysplasia. In the USA, abnormal PAP smears are currently graded using the standardized Bethesda Reporting System, now revised (Table 16.2).[121] HPV has been noted to be the most common sexually transmitted disease in adolescents.[122] The incidence of HPV infection in the adolescent population is undetermined, but has been reported to be present in 15–38% of sexually active adolescents.[122] HPV types 6 and 11 are associated with external condyloma accuminata, and HPV types 16, 18, 31, 33 and 35 are associated with flat condyloma and cervical disease. Cervical disease has been associated with a number of risk factors in adolescents, including early age at first coitus, multiple sexual partners, smoking, contraceptive method and HPV infection.[122]

Recent studies have suggested that patients with SLE are predisposed to cervical dysplasia.[117–120] One study indicated that adult patients with SLE had a higher incidence of cervical atypia than did controls.[117] There was no difference in the patients with SLE with regard to treatment with cytotoxic drugs. Colposcopy revealed three cases (23%) of cervical intraepitheal neoplasia (CIN 1–3). Another study found that patients treated with cyclophosphamide had an increased rate of cervical atypia, especially when combined with azathioprine.[118] Finally, one study has found an increased risk of high-grade cervical lesions in women with SLE, particularly when

---

Table 16.2   The Bethesda System II for reporting cervical/vaginal cytologic diagnoses[121]

1. Adequacy of specimen
2. General categorization
3. Descriptive changes:
   (a) benign cellular changes
       infection or reactive changes
   (b) epithelial cell abnormalities
       (i) squamous cell:
           − ASCUS (favours either dysplastic or reactive process)
           − low-grade squamous intraepithelial lesion (cellular changes of HPV; mild dysplasia (CIN 1))
           − high-grade squamous intraepithelial lesion (moderate dysplasia (CIN 2); severe dysplasia (CIN 3); carcinoma in situ (CIN 3))
           − squamous cell carcinoma
       (ii) glandular cell
           − benign
           − AGUS
           − malignant
4. Other malignant neoplasms
5. Hormonal evaluation for vaginal smears only

AGUS, atypical glandular cells of undetermined significance; ASCUS, atypical squamous cells of undetermined significance; CIN, cervical intraepithelial neoplasia; HPV, human papilloma virus.

treated with immunosuppressive agents.[119] These studies recommend regular PAP smears in patients with SLE to screen for these complications. This would seem particularly prudent in an adolescent population at high risk for HPV disease.

Pubertal or menarchal delay, menstrual irregularities, genital lesions and infections are other indications for gynaecological evaluation in teenagers with rheumatic diseases. Vaginal candidiasis may be increased in some patients especially those given steroids and immunosuppressives. Although there were concerns that commonly used drugs for the treatment of arthritis, especially methotrexate, might cause delayed menarche, recent data suggest that mean age of menarche in this population is normal. This has been attributed to better disease control, which minimizes the negative impact of chronic inflam-

mation on puberty.[123] However, menstrual abnormalities are common with young women with SLE treated with cyclophosphamide as well as high-dose corticosteroids.[114,124] Oligomenorrhoea and amenorrhoea have been reported in cyclophosphamide-treated patients and is reported to be somewhat dependent on dose, and perhaps method of administration.[124] Return of normal cycles usually occurs several months after treatment has been discontinued. However, rarely, permanent amenorrhoea with total ovarian destruction has been reported.[125]

Genital ulceration is one of the diagnostic criteria for Behçet's syndrome.[126,127] This is a multisystem disease primarily of adults, but onset during adolescence and childhood has been reported. Clinical manifestations include aphthous stomatitis, genital ulcers, uveitis, skin lesions, as well as gastrointestinal lesions, arthritis, and central nervous system lesions. One study has demonstrated that genital ulcers are rare in SLE and that the diagnosis of Behçet's syndrome should be strongly considered in patients who present with this problem.[128] The aetiology is not known; for mild cases, symptomatic therapy is adequate. For patients with more active disease whose sight is threatened or those with persistent disabling oral/genital ulcerations, treatment may include corticosteroids and/or immunosuppressive agents.

Reiter's syndrome involves genital lesions as well, and may have its onset during puberty with the advent of sexual activity.[129] This postinfectious arthritis is characterized by urethritis, conjunctivitis/uveitis and mucocutaneous lesions. It can occur following a number of sexually transmitted infections and enteric infections. Sexually transmitted organisms include *Chlamydia trachomatis* and *Ureaplasma urealyticum*. The illness has a significant male predominance and is associated with human leucocyte antigen (HLA) B27. There are no specific laboratory tests and the diagnosis is made on clinical criteria. It may be classified as a postinfectious (sterile) reactive arthritis, but recent studies have been successful in identifying *Chlamydia* and *Ureaplasma* in some cases.[129] In addition, through immunohistochemical techniques, various microbial antigens (e.g. *Chlamydia*, *Yersinia* and *Salmonella*) have been identified in the synovium of affected patients, although the accuracy and significance of these findings have been challenged. Antimicrobial treatment is indicated for diagnosed sexually transmitted diseases. Most studies advocate a short course of treatment according to standard Center for Disease Control (CDC) guidelines; however, some advocate longer treatment courses for patients with Reiter's syndrome.[129] The course is usually self-limited; however, some patients can have persistent disease activity with the arthropathy. Recent data suggest that, with the likelihood that subclinical infection persists in some individuals, a 3-month course of antibiotic therapy may be beneficial in patients with reactive arthritis and Reiter's syndrome.[129]

Contraception and pregnancy

Most young women with rheumatic disease maintain their ability to become pregnant. With few exceptions, disease and medication effects do not produce infertility. One-third of young women with chronic arthritis in childhood have children by their mid-20s, which is no different from unaffected females.[88,130] Similar to adult rheumatoid arthritis, JCA improves during pregnancy in most patients,[131] but may flare during the post-partum period in more than 50% of patients.[131] Delivery may be more difficult in young women with chronic changes from arthritis due to hip, knee or spine involvement. Caesarean sections are performed with increased frequency in chronic arthritis patients, usually due to mechanical restrictions to vaginal delivery.[131]

Young women with SLE also have normal rates of conception, but may have disease exacerbations during pregnancy or immediately post-partum.[132] Whether the rate of flare differs between pregnant and non-pregnant woman remains controversial. Autoantibodies to Ro (SS-A) and La (SS-B) cross the placenta and, in approximately 1 in 20 cases, cause neonatal lupus and/or congenital heart block in the child.[133] High titres of IgG anticardiolipin antibodies in the mother are associated with an increased risk of fetal loss.[134] Rare cases of presumed transplacentally induced fetal antiphospholipid syndrome have been reported.[135] Disease effects on the fetus, potential pregnancy effects on the disease process and teratogenic effects of rheumatological medication all emphasize the need for contraception and pregnancy planning in young women with chronic rheumatic disease.

The issue of sexual activity and appropriate contraception is a difficult topic for adolescents in general, and especially adolescents with chronic illnesses such as rheumatic disease. Teenage sexual activity is a major problem in our culture, and the early initiation of teenagers into sexual activity exposes them to a host of health problems. These include unintended pregnancy, leading either to a birth or abortion, increased infant and maternal morbidity and mortality with these pregnancies, and sexually transmitted diseases, including HIV infection.

Few teenagers in the USA complete adolescence without having sex.[136,137] The average age of first sexual intercourse is 16 years in males and 17 years in females.[138] Many do not use contraception, and the younger the individual the less likely they are to do so.[136,137] The average teenager waits 1 year after initiating sex to obtain birth control.[137] There are more than one million teenage pregnancies per year in the USA, with 47% having babies, 40% having abortions and 13% suffering miscarriages.[137] Sexually transmitted diseases are also common, especially human papilloma virus, herpes genitalis and *Chlamydia trachomatis*.

There are few data regarding the sexual activity of chronically ill adolescents, and specifically teenagers with rheumatological disease (reviewed in detail in Chapter 15). Sexual activity in women aged 19–37 years who have had arthritis is similar to that of their peers, but is less for men when compared to age-matched groups.[139] Although the rates of sexual activity may differ in teenagers with JCA, such differences are probably not significant in practice.[138] Thus health professionals caring for these teenagers need to consider the issue of appropriate contraception. In addition, the side-effects of these contraceptives need to be taken into consideration in light of the chronic condition of these patients.

The barrier methods of contraception (e.g. condoms, spermicides and the diaphragm) offer significant advantages for these patients.[138] These are safe for all patients, although some teenagers might have dexterity difficulties with their use and latex allergies can be related to condom use.[138] Their effectiveness is not always satisfactory when used alone, especially by teenagers, but they are very effective when used in combination (e.g. condoms and spermicidal foam). Indeed, condoms are always recommended for use during sex to prevent the spread of sexually transmitted diseases, including HIV. The intrauterine device (IUD) is not regularly recommended for adolescents because of the increased potential for pelvic inflammatory disease.

Hormonal contraception is normally recommended for adolescents regularly having sex.

Methods include the combined oral contraceptives, quarterly DMPA and levonorgesterol subdermal implants. They are considered very safe and effective for healthy teenagers. There are some concerns, however, about their safety in patients with rheumatological conditions, especially SLE.[138,140] The usual practice has been to avoid the use of combination oral contraceptives in patients with SLE.[138,140,141] Reviews of the contraceptive practices in patients with SLE have demonstrated a significantly lower use of combined oral contraceptives as compared with a control population of women.[141–143] Some of these concerns centre around the possible role of oestrogens in the activity of SLE. There is some evidence that oestrogen increases disease activity.[141,142] This evidence includes the female predominance of the disease, the increase in incidence after puberty and the exacerbation seen during pregnancy.[141] Anecdotal experience suggests exacerbations occur pre-menstrually in some girls.[141] In addition there are reports of hormonal treatments inducing the development of antinuclear antibodies and possibly inducing or exacerbating the disease itself, although the associations are controversial.[141] Indeed, in some patients combined oral contraceptives may alleviate symptoms and disease activity, especially if they have cyclic flares of their disease associated with the menstrual cycle.[141] Another concern is the association of combined oral contraceptives with thromboembolism. Most studies have concentrated on the role of oestrogens in the development of thromboembolism. A progestational effect has also been hypothesized, but is controversial.[141] One study has demonstrated that the risk of deep venous thrombosis in patients with SLE on combined oral contraceptives was slightly increased compared with controls.[142] In contrast, others have suggested that oral contraceptives could be used to preserve fertility in patients with SLE treated with cyclophosphamide.[141] This has been done in patients with Hodgkin's disease with some success.[116] However, its use in patients with SLE continues to remain controversial, as combined oral contraceptives have been shown to possibly cause an increase in disease activity in patients with renal disease, and these are the typical patients who require treatment with cyclophosphamide.[141]

The progestin only 'mini-pill' has been used in patients with SLE with some limited success.[142] However, menstrual irregularities seem to limit its acceptance and usefulness. Quarterly DMPA has been suggested as an alternative for chronically ill females, including those with SLE.[144,145] Menstrual irregularities can also occur with its use, but are usually self-limited.[142] Indeed, approximately 66% of young women regularly using this method will cease menses with regular use. The package labelling for DMPA indicates a concern about the risk of thromboembolism, but this has not been shown in clinical practice.[144] Implanted levonorgesterol could also have indications and advantages, although implantation and especially removal issues limit its use.

Patients with adolescent-onset arthritis have special concerns regarding contraception. Severe disability might limit the usefulness of barrier methods due to the finger dexterity or hip/knee range of motion required for insertion and removal.[139] Condoms would, of course, be indicated. It has been previously suggested that oral contraceptives might be beneficial in the treatment of rheumatoid arthritis because of the remission sometimes seen in pregnancy. Although it seems that concomitant use of oral contraceptives might protect patients from developing rheumatoid arthritis, they have not been shown to be clinically useful in the treatment of active disease.[146,147]

Discussions about sexual activity and contraception should be initiated as soon as is appropriate. When contraception fails, the pregnancy must be addressed directly to avoid or minimize disease– and medication-related complications. In all such patients, we recommend discontinuation of NSAIDs, except possibly low-dose aspirin, and SAARDs. Prednisone and methyl-prednisolone may be continued as indicated, as placental metabolism of these glucocorticoids minimizes drug delivery to the fetus.[109] Other drugs such as antihypertensives may need to be changed to decrease pregnancy and fetal risks.

Increased morbidity and prematurity are associated with pregnancy in teenagers. These concerns are increased in the pregnant teenager with SLE, since disease exacerbations are reported in many such individuals.[132] Therefore, close clinical and laboratory evaluations are imperative. High risk obstetricians must be a part of the team managing such a patient. Baseline laboratory studies should include urinalyses, complete blood counts, C3, C4 and anti-double stranded DNA, Ro (SS-A), La (SS-B) and antiphospholipid antibodies. Anti-double stranded DNA titres and C3 levels are helpful in monitoring disease activity during the course of the pregnancy, and may help differentiate pre-eclampsia from SLE exacerbation. If the antiphospholipid antibodies are positive, low-dose aspirin should be prescribed throughout the pregnancy. A history of prior recurrent fetal demise should be managed with full anticoagulation; this may be achieved with daily subcutaneous self-administration of heparin.[148] If Ro and/or La antibodies are present, fetal echocardiography should be planned for the second trimester to screen for potential cardiac and conduction abnormalities in the baby.[135] A more detailed review of pregnancy in adolescents with rheumatic disease is provided in Chapter 15.

SUMMARY

Autoimmune diseases frequently begin during or shortly after puberty. We have reviewed the potential interaction of developmental immunology and normal pubertal development with these illnesses. The interrelationship of the disease processes, medications and neuropsychosocial functioning of adolescents has been presented as well. Normal adolescent issues regarding growth, difference from peers and gynaecological concerns, such as pregnancy, contraception and health maintenance, have been reviewed and placed in the context of teenagers with chronic rheumatic disease. Research into these issues has been scant, and further work is indicated to better understand the relationship between puberty and adolescent rheumatic diseases.

REFERENCES

1. Neinstein LS, Kaufman FR. Normal physical growth and development. In: *Adolescent Health Care, A Practical Guide* (Neinstein LS, ed), 3rd edn. Williams & Wilkins: Baltimore, 1996:3–39.
2. Grumbach MM, Roth JC, Kaplan SL et al. Hypothalamic–pituitary regulation of puberty in man: evidence and concepts derived from clinical research. In: *Control of the Onset of Puberty* (Grumbach MM, Grave GD, Mayer FE, eds). Wiley: New York, 1974:115–16.
3. Kulin HE, Muller J. The biological aspects of puberty. *Pediatr Rev* 1996; **17**:75–86.
4. Copeland KC. Variations in normal sexual development. *Pediatr Rev* 1986; **8**:47–54.
5. Tanner JM. *Growth At Adolescence*, 2nd edn. Blackwell Scientific: Oxford, 1962.
6. Rosen DS. Pubertal growth and sexual maturation for adolescents with chronic illness and disability. *Pediatrician* 1991; **18**:105–20.
7. Polito CG, Strano AN, Olivieri M et al. Growth retardation in non-steroid treated juvenile rheumatoid arthritis. *Scand J Rheumatol* 1997; **26**:99–103.
8. Bernstein BH, Stobie D, Singsen BH et al. Growth retardation in juvenile rheumatoid arthritis. *Arthritis Rheum* 1977; **20**:212–16.
9. Hashkes PJ, Lovell DJ. Why are children with juvenile rheumatoid arthritis small? In: *Controversies in Rheumatology* (Isenberg DA, Tucker LB, eds). Martin Dunitz: London, 1997:139–53.
10. White PH. Growth abnormalities in children with JRA. *Clin Orthop Rel Res* 1990; **259**:46–51.
11. Bacon MC, White PH, Raiten DJ et al. Nutritional status and growth in JRA. *Sem Arthritis Rheum* 1990; **20**:97–106.
12. Henderson CJ, Lovell DJ. Assessment of protein energy malnutrition in children and adolescents with juvenile rheumatoid arthritis. *Arthritis Care Res* 1989; **2**:108–13.
13. Ansell BM, Bywaters EGL. Growth in Still's disease. *Ann Rheum Dis* 1956; **15**:295–319.
14. Bitnum S, Daeschner CW, Travis LB et al. Dermatomyositis. *J Pediatr* 1964; **64**:101–24.
15. Cassidy JT, Petty RE. *Textbook of Pediatric Rheumatology*, 3rd edn. Churchill Livingstone: New York, 1994.
16. Uziel Y, Krafchik BR, Silverman ED et al. Localized scleroderma in childhood: a report of 30 cases. *Semin Arthritis Rheum* 1994; **23**:328–40.
17. Hatzis JA, Stratigos AJ, Dimopoulou JC et al. Linear scleroderma with severe leg deformity. *Australasian J Dermatol* 1992; **33**:155–7.
18. Ostrov BE. Nutrition and pediatric rheumatic diseases. Hypothesis: cytokines modulate nutritional abnormalities in rheumatic diseases. *J Rheumatol* 1992; **19**(suppl 33):49–53.
19. Rosen DS. Pubertal growth and sexual maturation for adolescents with chronic illness or disability. *Pediatrician* 1991; **18**:105–20.
20. Bennett AE, Silverman ED, Miller JJ, Hintz RL. Insulin-like growth factors I and II in children with systemic onset juvenile arthritis. *J Rheumatol* 1988; **13**:655–8.
21. Allen RC, Jimenez M, Cowell CT. Insulin-like growth factor and growth hormone secretion in juvenile chronic arthritis. *Ann Rheum Dis* 1991; **50**:602–6.
22. Preece MA, Law CM, Davies PS. The growth of children with chronic pediatric disease. *Clin Endocrinol Metabolism* 1986; **15**:453–77.
23. Davies UM, Rooney M, Preece MA et al. Treatment of growth retardation in juvenile chronic arthritis with recombinant human growth hormone. *J Rheumatol* 1994; **21**:153–8.
24. Svantesson H. Treatment of growth failure with human growth hormone in patients with juvenile chronic arthritis. A pilot study. *Clin Exp Rheumatol* 1991; **9**(suppl 6):47–50.
25. Butenandt O. Rheumatoid arthritis and growth retardation in children: treatment with human growth hormone. *Eur J Pediatr* 1979; **130**:15–28.
26. Simon S, Whiffen J, Shapiro F. Leg length discrepancies in monoarticular and pauciarticular JRA. *J Bone Joint Surg* 1981; **63A**:209–15.
27. Blasberg B, Lowe AA, Petty RE et al. Temporomandibular joint disease in children with juvenile rheumatoid arthritis. *Arthritis Rheum* 1987; **30**:S27.
28. Mayro RF, DeLozier JB, Whitaker LA. Facial reconstruction considerations in rheumatic diseases. *Rheum Dis Clin North Am* 1991; **17**:943–69.
29. Hensinger RN, DeVito PD, Ragsdale CG. Changes in the cervical spine in juvenile rheumatoid arthritis. *J Bone Joint Surg* 1986; **68A**:189–98.
30. Christianson HB, Dorsey CS, O'Leary PA et al. Localized scleroderma. A study of 235 cases. *Arch Dermatol* 1956; **74**:629–39.
31. Falanga V, Medsger TA, Reichlin M, Rodnan GP. Linear scleroderma. *Ann Intern Med* 1986; **104**:849–57.

32. Tucker LB, Sadeghi-Nejad A, Schaller JG. The association of acquired lipodystrophy with juvenile dermatomyositis. *Arthritis Rheum* 1990; **33**:D76.

33. Bowyer SL, Blane CE, Sullivan DB et al. Childhood dermatomyositis: factors predicting functional outcome and development of dystrophic calcification. *J Pediatr* 1983; **103**: 882–8.

34. Fuchs D, Fruchter L, Fishel B et al. Colchicine suppression of local and systemic inflammation due to calcinosis universalis in chronic dermatomyositis. *Clin Rheumatol* 1986; **5**:527–30.

35. Palmieri GM, Sebes JI, Aelion JA et al. Treatment of calcinosis with diltiazem. *Arthritis Rheum* 1995; **38**:1646–54.

36. Mongey AB, Hess EV. Autoimmunity and the environment. *Res Staff Phys* 1995; **41**:31–40.

37. Atkinson JP. Some thoughts on autoimmunity. *Arthritis Rheum* 1995; **38**:301–5.

38. Sandyk R. Multiple sclerosis: the role of puberty and the pineal gland in its pathogenesis. *Intl J Neurosci* 1993; **68**:209–25.

39. Beeson PB. Age and sex associations of 40 autoimmune diseases. *Am J Med* 1994; **96**:457–62.

40. Weigle WO. Effects of aging on the immune system. *Hospital Prac* 1989; **Dec**:112–19.

41. Pacheco SE, Shearer WT. Laboratory aspects of immunology. *Pediatr Clin North Am* 1994; **41**:623–55.

42. Buckley RH, Dees SC, O'Fallon WM. Serum immunoglobulins. I: Levels in normal children and in uncomplicated childhood allergy. *Pediatrics* 1968; **41**:600–11.

43. Gerrard JW, Ko CG, Dalgleish R, Tan LK. Immunoglobulin levels in white and Metis communities in Saskatchewan. *Clin Exp Immunol* 1977; **29**:447–56.

44. Cooper MD. B lymphocytes. Normal development and function. *New Engl J Med* 1987; **317**:1452–6.

45. Lau YL, Jones BM, Yeung CY. Biphasic rise of serum immunoglobulins G and A and sex influence on serum immunoglobulin M in normal Chinese children. *J Pediatr Child Health* 1992; **28**:240–3.

46. Ambrosino DM, Black CM, Plikaytis BD et al. Immunoglobulin G subclass values in healthy black and white children. *J Pediatr* 1991; **119**:875–9.

47. Hochberg MC. Systemic lupus erythematosus. *Rheum Dis Clin North Am* 1990; **16**:617–39.

48. Erkeller-Yuksel FM, Deneys V, Yuksel B et al. Age related changes in human blood lymphocyte populations. *J Pediatr* 1992; **120**:216–22.

49. Hirokawa K, Utsuyama M, Kasai M et al. Understanding the mechanism of the age-change of thymic function to promote T cell differentiation. *Immunol Lett* 1994; **40**:269–77.

50. Hirokawa K, Utsuyama M, Kasai M, Kurashima C. Aging and immunity. *Acta Pathol Jpn* 1992; **42**:537–48.

51. Elkon KB. Apoptosis and systemic lupus erythematosus. *Lupus* 1994; **3**:1–2.

52. Fulop T. Signal transduction changes in granulocytes and lymphocytes with aging. *Immunol Lett* 1994; **40**:259–68.

53. Kay MM. An overview of immune aging. *Mech Aging Dev* 1979; **9**:39–59.

54. Timmerman JJ, Van der Woude IJ, Vangijlswijk-Janssen DJ et al. Differential expression of complement components in human fetal and adult kidneys. *Kidney Int* 1996; **49**:730–40.

55. Yonemasu K, Kitajima H, Tanabe S et al. Effect of age on C1q and C3 levels in human serum and their presence in colostrum. *Immunology* 1978; **35**:523–30.

56. Hanson LA, Soderstrom R, Avanzini A et al. Immunoglobulin subclass deficiency. *Pediatr Inf Dis J* 1988; **7**(suppl 5):S17–21.

57. Sneller MC, Strober W, Eisenstein E et al. New insights into common variable immunodeficiency. *Ann Intern Med* 1993; **118**:720–30.

58. Conley ME, Parlk CL, Douglas SD. Childhood common variable immunodeficiency with autoimmune disease. *J Pediatr* 1986; **108**:915–22.

59. Atkinson JP. Complement deficiency: predisposing factor to autoimmune syndromes. *Clin Exp Rheum* 1989; **7**(suppl 3):95–101.

60. Johnston A, Auda GR, Kerr MA et al. Dissociation of primary antigen–antibody bonds is essential for complement mediated solubilization of immune precipitants. *Mol Immunol* 1992; **29**:659–65.

61. Mathe G. Immunity aging. I. The chronic perduration of the thymus acute involution at puberty? Or the participation of the lymphoid organs and cells in fatal physiologic decline? *Biomed Pharmacother* 1997; **51**:49–57.

62. Masi AT, Feigenbaum SL, Chatterton RT. Hormonal and pregnancy relationships to rheumatoid arthritis: convergent effects with immunologic and microvascular systems. *Semin Arthritis Rheum* 1995; **25**:1–27.

63. Grossman CJ. Possible underlying mechanisms

of sexual dimorphism in the immune response, fact and hypothesis. *J Steroid Biochem* 1989; **34**:241–51.

64. Grossman CJ. Interaction between gonadal steroids and the immune system. *Science* 1985; **227**:257–61.

65. Waldhauser F, Ehrhart B, Forster E. Clinical aspects of melatonin action: impact of development, aging and puberty, involvement of melatonin on psychiatric disease and importance of neuroimmunoendocrine interactions. *Experientia* 1993; **49**:671–81.

66. Wilder RL. Neuroendocrine-immune interactions in autoimmunity. *Annu Rev Immunol* 1995; **13**:307–38.

67. Athreya BH, Rafferty JH, Sehgal GS, Lahita RG. Adrenohypophyseal and sex hormones in pediatric rheumatic diseases. *J Rheumatol* 1994; **20**:725–30.

68. Saldanha C, Touzas G, Grace E. Evidence for the anti-inflammatory effects of normal circulating plasma cortisol. *Clin Exp Rheumatol* 1986; **4**: 365–6.

69. Russell DH, Kibler R, Matrisian L et al. Prolactin receptors on human T and B lymphocytes. Antagonism of prolactin binding by cyclosporine. *J Immunol* 1985; **134**:3027–31.

70. McMurray RW, Allen SH, Braun AL et al. Longstanding hyperprolactinemia associated with systemic lupus erythematosus: possible hormonal stimulation of an autoimmune disease. *J Rheumatol* 1994; **21**:843–50.

71. Utsuyama M, Hirokawa K, Mancini C et al. Differential effects of gonadectomy on thymic stromal cells in promoting T cell differentiation in mice. *Mech Aging Dev* 1995; **81**:107–17.

72. Allen RC, Jimenez M, Cowell CT. Insulin-like growth factor and growth hormone secretion in JCA. *Ann Rheum Dis* 1991; **50**:602–6.

73. Neinstein LS, Juliani MA, Shapiro J. Psychological development in normal adolescents. In: *Adolescent Health Care, A Practical Guide* (Neinstein LS, ed), 3rd edn. Williams & Wilkins: Baltimore, 1996:40–5.

74. McAnarney ER. Social maturation. A challenge for handicapped and chronically ill adolescents. *J Adolesc Health* 1985; **6**:90–101.

75. Irwin CE, Millstein SG. Biopsychosocial correlates of risk-taking behaviors during adolescence. Can the physician intervene? *J Adolesc Health* 1986; **7**:82S–96S.

76. Kaplan ME, Friedman SB. Reciprocal influences between chronic illness and adolescent development. *Adolesc Med State Art Rev* 1994; **5**:211–21.

77. Ginsburg KS, Wright EA, Larson MG et al. A controlled study of the prevalence of cognitive dysfunction in randomly selected patients with systemic lupus erythematosus. *Arthritis Rheum* 1992; **35**:776–82.

78. Cappelli M, McGrath PJ, Heick CE et al. Chronic disease and its impact. The adolescent perspective. *J Adolesc Health* 1989; **10**:283–8.

79. Coupey SM, Cohen MI. Special considerations for the health care of adolescents with chronic diseases. *Pediatr Clin North Am* 1984; **31**:211–19.

80. Wolman C, Resnick MD, Harris LJ, Blum RW. Emotional well-being among adolescents with and without chronic conditions. *J Adolesc Health* 1994; **15**:199–204.

81. White PH. Psychosocial aspects of rheumatic disease in childhood and adolescence. *Adolesc Med State Art Rev* 1998; **9**:171–7.

82. Britto MT, Nash AA, Lovell DJ, Passo MH, Rosenthal SL. Substance use among adolescents with juvenile rheumatoid arthritis. *J Rheumatol* 1999; in press.

83. Kellerman J, Zeltzer L, Ellenberg L et al. Psychological effects of illness in adolescence. I. Anxiety, self-esteem, and perception of control. *J Pediatr* 1980; **97**:126–31.

84. Zeltzer L, Kellerman J, Ellenberg L et al. Psychological effects of illness in adolescence. II. Impact of illness in adolescents – crucial issues and coping styles. *J Pediatr* 1989; **97**:132–8.

85. Vandvik IH, Forseth KO. A bio-psychosocial evaluation of ten adolescents with fibromyalgia. *Acta Paediatr* 1994; **83**:766–71.

86. McAnarney ER, Pless IB, Satterwhite B, Friedman SB. Psychological problems of children with chronic juvenile arthritis. *Pediatrics* 1974; **53**:523–8.

87. Ungerer JA, Horgan B, Chaitow J, Champion GD. Psychosocial functioning in children and young adults with juvenile arthritis. *Pediatrics* 1988; **81**:195–202.

88. Miller JJ, Spitz PW, Simpson U, Williams GF. The social function of young adults who had arthritis in childhood. *J Pediatr* 1982; **100**:378–82.

89. Vandvik IH. Mental health and psychological functioning in children with recent onset of rheumatic disease. *J Child Psychiatry* 1990; **31**:961–71.

90. Ruperto N, Levinson JE, Ravelli A et al. Longterm health outcome and quality of life in American

and Italian inception cohorts of patients with juvenile rheumatoid arthritis. *J Rheumatol* 1997; **24**:945–52.

91. Peterson LS, Mason T, Nelson AM et al. Psychosocial outcomes and health status of adults who have had juvenile rheumatoid arthritis. *Arthritis Rheum* 1997; **40**:2235–40.

92. Box MCO, Smyth DP, Thomas AP. Health care of physically handicapped young adults. *Br Med J* 1988; **296**:1153–6.

93. Rapoff MA, Purviance MR, Lindsley CB. Educational and behavioral strategies for improving medication compliance in juvenile rheumatoid arthritis. *Arch Phys Med Rehab* 1988; **69**:439–41.

94. Rapoff MA. Compliance with treatment regimens for pediatric rheumatic diseases. *Arthritis Care Res* 1989; **2**:S40–7.

95. Lichtenstein DR, Syngal S, Wolfe MM. Nonsteroidal antiinflammatory drugs and the gastrointestinal tract. The double-edged sword. *Arthritis Rheum* 1995; **38**:5–18.

96. Cantor B, Tyler T, Nelson RM, Stein GH. Oligohydramnios and transient neonatal anuria: a possible association with the maternal use of prostaglandin synthetase inhibitors. *J Reprod Med* 1980; **24**:220–3.

97. Silveira LH, Hubble CL, Jara LJ et al. Prevention of anticardiolipin antibody related pregnancy losses with prednisone and aspirin. *Am J Med* 1992; **93**:403–10.

98. Beaufils M, Uzan S, Donsimoni R et al. Prevention of pre-eclampsia by early anti-platelet therapy. *Lancet* 1985; **i**:840–2.

99. Rimsza ME. Complications of corticosteroid therapy. *Am J Dis Child* 1978; **132**:806–10.

100. Cassidy JT, Hillman LS. Abnormalities in skeletal growth in children with juvenile rheumatoid arthritis. *Rheum Dis Clin North Am* 1997; **23**:499–521.

101. Markham A, Bryson HM. Deflazacort. A review of its pharmacologic properties and therapeutic efficacy. *Drugs* 1995; **50**:317–33.

102. Loftus J, Allen R, Hesp R et al. Randomized double-blind trial of deflazacort versus prednisone in juvenile chronic (or rheumatoid) arthritis: a relatively bone-sparing effect of deflazacort. *Br J Rheumatol* 1993; **32**(suppl):31–8.

103. Hyams JS, Carey DE. Corticosteroids and growth. *J Pediatr* 1988; **113**:249–54.

104. The Canadian Hydroxychloroquine Study Group. A randomized study of the effect of withdrawing hydroxychloroquine sulfate in systemic lupus erythematosus. *New Engl J Med* 1991; **324**:150–4.

105. Levy GD, Munz SJ, Paschal J et al. Incidence of hydroxychloroquine retinopathy in 1207 patients in a large multicenter outpatient practice. *Arthritis Rheum* 1997; **40**:1482–6.

106. Toth A. Reversible toxic effect of salicylazosulfapyridine on semen quality. *Fertil Steril* 1979; **31**:538.

107. Giannini EH, Brewer EJ, Kuzmina N et al. Methotrexate in resistant juvenile rheumatoid arthritis. *New Engl J Med* 1992; **326**:1043–9.

108. Schnabel A, Gross WL. Low-dose methotrexate in rheumatic diseases – efficacy, side effects and risk factors for side effects. *Semin Arthritis Rheum* 1994; **23**:310–27.

109. Bermas BL, Hill JA. Effects of immunosuppressive drugs during pregnancy. *Arthritis Rheum* 1995; **38**:1722–32.

110. Shaikov AV, Maximov AA, Speransky AI et al. Repetitive use of pulse therapy with methylprednisolone and cyclophosphamide in addition to oral methotrexate in children with systemic juvenile rheumatoid arthritis – preliminary results of a long-term study. *J Rheumatol* 1992; **19**:612–16.

111. Fox DA, McCune WJ. Immunosuppressive drug therapy of systemic lupus erythematosus. *Rheum Dis Clin North Am* 1994; **20**:265–99.

112. McCune WJ, Golbus J, Zeldes W et al. Clinical and immunologic effects of monthly administration of intravenous cyclophosphamide in severe systemic lupus erythematosus. *New Engl J Med* 1988; **318**:1423–31.

113. Reinhold-Keller E, Kekow J, Schnabel A et al. Influence of disease manifestations and antineutrophil cytoplasmic antibody titer on the response to pulse cyclophosphamide therapy in patients with Wegener's granulomatosis. *Arthritis Rheum* 1994; **37**:919–24.

114. Boumpas DT, Austin HA, Vaughan EM et al. Risk for sustained amenorhea in patients with systemic lupus erythematosus receiving intermittent pulse cyclophosphamide therapy. *Ann Intern Med* 1993; **119**:366–9.

115. Byrne J, Mulvihill JJ, Myers MH et al. Effects of treatment on fertility in long-term survivors of childhood or adolescent cancer. *New Engl J Med* 1987; **317**:1315–21.

116. Chapman RM, Sutcliffe SB. Protection of ovarian function by oral contraceptives in females receiving chemotherapy for Hodgkin's disease. *Blood* 1981; **58**:849–51.

117. Blumenfeld Z, Lorber M, Yoffe N, Scharf Y. Systemic lupus erythematosus: predisposition for uterine cervical dysplasia. *Lupus* 1994; **3**:59–61.

118. Ognenovski V, Farrehl J, Selvaggi S, McCune WJ. Increased cervical atypia in women with systemic lupus erythematosus treated with intravenous pulse cyclophosphamide. *Arthritis Rheum* 1996; **39**:S213.

119. Aguirre MA, Jimena PJ, Andres MD et al. Gynaecological abnormalities in women with systemic lupus erythematosus: a prospective controlled study. *Arthritis Rheum* 1996; **39**: S213.

120. Boukris SV, Menkes CJ, Charrier A et al. Risk of genital cancer in women with systemic lupus erythematosus. *Arthritis Rheum* 1996; **39**:S213.

121. Luff RD, Berek JS, Bibbo M et al. The Bethesda System for reporting cervical/vaginal cytologic diagnoses. *Acta Cytol* 1993; **37**:115–24.

122. Roye CF. Abnormal cervical cytology in adolescents: a literature review. *J Adolesc Health* 1992; **13**:643–50.

123. Henderson CJ, Lovell DJ, Passo MH. Onset of menarche in females with juvenile rheumatoid arthritis and healthy controls. Paper presented at Park City IV, March 1998, abstract T7.

124. Gonzalez-Crespo MR, Gonek-Reino GJJ, Merino R et al. Menstrual disorders in girls with systemic lupus erythematosus treated with cyclophosphamide. *Br J Rheumatol* 1995; **34**:737–41.

125. Miller JJ, Williams GF, Leissring JC. Multiple late complications of therapy with cyclophosphamide – including ovarian destruction. *Am J Med* 1971; **50**:530–5.

126. Ammann AJ, Johnson A, Fyfe G et al. Behçet syndrome. *J Pediatr* 1985; **107**:41–3.

127. Rakover Y, Adar H, Itamar T et al. Behçet disease: long-term follow-up of three children and review of the literature. *Pediatrics* 1989; **83**:986–91.

128. Fresko I, Yazici H, Isci H, Yurdakul S. Genital ulceration in patients with systemic lupus erythematosus. *Lupus* 1993; **2**:135.

129. Hughes RA, Keat AC. Reiter's syndrome and reactive arthritis: a current view. *Semin Arthritis Rheum* 1994; **24**:190–210.

130. Ostensen M. The effects of pregnancy on ankylosing spondylitis, psoriatic arthritis and JCA. *Am J Reprod Immunol* 1992; **28**:235–7.

131. Ostensen M. Pregnancy in patients with a history of juvenile chronic arthritis. *Arthritis Rheum* 1991; **34**:881–7.

132. Urowitz MB, Gladman DD, Farewell VT et al. Lupus and pregnancy studies. *Arthritis Rheum* 1993; **36**:1392–7.

133. Waltuck J, Buyon JP. Autoantibody associated congenital heart block: outcome in mothers and children. *Ann Intern Med* 1994; **120**:544–51.

134. Lynch A, Marlar M, Murphy J et al. Antiphospholipid antibodies in predicting adverse pregnancy outcome. A prospective study. *Ann Intern Med* 1994; **120**:470–5.

135. Tabbutt S, Griswold WR, Ogino MT et al. Multiple thromboses in a premature infant associated with maternal phospholipid antibody syndrome. *J Perinatol* 1994; **14**:66–70.

136. Spitz AM, Velebil P, Koonin LM et al. Pregnancy, abortion, and birth rates among US adolescents – 1980, 1985, and 1990. *JAMA* 1996; **275**:989–94.

137. Alexander CS, Guyer B. Adolescent pregnancy: occurrence and consequences. *Pediatr Ann* 1993; **22**:85–8.

138. Neinstein LS, Katz B. Contraceptive use in the chronically ill adolescent female. Part I. *J Adolesc Health Care* 1986; **7**:123–33.

139. Hill RH, Herstein A, Walters K. Juvenile rheumatoid arthritis: follow-up into adulthood – medical, sexual and social status. *Can Med J* 1976; **114**:790–6.

140. Neinstein LS, Katz B. Contraceptive use in the chronically ill adolescent female. Part II. *J Adolesc Health Care* 1986; **7**:350–60.

141. Petri M, Robinson C. Oral contraceptives and systemic lupus erythematosus. *Arthritis Rheum* 1997; **40**:797–803.

142. Julkunen HA, Kaaja R, Friman C. Contraceptive practice in women with systemic lupus erythematosus. *Br J Rheumatol* 1993; **32**:227–30.

143. Guerrero JS, Diaz JR, Peralta MM, Galindo MCC. Contraception in systemic lupus erythematosus, methods utilized by female patients. *Arthritis Rheum* 1997; **40**:S304.

144. Frederiksen MC. Depot medroxyprogesterone acetate contraception in women with medical problems. *J Reprod Med* 1996; **41**(suppl):414–18.

145. Kaunitz AM. Long-acting injectable contraception with depot medroxyprogesterone acetate. *Am J Obstet Gynecol* 1994; **170**:1543–9.

146. Brennan P, Bankhead C, Silman A, Symmons D. Oral contraceptives and rheumatoid arthritis: results from a primary care-based incident case-control study. *Semin Arthritis Rheum* 1997; **25**:817–23.

147. Koepsell T, Dugowson C, Voigt L. Preliminary

findings from a case-control study of the risk of rheumatoid arthritis in relation to oral contraceptive use. *Br J Rheumatol* 1989; **28**(suppl 1):41–5.

148. Rai R, Cohen H, Dave M, Regan L. Randomised controlled trial of aspirin and aspirin plus heparin in pregnant women with recurrent miscarriage associated with phospholipid antibodies (or antiphospholipid antibodies). *Br Med J* 1997; **314**:253–7.

17

Nutrition and the adolescent with rheumatic disease

Carol J Henderson, Barbara E Ostrov, Richard L Levine and Daniel J Lovell

INTRODUCTION

Physical growth and sexual maturation are prominent features of adolescence. All adolescents experience periods of acute self-consciousness during which they are extremely sensitive to 'difference' and are anxious about their progress through puberty. When this progression is disturbed by chronic disease, it is not only distressing to the teenager but may interfere with psychosocial development.[1] The common plea of these teenagers is to be treated according to their age rather than their appearance. It is essential for paediatricians and rheumatologists caring for children and adolescents to recognize and address growth and sexual development problems resulting from either the rheumatic disease or the treatment. This requires obtaining accurate measurements of weight, stature and sexual maturation at each visit, for early identification of potential abnormalities in pubertal development. The onset and progression of puberty varies considerably, and pubertal delay may be exaggerated and can occur more frequently in the face of a chronic illness.

The risks and benefits of all treatments considered should be weighed carefully to minimize their impact on growth. Growth-compromising treatments should be used with discretion, nutrition should be monitored for dietary adequacy, and nutritional supplementation should be considered when it is necessary. While in most instances abnormal growth and development can be explained adequately by the disease alone, other explanations must be carefully considered.[2] The identification of abnormal growth and maturation must always occur early and be corrected if possible before epiphyseal closure after which the window of opportunity for catch-up growth is lost.

This chapter contrasts recommended dietary needs and actual intake of healthy adolescents, summarizes publications about the observed nutritional status of children with rheumatic diseases, reviews nutritional concerns and approaches associated with steroid treatment, discusses dietary and disease-related aspects of osteoporosis, and reviews nutritional aspects of short stature that can occur in adolescents with a rheumatic disease.

DEVELOPMENT AND DIETARY NEEDS

The sequence of sexual maturation, growth patterns, nutritional requirements and food choices of adolescents can be characterized as diverse. The most consistent difference among adolescents is that the growth spurt in girls begins about 2 years before that in boys.

Accelerated growth or the adolescent growth spurt is closely linked to the process of sexual maturation. Timing of the growth spurt is influenced by many genetic and environmental factors. Growth and sexual maturation patterns of family members in past generations are generally predictive of those in subsequent generations. Both transform a child into an adult, and involve substantial changes in nutritional requirements. Good health and adequate nutrition during childhood are strong positive influences on the rate of growth before and during adolescence. When making nutritional recommendations for adolescents, many factors must be considered. Because of wide variations during pubescence, chronological age is an inadequate index of physical growth and, therefore, of nutritional requirements. A practical method of evaluating nutritional adequacy is by monitoring growth. Growth patterns can be tracked on standardized height and weight growth charts. These charts make it possible to compare the growth progress of an adolescent with others of the same age, gender and race via percentile rankings. By using growth charts, growth trends can be monitored over many years.

The onset of puberty is associated with an increased growth rate, changes in body composition, increased bone mineralization and altered physical activity levels. On average, girls reach their peak growth rate at about 11.5 years, and boys reach theirs at about 13.5 years. Most of the accelerated growth rate attained during pubescence lasts an average of 2–3 years, but may persist for 5–7 years before growth stops.[3]

Before puberty, there is little or no difference in the body composition of males and females, with fat constituting 15–20% of total body weight. During pubescence, girls show a striking increase in total body fat during sexual maturation, while boys have both an absolute and a relative decrease in total body fat. The most recent study to compare age of onset of menses in 53 Caucasian American females with juvenile rheumatoid arthritis (JRA, as defined in Chapter 5) and 50 healthy controls showed no significant difference in the mean age of menarche (12.7 and 12.5 years, respectively) (C Henderson, unpublished data). In this study the JRA and control population means for age of menarche were similar to current US statistics, which report the mean age (± standard deviation (SD)) of onset of menses as 12.9 (± 1.2) years for Caucasian females and 12.2 (± 1.2) years for African-American females.[4] The onset of menses is also closely linked to the growth process and will have a last-

ing impact on the adolescent female's nutritional requirements. One important nutritional implication of the start of menstruation is that the blood lost during each menstrual period contains iron that must be replaced by the diet.

Pre-adolescent growth in lean body mass is roughly linear, with boys having a slightly higher velocity. However, the growth spurt during puberty shows a tremendous sex difference, with both intensity and duration being greater in boys. A boy's nutritional needs at this time of life far exceed those of a girl.[5] Between the ages of 10 and 20 years, the average male lean body mass increases by 35 kg (range 27–62 kg), whereas females increase by only half as much (25–43 kg). The basal metabolic rate of pubescent males is higher than that of females, presumably because of their greater muscle mass. As the body grows, the amount of blood it contains must increase to keep pace with its increasing demands for oxygen. The ability to produce enough red blood cells depends on an adequate supply of iron from the diet.

NUTRITIONAL REQUIREMENTS AND RECOMMENDATIONS FOR THE HEALTHY ADOLESCENT

Few data are available on nutrient requirements that correlate with biological events during puberty. An adequate energy intake with high-quality protein is essential for optimal growth during puberty. The iron and calcium requirements of both males and females are of particular concern during adolescence.[6]

The keys to a healthy diet are variety, balance and moderation. Dietary guidelines for Americans include the following: eat a variety of foods; maintain healthy weight; choose a diet low in fat, saturated fat and cholesterol; choose a diet with plenty of vegetables, fruits and grain products; use sugars, salt and sodium in moderation.[7] Adherence to this prudent diet, including the incorporation of appropriate snacks, can provide a balanced diet that will meet the nutrient requirements of healthy teenagers.

For many nutrients, especially vitamins and minerals, few data are available based on measurements in adolescents. The nutritional health of America's youth is far better today than at any other time in the past. With the exception of iron and calcium deficiencies, overt nutrient deficiency diseases are not public health problems today as they were earlier in the century up until the 1940s. As problems of nutrient deficiency have diminished, they have been replaced by problems of dietary imbalance and excess. Dietary excesses of calories, sugar, fat, cholesterol, sodium and caffeine are common among adolescents.[8,9] Inadequate dietary intake of vitamins A, B$_6$ and folic acid, and minerals including iron, calcium and zinc are also evident, especially among teenagers of low socio-economic status and among females.[6]

Due to the concern that certain dietary habits established in adolescence may continue into adulthood, the combination of current dietary patterns and other factors could result in increased risk for the development of chronic disease, such as heart disease, osteoporosis and some types of cancer, in later life.

Recommended nutrient needs

Calories

Optimal growth requires adequate caloric and nutrient intake. It is often difficult to determine the exact calorie needs of an adolescent, as individual teenagers differ so much in size, activity level and growth rate. The US Recommended Dietary Allowance (RDA) of calories during adolescence is 2500–3000 calories per day for boys and 2200 calories per day for girls.[10] These estimates are based on the average caloric intakes of adolescents with average body weights and light activity levels. The RDA for caloric intake is best used as a guide, rather than a rigid standard. An appropriate way to determine whether an adolescent is getting an adequate amount of calories is to monitor their height and weight gain.

Macronutrients

Macronutrients include protein, carbohydrates and fats. Protein is essential for growth, development and maintenance of the body, and is also a source of energy. The RDA for protein varies with body weight, age and sex. Protein

should constitute a minimum of 7–8% of the total caloric intake in healthy teenager's diet.

Vitamins and minerals

During the adolescent years, the amount of vitamins and minerals required for growth and development increases. A well-balanced and varied diet generally provides an adequate supply of vitamins and minerals, making supplementation unnecessary. Many adolescents, however, have marginal or deficient intake of calcium, iron and folate because they consume inadequate amounts of vegetables, meat and dairy products. Folate is a B vitamin found primarily in green leafy vegetables, seeds, asparagus and beans. If deficient, low folate intakes can cause one form of anaemia. Folate deficiency is not uncommon in adolescents because the best food sources are often those not favoured by teenagers.

Calcium

Calcium intake during adolescence appears to affect skeletal calcium retention directly, and a calcium intake of up to 1600 mg/day in healthy adolescents may be required based on previous epidemiological, clinical and experimental studies.[11] In adolescent females at the time of puberty, bone mineral accretion is at a lifetime maximum and this represents the optimal time to maximize peak bone mass using calcium as an early preventive measure against the risk for developing osteoporosis. New recommended intakes for calcium were set by the US National Academy of Sciences in August of 1997. These values, referred to as Adequate Intakes (AIs), replaced the RDAs. The AI amounts are levels determined to maximize bone strength and prevent osteoporosis. The AI for males and females aged 9–18 years is 1300 mg calcium/day. Calcium is the nutrient most often consumed in inadequate amounts during teenage years, and girls have documented low calcium intake beginning as early as 11–12 years of age.[11] Mean calcium intake has been reported to decline with age. A recent study of about 900 healthy US adolescents documented a median calcium intake of 1016 mg/day for males and 676 mg/day for females. More than 75% of adolescent females and approximately 60% of males failed to meet the

RDA guidelines (1200 mg/day) for calcium.[12] Adolescent peer group influences on behaviour[3,5,12] and, for young women, societal pressures to be thin not only affect food intake,[6,12,13] but specifically reduce calcium intake due to intentional avoidance of dairy products.[12]

FOOD CUSTOMS AND CHOICES, BODY IMAGE, EATING BEHAVIOURS

By the time adolescence has arrived, teenagers have developed a set of attitudes, preferences, values and habits regarding food different from all other age groups, and these perspectives and actions stay with them as they move to adulthood. A variety of circumstances, including the amount of time family members allocate to food preparation and eating, activities and schedules of teenagers that conflict with family routines, busy schedules that result in 'eating on the go', peer influences and advertising influence the development of an adolescent's food customs and choices. Frequently these circumstances make for unfavourable food choices and patterns that hinder development of healthy nutrition habits.

Adolescents typically develop behavioural patterns that are often explained by a teenager's newly found independence, dissatisfaction with body image, search for self-identity, peer acceptance and conformity of lifestyle, and therefore become motivated to modify their diets in order to initiate change. Fear of becoming overweight can result in excessive restriction of intake or use of weight-loss products that can diminish growth. Many adolescent males desire enhanced muscle development, and secondarily will subscribe to the use of expensive, muscle-building supplements. These products are ineffective when adequate protein and calories are consumed in an adolescent's regular diet.

Some adolescents adhere to vegetarianism or extremely restrictive dietary regimens such as Zen macrobiotic diets that, when strictly adopted, can result in malnutrition, growth retardation and even death. Carefully planned vegetarian diets can provide adequate nutrition throughout the lifecycle. Careful attention must be given to specific nutrients, especially calcium, vitamins D and B_{12}, iron, zinc and sufficient calories to ensure adequate intake in adolescence. The principles of variety, balance and moderation apply equally to vegetarian and traditional diets.[14]

The prevalence of obesity is on the rise, and it is estimated that 10–25% of children and adolescents in North America are substantially overweight.[15] Inactivity and poor dietary habits are the most notable contributors to excess weight gain in adolescents. It is not uncommon for teenagers to skip meals, most often breakfast, and then snack to compensate for a missed meal. Snacks are typically chosen because they are accessible and convenient. They are frequently high in fat, have minimal vitamin and mineral density, and can easily make up 25% or more of daily caloric intake. Snacking does not have to be undesirable if the foods selected are healthful. It is often difficult to prescribe forms of exercise as a means by which obese adolescents with a rheumatic disease can increase energy expenditure. The amount and form of exercise should be individualized and prescribed according to the disease type, involvement and severity.

There is great temptation for obese adolescents to subscribe to 'miracle diets' to shed unwanted pounds. There is no 'quick fix' in order to overcome obesity. Successful weight reduction requires long-term lifestyle changes, including changes in food preferences and selection, exercise and attitude.

NUTRITION-RELATED ABNORMALITIES IN ADOLESCENTS WITH RHEUMATIC DISEASE

A number of studies have reported alterations in the nutritional status and abnormal dietary nutrient intake in adolescents with rheumatic disease.[16–25] Signs of malnutrition in adolescents with arthritis should not be unexpected. A variety of factors can affect nutritional status, including chronic inflammation, anorexia, reduced motility, medication and mechanical problems.

Observed nutritional status

The occurrence of protein-energy malnutrition (PEM) has been reported in 10–50% of those adolescents with arthritis.[16–19,25,26] In a non-random sample of Swedish girls aged 11–16 years with juvenile chronic arthritis (JCA, as defined in Chapter 5) and 28 controls, 19% of patients who had arthritis and 0% of controls were malnourished.[18] The patients with JCA had lower mid-arm circumference (MAC), serum albumin and prealbumin (PAB) levels and higher triceps skinfold (TSF) measures than did controls on a similar diet. These alterations were more pronounced in patients with active disease, and were only found in systemic or polyarticular involvement. Similar observations of lower MAC have been reported in other studies.[19,20] However, additional studies report no significant difference or below normal TSF measurements in patients with chronic arthritis compared to controls.[22,23] Warady et al[25] observed somatic muscle measurements that were less than the 50th percentile in over 50% of patients with arthritis, while subcutaneous fat stores were elevated.

Preliminary results from a small, randomly selected group of JRA patients demonstrated evidence of PEM in 47% of 19 patients; however, only 5% were below normal for TSF.[16] Similarly, 36% of 28 JRA patients were identified as malnourished.[19] Short half-life visceral proteins, PAB and retinol binding protein (RBP) were below normal in 37%, but the longer half-life protein, albumin, was normal in all subjects. Almost 20% of these patients believed to have no nutritional impairments by the managing rheumatology team were PEM, and required nutritional repletion. These findings underscore the potential for all types of patients with childhood-onset arthritis to develop PEM and the relative insensitivity of observable clinical stigmata.[19]

A word of caution is provided to the reader regarding the comparability of anthropometric findings documented in these studies. Several studies evaluated patients who were treated with corticosteroids, whereas other studies intentionally excluded corticosteroid-treated patients. As corticosteroids promote catabolism, those patients most likely to receive steroids for severe inflammation are also the ones most likely to have PEM.[24] In reports on the nutritional status of patients with juvenile idiopathic arthritis (JIA) or in rheumatic diseases that may require corticosteroid therapy, it is often difficult to discriminate between the possible effects of steroids and those due to the disease itself. The severity of inflammation is another crucial factor to bear in mind when evaluating nutritional status, especially in view of the variability of symptoms of patients with rheumatic disease.

In an attempt to isolate the effects of childhood-onset arthritis on nutritional status, Strano et al[22] studied a select group of 17 patients with active disease who had never received corticosteroids compared to 17 age- and sex-matched controls. Patients with systemic-onset arthritis had significantly lower values for height ($p < 0.05$), MAC ($p < 0.05$) and arm muscle area ($p < 0.01$), and in polyarticular subjects for arm muscle area ($p < 0.01$). No differences were detected between the patients and controls for TSF measures, and all anthropometric measurements were normal in pauciarticular patients.

Evaluation of the nutritional status in 15 Norwegian patients with JCA aged 12–14 years and 17 healthy controls demonstrated a decrease in serum concentrations of iron and zinc in polyarticular patients compared to controls ($p < 0.01$), and serum copper was increased ($p < 0.01$).[23] A reduction in serum iron and zinc was also observed in the patients with JCA assessed by Strano et al.[22] Biochemical abnormalities in systemic and polyarticular patients observed by Bacon et al[21] included low plasma levels of vitamins A and C, decreased serum albumin, PAB, RBP and zinc, and increased levels of copper and glutathione peroxidase activity. Johansson et al[18] reported a decrease in plasma selenium in patients with JCA compared to controls.

Dietary nutrient intake abnormalities

Nutrient intake and its relationship to nutritional status and body composition are additional concerns in patients with chronic arthritis. A study utilizing indirect calorimetry demonstrated that measured metabolic need for these patients was not greater than standard nutrient estimates based on age, sex and height.[16] Actual intake based on dietary analysis of a 3-day diet diary showed a median caloric intake of 285 kcal/day below the median measured metabolic need based on indirect calorimetry. Mean calorie and vitamin E intakes below the RDA were observed by Bacon et al[21] in patients with systemic-onset JRA. In a population of patients with arthritis who were mainly Hispanic, the combined mean caloric intake for all forms was 74% of the RDA.[17] Nutrient intake analysis revealed that the patients had mean calcium and iron intakes that were 50–80% of the RDA. In contrast, Strano et al[22] found no difference in calorie, zinc or copper intakes in patients with active arthritis compared to age- and sex-matched controls. Haugen et al[23] reported that dietary calcium intake was reduced in patients with JCA compared to controls ($p = 0.05$), in spite of slightly higher calorie and protein intakes in patients with arthritis. Moreover, the median intake of iron and zinc did not reach the RDA in either patients with arthritis or controls.

Anorexia

Anorexia, or poor appetite, that impedes routine adequate caloric intake, is a major nutritional problem in children and adolescents with chronic inflammatory illness and occurs most commonly in periods of increased articular or systemic inflammation. Although many factors are contributory, proinflammatory cytokines have been demonstrated to cause profound anorexia in experimental animals and humans,[26] and have been shown to be present in elevated amounts in children with arthritis.[27] The chronic arthritides are those in which the vast majority of nutritional investigations have been published and thus the majority of reported observations are in these diseases. Chronic inflammation dramatically alters what tissues account for losses in body weight. Weight loss due to inadequate intake in a healthy individual without an inflammatory component is approximately 90% from fat stores and 10% from lean mass stores. However, weight loss in the presence of underlying inflammation is accounted for by 50% loss in lean body mass and 50% from fat.[28] This inflammation-related anorexia is not only severe enough to alter body composition, but frequently serves as a primary contributor to poor growth and development in patients with idiopathic arthritis. Several studies document inadequate caloric intake in these patients compared to healthy controls or the RDA.[17,20,21,26]

Body composition abnormalities

Body composition abnormalities resulting in marked lean body mass wasting in the presence of normal or elevated subcutaneous fat reserves is a common observation in patients with JRA.[16,19,25] This is a likely result of inflammation shifting protein metabolism, inadequate dietary protein intake and disuse atrophy resulting from articular involvement in an extremity that can limit mobility and promote muscle weakening.[30] In order for muscles to grow, dietary protein and adequate supplies of minerals, particularly iron and zinc, are required. Nearly double the amount of protein, or 15–20% of total caloric intake, may be required to replete nutritionally an adolescent experiencing a decrease in lean body mass as a result of inflammation. Nutritional supplements that afford additional amounts of protein and calories can be useful only when taken in addition to an adequate, balanced diet in adolescents with a rheumatic disease who are attempting to replete lean body mass.

Physicians should warn against the use of creatine, a nutritional supplement advertised as a muscle-builder that is sold as a powder, capsules, candy and even chewing gum. Not unlike many other proclaimed 'dietary miracles', creatine may have serious negative effects. The creatine dosage recommended for athletes is typically in excess of 20 g/day, equivalent to the amount found in 20 8-oz steaks. In these high doses, creatine can contribute to dehydration because liquid is shunted into and retained in the muscle, therefore reducing the body's ability to cool down through the production of sweat. The safety of any dose and long-term efficacy of this unregulated dietary supplement has not been determined.

Obesity

Obesity can occur in adolescents with a rheumatic disease, independent of corticosteroid use. The observed frequency in a randomly selected population of patients with JIA was 19%, which is less than the observed 28% frequency of obesity reported in a national survey of healthy American school-aged children.[15] In patients with more severe rheumatic diseases, such as systemic lupus erythematosus (SLE), juvenile dermatomyositis (JDMS) and systemic vasculitis, systemic steroids are prescribed frequently and for a long time. Corticosteroids have a negative impact on many facets of an individual's nutritional status, including accelerated catabolism, negative calcium balance, growth retardation and weight gain. These developments are harmful; but each can be minimized or avoided, with persistent nutritional intervention initiated as soon as corticosteroids are prescribed. The initial instruction regarding adherence to a low sodium and reduced calorie diet should be arranged not only for the adolescent, but should also include all significant friends and family members interested and/or involved in providing support for the patient treated with corticosteroids. Continued ongoing, frequent nutrition counselling by a trained dietitian to provide new dietary suggestions and to instruct and implement additional behaviour and habit modification techniques (including self-monitoring, contracting and goal-setting) in an effort to minimize weight gain associated with moderate-to-large doses of corticosteroids is critical to minimize the weight gain associated with corticosteroid use.

Excessive weight gain due to corticosteroids and secondary complications including hypertension and hyperglycaemia can be circumvented if the dietary recommendations outlined above are implemented. The following provides an example: a newly diagnosed 12-year-old female with juvenile dermatomyositis initially received prednisone 1.5 mg/kg/day. Her pre-illness weight and height were recorded at the 50th percentile. This patient lost weight prior to diagnosis and regained the amount lost soon after initiation of corticosteroids. Her weight reached a plateau, and both weight and height remained between the 50th and 75th percentiles throughout the 2 years while continuing to receive corticosteroids. This was accomplished by providing nutrition counselling at each follow-up visit.

Anaemia

Anaemia is often present in children with arthritis[30,31] and its severity is usually correlated with the level of underlying inflammation. Patients with arthritis often demonstrate a moderate to severe normocytic hypochromic anaemia with a haemoglobin in the range 4–11 g/dl.[31] This anaemia is primarily a result of chronic inflammation resulting in sequestration of iron in the reticuloendothelial cells.[32] Iron deficiency anaemia may also develop because of poor dietary intake, which is reported to be common in adolescents, gastrointestinal blood loss secondary to medication, or preferential uptake of iron by inflamed synovial tissue.[32,33]

Anaemia occurs in approximately one-half of the children and teenagers with SLE and is usually typical of that seen in patients with JIA and other chronic diseases.[30] The cause of anaemia in SLE is often multifactorial and can be a result of blood loss, including menorrhagia and haemorrhage from the gastrointestinal tract related to ulceration and thrombocytopenia or to autoimmune haemolytic anaemia.

BONE MINERALIZATION

Developmental overview

During growth, bones and cartilage change in shape, proportion and microstructure. In the axial skeleton and extremities, bone develops by ossification of the pre-existing cartilage. As the chondrocytes proliferate, they migrate towards the ends of the bones, and then those cells closest to the middle of the bone ossify. These processes are influenced by, among other things, thyroxine, growth hormone and, during puberty, sex hormones. Chondrocytes synthesize cellular matrix, which is primarily made of collagen and proteoglycans, as well as the enzymes that have the ability to break down these components. Collagen strength and stability are maximized by cross-linking, which increases with advancing age.[34] Developmental changes also occur in the proteoglycans.[35] With increasing age, the proteoglycan aggregates get larger, with greater amounts of keratan sulphate and hyaluronic acid. At the same time, chondroitin sulphate levels fall.[36] Collagen and cartilage components are also antigenic, and may play a role in the development of autoimmune and degenerative joint diseases.[37] The age-related changes in these tissues may influence the distribution and clinical features of the childhood arthritides. The changes in the collagen and cellular matrix during the first two decades of life lead to decreased porosity and increased density of the bone.[38] In addition to increasing age, bone mineralization is also correlated with height and weight, and is dependent on genetic factors, nutrition, exercise and general medical health.

Natural history of bone mineralization in JIA

Calcium loss is common in patients with JIA, occurring early in the disease even in children not on corticosteroids as assessed from plain radiographs.[39] In the acute phase, bone loss occurs by resorption on the endosteal surface, resulting in diminished bone mass which can persist into adulthood.[39] In the older literature, generalized osteoporosis, pathological long bone fractures and vertebral crush fractures were reported in 15–26% of patients with chronic arthritis in studies using standard radiographic assessment.[40–41] However, significant osteopenia continues to be present in these patients. More recent studies that have measured both axial and appendicular bone mineral density (BMD) in patients with JIA have demonstrated significantly subnormal BMD and bone mineral content (BMC) levels in both the axial and appendicular skeleton.[42–45] In studies including older patients, peak bone mass was shown to be significantly decreased.[42,46]

Bone density has been assessed in normal children and those with chronic diseases.[47–50] A number of techniques have been employed, including single photon absorptiometry (SPA), dual photon absorptiometry (DPA) and, most recently, dual-energy x-ray absorptiometry (DEXA). DEXA is the best current method employed because of its low radiation, speed and accuracy. Biochemical markers of bone formation (bone-specific alkaline phosphatase, osteo-

calcin (OC) and carboxy terminal propeptide of type 1 procollagen) and bone resorption (plasma tartrate resistant acid phosphatase) can also be helpful in the evaluation of bone density.

A recent review by Cassidy and Hillman[49] has outlined the abnormalities in bone deposition in patients with chronic arthritis. Studies have demonstrated reduced bone mineral density in these patients. A number of factors influence the acquisition of bone mass in children with arthritis, and put them at risk for osteopenia. These factors include poor nutrition and inadequate dietary intake of calcium and vitamin D, diminished levels of activity secondary to disease activity, and the severity and effect of chronic inflammation. A number of studies have implicated circulating inflammatory mediators as an additional cause of osteopenia.[26,27]

Studies in children with chronic arthritis have demonstrated abnormalities in bone mineral acquisition. They have suggested that decreased bone formation is the primary problem, rather than increased resorption of bone. Appendicular cortical bone is predominantly affected, and there is a failure of patients to develop adequate skeletal mass, especially at puberty. Hopp et al[47] used DPA to measure bone density in 20 patients with JRA and compared them with 20 matched controls. Spinal bone density and total body BMD were similar in the prepubertal children, but significantly decreased in the postpubertal girls with JRA. In addition, this study suggested that the severity of the disease influences the accretion of bone mass. Hopp et al[48] repeated the scans in their patients and demonstrated a significant increase in BMD in patients after an improvement in their disease activity with intensive management. It is not known precisely why bone mineralization is affected by disease severity. A decrease in physical activity has been suggested, as has the influence of mediators of inflammation, such as cytokines. In addition, other studies have demonstrated low levels of OC, a marker of bone growth, and decreased BMC in patients with acute inflammation.[49,50] Normal OC levels and improved BMC are measured in children with successfully managed illness and in children with inactive disease. The sensitivity of OC levels in the face of corticosteroid treatment, however, has been questioned by Reeve et al.[51] They demonstrated that OC was a poor predictor of bone mineralization rates in glucocorticoid-treated JCA patients.

Cassidy and Hillman[49] have suggested that patients with chronic arthritis be monitored with DEXA scans to assess bone-mass accretion and growth. Data regarding the correct therapeutic interventions are lacking; however, improved exercise and nutrition would be important treatments. Reed et al[52] have studied the effect of 25-hydroxyvitamin D therapy in children with active JRA. They demonstrated normalization of serum OC levels and reduced urinary excretion of calcium in these patients. However, no change in bone density measurements was found after 6 or 12 months of supplementation. Longer duration of such interventions may prove beneficial. At the current time, aggressive treatment to suppress disease activity and inflammation appears to be the most successful mechanism to improve bone mass acquisition and prevent or modify the development of osteopenia in these patients.

Bone mineralization in JDMS and SLE

Abnormalities in BMD have also been detected in some children with JDMS[53] and SLE[53,54] In JDMS, corticosteroid effects, muscle atrophy and inactivity, development of calcinosis and abnormalities in OC have been implicated as potential causes.[55] In SLE, the use of glucocorticoids, disease activity and the presence of avascular necrosis are associated with increased risk of osteoporosis.[54] This complication has also been attributed to the effects of cytokines and inflammation.[55] In other studies, high-dose corticosteroids have not been found to play a role in SLE-associated osteoporosis.[54] Nonetheless, given the profound effects of corticosteroids on growth and bone density in children, glucocorticoid use should be minimized as much as possible, with early use of steroid-sparing agents in the management of these diseases.

Development of peak bone mass

As bones grow, their dimensions change and they alter the shape and size of the maturing body. Bone is the major reservoir for calcium, accounting for 99% of total body calcium. Almost half of the adult skeletal mass is formed during adolescence, and calcium accumulation normally triples during the pubertal growth spurt.[47,56,57] Maximal deposition of mineral in the skeleton during adolescence is important in order to offset the inexorable bone loss that accompanies ageing, especially in women. A critical factor in the development of osteoporosis is peak bone mass. As mentioned previously, optimal intake of calcium, the crucial mineral involved in bone growth, must be achieved in adolescence to ensure that bone development is not compromised by an inadequate supply of building material. It is unknown if the recommended calcium intake should be higher for adolescents with joint inflammation or corticosteroid use than for healthy teenagers. Peak calcium requirements occur during the first month of life and during the adolescent growth spurt.

By 24 months after menarche, adolescent females will have attained approximately 90–95% of their peak bone mass. A study of non-corticosteroid treated postpubertal females with JRA revealed that nearly 20% of these patients who had attained peak bone mass were osteopenic, based on the World Health Organization definition[58] (total body BMD z-score $\leq \sim 1.0$), compared with age-, race- and sex-matched healthy controls assessed using DEXA, and consequently were at increased risk for the development of osteoporosis (C Henderson, D Lovell, unpublished data). Osteopenia, or low bone density, is not a benign disorder. Numerous studies in adults have demonstrated that a decrease of 1 SD in BMD is associated with a 50–100% increase in the incidence of hip or spine fractures.[59–62] Due to the growth potential inherent in children and teenagers there is an opportunity to maximize attainment of adult peak mass, thus reducing the potential risk of developing osteoporosis.

The most commonly recognized modifiable factors related to suboptimal bone mass in adolescents are low body weight, inadequate calcium intake, inadequate mechanical forces on bones (frequently associated with decreased physical activity) and menstrual irregularities.[47,62] BMD is enhanced by weight-bearing physical activity and adequate vitamin D intake. Pubescent and postpubescent subjects of both genders have a lower level of activity than prepubescent children, suggesting that maturation may be an important correlate to a sedentary lifestyle. Puberty may be the transitional period from an active to an inactive way of life.[64] If a carryover of activity patterns does exist from the developmental years to adulthood, the low level of activity in adolescence can be expected to persist into adult years. This trend should be of concern, because a sedentary adult lifestyle has been clearly associated with increased morbidity (e.g. development of osteoporosis) and mortality, particularly due to coronary artery disease.

Although daily physical activity has not been quantitated in adolescent patients with arthritis, a quantifiable reduction in measured daily physical activity in prepubertal children with arthritis compared to healthy controls has been reported.[65] This decline in activity may also exist in adolescence as a result of the development of physical limitations associated with JIA, or imposed activity restrictions recommended by the managing physician that restrain levels of physical activity. This often denies participation in many organized sports that require strenuous weight-bearing activity in order to avoid excessive mechanical stress on the joints.

Medication effects in bone mineralization

Glucocorticoids are widely used in the treatment of some rheumatic diseases in adolescents. One of the most significant side-effects is osteoporosis and related fractures. Glucocorticoid associated bone loss is most obvious during the first 6 months of glucocorticoid use, affects trabecular bone more than cortical bone, and is related to both the dose and duration of therapy. It is probably true that there is no dose of corticosteroids that does not adversely affect bone mineralization. Alternate-day routines have been shown to have the same negative impact on bone mineralization as daily intake, and even inhaled steroids have been shown

to increase bone loss.[66] Glucocorticoids adversely affect bone mineralization by a number of mechanisms that result in both an increase in bone resorption and a decrease in bone formation. The reader is recommended to a number of recent reviews for additional information regarding this complex topic.[67–71]

Data from both adult and paediatric rheumatic disease patients suggest that corticosteroid-induced bone loss can be prevented. As always, the lowest dose of corticosteroids should be used and, unlike other side-effects, changing to an alternate-day schedule offers little benefit. We endorse the recommendations of the American College of Rheumatology Task Force on Osteoporosis Guidelines that call for a total daily calcium intake of 1500 mg/day, and 25-hydroxyvitamin D 400 IU/day,[66] based on studies in adults. Warady et al[72] showed in a cross-over study of 10 adolescent corticosteroid-treated patients with rheumatic disease and osteoporosis, that daily intakes of 1000 mg calcium and 400 IU vitamin D resulted in a mean improvement of 11% in lumbar spine bone mineral density measurements in 6 months ($p \leq 0.02$). When these same patients were withdrawn from the calcium and vitamin D therapy, 7/10 demonstrated a decline in lumbar spine BMD. The age range of the patients in this study was 10.9–18.0 years – essentially an adolescent population. Studies suggest that treatment with calcium and vitamin D supplements alone is sufficient for many patients when on corticosteroids to avoid excessive bone loss. However, not all will respond, and serial measurements of bone mineralization are recommended. Recommendations for treatment of adolescents not responding to calcium and vitamin D are difficult, since only a few, small, open, short-term studies of pharmacological approaches to increasing bone mineral density in children and adolescents have been published.[35] Controlled trials in paediatric patients will need to be performed before treatment recommendations can be made. Certainly, the bone physiology in children and adolescents is much different than that in postmenopausal women, on whom the vast majority of published trials of osteoporosis treatments have been performed.

Methotrexate has been shown to have an inhibitory effect on osteoblasts in vitro,[73] and children with cancer treated with high-dose methotrexate have demonstrated clinically important demineralization.[74] However, studies of BMD in patients with chronic arthritis have failed to demonstrate any significant negative effect of methotrexate on bone mineralization.[42,43,45,46]

SHORT STATURE

Data on growth in adolescents with arthritis has been reported in several long-term observational studies in hospitalized patients or subjects followed in a tertiary centre. Selection biases of patients for these studies most likely resulted in those with more severe disease being seen in these settings, and thus biasing results toward greater observed growth disturbances. In an investigation of 433 hospitalized German children followed, on average, for 15 years over the period 1952–1979, 10% of 209 patients with systemic-onset JCA were below the third percentile for height.[75] Epiphyseal lines were reported as closed in the majority of patients; therefore, their reported height was representative of their adult stature. Svantesson et al[76] followed 33 hospitalized Swedish patients with systemic-onset JCA for 4–24 years (median 10 years). Thirteen patients were reported to be growth retarded, having heights more than 3 SD below the normal mean. All 13 patients were treated with daily corticosteroids for 4 years or more, and 12 of the 13 patients experienced onset of disease before the age of 5 years.

A recent community-based study was designed to determine the natural history and outcome of 133 patients with JCA, utilizing five counties in south-west Sweden, having followed the patients until they reached a median age of 17.7 years.[77] Patients were born between 1968 and 1972 and were studied between 1992 and 1994. Systemic-onset disease was reported in 3.2% of patients, and 29% had polyarticular-onset disease. While 49% continued to have active disease requiring medication, no patients were more than 2 SD below the age-matched comparable population in height. In a cross-sectional study conducted by Hashkes and Lovell,[78] 103 consecutive outpatients with JRA seen in a tertiary centre were evaluated.[79] Disease onset was systemic in 20.4% of patients, polyarticular in 38.8% and pauciarticular in 40.8%. Overall, 16% of the patients were at or below the 5th percentile for height ($p = 0.03$) compared with the normal population. Less than 8% of patients were receiving corticosteroids at the time of assessment, and 28% had received corticosteroids in the past. When comparing the means for height among disease-onset subtypes, JRA patients with systemic onset were significantly shorter than patients with polyarticular- and pauciarticular-onset disease. These two studies confirm previous findings regarding the association of short stature to systemic-onset disease and corticosteroid therapy. However, they do not concur with previous studies that routinely reported that the height of polyarticular- and pauciarticular-onset disease patients fell at or below 3 SD of the mean compared to normal subjects.

Chronic undernutrition seems to be a major contributor to the growth observed in patients with arthritis. In five patients with persistent moderate to severe protein and caloric malnutrition, poor dietary intake despite intensive efforts to maximize volitional oral intake, and significant growth failure, nutritional repletion was accomplished by a combination of nocturnal nasogastric tube feedings and daytime volitional oral intake. The results were remarkable. During the 6 months before the nocturnal nasogastric feedings, on average, the five patients were losing 0.22 kg/month and height velocity was 0.15 cm/month. During the 6 months after initiation of nocturnal tube feedings, the patients averaged a gain of 0.8 kg/month ($p < 0.05$) and the height velocity was 1.62 cm/month ($p < 0.05$). Patients tolerated the nocturnal tube feedings without complications.[79] However, the primary stimulus for the malnutrition was the anorexia and metabolic alterations secondary to the chronic inflammation of chronic arthritis. This nutritional repletion did not improve the inflammatory status (nor did it worsen the inflammation, as was the concern of some), and thus these patients used the nocturnal tube feeds for months to years. This was a small sample of patients, and more experience is needed before a general recommendation is appropriate. However, nocturnal enteral feedings have resulted in significant improvements in growth in other paediatric chronic inflammatory conditions such as inflammatory bowel diseases,[80] chronic renal disease[81] and cystic fibrosis.[82]

SUMMARY

Several observations and conclusions follow from this review of nutritional issues in adolescents with rheumatic disease. Adolescence is indeed a critical time for growth in a number of areas that are directly influenced by nutritional intake, linear growth and bone mineralization. Published studies relating to nutritional issues exist for children with chronic arthritis, but are scarce or non-existent for the other childhood rheumatic diseases, and this remains an important void in our clinical understanding in paediatric rheumatology. The available information supports an important and effective role for nutritional evaluation of all patients with chronic arthritis, early and ongoing nutritional intervention to prevent or minimize excessive weight gain associated with glucocorticoid use, and the role of calcium and vitamin D supplementation in the prevention or treatment of glucocorticoid-induced bone mineral loss.

REFERENCES

1. Gross RT, Duke PM. The effect of early versus late physical maturation on adolescent behavior. *Pediatr Clin North Am* 1980; **27**:71–7.
2. Rosen DS. Pubertal growth and sexual maturation for adolescents with chronic illness or disability. *Pediatrician* 1991; **18**:105–20.
3. Fung T, Anyan WA Jr. Adolescence: life in the fast lane. In: *The Yale Guide to Children's Nutrition* (Tamborlane WV, ed), 1st edn. RR Donnelley: Harrisonburg, 1997:64–73.
4. Herman-Giddens ME, Slora EJ, Wasserman RC. Secondary sexual characteristics and menses in young girls seen in office practice: a study from the pediatric research in office settings network. *Pediatrics* 1997; **99**:505–12.
5. Dwyer JT. Nutrition and the adolescent. In: *Textbook of Pediatric Nutrition* (Suskind RM, Lewinter-Suskind L, eds), 2nd edn. Raven: New York, 1993:257–64.
6. Story M, Heald F, Dwyer J. Adolescent nutrition: trends and critical issues for the 1990s. In: *Call to Action/Better Nutrition for Mothers, Children, and Families*, National Center for Education in Maternal and Child Health: Washington, DC, 1990:169–89.
7. US Department of Agriculture and US Department of Health and Human Services, Dietary Guidelines Advisory Committee. *Report of the Dietary Guidelines Advisory Committee on the Dietary Guidelines for Americans.* Human Nutrition Information Service, US Department of Agriculture: Hyattsville, MD, 1990.
8. US Department of Health and Human Services. *Surgeon General's Report on Nutrition and Health.* Government Printing Office; Washington, DC, 1978, Publication No 88–50210.
9. Ellison RC, Singer MR, Moore LL et al. Current caffeine intake of young children: amount and sources. *Res Professional Briefs* 1995; **95**:802–4.
10. National Research Council. *Recommended Dietary Allowances.* National Academy of Science: Washington DC, 1989.
11. Matkovic V. Calcium and peak bone mass. *J Intern Med* 1992; **231**:51–160.
12. Barr SI. Associations of social and demographic variables with calcium intakes of high school students. *J Am Diet Assoc* 1994; **94**:260–266.
13. The Weight-Control Information Network. *1 Win Way.* Bethesda, MD 20892–3665, 1-800-WIN-8098, WINNIDDK@aol.com.
14. Gay L. Not all vegetarians are created equal. In: *The Yale Guide to Children's Nutrition* (Tamborlane WV, ed), 1st edn. RR Donnelly: Harrisonburg, 1997:84–7.
15. Gortmaker S, Dietz W, Sobol A et al. Increased pediatric obesity in the United States. *Am J Dis Child* 1987; **141**:535–40.
16. Lovell DJ, Gregg D, Heubi J, Levinson JE. Nutritional status in juvenile rheumatoid arthri-

tis (JRA) – an interim report. *Arthritis Rheum* 1986; **29**:S67.

17. Miller ML, Chacko JA, Young EA. Dietary deficiencies in children with juvenile rheumatoid arthritis. *Arthritis Care Res* 1989; **2**:22–4.

18. Johansson U, Portinsson S, Akesson A et al. Nutritional status in girls with juvenile chronic arthritis. *Hum Nutrit Clin Nutrit* 1985; **40C**:57–67.

19. Henderson CJ, Lovell DJ. Assessment of protein-energy malnutrition in children and adolescents with juvenile rheumatoid arthritis. *Arthritis Care Res* 1989; **2**:108–13.

20. Mortensen AL, Allen JR, Allen RC. Nutritional assessment of children with juvenile chronic arthritis. *J Paediatr Child Health* 1990; **26**:335–8.

21. Bacon MC, White PH, Raiten DJ et al. Nutritional status and growth in juvenile rheumatoid arthritis. *Semin Arthritis Rheum* 1990; **20**:97–106.

22. Strano CG, Polito C, Alessio M et al. Nutritional status in active juvenile chronic arthritis not treated with steroids. *Acta Paediatr* 1995; **84**:1010–13.

23. Haugen MA, Hoyerall HM, Larsen S et al. Nutrient intake and nutritional status in children with juvenile chronic arthritis. *Scand J Rheumatol* 1992; **21**:165–70.

24. Di Toro R, Polita C. Nutrition in juvenile rheumatoid arthritis. *Nutr Res* 1997; **17**:741–58.

25. Warady BD, McLemmon SP, Lindsley CB. Anthropometric assessment of patients with juvenile rheumatoid arthritis. *Top Clin Nutr* 1989; **4**:7–14.

26. Henderson CJ, Lovell DJ. Nutritional aspects of juvenile rheumatoid arthritis. In: *Rheumatic Disease Clinics of North America* (Parish RS, ed), WB Saunders Co.: Philadelphia, 1991.

27. Martini A, Ravelli A, Notarangelo LP. Enhanced interleukin-1 and depressed interleukin-2 production in juvenile arthritis. *J Rheumatol* 1986; **13**:598–603.

28. Mascioli EA, Blackburn GL. Nutrition and rheumatic diseases. In: *Textbook of Rheumatology* (Kelly WN, Harris ED, Ruddy S et al, eds), 1st edn. WB Saunders: Philadelphia, 1985:352–60.

29. Brewer EJ, Giannini EH, Person DA. *Juvenile Rheumatoid Arthritis*. WB Saunders: Philadelphia, 1982.

30. Cassidy JT, Petty RE. *Textbook of Pediatric Rheumatology*. Churchill Livingstone: New York, 1990.

31. Craft AW, Eastham EJ, Bell JI. Serum ferritin in juvenile chronic polyarthritis. *Ann Rheum Dis* 1977; **36**:271.

32. Giodano N, Floravanti A, Sancasciani S et al. Increased storage of iron and anaemia in rheumatoid arthritis: usefulness of deferoxamine. *Br Med J* 1984; **289**:961–2.

33. Lloyd KN, Williams P. Reaction to total dose infusion of iron dextran in rheumatoid arthritis. *Br Med J* 1970; **11**:323–5.

34. Weiss JB, Sedowofia, Jones C. Collagen degradation: a defended multienzyme system. In: *Biology of Collagen* (Viidik A, Vuust J, eds). Academic Press: London, 1978.

35. Fedarko NS, Vetter UK, Weinstein S, Robey PG. Age related changes in hyaluronan, proteoglycan, collagen, and osteonectin synthesis by human bone cells. *J Cell Physiol* 1992; **151**:215–27.

36. Karube S, Shoji H. Compositional changes of glycosaminoglycans of the human menisci with age and degenerative joint disease. *J Jpn Orthop Assoc* 1982; **56**:51–7.

37. Champion BR, Reiner A, Roughley PJ, Poole AR. Age related changes in the antigenicity of human articular cartilage proteoglycans. *Collagen Rel Res* 1982; **2**:45–60.

38. Robey PG. The biochemistry of bone. *Endocrinol Metab Clin North Am* 1988; **18**:859–79.

39. Pachman LM, Poznanski AK. Juvenile rheumatoid arthritis. In: *Arthritis and Allied Conditions*, 12th edn. Lea & Febiger: Malvern, 1993.

40. Elsasser U, Willkins B, Hesp R. Bone rarefaction and crush fractures in juvenile chronic arthritis. *Arch Dis Child* 1982; **57**:377–80.

41. Martel W, Holt JF, Cassidy JT. Radiologic manifestations of juvenile rheumatoid arthritis. *Am J Roentgenol* 1962; **88**:400–24.

42. Hickman PL, Johnson L, Lorrens C et al. Skeletal maturation and bone mineral metabolism in children with juvenile rheumatoid arthritis. *Arthritis Rheum* 1993; **35**:S54.

43. Fantini F, Beltrametti P, Gallazzi M et al. Evaluation by dual-photon absorptiometry of bone mineral loss in rheumatic children on long term treatment with corticosteroids. *Clin Exp Rheumatol* 1991; **9**(suppl 6):21–8.

44. Henderson C, Lovell DJ. Bone mineral content in juvenile rheumatoid arthritis – pilot project results. *Arthritis Rheum* 1991; **34**:S239.

45. Lovell DJ, Henderson CJ, Specker B et al. Relationship of total body bone mineral density and physical activity in JRA – a controlled study using dual energy X-ray absorptiometry (DEXA). *Arthritis Rheum* 1992; **35**:S57.

46. Ott SM. Attainment of peak bone mass. *J Clin Endocrinol Metab* 1990; **71**:1082A–C.
47. Hopp R, Degan J, Gallagher C et al. Estimation of bone mineral density in children with juvenile rheumatoid arthritis. *J Rheumatol* 1991; **18**:1235–9.
48. Cassidy JT, Langman CB, Allen SH, Hillman LS. Bone mineral metabolism in children with juvenile rheumatoid arthritis. *Rheum Dis Pediatr Clin North Am* 1995; **42**:1017–29.
49. Cassidy JT, Hillman LS. Abnormalities in skeletal growth in children with juvenile rheumatoid arthritis. *Rheum Dis Clin North Am* 1997; **23**:499–521.
50. Pepmueller PH, Cassidy JT, Allen SH, Hillman LS. Bone mineralization and bone mineral metabolism in children with juvenile rheumatoid arthritis. *Arthritis Rheum* 1996; **39**:746–57.
51. Reeve J, Loftus J, Hesp R et al. Biochemical prediction of changes in spinal bone mass in juvenile chronic (or rheumatoid) arthritis treated with glucocorticoids. *J Rheumatol* 1993; **20**:1189–95.
52. Reed A, Haugen M, Pachman LM, Langman CB. 25-Hydroxyvitamin D therapy in children with active juvenile rheumatoid arthritis: short-term effects on serum osteocalcin levels and bone mineral density. *J Pediatr* 1991; **119**:657–60.
53. Castro TCM, Hilaro MOE, Szejnfeld VL et al. Reduced bone mineral density in juvenile SLE and JDMS. *Arthritis Rheum* 1997; **40**:S190.
54. Petri M. Musculoskeletal complications of SLE in the Hopkins lupus cohort: an update. *Arthritis Care Res* 1995; **8**:137–45.
55. Kalla AA, Fataar AB, Jessop SJ, Bewerunge L. Loss of trabecular bone mineral density in SLE. *Arthritis Rheum* 1993; **36**:1726–34.
56. Matkovic V. Calcium metabolism and calcium requirements during skeletal modeling and consolidation of bone mass. *Am J Clin Nutr* 1991; **54**(suppl):2455–605.
57. Kreipe RE. Bones of today, bones of tomorrow. *Am J Dis Child* 1992; **146**:22–5.
58. Alexeyva L, Burkhardt P, Christiansen C et al. Assessment of fracture risk and its application to screening for postmenopausal osteoporosis. *WHO Tech Rep Ser* 1994; **834**:1–129.
59. Johnston CC, Slemenda CW, Melton LJ. Clinical use of bone densitometry. *N Engl J Med* 1991; **324**:1105–9.
60. Washnick RD, Ross PD, Davis JW et al. A comparison of single and multi-site BMC measurements for assessment of spine fracture probability. *J Nucl Med* 1989; **30**:1166–71.
61. Hui SL, Slemenda CS, Johnson CC. Baseline measurement of bone mass predicts fracture in white women. *Ann Intern Med* 1989; **111**:355–61.
62. Cummings SR, Black SM, Nevitt MC et al. Appendicular bone density and age predicts hip fracture in women. *JAMA* 1990; **263**:665–8.
63. Matkovic V, Fonatan D, Tominac C et al. Factors that influence peak bone mass formation: a study of calcium balance and the inheritance of bone mass in adolescent females. *Am J Clin Nutr* 1990; **52**:878–88.
64. Janz KF, Golden JC, Hansen JR et al. Heart rate monitoring of physical activity in children and adolescents: the Muscatine Study. *Pediatrics* 1992; **89**:256–68.
65. Henderson CJ, Lovell DJ, Specker BL et al. Physical activity in children with juvenile rheumatoid arthritis: quantification and evaluation. *Arthritis Care Res* 1995; **8**:14–119.
66. American College of Rheumatology Task Force on Osteoporosis Guidelines. Recommendations for the prevention and treatment of glucocorticoid-induced osteoporosis. *Arthritis Rheum* 1996; **39**:791–1801.
67. Luckert BP, Raisz LG. Glucocorticoid-induced osteoporosis. *Rheum Dis Clin North Am* 1994; **20**:630–51.
68. Lane NE, Mroczkowski PJ, Hockberg MC. Prevention and management of glucocorticoid-induced osteoporosis. *Bull Rheum Dis* 1995; **44**:1–4.
69. Dequeker J, Westhovens R. Low dose corticosteroid associated osteoporosis in rheumatoid arthritis and its prophylaxis and treatment: bones of contention. *J Rheumatol* 1995; **22**:1013–19.
70. Hahn BH. Glucocorticoid-induced osteoporosis. *Hosp Pract* 1995; **30**:49–9, 52–6.
71. Gulko PS, Mulloy AL. Glucocorticosteroid-induced osteoporosis: pathogenesis, prevention and treatment. *Clin Exp Rheumatol* 1996; **14**:199–206.
72. Warady BD, Lindsley CB, Robinson RG, Lukert BP. Effects of nutritional supplementation on bone mineral status of children with rheumatic diseases receiving corticosteroid therapy. *J Rheumatol* 1994; **21**:530–5.
73. May KP, West SG, McDermott MT, Huffer WE. The effect of low-dose methotrexate on bone metabolism and histomorphometry in rats. *Arthritis Rheum* 1994; **37**:201–6.
74. Gnudis, Butturinil, Ripamonti C, Avella M et al. The affects of methotrexate (MTX) on bone: a densitometric study conducted on 59 patients

with MTX administered at different doses. *Ital J Orthop Traumatol* 1998; **14**:227–31.

75. Stoeber E. Prognosis in juvenile chronic arthritis. Follow-up of 433 chronic rheumatic children. *Eur J Pediatr* 1981; **135**:225–8.

76. Svantesson H, Akesson A, Eberhardt K, Elborgh R. Prognosis in juvenile rheumatoid arthritis with systemic onset. *Scand J Rheumatol* 1983; **12**:139–44.

77. Anderson-Gäre B, Fasth A. The natural history of juvenile chronic arthritis: a population based cohort study II. Outcome. *J Rheumatol* 1995; **22**:308–19.

78. Hashkes P, Lovell DJ. Why are children with juvenile rheumatoid arthritis small? In: *Current Controversies in Rheumatology* (Isenberg D, Tucker, eds). Dunitz: London, 1997:139–153.

79. Woo P, White PH, Ansell BM. *Paediatric Rheumatology Update*. Oxford University Press: Oxford, 1990.

80. Kelts DG, Grand RJ, Shen G et al. Nutritional basis of growth failure in children and adolescents with Crohn's disease. *Gastroenterology* 1979; **76**:720–7.

81. Rizzoni G, Broyer M, Guest G et al. Growth retardation in children with chronic renal disease: scope of the problem. *Am J Kidney Dis* 1986; **7**:256–61.

82. Shepard RW, Holt TL, Thomas BJ et al. Nutritional rehabilitation in cystic fibrosis: controlled studies of effects on nutritional growth retardation, body protein turnovers and course of pulmonary disease. *J Pediatr* 1986; **109**:788–94.

Leaving home – preparing the adolescent with arthritis for coping with independence in the adult rheumatology world

Patricia A Rettig and Balu H Athreya

INTRODUCTION

Adolescents with chronic disease often make their way into the adult health-care system in an unplanned, uncoordinated fashion. This may lead to young adults dropping out of this system and using medical care only for emergencies or in an episodic fashion. There is a need for paediatric health professionals to support the transition of adolescents with rheumatic diseases into the adult rheumatology world in a supportive, planned environment.

In the context of health care, transition is defined as the 'purposeful, planned movement of adolescents and young adults with chronic physical and medical conditions from child-centered to adult-oriented health care systems'.[1] The optimal goal of transition is to provide coordinated, uninterrupted health care that is age-appropriate and which addresses the developmental issues of this age period. For adolescents with rheumatic conditions, participation in an organized transition programme is ideal. In the absence of such an organized programme there should be a clear transition plan (Table 18.1). A comprehensive plan will promote self-care and independence, and also pave the path for a smooth transfer to the internist-rheumatologist.[2]

The focus of this chapter is the role of the physician and the allied health professionals in preparing the adolescents proactively for transition. Topics to be discussed include barriers to and benefits of a planned transitional process, models of transitional programmes that have been attempted, and key principles of transitional services. In addition, the need for primary-care services, training of paediatric and adult care providers, and the need for research in transition programmes are explored.

PERSPECTIVE ON TRANSITION ISSUES

Over the past 25 years, advances in medical sciences have resulted in increasing survival of children with diseases which were once considered fatal, such as leukaemia and congenital heart diseases. Children with various genetic and metabolic diseases may also survive into adulthood. Children with rheumatic diseases may enter adulthood with significant functional disabilities that impact on their acquisition of developmental skills and goals.[3] In addition to physical and functional disabilities, these children also carry greater psychosocial and financial burdens.[4]

The global trend in increasing survival of children with chronic illness and disability has resulted in greater attention to transitional services at an international level.[5] In the USA

Table 18.1   An example of a transition intervention plan

1. Assess level of independence in health care:
   (a) adolescent completes transition skills checklist (Figure 18.1)
   (b) encourage continuous progression of accomplishment in each area
   (c) educate about illness, treatment, self-care
2. Promote transition process:
   (a) set early, clear, realistic expectations about transfer
   (b) discuss differences between paediatric and adult health care
   (c) encourage 'teen visits' at appointments (see Table 18.2)
   (d) discuss issues of timing and readiness to transfer
   (e) discuss options in choosing a physician or medical centre
3. Address developmental transition issues:
   (a) identify concerns and need; counsel and refer as needed
   (b) utilize knowledgeable professionals, community resources
4. Prepare for actual transfer of care:
   (a) choose, preferably meet, the adult physician and providers
   (b) paediatric and adult providers relay medical information
   (c) transfer of written medical records
   (d) make appointment; proceed with transfer of care
5. Evaluation:
   (a) assessment of satisfactory transition
   (b) follow up with phone call

government agencies and health-service providers have convened national and international conferences on this subject. Rosen[6] provides a succinct summary of the major activities and leading references on the transition movement in the following excerpt:

This transition, from pediatric to adult-centered care, has been debated in the literature,[7–9] explored in national conferences[10,11] modeled in demonstration and service projects,[12,13] and codified in guidelines and standards of care.[14,15] Nevertheless, despite some momentum over the past several years, there has been far too little progress in ensuring that adolescents and young adults with special health care needs, have suitable pathways for transition to adult care.

Most health professionals agree with the need for age-appropriate care for young adults. Yet, there are very few services for adolescents to transition to adult care. A number of countries have tried to develop transition services for adolescents with chronic diseases. Depending on the nationwide system of health-care delivery and financing of health care in these countries, there are a number of barriers to the transition process.[16]

Barriers to transition

Barriers to transition can be grouped into two categories: individual issues associated with the adolescent and his or her family; and systems of health-care delivery and finances.

Adolescents and parents who have a long-standing relationship and trust in their paediatric providers may have a difficulty with the idea of transferring to adult care.[12] Moreover, teenagers with severe disease, delayed maturity, dependency on parents, or history of poor adherence to treatment regimes are at risk of difficult transition to adult care.[17,18] Likewise, parents who encourage dependence and are overprotective will inhibit the adolescent's progress in transition.

In one study on adolescents and young adults with sickle cell disease,[19] when asked what their concerns were in transferring care to adult health providers, responses included: concerns about being treated as an adult, ability to pay for medical care, and whether adult providers

	Plan to start	Will practice and discuss	Can do it independently	Plan: who, what, how often, comments
1. Describes illness/impact on life				
2. Discuss concern/issues about transfer				
3. Understand differences between paediatric and adult care				
4. Prepares questions and speaks up at medical visit				
5. Participates in 'teen visit'				
6. Takes own medications at right time				
7. Knows all medications, doses, and keeps list in wallet				
8. Knows health provider's phone numbers and emergency numbers and keeps in wallet				
9. Keeps 'diary' information (BP, wt, medication changes)				
10. Schedules own medical appointments				
11. Calls for and gets prescription refilled, lab. results, etc.				
12. Calls to report change in illness, new symptoms, concerns				
13. Knows insurance and has plans for continuous medical coverage after transfer				
14. Continues primary care visits – plans for primary care after transfer				
15. Obtains sexual/reproductive health information and appointments				
16. Independent with dressing, bathing, chores – uses devices for ADLs if needed				
17. Discusses how drugs, alcohol, cigarettes affect illness and medication toxicities				
18. Contacts resources/agencies, i.e. vocational rehabilitation, driving, college office for students with disabilities, financial aid, etc.				
19. Discusses and plans for good time to transfer care				
20. Chooses an internist				
21. Makes appointment with internist				

Physician ——————————— Address———————————————————

Phone Number ——————————— First Appointment Date ———————————

Figure 18.1 Transition skills checklist. ADL, activities of daily living; BP, blood pressure.

would understand how their disease affects them as individuals. When parents were asked similar questions, they expressed worries about internist's understanding of the disease, and also about their children's ability to be responsible for their own care.

The health-care system presents other potential barriers. Paediatricians may be hesitant to let go of the patients that they have cared for for many years. Internists may be unfamiliar with some of the specific paediatric diseases, details of the past medical history, and of developmental issues specific to the adolescent age group. Moreover, parents and adolescents may be ill-prepared for the substantial differences in the care of patients by paediatricians and internists.[1,6] Paediatric providers use a family-centred, team approach in which care is coordinated and support services are provided. However, paediatric providers are also known to coddle their patients and their families, leading to dependence and high expectations of providers.

In adult settings, the adolescent and young adult are expected to participate actively in management decisions with the physician. The doctor–parent–patient relationship in paediatric care is reconfigured to a doctor–patient relationship in adult care.[6]

In the USA, financing health-care and related services may be a problem for older adolescents and young adults, many of whom are underinsured or uninsured. Because of age, many lose their parent's insurance coverage. They may be unable to get their own insurance because of exclusion clauses for pre-existing conditions. Inadequate public funding and lack of employment benefits add to the financial problems experienced by young adults.[20] In the USA the existing system is complex, fragmented and confusing for families of adolescents. For example, a vast discrepancy exists among states regarding public funding sources, eligibility criteria and types of service funded, and age limit for services.[21]

During the adolescent years, paediatric providers can be sensitive and supportive of families faced with these issues and provide education on the benefits of transition.

Benefits of transition plans

Planning for transition to adult care sends the message to the adolescent that independence and self-mastery of one's health care is expected. Transition planning promotes the development of skills in communication, decision-making, assertiveness, and self-care in the adolescent. Therefore, sense of control and independence in health care are enhanced.[1,14] Critical issues such as reproductive health, substance use, independent living and risk-taking behaviours can be addressed. Referrals can be made to appropriate community agencies, such as vocational rehabilitation and adaptive driving schools. With transition of health care to the adult setting, the focus is on the 'emerging adult rather than the older child.'[1,14]

Transition planning promotes continuity of specialty care and prevents gaps in services. When a young adult does not 'connect' to the adult provider, preventable sequelae and disease complications may occur. Transition planning can prevent haphazard and crisis care in emergency rooms. In addition, transferring to the internist rheumatologist when the adolescent is well and involved in the change has a better medical and psychological outcome than being forced to move during a time of crises.[22]

CURRENT MODELS OF TRANSITION PROGRAMME

Several models of transition have been described and they generally fall into four categories:[21]

- *Disease-focused model*, whereby a young person moves from a paediatric subspecialist to an internist subspecialist at a different site. In this model, certain professionals (e.g. social workers and/or nurses) provide continuity across all settings.
- *Adolescent-focused model*, whereby a young person moves from paediatric to adolescent and, subsequently, to adult health-care services. In this model, there is a core team of health-care providers that includes disease

subspecialists. The care is coordinated by primary care and adolescent health specialists.

- *Primary-care model*, which uses the family physician (or general practitioner) as the care coordinator. Paediatric subspecialists serve as consultants for children and internists serve a parallel role for adults with disabling conditions. Likewise, other disciplines can participate in either consultative or core team roles, depending on the needs of the young person and his or her family.
- *Single-site models*, where the adolescent moves from paediatric to adult care, but remains in the same clinical site. In this model, service providers, such as the nurse or social workers, remain the same, but the specialist changes as the adolescent matures.

In rheumatology, a disease-focus model that involves a nurse and social worker has been described.[2] Key to the success of this programme was the involvement of a committed internist rheumatologist who was knowledgeable about the unique needs of adolescents and young adults. In addition, the strength of this rheumatology transition programme included the close proximity of the paediatric and adult hospitals, a strong paediatric rheumatology team with a shared philosophy in how to implement transition, collaborative efforts with the internist rheumatologists, an active adolescent group in the paediatric centre, and government funding. However, when the grant funding that supported the programme was lost, an alternative and less costly programme evolved. In the new programme, the internist rheumatologist saw adolescents jointly with the paediatric rheumatologist and nurse specialist on several occasions at the paediatric site prior to the actual transfer. The internist came to the paediatric site once a month.

PRINCIPLES OF TRANSITIONAL SERVICES

Transition of adolescents to adult health-care services can occur either through a formalized programme or, in the absence of a programme, by implementing a comprehensive transition plan (Table 18.1). With either approach, the following principles can guide the planning process:

- Transition is a gradual, individualized process, not an event.
- Transition involves the entire family.
- Transition planning should begin at diagnosis.
- A transition plan that includes goals for independence and self-care should be developed, and revised as necessary.
- The plan should incorporate clear expectations, education, and recognition of the adolescent's increasing independence, capacity for decision-making, and need for empowerment.
- Paediatric providers must prepare themselves for letting go of long-term relationships.
- Parents must be supported as their roles change.
- Coordination between paediatric and adult providers, between primary and specialty providers, and among health-care, educational, vocational and social service systems is essential.

With these guidelines, a transition plan can be implemented, and a tool such as the transition skills checklist (Figure 18.1), can help the young teenager track his or her own progress. A list of resources that may be of use to health-care providers is given in Appendix 1.

The teenager should be encouraged to communicate directly during phone calls and clinic visits with health professionals. When ready, he or she can spend a portion of the visit (or 'teen visits' as we call them) with the health-care providers, separate from their parents (Table 18.2). This will promote communication of sensitive issues and preparation for adult health care.

TIMING OF TRANSFER OF CARE

The age range for transfer may start at age 17 years. However, timing of the actual transfer of care depends upon a number of factors. Chronological age is only one variable. Other considerations include maturational level,

---

Table 18.2   Principles of 'teen visits'

- Teenager is able to discuss concerns about disease and sensitive, confidential issues with provider
- Teenager feels more control over health and future
- Reason for visits made clear with acknowledgment of potential initial difficulty for the teenager and parent
- Parents always included as part of visit, usually at end of visit to discuss treatment plan and parent's questions
- 'Teen visits' serve as practice for adult health-care visits
- Provider's approach is always supportive and includes bi-directional communication strategies[27] such as:
  - (a) asking ('Is there anything that you have a question about?')
  - (b) posing hypothetical situations ('Some teenagers with (disease) worry about . . . ; do you ever worry about this?')
  - (c) problem-solving ('What might you do if your friends are drinking alcohol at a party?')

---

medical status, availability of internist and other medical specialists, self-care skills, transitional issues, and the adolescent's readiness to transfer. For example, transition will be difficult at a time when the disease is flaring, when new treatments are being started, or at the time of leaving home for college/university. If transition occurs too early or when the adolescent is not prepared or ready, poor adherence to the medical regimen or poor continuity of care can occur. Adolescents and families need to have ongoing discussions with the paediatric providers regarding the best time for the transfer to occur. When transition is a known expectation from the time of diagnosis, it is easy for all participants to move towards that goal with a prepared plan.

Three additional areas of importance should be considered in order to create more responsive transition services: the role of the primary-care provider, training of paediatric and adult health-care providers, and research in transition.

Primary health care in the adolescent with rheumatic disease

Most adolescents with chronic disease regard their subspecialist as their personal physician; however, less than one-third actually address primary-care issues with the subspecialist. In fact, up to 40% of adolescents with major chronic illness have reported no source of primary care.[23] Although paediatric rheumatologists have traditionally worked well with primary-care physicians, primary care is often non-existent for the adolescent age group. In the USA, systems of managed care have forced the primary-care providers to play a significant role in the use and coordination of care.

Teenagers with chronic illness and disability report more age-related concerns than their non-disabled peers. These include: acne, headaches, insomnia, alcohol and drug use, anxiety, worry about height and weight, menstruation problems, contraceptive use, and reproductive health.[23] Learning to use primary care to address these issues as an adolescent can foster optimal usage of primary-care physicians for non-rheumatological problems and preventive medical care by the emerging young adult.

Genetic counselling is an important component of transition services. For example, health professionals can discuss the significance of human leucocyte antigen (HLA) B27 with young adults who have ankylosing spondylitis and are planning a family. With recent developments in histocompatibility typing as it relates to rheumatic diseases and molecular genetics, primary physicians of the future may be expected to have a wealth of knowledge in genetics and in counselling.[24] Moreover, the primary-care provider of the future will have an increasing role as advocate, family counsellor and care coordinator, and will be expected to work with schools, community agencies and public health agencies.[25]

TRANSITION AND TRAINING ISSUES

More providers – both paediatric and adult – could benefit from increased understanding of adolescent issues. A survey of 3066 physicians and allied health professionals in the USA revealed major deficits in their knowledge of and skills in adolescent health care, including care for youth with disabilities.[26] Many training programmes for internist rheumatologists include clinical rotations in paediatric rheumatology. Besides learning about manifestation and treatment of paediatric disease, the internist has the opportunity to gain understanding about both the adolescent's struggle for increased independence and the parent's anxiety. Likewise, if paediatric providers spend some time training with internists, they may be better equipped in preparing adolescents and their families for adult care. However, reciprocal education specific to training in transitional care is uniformly lacking in medical education.[1] Certainly, developing collaborative relationships in clinical training, education and research among adult and paediatric rheumatologists can only be beneficial in forwarding the transition process for adolescent patients.

OUTCOME CRITERIA AND RESEARCH

Although a number of models of transition services have been developed, there has been little research on the impact or efficacy of transitional services.[1–5] In adolescents with rheumatic disease, rates of referral and long-term follow-up within the transitioned health system were demonstrated to improve greatly with a formalized transition programme.[2]

Success in transition of adolescents with rheumatic disease could be measured using several outcome criteria such as: accomplishment of self-care skills; disease severity and complications; functional status; continuity of care; long-term follow-up with subspecialists and the primary-care physician; quality of life and well-being; employment and education levels; maintenance of insurance coverage and financial stability; participation in young adult education or support programmes (e.g. career planning workshops, if available); independent-living achievements, including driving; and collaboration demonstrated between paediatric and adult providers.

The Society for Adolescent Medicine outlines potential areas for research in their position paper on transition.[1] This includes the following research questions: Compared to adolescents without a transition programme, do adolescents who move from child-centred to adult health care via a transition programme have increased adult health visits and fewer medical complications? Do these adolescents have better social–emotional adjustment, better optimism about their future, and greater satisfaction with their health care? The position paper concludes that it is 'critically important that we promote discussion of transition issues, development of transition programs, and thoughtful evaluation of such programs. If we are to help adolescents with chronic conditions develop to their fullest capacity, we must understand what works and why'.[1]

REFERENCES

1. Blum WM, Garell D, Hodgman DH et al. Transition from child-centered to adult health-care systems for adolescents with chronic conditions: a position paper of the Society of Adolescent Medicine. *J Adolesc Health* 1993; **14**:570–6.
2. Rettig P, Athreya BH. Adolescents with chronic disease: transition to adult health care. *Arthritis Care Res* 1991; **4**:174–80.
3. White P. Success on the road to adulthood: issues and hurdles for adolescents with disabilities. *Rheum Dis Clin North Am* 1997; **23**:697–707.
4. Newacheck P, Taylor WR. Childhood chronic illness: prevalence, severity, and impact. *Am J Public Health* 1992; **82**:364–71.
5. Conference proceedings. Moving on: transition from pediatric to adult health care. *J Adolesc Health* 1995; **17**:3–36.

6. Rosen D. Between two worlds: bridging the cultures of child health and adult medicine. *J Adolesc Health* 1995; **17**:10–16.

7. Fulginiti VA. What is pediatrics? Prenatal medicine to young adult care. *Am J Dis Child* 1992; **146**:17–18.

8. Garson A. The science and practice of pediatric cardiology in the next decade. *Am Heart J* 1987; **114**:462–8.

9. Barbero GJ. Leaving the pediatrician for the internist. *Ann Int Med* 1982; **96**:673–4.

10. Magrab PR, Miller HEC. *Surgeon General's Conference. Growing Up and Getting Medical Care: Youth with Special Health Care Needs* (Magrab PR, Millar HEC, eds). National Center for Networking Community-Based Services: Washington, DC, 1989.

11. Reaman GH, Bonfiglio J, Krailo M et al. Cancer in adolescent and young adults. *Cancer* 1993; **71**(suppl):3206–9.

12. Shidlow DV, Fiel SB. Life beyond pediatrics: transition of chronically ill adolescent from pediatric to adult care systems. *Med Clin North Am* 1990; **74**:1113–20.

13. Court JM. Outpatient-based transition services for youth. *Pediatrician* 1991; **18**:150–6.

14. *Moving on: Transition from Child-centered to Adult Health Care for Youth with Disabilities.* US Department of Health and Human Services, Public Health Service, Health Resources and Services Administration, Maternal and Child Health Bureau: Washington, DC, 1992:1–20.

15. Cystic Fibrosis Center Committee and Guidelines Subcommittee. Cystic Fibrosis Foundation guidelines for patient services, evaluation, and monitoring in cystic fibrosis centers. *Am J Dis Child* 1990; **144**:1311–12.

16. Bowes G, Sinnema G, Suris JC, Buhlmann U. Transition health services for youth with disabilities: a global perspective. *J Adolesc Health* 1995; **17**:23–31.

17. Rosen D. Transition to adult healthcare for adolescents and young adults with cancer. *Cancer* 1993; **71**(suppl):3411–14.

18. Baker KL, Coe LM. Growing up with a chronic condition: transition to young adulthood for the individual with cystic fibrosis. *Holistic Nursing Practice* 1993; **8**:8–15.

19. Telfair J, Myers J, Drezner S. Transfer as a component of the transition of adolescents with sickle cell disease to adult care: adolescent, adult, and parent perspectives. *J Adolesc Health* 1994; **15**:558–65.

20. McManus P. Adolescents and young adults with special health care needs: the challenges for financing. In: *Surgeon General's Conference. Growing Up and Getting Medical Care: Youth with Special Health Care Needs* (Magrab PR, Millar HEC, eds). National Center for Networking Community-Based Services: Washington, DC, 1989.

21. Blum RW. Summary of Conference Recommendation. Moving on: transition from pediatric to adult health care. *J Adolesc Health* 1995; **17**:6–9.

22. White P. Future expectations: adolescents with rheumatic diseases and their transition into adulthood. *Br J Rheumatol* 1996; **35**:80–3.

23. Carroll G, Massarelli E, Opzoomer A et al. Adolescents with chronic disease: are they receiving comprehensive health care? *J Adolesc Health Care* 1983; **4**:261–5.

24. Collins FS. Preparing health professionals for the genetic revolution. *JAMA* 1997; **278**:1285–6.

25. Kelly A. The primary care providers role in caring for young people with chronic illness. *J Adolesc Health Care* 1995; **4**:261–5.

26. Blum RW, Bearinger LH. Knowledge and attitudes of health professionals towards adolescent health care. *J Adolesc Health Care* 1990; **11**:289–94.

27. Schubiner H, Eggly S. Strategies for health education for adolescents patients: a preliminary investigation. *J Adolesc Health* 1995; **17**:37–41.

APPENDIX 1

The following are some useful health-care transition resources:

American Juvenile Arthritis Organization (AJAO)
AJAO/Arthritis Foundation
P.O. Box 7669
Atlanta, GA 30357-9669
USA

Tel. (800) 283-7800

Resources:
- *Decision Making for Teenagers with Arthritis* (1996)
- AJAO National and Regional Conferences for families and professionals.

National Center for Youth with Disabilities
University of Minnesota
P.O. Box 721
420 Delaware Street, S.E.
Minneapolis, MN 55455
USA

Tel. (612) 626-2931

Resources:
- *Transitional Planning for the 21st Century: A Call to Action* (1995)
- bibliographic database
- technical assistance
- newsletters, other publications on transition.

On TRAC – Taking Responsibility for Adolescent/Adult Care
British Columbia Children's Hospital
Room 2 D20 4480 Oak Street
Vancouver, B.C.
Canada 3V4

Tel. (604) 875-3472

Resources:
- annotated bibliography
- workshops, training, and consultation.

Parent Training and Information Center
PACER Center, Inc.
4826 Chicago Avenue South
Minneapolis, MN 55412
USA

Tel. (612) 827-2966

Resources:
- *Speak Up for Health* (handbook for parents)
- *Living Your Own Life* (handbook for teenagers with disabilities).

Index